Vitamins: Their Role in the Human Body

Vitamins

Their Role in the Human Body

G.F.M. Ball
Consultant, London, UK

Blackwell
Science

Editorial offices:
Blackwell Publishing Ltd, 9600 Garsington Road, Oxford OX4 2DQ, UK
  Tel: +44 (0)1865 776868
Blackwell Publishing Professional, 2121 State Avenue, Ames, Iowa 50014-8300, USA
  Tel: +1 515 292 0140
Blackwell Publishing Asia Pty Ltd, 550 Swanston Street, Carlton, Victoria 3053, Australia
  Tel: +61 (0)3 8359 1011

First published 2004

Library of Congress Cataloging-in-Publication Data is available

ISBN 0-632-06478-1

A catalogue record for this title is available from the British Library

Set in 10/12 pt Minion
by Sparks, Oxford, UK – www.sparks.co.uk
Printed and bound in India
by Gopsons Paper Ltd, Noida

The publisher's policy is to use permanent paper from mills that operate a sustainable forestry policy, and which has been manufactured from pulp processed using acid-free and elementary chlorine-free practices. Furthermore, the publisher ensures that the text paper and cover board used have met acceptable environmental accreditation standards.

For further information on Blackwell Publishing, visit our website:
www.blackwellpublishing.com

To the memory of Mariah Margaret Ball

Contents

Foreword

The thirteen vitamins that are essential for an adequate human diet are staggeringly diverse in their structures, chemical properties and functions, but they have, by and large, all arrived at a similar juncture in their evolving recognition and understanding. Fifty to a hundred years ago, the main research emphasis was on isolation, structural determination, basic biochemical properties and functional significance. As George Ball's new book demonstrates, the quest for their functional significance is still continuing and is by no means yet complete. However, the recent focus on their public health significance has shifted from a relatively straightforward concern with the prevention and cure of overt deficiency diseases towards more subtle functional properties, often linked to those medical conditions that are not obviously vitamin-dependent.

An example is folate, a generic group of compounds which includes folic acid. When discovered, its medical significance was in the prevention of megaloblastic anaemia in pregnant women in developing countries such as India. Today, the focus has shifted towards the avoidance of neural tube defects (spina bifida, anencephaly) in western countries and the reduction of hyperhomocysteinaemia, which is considered to be a precursor, predictor, and likely causative agent for vascular diseases, including some dementias. There are recent indications that folate may influence cancer risk, especially for bowel cancers. Paradoxically, whereas anti-folate drugs are frequently used to treat existing cancer, poor folate status may be a risk factor for development of new cancers, perhaps by compromising DNA repair mechanisms. None of these implications of folate status were recognized before the final decades of the twentieth century, and they are still being researched and refined.

Another recently emergent research topic has involved the so-called 'antioxidant' vitamins, principally vitamins C and E, perhaps better described as 'redox modulators', because they can act as pro-oxidants as well as antioxidants. Risk of developing degenerative diseases such as vascular disease, cancers and eye diseases (cataract, macular degeneration) has been linked to these 'protective' nutrients via animal and tissue culture model studies and epidemiological associations. The removal of oxygen-derived reactive free radicals seems generally beneficial and desirable, and is performed efficiently by these micronutrients. Just how important this is for human health remains controversial, as is the question, how far we now need to go 'beyond deficiency' and 'toward enhanced and optimal protection' against noxious agents in the environment and those derived from our own metabolic processes.

The fat-soluble vitamins have likewise proved equally elusive, with respect to the breadth of their functional implications. Thus, until a couple of decades ago, vitamin A was seen as the anti-xerophthalmia, anti-keratomalacia vitamin, preventing blindness in children in poor, developing countries. Then its role in preventing severe morbidity and mortality from infectious diseases was recognized, and this soon assumed dominance. Now, new roles for vitamin A in gap-junction cell–cell communication and on cell-signalling are recognized, revealing a potential role for retinoids in the treatment of cancer. Derivatives of vitamin D, the 'sunshine vitamin' which prevents rickets and osteomalacia, also have therapeutic potential for cancer. Vitamin K, which is used clinically to prevent haemorrhagic disease in breast-fed babies, now assumes important new significance for osteoporosis and arterial calcification.

All these newly discovered roles for individual vitamins have serious implications for recommended dietary amounts and for public health food policies. In the UK, government recommendations for 'reference' (or recommended) nutrient intakes have traditionally been linked to the avoidance of deficiency diseases. New evidence for subtle, unexpected functional advantages of increased intakes, coupled with the realization that genetic and lifestyle diversity – especially the genetic diversity associated with common enzyme polymorphisms – has tended to increase the level of controversy about the exact aims of dietary recommendations. It is a frustrating fact that almost every expert committee, in every country, has a different set of dietary recommendations.

Another area where the information available varies greatly in quality and quantity is the characterization of population dietary intakes and biochemical status parameters. In the UK, we are fortunate in having a recent set of National Diet and Nutrition surveys, which have enabled us to determine which subgroups of the British population are at risk for inadequate nutrient intakes and which status parameters are appropriate. This survey work is admittedly expensive and time-consuming, but such information is of vital importance for the effective targeting of public health interventions to combat deficiency and to optimize intakes in the population.

The other end of the nutrient intake spectrum is that of excessively high intakes, with the attendant risk of tissue overload and toxicity. The increasing availability and sales of over-the-counter vitamin supplements in the UK renders this hazard increasingly problematic. Whereas the toxicity of high in-takes of vitamins A or D is well known, perhaps one should also be concerned about high intakes of other vitamins. Thus: can high intakes of folic acid mask incipient pernicious anaemia? – or perhaps increase the growth rate of any pre-existing tumours? For governments, it is vital to decide when and how to make vitamin fortification of foods mandatory, voluntary or forbidden.

Our perception of what is the minimum intake to achieve adequacy tends to be higher than it once was, yet our perception of the maximum intake that is compatible with adequate safety is lower, so the 'safe range' is becoming ever narrower. This safe (or optimal) range may vary between individuals (e.g. with genotype and enzyme polymorphisms) and with lifestyle variations. Will it perhaps be necessary to tailor nutrient recommendations to specific individuals and/or specific lifestyles in the future?

George Ball's book has drawn together much of the scientific information about vitamin function that is scattered throughout the literature. Our next challenge will be to harness this invaluable knowledge effectively, for the benefit of individuals and of populations.

C. J. Bates
Head of Micronutrient Status Research (retired)
Medical Research Council
Human Nutrition Research
Cambridge, UK

Preface

Vitamins are involved in many branches of biology. To facilitate an understanding of their mode of action I have included background chapters on physiology and functional anatomy, biochemistry, immunology and the genetic control of protein synthesis. A glossary provides rapid access to some of the lesser-known terms.

The information presented in this book is not set in stone. Some information is controversial and current concepts are likely to change in the near or distant future as new knowledge comes to light. The truth, or as near as we can approach it, can only be arrived at by consensus from different research groups using different experimental approaches and perhaps working from different viewpoints.

George F. M. Ball

1
Historical Events Leading to the Establishment of Vitamins

1.1 Introduction

The vitamin story does not unfold in an orderly chronological fashion. Investigations were long-term and conducted on different aspects in different parts of the world, making it impossible to pinpoint dates of specific discoveries. Those dates which are given are those of publications that we now recognize as ground-breaking. At the same time, much of the published work was overlooked or not accepted until decades later. The poor dissemination of knowl- edge, attributable in part to lack of communication and transport, meant that an investigator was often completely oblivious of another's work in a distant country. Moreover, the vitamin pioneers were unwit- tingly dealing with a hitherto unknown concept – a disease caused by a nutritional deficiency. They faced huge obstacles in getting their work accepted by the medical establishment, which adhered tenaciously to the belief that diseases must have a positive aetiology. Some investigators achieved fame, a few being award- ed the Nobel Prize (Table 1.1), and their names live on

Table 1.1 Nobel Prizes for research into vitamins.

Year	Category	Nobel Laureates and their scientific achievements
1929	Physiology or medicine	Christiaan Eijkman: for discovering that a diet consisting mostly of polished rice causes polyneuritis (a form of beriberi) in chickens.
		Frederick Hopkins: for establishing that artificial diets composed solely of purified proteins, fats, carbohydrates, mineral salts and water are insufficient for normal animal growth; 'accessory substances' (now known as vitamins) are essential.
1934	Physiology or medicine	George Whipple, George Minot and William Murphy: for treating pernicious anaemia patients with dietary liver.
1937	Physiology or medicine	Albert Szent-Györgyi: for isolating vitamin C.
1937	Chemistry	Walter Haworth: for determining the structure of vitamin C and synthesizing it.
		Paul Karrer: for his research into carotenoids, flavins and vitamin A; accomplished the total synthesis of riboflavin.
1938	Chemistry	Richard Kune: for his research into carotenoids and vitamins of the B complex.
1943	Physiology or medicine	Carl Dam: for discovering vitamin K.
1964	Chemistry	Dorothy Hodgkin: for determining the structure of vitamin B_{12}.
1967	Physiology or medicine	George Wald: for determining the role of vitamin A in the biochemistry of vision.

in encyclopaedias and textbooks. The excellent work of many other scientists, however, was never given the recognition it deserved and prophecies which turned out to be correct were largely ignored. This chapter aims to give some idea of the scale of the vitamin pioneers' intellectual and practical achievements and also their exceptional perseverance. Additional information about the nature of nutritionally related diseases and the discovery of specific vitamins is provided within each relevant chapter.

The discovery of vitamins has developed along two parallel lines of enquiry; namely, (1) studies of the aetiology of nutritionally related diseases, and (2) studies of the effects of formulated diets.

1.2 Early studies of nutritionally related diseases

For centuries in the past, certain populations in the world were subjected to the ravages of four particular diseases with well-characterized symptoms: these diseases are beriberi, scurvy, pellagra and rickets. Progress in the aetiology of these diseases was hindered by the dogged belief that a disease must be caused by a positive factor, i.e. a microorganism or a toxin. The medical authorities could not envisage that a disease could be caused by a lack of something in the diet. Although the aetiologies were not understood until the early part of the twentieth century, dietary cures were known much earlier among certain people.

1.2.1 Beriberi

The first clinical description of beriberi is attributable to a Dutch physician, Jacobus Bonitus, while working in Java in 1642. No remedies for beriberi were known until 1882 when Admiral Kanehiro Takaki, Director-General of the Medical Department of the Japanese Navy, showed the disease to have a dietary origin. By simply increasing the allowance of vegetables, fish, meat and barley in a diet consisting predominantly of polished (milled) rice, Takaki was able to prevent the disease. Furthermore, Takaki managed to persuade the Japanese authorities to change the standard naval ration to one with a higher protein content. The beriberi problem in the Japanese Navy disappeared almost entirely following the change. Takaki ascribed his success to the increase in the nitrogen to carbon

ratio of the diet. This explanation was not accepted by the medical establishment who, finding no causative microorganism, switched their attention to searching for a toxin.

In 1886, the Dutch government sent Christiaan Eijkman, a physician, to Batavia on the island of Java in the Dutch East Indies (now Djakarta, the capital of Indonesia) to join a research team in the investigation of beriberi. The disease was rampant among the native soldiers and also among the island's prisoners. Because of its epidemic character, beriberi was assumed to have a bacterial origin and the scientists thought that they had isolated the causative micrococcus from the tissues of sufferers. They believed that the bacteria were floating in the damp air of barracks and prisons, so that ventilation and disinfection were the appropriate preventive actions.

Eijkman tried to infect rabbits and then monkeys with the micrococcus but the animals showed no signs of disease. Switching to chickens, because they were more economical both to buy and maintain, Eijkman noted that control birds as well as injected birds developed a paralytic disease, which he named polyneuritis gallinarum. The disease was characterized by an unsteady gait leading to an inability to stand and culminating in death. Autopsies revealed degeneration of peripheral nerves, most conspicuously in the limbs, that resembled nerve degeneration seen in the autopsies of people who had died from beriberi. Thinking that infection had spread from injected birds to control birds, Eijkman set up another site, remote from the first, to investigate whether chickens would remain healthy unless deliberately infected. Then a surprising thing happened: the chickens at the original site began to recover and there were no new deaths.

Eijkman, at first perplexed, then found out that, during the five months in which the disease had been developing, the chickens had been fed cooked rice from the military hospital. Before and after this period, the birds had been fed feed-grade uncooked rice. Eijkman performed a controlled experiment which showed that the cause of the disease was associated with the cooked rice diet. His explanation was that 'cooked rice favoured conditions for the development of microorganisms in the intestinal tract, and hence for the formation of a poison causing nerve degeneration'.

Eijkman turned his attention to the difference between hospital rice and the raw rice normally used for the chicken feed. The latter had been crudely pounded to remove most of its outer husk, but the adhering pericarp or 'silverskin' (also known as rice polishings) was still attached. The hospital rice, on the other hand, had been further processed by polishing to remove its silverskin. The important difference between the two types of rice seemed therefore to be the presence or absence of the silverskin layer. Eijkman proposed two theories. In the first theory, the polished rice might cause disease because, once its protective skin has been removed, pathogens have easier access to the starchy endosperm and can multiply there during storage. In the second theory, the silverskin contains substances indispensable to life and health that are absent or occur in too low concentrations in the underlying grain. Eijkman tested the first theory by feeding four chickens uncooked polished rice freshly processed each day. Two of the birds developed the polyneuritis, making this theory the less likely. At the end of many experiments, Eijkman's tentative hypothesis was that the rice polishings contributed an antidote to a nerve poison produced by the fermentation of starch in the chicken's crop.

Having shown the association of avian polyneuritis with polished rice, Eijkman still had no evidence that the polyneuritis and human beriberi had a common origin. He therefore encouraged a medical colleague, A. G. Vorderman, who was the inspector of prisons, to study the relation between the incidence of beriberi in the many prisons in the Dutch East Indies and the diet and hygienic condition of the prisoners. It was standard practice to supply a given prison with a particular type of rice, therefore the inmates were ideal subjects for a controlled feeding trial. The statistics of this study dealt with no less than 279 621 individuals, all of them prisoners at different times. In 37 prisons, unpolished rice was supplied; only one of these prisons developed beriberi. In 13 prisons the rice supplied was polished mixed with unpolished; in six of them beriberi developed. Out of 51 prisons where polished rice was supplied, as many as 38 developed cases of the disease. From these data it was calculated that for each 10 000 of the prison population there was only one case among those eating unpolished rice, 416 on the mixed rice diet, and 3900 on polished rice. There was no significant correlation with the age of the inmates, the ventilation of their accommodation or degree of overcrowding.

Despite all of Eijkman's efforts, beriberi was still considered to be the result of some kind of infection and rice was still regarded as a possible carrier of bacterial toxins. After Eijkman left Java on the grounds of ill-health, plans to use unpolished rice for all prisons in the Dutch East Indies were cancelled. Eijkman's successor Grijns at the laboratory in Batavia extracted a water-soluble 'polyneuritis preventive factor' from rice polishings and in a paper published in 1901 he correctly concluded (the first to do so) that beriberi is the result of a dietary lack of an essential nutrient.

1.2.2 Scurvy

A decoction of spruce or pine needles was known in Sweden to cure scurvy at least as early as the sixteenth century, and North American Indians demonstrated a similar elixir to the French explorer Jacques Cartier in 1535. Ships' crews of the East India Company had been using lemon juice to combat scurvy from 1601 onward at the instigation of Sir James Lancaster. However, this knowledge was not publicised and scurvy was still the scourge of sailors enduring long sea voyages. In 1734, Bachstrom stated his belief that 'this evil is solely owing to a total abstinence from fresh vegetable food, and greens; which is alone the primary cause of the disease'.

The first recorded experiment on the cause and cure of scurvy in humans was performed in 1747 on board H.M.S. *Salisbury* by the Scottish naval physician James Lind. Twelve sailors with scurvy were divided into six pairs and each pair was given a different daily concoction in addition to a common diet. Two fortunate patients were each given two oranges and one lemon every day; only these two recovered, thus demonstrating the efficacy of oranges and lemons. In Lind's *A Treatise of the Scurvy* published in 1757, Lind stated that 'greens or fresh vegetables, with ripe fruits, are the best remedies' and 'the difficulty of obtaining them at sea, together with a long continuance in the moist sea air' are the true causes of scurvy at sea. Although he was mistaken as to the bad effects of salt water and salt air, Lind's powers of observation led him to discover the true cause of scurvy and many of the factors influencing its occurrence.

Captain James Cook maintained a healthy crew by stopping frequently to take on fresh fruit and vegetables during his 1772–1775 voyages around the world.

The Royal Navy, on the other hand, refused to accept Lind's findings and countless sailors succumbed to scurvy for several years to follow.

Lind devoted his energies to securing a regular issue of lemon juice in the Royal Navy, but it was not until 1795 that success was finally achieved. The argument for issuing lemon juice was reinforced by a report in the previous year of a 23-week voyage, during which each seaman received two-thirds of an ounce of lemon juice daily: the crew remained entirely free from scurvy. The scheduled allowance for the sailors in the Navy was fixed at 1 ounce of lemon juice (often called 'lime juice') after two weeks at sea. The consequences of the new regulations were startling and by the beginning of the nineteenth century scurvy in the British Navy had disappeared.

The modern era of research into scurvy, leading to the discovery of vitamin C, began in 1907 when Holst and Frölich reported from Christiana (now Oslo) that the disease could be produced experimentally in guinea pigs. It was Holst and Frölich's original intention to find a suitable mammalian species for studying beriberi, following Eijkman's experiments with chickens. When the guinea pigs were fed a specially prepared cereal-based diet, the animals developed not the expected signs of beriberi, but rather the characteristic signs of scurvy, namely loss of body weight, loosening of teeth, haemorrhages in all parts of the body, and severe bone lesions. Supplementation of the basal cereal diet with fresh vegetables and fruit had a protective and curative action. This important discovery led Chick and Hume in 1919 to develop a bioassay, using the guinea pig, for testing antiscorbutic activity in biological materials. The decision by Holst and Frölich to use guinea pigs was fortuitous as we now know that the more usual laboratory rodents (rats and mice) are not rendered scorbutic when deprived of dietary vitamin C.

From 1910, Zilva and his associates at the Lister Institute in London were engaged in studying the chemical nature of the antiscorbutic factor. Two great obstacles to progress were the instability of the vitamin and the difficulty of guiding the required chemical steps by biological assays. Assay periods were 13 weeks, later shortened to 8 weeks. By 1927, Zilva had obtained syrupy concentrates of the antiscorbutic substance from the juice of lemons and shown them to possess strong reducing properties. The reducing power appeared to be associated with the antiscor-

butic activity, and yet freshly oxidized solutions still retained their activity. This apparent anomaly was resolved by Tillmans who correctly deduced that the antiscorbutic factor was responsible for the reducing properties of the lemon juice concentrates, and that both oxidized and reduced forms of the reducing substance possessed antiscorbutic activity. Drummond's proposal to name the antiscorbutic factor 'vitamin C' was accepted in 1922.

In September 1931, C. G. King and W. A. Waugh at the University of Pittsburgh obtained a crystalline product from lemon juice that exhibited antiscorbutic activity. They prepared to publish their findings, but press reports then appeared that Rygh at the University of Oslo had identified vitamin C as methyl*nor*narcotine. King and Waugh deferred their manuscript until they tested Rygh's claim and found it to be spurious.

Meanwhile, Albert Szent-Györgyi was investigating redox systems in plants and animals for his Ph.D. degree at Cambridge University, England. In 1927 he isolated from the adrenal cortex of oxen, and also from cabbage and paprika, a crystalline, optically active, acidic substance with the empirical formula $C_6H_8O_6$. This substance was a strong reducing agent and gave colour tests characteristic of sugars, therefore Szent-Györgyi designated it as a 'hexuronic acid'. Later, in his native country Hungary, Szent-Györgyi suspected that hexuronic acid might be vitamin C, but he did not have the practical experience in his laboratory to test it with the guinea pig assay. Then fate intervened. Joseph Svirbely, who had only recently left King's laboratory in Pittsburgh, turned up at Szent-Györgyi's laboratory in Szeged to offer his services. Szent-Györgyi asked Svirbely to test hexuronic acid for vitamin C activity and after one month the result was evident: hexuronic acid was indeed vitamin C. Szent-Györgyi and Svirbely's note in *Nature*, April 1932, appeared two weeks after King and Waugh's deferred paper in *Science* (neither of these publications carried a date of receipt). A sample of hexuronic acid prepared from adrenal glands by E. C. Kendall using new and very different procedures was found to be identical to King's vitamin C preparation from lemons.

1.2.3 Pellagra

Pellagra was unknown in Europe until the 1730s, when it was described in Spain by Gaspar Casal. It appeared at around the time that maize was brought to Spain by Columbus from his voyages to America. The disease spread from Spain into France and Italy and eastward with the cultivation of maize and its use as a staple foodstuff. Great epidemics occurred in North Africa, especially in Egypt, later spreading to other parts of Africa. It was widely held that pellagra was in some way associated with spoiled maize and this led investigators on a false trail looking for an infectious or toxic agent. Pellagra first became prominent in the USA in 1907, affecting many poor families in the Midwest and Southern States. Hundreds of thousands of victims suffered 'the 3-Ds' – dermatitis, diarrhoea and dementia. The widespread nature of the disease and its association with poverty fuelled the belief that it was infectious, perhaps spread by an insect vector.

By 1912, pellagra had become a matter of grave national concern in the USA, with death rates up to 10 000 per year. In 1914 Joseph Goldberger, a bacteriologist with the US Public Health Service, was assigned the task of identifying the cause of pellagra. He noted the association of the disease with poor diet and was able to cure the disease and prevent recurrences in orphans and hospital patients by adding liberal amounts of milk and eggs to the institutional diets. Goldberger's next objective was to produce pellagra in previously healthy human subjects by feeding them a pellagragenic diet. The opportunity came in 1915 when a group of twelve convicts volunteered to undergo the experiment in return for pardons upon its completion. The diet consisted of corn (maize) meal, grits, cornstarch, wheat flour, rice, cane syrup, sugar, sweet potatoes, small amounts of turnip greens, cabbage and collards, and a liberal portion of pork fat. After six months on this diet, six of the eleven remaining volunteers had developed pellagra. Goldberger concluded in his report that 'Pellagra may be prevented completely by a suitable diet without intervention of any other factor, hygienic or sanitary.' He also considered the possibility that the lack of a hitherto unknown factor in the diet was responsible for the disease.

In the meantime, another group, the Thompson–McFadden Commission, had tried to produce pellagra in monkeys and baboons by injecting them with blood, urine, cerebrospinal fluid and tissue filtrates from patients with pellagra. The results were entirely negative and the Commission reported that infection had not been demonstrated, no insect vector had been found, and no relation between maize and the disease had been noted. Even so, much emphasis was laid on the poor sanitation of the communities investigated. There was still a question mark over whether humans could be infected with the disease.

It was Goldberger and 15 courageous colleagues who finally put paid to the infection dogma. They injected themselves with blood, swabbed their throats with nasopharyngeal secretions and swallowed the excreta and epidermal squames from patients severely ill with pellagra. During the following six months not one of these 16 scientists became ill.

1.2.4 Rickets

Much of the pioneering work on the aetiology of rickets should be accredited to the eminent French physician Armand Trousseau during the 1830s. Trousseau called attention to the experiments of Jules Guérin, published in 1838. Weaned puppies were placed in a dark basement and fed raw meat while their littermates were given a varied diet in a normal environment. After a few weeks the meat-fed animals exhibited all the classic signs of advanced rickets, in contrast to the littermates which showed no signs of rickets. A similar experiment conducted on young pigs given no access to animal fats or to sunlight gave analogous results. This led Trousseau to postulate that rickets was due in part to deficient diets. Trousseau also postulated that cod-liver oil, which had been demonstrated to cure rickets in children, was acting as a fat containing unknown beneficial dietary factors, rather than acting as a specific drug. He recognized that 'good general alimentation' is of prime importance in the aetiology of rickets as well as the beneficial effects of sunshine. Unfortunately, these experiments were ignored and forgotten by 1900. Most medical authorities at the time advocated the development of a vaccine in the belief that rickets was a chronic infectious disease. They dismissed cod-liver oil as a useless 'quack' remedy.

In 1918, Sir Edward Mellanby in Great Britain undertook the study of rickets, starting again at the same point as Guérin 80 years before. Mellanby produced rickets in puppies by raising them without the benefit of sunlight or UV radiation, and feeding them a high-cereal, low-fat diet in which white bread was replaced by unrefined oatmeal. Mellanby further showed that the addition of cod-liver oil or butterfat to the feed prevented rickets. This clearly showed that rickets was a nutritional disease, and cod-liver oil or butterfat contained a factor that prevented it.

In 1922 McCollum and associates published the results of experiments designed to determine whether the antirachitic factor in cod-liver oil was identical to or distinct from the previously discovered vitamin A. They found that cod-liver oil retained its antirachitic properties after destruction of the vitamin A by heating and aeration. Thus, in addition to vitamin A, cod-liver oil contained a new fat-soluble vitamin, which McCollum later (1925) called 'vitamin D'. Zucker and co-workers in 1922 found that vitamin D was present in the unsaponifiable fraction of cod-liver oil, and suggested that it was closely related to cholesterol.

1.3   Experiments on formulated diets

In the meantime, research was under way into what constituted a physiologically complete diet. Lunin, a pupil of the Swiss biochemist Bunge, first showed in 1882 that laboratory animals failed to thrive when kept on an artificial diet comprising the then known constituents of food (fat, protein, carbohydrate, mineral salts and water) in purified form. Taking a similar approach of using isolated purified food ingredients, Pekelharing formulated a baked product containing only casein, albumin, rice flour, lard and a mixture of all the salts which ought to be found in food. When this product, plus water to drink, was provided as food for mice, the mice failed to grow and died. When other mice were provided with the same meal, but with milk to drink instead of water, they kept in good health. Pekelharing concluded in 1905 that 'There is an unknown substance in milk, which, even in very small quantities, is of paramount importance to nutrition. If this substance is absent, the organism loses the power properly to assimilate the well-known principal parts of food, the appetite is lost and, with apparent abundance, the animals die of want. Undoubtedly, this substance not only occurs in milk, but in all sorts of foodstuffs, both of vegetable and animal origin.' Stepp from 1909 to 1913 provided mice with a natural complete foodstuff (milk and bread) from which he had removed certain constituents by means of alcohol-ether extraction. He discovered thereby that milk and other foods contained some unknown alcohol-soluble dietary factor indispensable for life. As no-one had yet succeeded in isolating the factor,

there was no proof of its existence and many doubts were raised concerning the validity of Pekelharing's conclusions. One school of thought was that the animals failed because of the mere monotony of the diet, or its lack of palatability, or to the absence of flavouring substances. Others thought that the cause was to be found in insufficient consumption or failure of absorption.

That a monotonous and unaccustomed food may be used successfully over long periods of time without ill-effects was proved by the experiments of Falta and Noeggerath, published in 1905. They maintained rats successfully for six months or more on monotonous diets of milk, milk powder or lean horsemeat.

We now turn to the work of Sir Frederick Hopkins in England. He fed young rats on an artificial food mixture containing caseinogen, starch, cane sugar, lard and inorganic salts. When these constituents were given in their crude condition, they were apparently adequate to maintain life and a certain amount of growth. When, however, they were subjected to careful purification, growth invariably ceased within a comparatively short time, and the rats died. By carefully determining the total energy consumption of his test rats, Hopkins was able to show that this failure was not due to an insufficient food intake. They ceased, in fact, to grow at a time when they were consuming food in more than sufficient quantity to maintain normal growth. Cessation of growth took place before any failure in appetite. Any effects upon the appetite must therefore have been secondary to a more direct effect upon growth processes. In his classic paper (Hopkins, 1912), Hopkins suggested the term 'accessory factors' for the missing nutrients, postulating that their necessity is a consequence of physiological evolution. Hopkins' work was the first to attract general attention to the existence of the hitherto unrecognized growth-promoting substances.

Casimir Funk, a Polish biochemist working at the Lister Institute in London, set out to isolate the anti-beriberi factor from rice polishings and obtained a biologically active, crystalline substance with the chemical properties of an amine. Funk believed that he had isolated the pure factor, but it was later realized that he had not. In 1912 Funk published a review of the existing knowledge of the diseases caused by nutritional errors (Funk, 1912). He proposed that beriberi, scurvy, pellagra and possibly rickets were caused by the absence from the diet of 'special substances which are of the nature of organic bases, which we will call vitamines'. His new word 'vitamine' was derived from *vita* (meaning life in Latin) and amine. Funk postulated the existence of an anti-beriberi vitamine, an anti-scurvy vitamine, probably an anti-pellagra vitamine and possibly an anti-rickets vitamine. Later, in 1922, Funk wrote, 'I must admit that when I chose the name vitamine I was well aware that these substances might later prove not to be of an amine nature. However, it was necessary for me to choose a name that would sound well and serve as a catch-word.'

The year 1912 was a landmark in the history of vitamins and heralded a new era in vitamin research. Hopkins' celebrated paper and Funk's review, published a few months earlier, attracted world-wide attention and, finally, a general acceptance of the existence of vitamins. In his review Funk commented, 'There is perhaps no other subject in medicine where so many contradictions and inexact statements were made, which, instead of advancing the research, retarded it by leading investigators in a wrong direction.'

The importance of the pioneering experiments of Eijkman and of Hopkins was finally recognized by the award to them jointly of the Nobel Prize for Physiology or Medicine in 1929.

1.4 Naming of the vitamins

By 1915, Osborne and Mendel and also McCollum and Davis had between them distinguished two types of accessory factors based on their solubilities and called them 'fat-soluble A' and 'water-soluble B'. Fat-soluble A was present in butterfat and egg yolk; a deficiency of this substance produced an infectious eye disease (xerophthalmia) and growth retardation in young rats. Water-soluble B was present in wheat germ and milk powder; its deficiency produced the avian form of beriberi in pigeons. In 1920, the terminal '-e' was dropped from the word 'vitamine' and fat-soluble A and water-soluble B were renamed vitamin A and vitamin B, respectively. The anti-scurvy factor was named vitamin C. For some time it was considered probable that the anti-rickets factor might be identical with vitamin A, since those foods which protected against experimental rickets were generally the same as those rich in vitamin A. Later, however, differences in distribution and chemical properties were established, and the anti-rickets factor was designated vitamin D. In 1922 Evans and Bishop discovered an anti-sterility factor necessary for successful reproduction in the rat; this factor was later named vitamin E. An anti-haemorrhagic factor for chicks reported in 1935 by Dam was later named vitamin K.

Vitamin B eventually proved to be a mixture of compounds having different chemical and physiological properties. This mixture is referred to today as the 'vitamin B complex' in accordance with the original nomenclature. The components of the vitamin B complex were originally designated arbitrarily as vitamins B_1, B_2, B_3, B_4, etc.

Gaps in the present alphabetical and numerical designations can be explained by the fact that several nutritional factors originally claimed to be vitamins turned out not to be vitamins after all, or were identical to another vitamin. Later, when the vitamins had been isolated and chemically characterized, they were given names according to the class of chemical compounds to which they belong. The last vitamin to be discovered was vitamin B_{12}, which was isolated in crystalline form from liver in 1948.

Further reading

Carpenter, K. J. & Sutherland, B. (1995) Eijkman's contribution to the discovery of vitamins. *Journal of Nutrition*, **125**, 155–63.
Chick, H. (1953) Early investigations of scurvy and the antiscorbutic vitamin. *Proceedings of the Nutrition Society*, **12**, 210–18.
Sydenstricker, V. P. (1958) The history of pellagra, its recognition as a disorder of nutrition and its conquest. *American Journal of Clinical Nutrition*, **6**, 409–14.

References

Funk, C. (1912) The etiology of the deficiency diseases. *Journal of State Medicine*, **20**, 341–68.
Hopkins, F. G. (1912) Feeding experiments illustrating the importance of accessory factors in normal dietaries. *Journal of Physiology*, **44**, 425–60.

2
Nutritional Aspects of Vitamins

2.1 Definition and classification of vitamins

Vitamins are a group of organic compounds which are essential in very small amounts for the normal functioning of the body. Thirteen vitamins are recognized in human nutrition and these have been classified, according to their solubility, into two groups. The fat-soluble vitamins are represented by vitamins A, D, E and K; also included are the 50 or so carotenoids that possess varying degrees of vitamin A activity. The water-soluble vitamins comprise vitamin C and the members of the vitamin B group, namely thiamin (vitamin B_1), riboflavin (vitamin B_2), niacin, vitamin B_6, pantothenic acid, biotin, folate and vitamin B_{12}. Vitamins have widely varying biochemical and physiological functions and are broadly distributed in natural food sources.

For several of the vitamins, biological activity is attributed to a number of structurally related compounds known as vitamers. The vitamers pertaining to a particular vitamin display, in most cases, similar qualitative biological properties to one another, but, because of subtle differences in their chemical structures, exhibit varying degrees of potency.

It is often stated that vitamins cannot be produced in the body and must, therefore, be supplied in the diet. This statement is valid for many of the vitamins, but is not strictly true for others. For example, vitamin D can be formed in the skin upon adequate exposure to ultraviolet radiation; vitamin K is normally produced in sufficient amounts by intestinal bacteria; and niacin can be synthesized *in vivo* from an amino acid precursor, L-tryptophan. With the possible exception of vitamins D and K, vitamins must be supplied by the diet because they cannot be produced in adequate amounts by the human body. Plants have the ability to synthesize most of the vitamins and serve as primary sources of these dietary essentials.

2.2 Nutritional vitamin deficiency

In countries where diets are unbalanced and inadequate, or where there are particular dietary customs, certain typical disease patterns have been shown to be due to vitamin deficiency. Examples of the most commonly observed diseases are xerophthalmia, rickets, beriberi, pellagra and scurvy, which result from deficiencies of vitamin A, vitamin D, thiamin, niacin and vitamin C, respectively. Deficiency of a single member of the vitamin B group is rare in humans because these vitamins are largely found together in nature, and foodstuffs lacking in one member of the complex are likely to be poor in the others. Moreover, the overt manifestations of deficiency of this group overlap to some extent.

Subclinical deficiency and marginal deficiency are synonymous terms used to describe conditions in individuals who are not clinically nutrient deficient, but who appear to be close to it. An alternative and perhaps better term proposed by Victor Herbert in 1990 is 'early negative nutrient balance', which is used when laboratory measurements indicate that an individual is losing more of a nutrient than is being absorbed.

By reference to the sequence of events in the development of vitamin deficiency, Pietrzik (1985) emphasized the importance of preventing functional metabolic disturbances that can evolve into overt clinical symptoms. This sequence can be subdivided into six stages as follows.

- **Stage 1** Body stores of the vitamin are progressively depleted. A decreased vitamin excretion in the urine is often the first sign. Normal blood levels are maintained by homeostatic mechanisms in the very early stages of deficiency.
- **Stage 2** The urinary excretion of the vitamin is further decreased and vitamin concentrations in the blood and other tissues are lowered. A diminished concentration of vitamin metabolites might also be observed.
- **Stage 3** There are changes in biochemical parameters such as low concentrations of the vitamin in blood, urine and tissues, and a low activity of vitamin-dependent enzymes or hormones. Immune response might also be reduced. Non-specific subclinical symptoms such as general malaise, loss of appetite and other mental changes appear.
- **Stage 4** The biochemical changes become more severe and morphological or functional disturbances are observed. These disturbances might be corrected by vitamin dosing in therapeutic amounts within a relatively short time or vitamin supplementation in amounts of (or exceeding) the recommended dietary allowances over a longer period. Malformation of cells is reversible at this stage.
- **Stage 5** The classical clinical symptoms of vitamin deficiency will appear. Anatomical alterations characterized by reversible damage of tissues might be cured in general by hospitalization of the patient. In most cases there are deficiencies of several nutrients

and a complicated dietetic and therapeutic regimen has to be followed.
- **Stage 6** The morphological and functional disturbances will become irreversible, finally leading to death in extreme cases.

From the health point of view, Pietrzik (1985) proposed that the borderline vitamin deficiency is represented by the transition from the third to the fourth stage.

The causes of nutritional vitamin deficiency are any one or combination of the following: inadequate ingestion, poor absorption, inadequate utilization, increased requirement, increased excretion and increased destruction in the body. The capacity to store vitamins in the body is another aspect to be considered: humans can store thiamin for only about two weeks, whereas vitamin B_{12} can be stored for several years. Other factors that contribute to nutritional vitamin deficiency are listed in Table 2.1.

Table 2.1 Causes of vitamin deficiency. From Marks (1975).

Due to	Caused by
Primary food deficiency	Crop failure
	Food storage losses
Diminished food intake	Poverty and ignorance
	Loss of appetite
	Apathy
	Food taboos and fads
	Pregnancy sickness
	Dental problems
	Chronic disease
Diminished absorption	Absorption defect diseases
	Parasitic infections
	Malignant diseases
Increased requirements	Increased physical activity
	Infections
	Pregnancy and lactation
	Drug therapy
	Vitamin imbalance
	Rapid growth
Increased losses	Excessive sweating
	Diuresis
	Lactation

2.3   Stability and bioavailability of vitamins

2.3.1   Stability

Vitamin stability is an important issue when considering the nutritional value of a food. Processing and storage losses depend upon conditions such as pH, temperature and moisture content. Niacin and biotin are relatively stable, but the other water-soluble vitamins are labile to varying extents and under different conditions. Riboflavin is notoriously susceptible to decomposition by light. During domestic cooking the water-soluble vitamins are easily leached out into the cooking water or exuded from meat, but are not lost if the cooking fluids are consumed. In the case of vitamin C, rapid heat treatment, such as the blanching of fruits and vegetables or the pasteurization of fruit juices, actually serves to prevent vitamin losses during post-processing storage by inactivating enzymes that promote the direct oxidation of ascorbic acid.

2.3.2   Bioavailability

The term 'bioavailability', as applied to vitamins in human nutrition, refers to the proportion of the quantity of vitamin in the food ingested that undergoes intestinal absorption and utilization by the body. Utilization encompasses transport of the absorbed vitamin to the tissues, cellular uptake and the subsequent fate of the vitamin. The vitamin may be converted to a form which can fulfil some biochemical function. Alternatively, the vitamin may be metabolized within the cell to a nonfunctional form for subsequent excretion or simply stored within the cell for future use. Any definition must be viewed as an operational definition within the context of the method used to determine bioavailability.

Bioavailability should not be confused with nutrient stability. Whereas food processing can result in the loss of a labile vitamin, the bioavailability of the remaining amount of vitamin is not necessarily altered. Bioavailability is influenced by a diverse range of interacting parameters and therefore the amount of bioavailable vitamin in a diet or individual food can vary considerably.

Absorption of a vitamin depends on the chemical form and physical state in which the vitamin exists within the food matrix. These properties may be influenced by the effects of food processing and cooking, particularly in the case of niacin, vitamin B_6 and folate. In foods derived from animal and plant tissues, the B-group vitamins occur as their coenzyme derivatives, usually associated with their protein apoenzyme. In addition, niacin in cereals and vitamin B_6 in certain fruits and vegetables occur largely as bound storage forms. In milk and eggs, which are derived from animal secretions, the B-group vitamins occur, at least to some extent, in the underivatized form, a proportion of which is associated with specific binding proteins. Vitamins that exist naturally as chemically bound complexes with some other material in the food matrix exhibit lower efficiencies of digestion and absorption compared with the free (unbound) vitamin ingested, for example, in tablet form.

Certain dietary components can retard or enhance a vitamin's absorption, therefore the composition of the diet is an important consideration. For example, the presence of adequate amounts of dietary fat is essential for the absorption of the fat-soluble vitamins. Carotenoids exhibit low bioavailability relative to vitamin A due to the poor digestibility of fibrous plant material. Other ingested substances such as alcohol and drugs may interfere with the physiological mechanisms of absorption.

Biological factors can influence the absorption of a vitamin from a particular food or diet. For example, the absorption mechanism in intestinal epithelium can be adapted physiologically to meet changing metabolic requirements and food deprivation. Malabsorption may occur in the presence of gastrointestinal disorders or disease. Other general factors that influence absorption include the plane of nutrition, metabolic requirements, age and state of health.

It is impracticable to determine true or absolute bioavailability, and therefore almost all methods for determining vitamin bioavailability in foods yield a measurement of relative bioavailability. This is the observed response obtained when the animal is fed the test food or diet expressed as a percentage of the response obtained by feeding a reference material of high bioavailability. Rats or chicks have been used extensively as experimental animals, but these animal studies are now thought to have relatively little value in predicting vitamin bioavailability for humans. This is because of problems such as intestinal synthesis of water-soluble vitamins by gut microflora, coprophagy (faecal recycling) and metabolic differences between animals and humans. The main emphasis nowadays in the field of nutrient bioavailability has turned to the use of protocols with human subjects in order to avoid the uncertain relevance of animal models (Gregory, 1988).

2.4   Vitamin requirements

Metabolic processes must respond to the immediate needs of the body and therefore vitamin requirements are subject to continuous variation between certain limits. The Food and Nutrition Board of the Institute of Medicine in the United States defines a requirement as the lowest continuing intake level of a nutrient that, for a specific indicator of adequacy, will maintain a defined level of nutriture in an individual. A Recommended Dietary Allowance (RDA) of a nutrient is the average daily dietary intake level that is sufficient to meet the requirement of nearly all (97 to 98 per cent) apparently healthy individuals in a particular life stage and gender group. The RDA is derived from an Estimated Average Requirement (EAR), which is an estimate of the intake at which the risk of inadequacy to an individual is 50 per cent. RDAs have been published for vitamins A, D, E and K, thiamin, riboflavin, niacin, vitamin B_6, folate, vitamin B_{12} and vitamin C (National Research Council, 1989). In the case of pantothenic acid and biotin, there is insufficient evidence to calculate an EAR and a reference intake called an Adequate Intake (AI) is provided instead of an RDA (Institute of Medicine, 1998). The AI is a value based on experimentally derived intake levels or approximations of observed mean nutrient intakes by a group (or groups) of apparently healthy people.

Further reading

Bates, C. J. & Heseker, H. (1994) Human bioavailability of vitamins. *Nutrition Research Reviews*, 7, 93–127.
Goldsmith, G. A. (1975) Vitamin B complex. Thiamine, riboflavin, niacin, folic acid (folacin), vitamin B_{12}, biotin. *Progress in Food and Nutrition Science*, 1, 559–609.

References

Gregory, J. F. III (1988) Recent developments in methods for the assessment of vitamin bioavailability. *Food Technology*, 42(10), 230, 233, 235, 237–8.
Institute of Medicine (1998) *Dietary Reference Intakes for Thiamin, Riboflavin, Niacin, Vitamin B_6, Folate, Vitamin B_{12}, Pantothenic Acid, Biotin and Choline*. National Academy Press, Washington, DC.
Marks, J. (1975) *A Guide to The Vitamins. Their Role in Health and Disease*. MTP Press, Lancaster.
National Research Council (1989) *Recommended Dietary Allowances*, 10th edn. National Academy Press, Washington, DC.
Pietrzik, K. (1985) Concept of borderline vitamin deficiencies. *International Journal for Vitamin and Nutrition Research*, Suppl. 27, 61–73.

3
Background Physiology and Functional Anatomy

Key discussion topics

Key discussion topics

- Physiological concentrations of water-soluble substances (apart from small uncharged solutes) require carrier-mediated transport mechanisms in order to pass through the lipid bilayer of cell membranes.
- The passage of substances through a cell membrane against a concentration gradient requires active transport with the expenditure of metabolic energy.
- The physiology of intestinal glucose absorption has been extensively studied and forms a basis for understanding the absorption of water-soluble vitamins.
- For micronutrients to enter brain cells from blood, they must (1) enter the extracellular space of the brain through the blood–brain barrier or (2) enter the cerebrospinal fluid via the choroid plexus.

- Most sites of known mechanisms of placental transport are localized to the microvillous and basal plasma membranes of the syncytiotrophoblast.
- G proteins act as molecular switches in relaying the signal from activated receptors on the cell surface to effector enzymes that catalyse the generation of second messengers such as cyclic AMP.
- Bone is a dynamic living tissue that is constantly being destroyed and renewed in order to maintain its strength.
- Inhibiting the flow of growth-controlling factors through gap junctions leads to neoplastic transformation of cells and the formation of cancerous tumours.

3.1 Movement of solutes across cell membranes and epithelia

An epithelium is a sheet of closely apposed cells that forms a boundary at the interface of the body and its external environment or between fluid compartments within the body. The epithelium rests on a thin sheet of an extracellular matrix, the basal lamina, that is rich in mucopolysaccharides. We are concerned with epithelia that can perform vectorial (transepithelial) transport of solutes, such as the epithelia of the small intestine, kidney and liver. Vectorial transport regulates the volume and/or composition of body-fluid compartments by absorption or secretion.

3.1.1 Epithelial cell structure

The plasma membrane

Individual animal cells of all types are enveloped by a plasma membrane composed of a lipid bilayer about 5 nm thick with globular proteins either partially embedded in it or attached to the outer or inner surface (Fig. 3.1). The lipids are represented by phospholipids, glycolipids and cholesterol, all of which are amphipathic, i.e. having both hydrophilic and hydrophobic portions. The phospholipids are predominantly phosphoglycerides, which have a glycerol backbone; sphingomyelin, a phospholipid which lacks a glycerol moiety, is a common constituent. The phospholipids are organized into a bilayer, only two molecules thick,

with polar heads facing outward toward the aqueous environment and fatty acid tails forming a hydrophobic interior. Each phospholipid layer in this lamellar structure is called a leaflet. The molecular arrangement of the phospholipids represents the stable state of minimum free-energy expenditure and is due to a maximization of hydrophilic and hydrophobic interactions. Glycolipids are distinguished from phospholipids by the presence of one or more sugar residues at the polar head group. Cholesterol contributes to the membrane fluidity whilst also providing mechanical stability. The cholesterol molecules are orientated in the bilayer with their hydroxyl group close to the polar heads of the phospholipids and glycolipids. This leaves the distal portions of the phospholipid/glycolipid fatty acid tails free and relatively flexible.

The plasma membrane regulates the movement of substances across the impervious lipid bilayer by virtue of its property of selective permeability. This property is attributed to the protein constituents of the membrane. Membrane proteins can be classified into two broad categories – integral and peripheral – according to how they interact with the lipid bilayer. Integral membrane proteins are amphipathic molecules whose hydrophobic regions are embedded within the lipid bilayer and hydrophilic regions are exposed at the membrane's surface. Almost all are transmembrane proteins that span the bilayer in a weaving fashion and account for most membrane-associated receptors and transporters and certain enzymes. Most

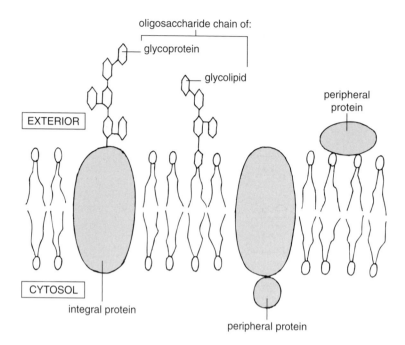

oligosaccharide chain of:

glycoprotein

glycolipid

peripheral protein

EXTERIOR

CYTOSOL

integral protein

peripheral protein

Fig. 3.1 Schematic diagram of a typical plasma membrane. (Cholesterol molecules not shown.) The lipid bilayer consists of two leaflets of phospholipid molecules whose fatty acid tails form the hydrophobic interior of the bilayer; their polar hydrophilic head groups line both surfaces. Integral proteins mostly span the bilayer. Peripheral proteins are associated with the membrane by protein–protein and lipid–protein interactions. Chains of sugar residues (oligosaccharides) bind to membrane proteins and also to lipids, forming glycoproteins and glycolipids, respectively.

of the integral membrane proteins are glycoproteins, whose chains of sugar residues invariably protrude to the outside of the cell. These chains, together with those of membrane glycolipids and other structures called proteoglycans, form a carbohydrate coat at the cell surface called the glycocalyx. Peripheral membrane proteins function almost entirely as enzymes. They do not interact with the hydrophobic interior of the lipid bilayer, but instead are bound ionically to the membrane's outer or inner surface. Binding is either indirectly to an integral membrane protein or directly to the polar head of a phospholipid.

The junctional complex

Each epithelial cell is adjoined with its neighbour by a junctional complex, which comprises three specialized attachment sites: the tight junction (zonula occludens), an intermediate junction (zonula adherens) and a desmosome (macula adherens) (Fig. 3.2). The tight junction constitutes a gasket encircling the apical end of each epithelial cell and separating the luminal fluid from the fluid in the lateral intercellular space. If the epithelium is visualized as a six-pack of beer, with the cans representing the cells, the sheet of plastic holding the cans together corresponds to the tight junction. The intermediate junction is an

adhesive band that also completely encircles the cell. Desmosomes are found all over the basolateral membrane and are sites of attachment to filaments of the cytoskeleton.

The cytoskeleton

The cytoskeleton forms an internal framework of protein filaments supporting the large volume of cytoplasm. The three principal types of protein filaments – intermediate filaments, microtubules and actin filaments – are connected to one another, and their functions are co-ordinated.

Intermediate filaments are tough, rope-like structures that provide mechanical stability to cells and tissues. Microtubules are long, stiff, hollow cylinders composed of polymerized tubulin molecules. Besides providing structural support for the cell, microtubules act as lines of transport for the organized movement of mitochondria and other membranous organelles to desired locations within the cell. They also facilitate delivery of transport vesicles from the Golgi complex to the apical membrane in epithelial cells, and become associated with the centrioles and chromosomes to form the spindle during mitosis and meiosis. The movement of organelles is facilitated by specialized motor proteins which use the energy derived from

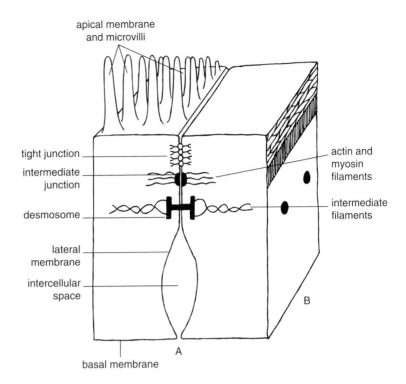

apical membrane
and microvilli

tight junction

intermediate
junction

desmosome

lateral
membrane

intercellular
space

basal membrane

actin and
myosin
filaments

intermediate
filaments

B

A

Fig. 3.2 Diagram of the epithelial junctional complex shown in (A) cross-section and (B) face view. Tight junctions and intermediate junctions both form continuous zonular structures circumscribing the cell apex. Desmosomes resemble spot welds between the lateral plasma membranes.

the hydrolysis of adenosine triphosphate (ATP) to drag organelles along the microtubule. When cells are treated with colchicine (an alkaloid that inhibits the polymerization of tubulin molecules), organelles change their location. When the drug is removed, the organelles return to their original position. The normal position of an organelle is thought to be determined by a receptor protein on the cytosolic surface of its membrane that binds a specific motor protein.

A terminal web composed of ordered arrays of actin filaments and associated proteins underlies and supports the microvilli of brush-border-type epithelial cells such as the intestinal absorptive cell (see Section 3.3.1). Within each microvillus is a core of actin filaments whose roots interdigitate with filaments of the terminal web (Fig. 3.3). Different sets of filaments within the terminal web are closely associated with the three components of the junctional complex. Of particular interest is a circumferential band of contractile filaments known as the perijunctional actomyosin ring, which is located at the level of the intermediate junction.

The microvillous core is attached laterally to the apical membrane by cross-filaments (Fig. 3.3).

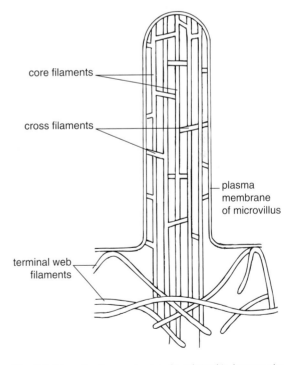

core filaments

cross filaments

plasma
membrane
of microvillus

terminal web
filaments

Fig. 3.3 Schematic diagram showing the relationship between the various filament systems in the brush-border region of intestinal epithelial cells (enterocytes).

These filaments are composed of a 110-kDa protein–calmodulin complex belonging to a family of mechanoenzymes known as myosin I, and is specifically known as 'brush border myosin I'. Like the well-known myosin of skeletal muscle, myosin I is an ATPase, capable of transducing energy stored in ATP into motion along actin filaments. Because of its cellular location, it can be envisaged that brush border myosin I produces force on the apical membrane relative to the actin filaments in the core bundle.

Tight junctions

A tight junction appears by transmission electron microscopy of thin sections as a series of discrete sites of apparent fusion involving the outer leaflet of the lateral plasma membrane of adjacent cells. A more detailed picture is obtained by examination of cells prepared by freeze-fracturing. In freeze-fracture replicas the apparent membrane fusion sites are evident as branching linear arrays of strands on the P face and complementing grooves on the E face. It seems that at the apparent fusion sites there are pairs of strands, offset with respect to each other, with one being contributed by each cell. Each strand may be composed of large aggregates of occludin molecules.

A proposed model for the molecular organization of tight junctions is shown in Fig. 3.4. Occludin molecules spanning the membrane of one cell interact with complementary domains on occludin molecules from adjacent cells, thereby forming the barrier portion of the tight junction. Another protein, named ZO-1 (zonula occludens 1), connects occludin to actin filaments of the cytoskeleton through spectrin II and cingulin. Contraction of the actin cytoskeleton (possibly the perijunctional actomyosin ring) or changes in the phosphorylation state of ZO-1 or any other tight junction-associated protein could cause conformational changes in these proteins that would affect their interactions with occludin and alter the tight junction barrier. In this regard, the ZO-1 multiprotein complex could be a target for second messengers. For example, Duffey et al. (1981) observed a reduced ionic permeability across the tight junction and a reorientation of the junctional strands when amphibian gall bladder epithelium was exposed to adenosine 3′,5′-cyclic monophosphate (cyclic AMP).

Tight junctions of intestinal epithelia are much more permeable to potassium ions (K^+) and so-

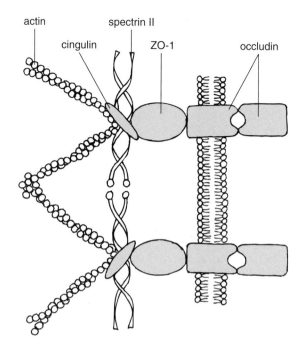

Fig. 3.4 Molecular organization of tight junctions. The transmembrane-spanning protein occludin is shown binding complementary domains on occludin molecules in an adjacent cell. Cytoplasmic domains of occludin are bound to ZO-1 and its associated multiprotein complex. This ZO complex is linked to the actin cytoskeleton through spectrin II and cingulin. Reproduced, with permission, from Ballard et al. (1995), *Annual Review of Nutrition*, Volume 15, pp. 35–55, ©1995 by Annual Review (www.annualreviews.org).

dium ions (Na^+) than to chloride ions (Cl^-). This cation selectivity has been explained by the tight junctions being lined with hydrated negative charges that discriminate against the passive movement of anions (Cereijido et al., 1978). The permeability of an epithelium to inorganic ions seems to be directly proportional to the transepithelial electrical resistance, measured by placing microelectrodes on either side of the epithelium. Because plasma membrane resistances are, in most cases, relatively high, transepithelial resistance values reflect the resistance to current flow through the tight junction, and hence its ionic permeability. Different epithelia exhibit a wide range of resistance values, depending on the physiological requirements of the tissue. The transepithelial resistance correlates with the number of freeze-fracture strands in the tight junctions of various epithelia. For example, the low resistance (6 ohm cm^{-2}) epithelium of the mammalian renal proximal convoluted tubule has only a single continuous strand whereas the high resistance (>2000 ohm cm^{-2}) epithelium of the toad urinary bladder has more than eight strands lying in parallel. This correlation suggests that the strands represent the functionally important elements of the tight junction.

Gap junctions

While individual cells are capable of maintaining their own functions, the co-ordination of cellular activities within a tissue depends on the exchange of information among constituent cells. Neural and endocrine co-ordination are ways to achieve this goal, but these involve long-range interactions. Intercellular communication can be achieved directly via the connecting channels of gap junctions. Gap junctions are plasma membrane structures formed at points of contact between two similar cells. As viewed by electron microscopy, they appear as clusters of particles (connexons) embedded in the plasma membrane. These clusters are present at very high density (~10^4 gap junctions μm^{-2}) and are referred to as gap junctional plaques (Musil & Goodenough, 1991). An individual connexon is formed from six subunits of transmembrane proteins of the connexin family. Each connexon is tightly joined to an identical connexon within the plasma membrane of the adjacent cell. As shown in Fig. 3.5, the paired connexons form water-filled pipes (usually referred to as channels) which permit the ready diffusion of cytoplasmic ions and molecules from cell to cell. The pore size of the mammalian gap junction is such that it excludes molecules larger than approximately 1000 daltons. Diffusible molecules include most sugars, amino acids, nucleotides, vitamins and 'messenger' molecules such as cyclic AMP.

One function of intercellular communication may be to maintain cellular homeostasis through the exchange of ions, metabolites and water. In electrically active cells such as neurons, cardiocytes and smooth muscle cells, gap junctions serve as electrical synapses for the rapid conduction of action potentials. In other cells, intercellular communication may co-ordinate tissue responses to hormones through the exchange of second messenger ions or molecules between hormone-stimulated cells and non-stimulated cells. Intercellular communication is also important in the

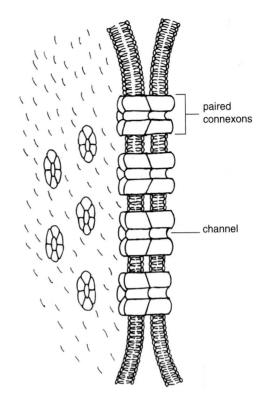

Fig. 3.5 Diagram of a possible structure of a gap junction. The connexons within the plasma membranes of adjacent cells form a channel allowing intercellular communication. Reproduced, with permission, from Patricia J. Wynne.

regulation of mitotic cell proliferation. Many types of cancer cell have a decreased capacity for intercellular communication and a decreased number of gap junctions. This loss of intercellular communication has been correlated with the degree of malignancy of the neoplasm (Klaunig & Ruch, 1990).

Increasing concentrations of intercellular calcium ions (Ca^{2+}) causes a progressive decrease in gap junction permeability by a channel closure mechanism that resembles the shutter in a camera. This channel closure may be mediated by the protein calmodulin, which binds to gap junction proteins in the presence of Ca^{2+}. The Ca^{2+}-activated calmodulin may directly induce the conformational change in the gap junction protein(s) that results in channel occlusion (Peracchia & Bernardini, 1984). Calcium ions trigger channel closure whenever it is necessary to isolate a damaged cell.

3.1.2   Membrane fluidity

An artificial bilayer composed of a single type of phospholipid changes abruptly from a highly ordered gel-like state to a more mobile fluid when the temperature is raised. This change of state is called a phase transition and is due to increased motion about the C–C bonds of the fatty acid chains. The narrow temperature range over which the gel-like fluid transition takes place is known as the 'transition temperature'. The lipid bilayer is in a more fluid state when the fatty acid chains of the phospholipids or glycolipids are not tightly packed (Fig. 3.6). This condition is favoured when the chains are unsaturated and of shorter length. *Cis* double bonds produce kinks in the fatty acid chains that makes them more difficult to pack, and a shorter chain length reduces the tendency of the hydrocarbon chains to interact with one another. The addition of cholesterol restricts the C–C movements of the part of the fatty acid chains situated closest to the polar heads of the phospholipids, but it separates the flexible tails of the fatty acids and causes the inner regions of the bilayer to become slightly more fluid.

The fluidity of the lipid bilayer allows individual constituent phospholipids to diffuse laterally within their own monolayer, but they are always orientated with their polar heads facing outwards. Integral membrane proteins also float quite freely, but tend to be restricted to a limited area of the membrane. The restrictions are imposed by tight junctions acting as barriers, linkage to cytoskeletal proteins, and aggregation of membrane proteins with each other. Such restrictions give rise to a 'patchwork' of membrane domains, each exhibiting a different protein composition and function.

It is essential for many membrane functions that a precise fluidity of cell membranes be precisely maintained. Certain membrane transport processes and enzyme activities, for example, can be shown to cease when the viscosity of the plasma membrane is experimentally increased beyond a threshold level. Membrane fluidity provides the required motional freedom of the phospholipid molecules, allowing integral proteins to undergo conformational changes associated with their function. By synthesizing a diverse array of phospholipids intercalated with cholesterol, cells maintain an appropriate fluidity of their plasma membranes, as well as of all subcellular membranes.

3.1.3   Elementary principles of bioelectricity

Some basic electrical principles
The removal of electrons from a neutral body results in a positive charge, as when one electron is removed from the neutral sodium atom to form a sodium ion. The practical unit for measuring charge is the coulomb, which equals 6.2×10^{17} electrons. An electric field exists in the space around a charge and extends to infinity. In order to move a charge against the field, work must be performed. In experimental work, the difference in potential between two points is defined as the work necessary to move a unit charge from one

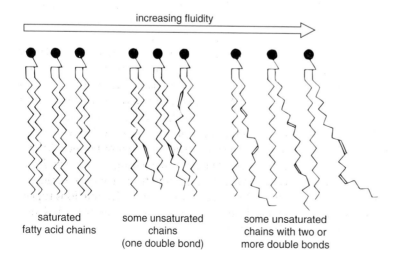

increasing fluidity

saturated
fatty acid chains

some unsaturated
chains
(one double bond)

some unsaturated
chains with two or
more double bonds

Fig. 3.6 Diagram showing that regions of the plasma membrane are in a more fluid state when phospholipids or glycolipids with unsaturated hydrocarbon chains are present than when the lipid chains are fully saturated. Enhanced fluidity is a consequence of kinks formed at double bonds in the hydrocarbon chains, which allow greater lateral mobility of these and associated molecules within their own monolayers. Reproduced, with permission, from Avers (1986), *Molecular Cell Biology* (©1986), Addison Wesley Longman.

point to the other. The practical unit of electrical potential difference is the volt, which is the potential difference against which 1 joule of work is done in the transfer of 1 coulomb.

A difference in potential is associated with a flow of current in a medium. The current can be charge-carrying ions in solutions of electrolytes. The current flow requires energy since it encounters resistance in the medium. In order to produce electrical currents, special sources of electrical energy are available, such as the battery and generator. Such sources of energy are said to produce an electromotive force. In solution, electrical energy is produced by chemical reactions which result in the separation of positive and negative charges at electrodes. Such separation of charge itself constitutes a form of stored energy which manifests as a difference in electrical potential.

Movement of an ion in a solution in which a potential difference is present requires work to be done with or against two forces: the electric field and any concentration difference in the ion.

The membrane potential

A potential difference exists across plasma membranes that makes the inside of the membrane electrically negative and the outside positive. The magnitude of this membrane potential is influenced by the composition of the fluid bathing the membrane. When mucosal strips of rabbit ileum are bathed by a physiological electrolyte solution, the membrane potential across the brush border averages –36 mV (cell interior negative) (Rose & Schultz, 1971). We will see that the membrane potential plays an essential role in the transport of substances across the membrane.

Figure 3.7 shows very simply how a membrane potential is established. The membrane separating the two aqueous compartments is permeable to K[+] but not to anions. The K[+] concentration of the intracellular compartment is 10-fold that of the extracellular compartment. Potassium ions tend to diffuse by random motion in both directions across the membrane. However, because the K[+] concentration is initially higher in the intracellular compartment, there is greater net movement of K[+] from inside to outside. This diffusion of K[+] down the concentration gradient, unaccompanied by anions, produces separation of charge and therefore the membrane becomes electrically charged, with the inside negative with respect to

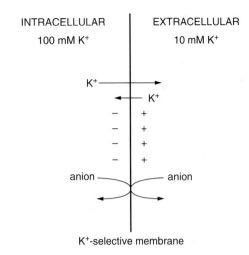

Fig. 3.7 Diagram showing the principle of how a membrane potential is established. A membrane separates two compartments. The left (intracellular) compartment contains 100 mM K[+] and the right (extracellular) compartment contains 10 mM K[+]. The membrane is freely permeable to K[+] but not to the accompanying anion. Net K[+] movement from left to right creates a membrane voltage, left side negative. This build-up of electronegativity will tend to retard the movement of K[+] from left to right until further net movement is prevented. The membrane voltage at this point defines the membrane potential.

the outside. This build-up of electronegativity along the inside of the membrane will tend to retard the outward diffusion of K[+]. The membrane potential is the point at which the electric potential across the membrane becomes great enough to prevent further net diffusion of K[+] to the exterior, despite the high K[+] concentration gradient.

In an actual plasma membrane, the membrane potential is established in a similar manner by an interaction between permanently open potassium leak channels and a sodium-potassium pump located in the membrane. As described later, K[+] is pumped into the cell in exchange for the outward removal of Na[+], creating the high intracellular concentration of K[+]. The net outward diffusion of K[+] through the potassium leak channels down the concentration gradient generates the inside-negative membrane potential aided by a small contribution by the sodium-potassium pump. Membranes are not in fact solely permeable to K[+]; they are also permeable to Cl[-], and are not totally impermeable to Na[+].

The separation of electric charges that creates the membrane potential occurs only in the immediate vicinity of the membrane, therefore the bulk of the cytosol and extracellular fluid remains electrically neutral. The charge separation involves only a minute fraction of the total number of positive and negative charges that exist in the cell, so ion concentrations are practically unaffected.

3.1.4 Protein-mediated membrane transport systems

The term 'transport' refers to solute translocation that is mediated by a transmembrane protein (transporter). Most transporters are multisubunit protein complexes made up of identical or structurally similar polypeptides held together noncovalently. Transporters exert their effect through a change in their three-dimensional shape (conformational change), and it is this change that limits the rate of transport. Each transporter is responsible for the translocation of a specific type of molecule, or a group of closely related molecules. Specificity is imparted by the tertiary and quaternary structures of the transporter molecule – only if a solute's spatial configuration fits into the protein will the solute be transferred across the membrane. The rapidity of protein-mediated transport is due to the fact that the transported molecules are prevented from entering the hydrophobic core of the membrane bilayer, and are therefore not slowed down.

Transporters fall into two main classes: carriers and ion channels. Ion pumps are a type of carrier protein that is also an enzyme.

Dozens of different transport proteins have been identified. Some of these proteins, called uniporters, transport a single substance from one side of a membrane to the opposite side. Others couple the movement of two substances to one another. When two coupled substances are moved in the same direction, the transport protein is called a symporter; if the two substances are moved in opposite directions, the protein is termed an antiporter. While channel proteins are always uniporters, carrier proteins can be uniporters, symporters or antiporters.

The movement of ions across the plasma membrane is also mediated by transport proteins. Symporters and certain antiporters co-transport ions together with specific small molecules, whereas ion channels, ion pumps and certain antiporters transport only ions. In all cases, the rate and extent of ion transport

across membranes is influenced not only by the ion concentration gradient, but also by the membrane potential. The combination of the ion concentration gradient and the membrane potential is referred to as the electrochemical gradient.

Carriers

At physiological concentrations, the translocation of several water-soluble vitamins (thiamin, riboflavin, pantothenic acid, biotin and vitamin C) across cell membranes takes place by carrier-mediated transport.

The interaction of a transportable substrate with its carrier is characterized by saturation at high substrate concentration, stereospecificity and competition with structural analogues. These properties are shared by the interaction of a substrate and an enzyme, thus the carrier may be considered as a specialized membrane-bound enzyme. Figure 3.8 shows the relationship between substrate concentration and the rate of carrier-mediated substrate transport. The terms V_{max} and K_m (Michaelis constant) can be used to describe the kinetics of carrier-mediated transport. The maximum rate of transport (V_{max}) is the point at which all of the available binding sites on the carrier are occupied by substrate – a further increase in the substrate concentration has no effect on the transport rate. V_{max} values are expressed in pmoles of substrate per mg protein during a specified period (min). Each carrier protein has a characteristic binding constant (K_m) for its substrate. K_m is defined as the concentration of substrate (expressed in units of molarity, mM)

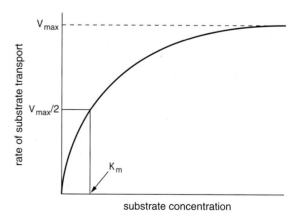

Fig. 3.8 Relationship between substrate concentration and the rate of carrier-mediated substrate transport.

at which half of the available carrier sites are occupied and is independent of the amount of carrier. Experimentally, K_m is determined from the graph shown in Fig. 3.8 and is the substrate concentration that corresponds to $V_{max}/2$. The lower the value of K_m, the greater the affinity of the carrier for its substrate and the greater the transport rate. When two substrates are transported simultaneously on the same carrier, the observed K_m for one of them will be an 'apparent K_m' and will depend on the concentration of the second substrate (Kimmich, 1981).

The term 'carrier' is a misnomer because it implies that the protein is mobile and ferries the transported substrate from one side of the membrane to the other. This was once thought to be the case, but it is now known that it is the conformational change which brings about substrate translocation. A carrier must undergo a conformational change in every transporting cycle and transports molecules at a rate of 10^2–10^4 per second.

Ion channels

Ion channels are integral membrane proteins that allow small specific inorganic ions, mainly Na$^+$, K$^+$, Ca^{2+} or Cl$^-$, to diffuse rapidly down their electrochemical gradients across the plasma membrane. The proteins form a narrow water-filled pore across the membrane through which ions can pass in single file at rates of 10^6–10^8 per second – very much faster rates than transport mediated by carrier proteins. The pore creates a direct link between the cytosol and the cell exterior, and therefore there is no need for solute binding. Ionic diffusion through channels may exhibit saturation, but usually only when concentrations are well beyond the physiological range.

Ion channels are highly selective and can distinguish, among ions of the same charge, those whose diameters differ by less than 0.1 nm. Selectivity results from the characteristics of the hydrophilic pore in the protein, namely its diameter, its shape and the nature of the electrical charge along its inside surface. Some ion channels in nerve and muscle membranes are 100 times more permeable to K$^+$ than to Na$^+$, even though sodium ions are actually smaller than potassium ions.

Many types of ion channel are responsible for the electrical excitability of muscle cells, and they mediate most forms of electrical signalling in the nervous system. These types are usually closed, opening only in response to specific stimuli and closing rapidly and spontaneously within milliseconds of having opened. Such channels are called gated channels, where the gate is the part of the channel protein that undergoes conformational change during opening and closing. One gating episode allows the channel to be in the transporting mode for as long as it remains open. A single ion channel operates in an all-or-nothing fashion – the gate is either open or closed. Gated channels may open in response to changes in the membrane potential (voltage-gated channels), to mechanical stress (mechanically gated channels) or to a ligand binding to a cell-surface receptor (ligand-gated channels). The ligand can be either an extracellular mediator – specifically, a neurotransmitter – or an intracellular mediator, such as an ion or a nucleotide.

Ion pumps

Ion pumps are transmembrane proteins that transport inorganic ions such as Na$^+$, K$^+$, Ca^{2+} and H$^+$ in or out of epithelial cells. The energy that drives the pump is obtained directly from the hydrolysis of metabolically derived ATP by an ATPase that is inherent to the pump. The ATPase attacks the high-energy terminal phosphate bond of ATP, forming adenosine diphosphate (ADP). The liberated phosphate is transferred to a specific phosphorylation site in the protein, forming a high-energy acyl phosphate bond. Hydrolysis of this bond provides the energy required to elicit a conformational change in the protein, making the bound ion accessible to the opposite side of the membrane.

There are three principal classes of ATP-driven ion pumps, namely P, F and V. Included in the P class are the Na$^+$–K$^+$-ATPase (sodium pump) and several Ca^{2+}-ATPases (calcium pumps). All known members of the F and V classes transport only protons (hydrogen ions, H$^+$).

3.1.5 Movement of solutes across cell membranes

The plasma membrane constitutes a selective barrier to the movement of molecules and ions between the extracellular and intracellular fluid compartments. Although fat-soluble substances, water and small uncharged polar solutes can simply diffuse through the membrane, ions and water-soluble molecules having five or more carbon atoms cannot do so. Most biologically important substances (e.g. glucose, essential amino acids, water-soluble vitamins and certain inorganic ions) are translocated across the plasma membrane by means of transporting membrane proteins at rates that are sufficiently rapid to sustain essential metabolic processes.

The movement of substances across cell membranes can take place either passively, without the expenditure of metabolic energy or by active transport, which involves 'uphill' movement of substances from a region of lower concentration to one of higher concentration with the expenditure of metabolic energy. We will encounter two types of passive movement – simple diffusion and facilitated diffusion – and two types of active transport – primary and secondary active transport. We will also encounter receptor-mediated endocytosis, which is an energy-dependent mechanism by which macromolecules can enter cells without actually crossing the plasma membrane.

Simple diffusion

The most straightforward mechanism for moving substances across cell membranes or within the cell itself is simple diffusion. Diffusion is the random movement of substances that ultimately results in their equal distribution. All molecules and ions in liquids or in gases undergo continual random jumping movements, driven by their inherent thermal energies, and are continually colliding with one another. These movements (collectively known as Brownian motion) and the impact of the collisions between individual molecules causes the displacement of molecules from one location to another. If two solutions of a particular solute at different concentrations are separated by a permeable membrane, solute molecules will migrate unaided along the concentration gradient from the region of higher concentration to the region of lower concentration. Eventually, the molecules will be equally distributed throughout the area that encloses them – a state of equilibrium. At equilibrium, individual molecules will continue to migrate randomly back and forth across the membrane, but there will be no *net* migration of molecules across the membrane.

The net rate of diffusion of a solute across a cell membrane depends on the permeability of the membrane and the pressure difference across the membrane. In the case of an uncharged solute, the sole driving force is the difference in solute concentration between the two sides of the membrane. (Note that an uncharged solute refers to a molecule that bears no net electrical charge; this includes solutes that have an equal number of positive and negative charges.) In the case of permeating ions, the driving force is the electrochemical gradient, which is a combination of the concentration difference and the membrane potential. Because the inside of the plasma membrane is negative with respect to the outside, the membrane potential favours the entry of cations into the cell, but opposes the entry of anions.

Lipid-soluble molecules readily pass through the plasma membrane by dissolving in the lipid matrix and diffusing through the lipid bilayer. Water and small uncharged water-soluble molecules, which have little affinity for the lipid matrix, can pass unhindered through some membrane protein molecules via narrow aqueous channels of no more than 0.5–1.0 nm diameter. Charged molecules, because of their shell of water molecules, are insoluble in the lipid bilayer and too big to pass through the narrow aqueous channels. However, specific inorganic ions can diffuse through membranes via ion channels, as previously discussed.

Facilitated diffusion

Facilitated diffusion refers to the carrier-mediated diffusion of molecules across the plasma membrane. Substances translocated in this way cannot usually pass through the membrane without the aid of a specific carrier protein. As in simple diffusion, the driving force is the concentration gradient between the inside and the outside of the cell. When the concentrations of solutes on the two sides of the membrane are equal, the carrier-mediated flow in both directions will also be equal. That is, net transport will cease when the solute distribution is equilibrated. Facilitated diffusion differs from simple diffusion in that it exhibits the characteristic properties of carrier-mediated processes, i.e. saturation kinetics, susceptibility to competitive inhibition and solute specificity.

The classic example of facilitated diffusion is glucose transport across the plasma membrane of erythrocytes. The glucose concentrations in erythrocytes are much lower than those in the extracellular fluid because the sugar is rapidly metabolized by these cells after gaining entry. The glucose transporter (a uniporter) contains a single glucose-binding site and alternates between two conformational states, one facing the exoplasmic (outside) surface of the membrane and the other facing the cytoplasmic (inside) surface. Only the thermal energy of the system is required for the conformational change to take place. A molecule of extracellular glucose binds to the outward-facing site, which then reorientates to face the inside of the cell. After release of the glucose into the cell interior, the transporter (without a bound glucose molecule) undergoes the reverse conformational change to re-create the outward-facing binding site.

The facilitated diffusion of glucose in erythrocytes occurs at a rate that is at least a hundred times faster than that predicted for simple diffusion. Specificity is high: for example, the K_m for the transport of the non-biological L-isomer of glucose is >3000 mM (cf. 1.5 mM for D-glucose).

Primary active transport

Primary active transport is a transport process that is driven *directly* by metabolic energy. Such processes are carried out exclusively by ion pumps, such as the calcium pumps, the sodium pump and the proton pumps. Ion pumps are ATPases, which utilize the energy released by the hydrolysis of ATP.

Ca²⁺-ATPases (calcium pumps)

Ca^{2+}-ATPases (calcium pumps)
A calcium pump in the basolateral membrane of entero-cytes plays a major role in the vitamin D-regulated intestinal absorption of calcium (see Chapter 8).

The Na$^+$–K$^+$-ATPase (sodium pump)
In most cells the concentrations of K^+ and Na^+ are re-spectively higher and lower than their concentrations in the extracellular fluid. A high cytosolic concentra-tion of K^+ is essential to maintain the membrane potential, and the sodium concentration gradient is required for the active membrane transport of sugars, amino acids and certain water-soluble vitamins. The unequal distribution of K^+ and Na^+ is maintained by the sodium pump. The sodium pump is also re-quired to maintain osmotic balance and stabilize cell volumes: without its function most cells of the body would swell until they burst.

The sodium pump operates as an antiporter, ac-tively pumping Na^+ out of the cell against its steep electrochemical gradient and pumping K^+ in. The in-flux of K^+ helps to balance the negative charges carried by organic anions that are confined within the cell. Three sodium ions are moved for every two potas-sium ions. The net outward movement of positively charged ions constitutes an electrical current, creating a potential difference across the membrane, with the inside negative to the outside. This electrogenic effect of the pump, however, seldom contributes more than 10% to the membrane potential. The remaining 90% depends on the pump only indirectly, as previously discussed. In epithelial cells such as the intestinal absorptive cell, sodium–potassium pumping activity is confined to the basolateral domain of the plasma membrane; there is no such activity on the apical domain. The drug ouabain competes with K^+ for the same site on the exoplasmic surface of the sodium pump and specifically inhibits its action.

H$^+$-ATPases (proton pumps)
Proton pumps have been described in the membranes of various intracellular compartments concerned with endocytosis and potocytosis, such as clathrin-coated vesicles, plasmalemmal vesicles derived from caveolae, endosomes and lysosomes, where their function is to acidify the lumen (Mellman *et al.*, 1986; Anderson & Orci, 1988). The pumping of protons across a vacuolar membrane from one compartment to another will generate an electrical potential across the membrane, and this will oppose further move-ment of protons. For proton movement to continue, there is an accompanying movement of an equal number of chloride anions in the same direction. A chloride transporter necessary for the maintenance of proton pump activity in clathrin-coated vesicles has been characterized (Xie *et al.*, 1989). Bafilomycin A₁, a macrolide antibiotic isolated from *Streptomyces* sp., specifically inhibits the V-type H$^+$-ATPase at na-nomolar concentration (Bowman *et al.*, 1988).

Secondary active transport

Whereas primary active transport is driven directly by metabolic energy, secondary active transport is *indirectly* linked to metabolic energy through a cou-pling of the solute to the movement of an inorganic ion (usually Na^+).

Secondary active transport provides the means whereby physiological amounts of monosaccharides, amino acids and several water-soluble vitamins in the intestinal lumen cross the epithelium of the small in-testine to gain access to the blood vessels; that is, the absorption of these substances. When sodium ions are transported out of enterocytes by the action of the ATP-dependent sodium pump at the basolateral membrane, an inward downhill concentration gradi-ent of sodium develops across the cell. This gradient represents a storehouse of energy because the excess sodium outside the cell is always attempting to diffuse back into the cell. The sodium concentration gradient drives the coupled transport of sodium and an accompanying substance from the intestinal lumen into the cell via the apical membrane. The coupled transport system is mediated by a carrier protein that has sites for both the sodium ion and the accompanying substance. If the accompanying substance is an anion (negative charge) and one anion is co-transported with one sodium ion (positive charge), the loaded carrier bears no net charge and responds solely to the sodium concentration gradient. If, however, the loaded carrier bears a net positive charge (e.g. a 2:1 ratio of Na^+ to anion$^-$), it is responsive to the negative membrane potential as well as the sodium concentration gradient; together these constitute the electrochemical gradient for sodium.

In co-transport (also called symport) the sodium moves down its concentration gradient or electrochemical gradient and the accompanying substance moves in the same direction. The absorption of glucose (Section 3.2.6) is an example of co-transport. In countertransport (also called antiport) the sodium and accompanying substance move in opposite directions. A typical antiporter is the sodium-calcium exchanger, which exchanges one calcium ion for every three sodium ions, and is important for extruding calcium ions from the cytosol of cardiac muscle cells. It may also play a minor role in the intestinal absorption of calcium by helping to transport cytosolic calcium across the basolateral membrane of the enterocyte.

Endocytosis and potocytosis

Endocytosis and potocytosis are mechanisms that cells use to import nutritious molecules from the extracellular environment. Both mechanisms are energy-dependent and tightly controlled. The principal function of endocytosis is to deliver macromolecules to lysosomes for hydrolytic processing or to transport them across polarized cells by transcytosis (Rodman et al., 1990). Pinocytosis refers to the trapping of a portion of the extracellular fluid during endocytosis. For the internalization of certain vital macromolecules in a minimum of extracellular fluid, receptor-mediated endocytosis provides much greater rates than ordinary endocytosis. Potocytosis describes the sequestration and transport of molecules and macromolecules by caveolae. Caveolae seal off from the plasma membrane, but remain separate from other endocytic compartments.

Receptor-mediated endocytosis

The various pathways of receptor-mediated endocytosis share one common feature: in each case receptor–ligand complexes are conveyed in coated pits and coated vesicles. However, there are differences in the routes that ligands and receptors follow after entering the cell. The model depicted in Fig. 3.9 is based on the endocytosis of plasma low-density lipoprotein (LDL) and other macromolecules in which the receptor recycles and the ligand is degraded. In this model, the macromolecular ligands bind to specific cell-surface receptors, which are transmembrane proteins. This binding triggers clustering of receptor–ligand complexes at specialized internalization sites known as coated pits. The 'coat' is formed entirely of the protein, clathrin, whose heavy and light chains are organized to form a network on the cytoplasmic face of the plasma membrane. The coated pits invaginate and pinch off to form intracellular coated vesicles enclosing the receptor–ligand complexes. This fusion of the ends of the coated pit membranes and pinching off of vesicles is ATP-dependent. Within the cytosol, the vesicles are uncoated by an ATP-dependent enzyme, after which they fuse with one another to form endosomes, whose contents are acidified by a proton pump. Within the endosomes the ligands dissociate from their receptors, and the ligands are carried further to lysosomes, where they undergo proteolysis. The receptors leave the endosomes, apparently via incorporation into the membrane of vesicles that bud off from the endosome surface, and are recycled to the cell surface to bind new ligand.

Potocytosis

Potocytosis utilizes membrane proteins to concentrate the molecules before internalization. The membrane proteins are anchored by glycosylphosphatidylinositol (GPI) chains and are organized into clusters within flask-shaped membrane invaginations known as caveolae. There are at least three distinct ways that the GPI-anchored proteins can concentrate molecules: namely, receptor-mediated, enzyme-mediated and carrier-mediated potocytosis (Anderson, 1993).

Folate uptake by certain cells takes place by receptor-mediated potocytosis in which the membrane protein is a specific receptor for 5-methyltetrahydrofolate. On

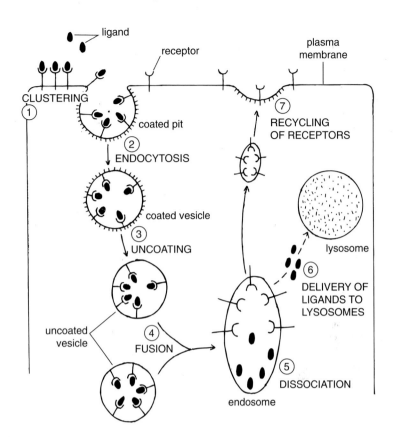

Fig. 3.9 Diagram showing the pathway of receptor-mediated endocytosis of LDL and other macromolecules. Ligand signifies the macromolecule to be internalized. Reproduced, with permission, from Avers (1986), *Molecular Cell Biology* (©1986), Addison Wesley Longman.

binding of the folate molecule to the receptor, the caveola closes and acidification of the caveola space by the action of a membrane proton pump causes the folate to dissociate from the receptor. The high concentration of folate in the caveola space creates a gradient that favours movement of folate across the membrane by facilitated diffusion. When the folate reaches the cytoplasm, it is covalently modified by the addition of multiple glutamic acid residues. The folylpolyglutamate is unable to diffuse out of the cell and is therefore trapped within the cytoplasm. The caveola then reopens thereby exposing the receptors for the next cycle (Anderson *et al.*, 1992).

Invagination of the plasma membrane to form caveolae is controlled by protein kinase C-α (PKC-α), which is constitutively present in the membrane. The membrane also contains a 90-kDa protein PKC-α substrate that, when phosphorylated, initiates invagination of the plasma membrane. Once the caveola has formed, the PKC-α activity declines. The 90-kDa protein is then dephosphorylated by a resident protein phosphatase which results in the return of the plasmalemmal vesicle to the cell surface. The kinase and phosphatase are targets for regulatory hormones such as histamine (Smart *et al.*, 1995).

3.1.6 Transepithelial movement of solutes and water

At many places in the body, substances must be translocated all the way through an epithelium instead of simply through the cell membrane. Movement of this type occurs, for example, through the epithelia of the intestine, renal tubules and choroid plexus. The vectorial nature of such movement is made possible by the polarity of the cell surface, whereby distinct sets of surface components (carriers, ion channels and ion pumps) are localized to separate plasma membrane domains. Transepithelial movement may involve concentrative active transport through the apical membrane domain and facilitated diffusion for the downhill exit through the basolateral membrane domain.

Molecules crossing a simple epithelium (one consisting of a single layer of cells) can do so by (1) a transcellular route, via the apical cell membrane, cytoplasm and basolateral cell membrane or (2) by a paracellular route or shunt pathway, via the tight junction and underlying lateral intercellular space, bypassing the cells. By selectively controlling the passive diffusion of ions and small water-soluble molecules through the shunt pathway, the tight junction maintains any gradients created by the activity of pathways associated with the transcellular route. In leaky epithelia having electrical resistances of <1000 ohm cm^{-2}, the shunt pathway is the major route for passive transepithelial flow. This is borne out by the work of Frizzell & Schultz (1972) who showed that at least 85% of passive ion flow across the fairly leaky epithelium of the small intestine takes the paracellular route.

It is well documented that the intestinal absorption of glucose increases the rate of water absorption. Active transepithelial co-transport of glucose and Na$^+$ is thought to drive water absorption by establishing a standing solute osmotic gradient across the enterocytes as illustrated in Fig. 3.10. This movement of water results in dilation of the lateral intercellular spaces.

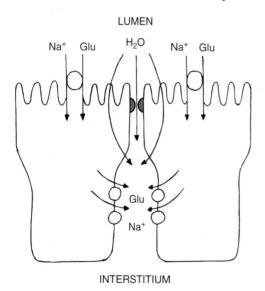

LUMEN

INTERSTITIUM

Fig. 3.10 The standing osmotic gradient theory for solute and water absorption. Glucose (Glu), accompanied by Na$^+$, is transported across the apical membrane into the enterocyte by secondary active transport. Glucose and Na$^+$ then move across the basolateral membrane into the lateral intercellular spaces by facilitated diffusion and primary active transport, respectively. Water then flows through the cells and/or tight junctions and into the lateral spaces in response to the osmotic gradient created by the transport of sodium and glucose. Reproduced, with permission, from Ballard *et al.* (1995), *Annual Review of Nutrition*, Volume 15, pp. 35–55, ©1995 by Annual Review (www.annualreviews.org).

3.2   The blood–brain, blood–cerebrospinal fluid and placental barriers

3.2.1   The blood–brain and blood–cerebrospinal fluid barriers

The brain must be protected from abrupt changes in the concentrations of circulating adrenaline and other neurally active substances which would interfere with synaptic communication, as well as from potentially toxic molecules that may find their way into the bloodstream. On the other hand, essential molecules such as glucose, amino acids and water-soluble vitamins must have access to the brain cells (neurons and glial cells). The blood–brain barrier serves to control the chemical composition of the extracellular fluid compartment of the brain, i.e. the interstitial fluid surrounding the brain cells which comprise the intracellular compartment. The cerebrospinal fluid bathes the exterior of the brain and spinal cord in the subarachnoid space and also fills the ventricles of the brain. The interstitial fluid and cerebrospinal fluid are separated by only a single layer of ependymal cells, which form the lining of the ventricles. These cells are loosely linked by gap junctions so that the ependymal layer allows interchange of solutes by simple diffusion between the two fluid compartments. Because of the leaky ependymal layer, a blood–cerebrospinal fluid barrier is also necessary to maintain a constant chemical environment for the brain cells. The surface area of this barrier is only about 0.02 per cent of the surface area of the blood–brain barrier. The relationship between the blood–brain and blood–cerebrospinal fluid barriers is shown in Fig. 3.11.

For a typical water-soluble vitamin to enter the extracellular space of brain or the cerebrospinal fluid, the circulating molecule must pass through the blood–brain and/or blood–cerebrospinal fluid barriers. Specialized transport systems are required for water-soluble vitamins to negotiate these barriers. The blood–brain barrier is due to high resistance tight junctions between adjacent endothelial cells of cerebral capillaries. The blood–cerebrospinal fluid barrier is due to tight junctions between epithelial cells of the choroid plexus. There is no anatomical barrier to the movement of substances between the cerebrospinal fluid and the extracellular space of the brain. Once inside the extracellular space, the molecules must pass through the plasma membrane of the brain cell itself before finally entering the cell.

Fig. **3.11** Relationship between the blood–brain and blood–cerebrospinal fluid barriers. Before water-soluble molecules in the blood can enter the brain cells, the molecules must enter the extracellular space of brain (the interstitial fluid surrounding the brain cells) or the cerebrospinal fluid which bathes the brain's surfaces. To enter the extracellular space from blood, the molecule must pass through the blood–brain barrier, while to enter the cerebrospinal fluid, the molecule must pass through the blood–cerebrospinal fluid barrier. There is no barrier to the movement of molecules between the extracellular space and the cerebrospinal fluid.

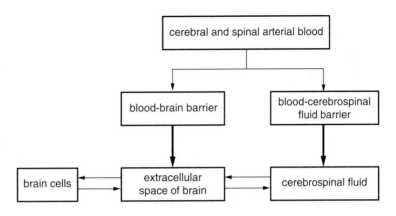

An important fact to be considered in brain nutrition is that the cerebrospinal fluid is constantly leaving the central nervous system and being replaced by new fluid; the total turnover time is about 6 hours. Thus there is a clear need for continuing transfer of essential nutrients from blood into cerebrospinal fluid and the extracellular space of brain.

The blood–brain barrier

The properties of the cerebral capillary endothelial cells account for the blood–brain barrier. The wall of a cerebral capillary is composed of endothelial cells surrounded by a basal lamina, similar to the walls of capillaries in peripheral tissues. Here, however, the similarities end. Whereas spaces between adjacent peripheral endothelial cells allow small molecules and ions to diffuse freely through the capillary wall, adjacent endothelial cells in cerebral capillaries abut against each other and the cells are completely sealed together by continuous tight junctions of high electrical resistance ($1000 \, \text{ohm cm}^{-2}$) or more). These high resistance junctions present an effective barrier, even to ions. This means that all substances entering or leaving the brain must pass through two plasma membranes and cytoplasm of the endothelial cells rather than between the cells. In addition, cerebral capillaries lack the fenestrations and vesicular transport systems found in peripheral capillaries, thus excluding the passage of small molecules and macromolecules via these routes.

Certain regions of the brain, accounting for less than 1 per cent of the brain volume, lack a blood–brain barrier. In these brain regions, neurons secrete hormones and other factors that require rapid and uninhibited access to the systemic circulation. These leaky regions are isolated from the rest of the brain by specialized cells called tanycytes.

Neurons in the brain do not abut directly upon capillaries except in certain special structures, e.g. parts of the hypothalamus. Usually they are separated from capillaries by the protoplasmic processes of astrocytes, a type of glial cell. The intervening astrocytes are therefore implicated in the exchange of materials between the blood and the nervous tissue. Around the capillary lies a virtual perivascular space occupied by another cell type, the pericyte. The functions of pericytes include the secretion of basal lamina components, the regulation of revascularization and repair, and the regulation of vascular tone in capillaries. The association between endothelial cells, pericytes and astrocytes is illustrated in Fig. 3.12.

The blood–brain barrier does not exclude the passage of small lipophilic molecules into the extracellular fluid compartment, as such molecules dissolve readily in the lipid components of plasma membranes. Water can also enter the brain by simple diffusion. Essential hydrophilic molecules that the brain consumes rapidly and in large quantities, such as glucose and amino acids, rapidly traverse the blood–brain barrier by means of facilitated diffusion. Similar carrier-mediated transport systems also move surplus substances out of the brain and into the blood.

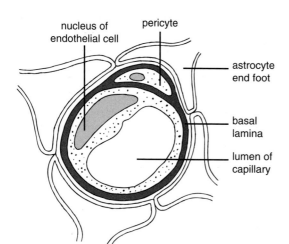

Fig. 3.12 The blood–brain barrier is imposed by the specialized endothelial cells of the cerebral capillaries. The diagram shows a cerebral capillary and associated cells in cross-section. A single endothelial cell can completely surround the lumen of a capillary. The capillary endothelium is encased within a basal lamina, which also houses pericytes. Almost completely enclosing the basal lamina are terminal processes (end feet) of astrocytes. Reproduced, with permission, from Rowland *et al.* (1991), in Kandel *et al.* (eds.) *Principles of Neural Science*, © 1991, McGraw-Hill Publishing Company.

The blood–cerebrospinal fluid barrier

The inner surfaces of the cranium and vertebral column are lined by three membranes called the meninges; from the outside inwards these are termed the dura mater, the arachnoid membrane and the pia mater. The dura mater consists of two layers – an outer layer of dense connective tissue containing numerous blood vessels and nerves, and an inner layer of dense fibrous tissue. The arachnoid membrane and pia mater are delicate nonvascular membranes covering the brain surface. These two membranes are separated by the subarachnoid space, which contains some of the cerebrospinal fluid. The arachnoid membrane forms an impermeable barrier between the blood supply of the dura mater and the cerebrospinal fluid in the subarachnoid space.

Projecting into the cavities of the brain ventricles are fronds of blood capillary networks collectively called the choroid plexus. The capillaries are surrounded by a single layer of epithelial cells continuous with the ventricular lining of ependymal cells (Fig. 3.13). Like the epithelial cells that line the intestine and other organs, the choroid epithelial cells are structurally polarized. The basolateral surfaces of the choroid epithelial cells are in contact with the blood plasma that filters through the leaky walls of the capillaries. The apical surfaces contain villi that extend into the ventricular cerebrospinal fluid. Adjacent choroid epithelial cells

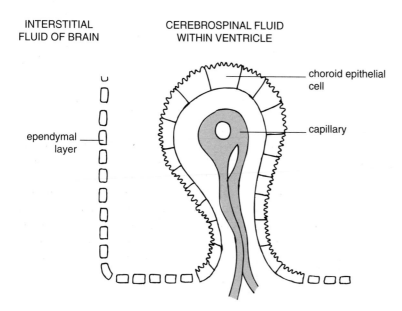

Fig. 3.13 The blood–cerebrospinal fluid barrier is imposed by tight junctions between epithelial cells of the choroid plexus. Water-soluble molecules cannot diffuse freely between the blood and the cerebrospinal fluid (CSF) because of the tight junctions. Certain molecules can pass through the epithelial cells from the blood into the CSF by active transport. Molecules entering the CSF can easily diffuse through the leaky ependymal layer into the interstitial fluid. Reproduced with permission of Carol Donner from Spector and Johanson (1989).

are sealed together by tight junctions that impede the passage of even small water-soluble molecules. These tight junctions constitute the blood–cerebrospinal fluid barrier of the choroid plexus.

The choroid plexus controls the one-way transfer of essential micronutrients that the brain needs in relatively small amounts over extended periods. Such substances include vitamin B_6, folate and ascorbic acid. Active transport mechanisms, mediated by carriers on the basolateral surface of choroid epithelial cells, extract micronutrients out of the blood and into the cells' cytoplasm. Once concentrated therein, the micronutrients are released into the cerebrospinal fluid through the apical cell surface, probably by facilitated diffusion.

Transport regulation

In many cases of carrier-mediated micronutrient transport from blood to brain, the K_m (the concentration of micronutrient at which the carrier system is half-saturated) is approximately equal to the normal concentration of micronutrient in the plasma. In other words, the system is already half-saturated when plasma concentrations are normal. In such cases, typified by thiamin, folate and ascorbic acid, an increase in plasma concentration will progressively decrease brain uptake as the carrier system approaches saturation. Nicotinamide, pantothenic acid and biotin are exceptions: they have K_m values that are much higher than their normal plasma concentration, creating the potential for high uptake by the brain (Spector, 1989).

3.2.2 The placental barrier

The placenta regulates the transport of nutrients from the maternal to the fetal circulation and also the transport of fetal metabolic waste products to the maternal circulation. Transport may be regulated intrinsically by cellular proteins or extrinsically by circulating hormones. Communication between the microvillous and basal membranes of the syncytiotrophoblast (see below) allow stimuli originating in the mother or fetus to regulate solute transport across the maternal- or fetal-facing membranes.

Cellular structure of the trophoblast

By the time the fertilized ovum has entered the uterus after its journey down the Fallopian tube, several cell divisions have occurred, and it consists of a mass of cells. A cavity appears within the cellular mass, after which it is called a blastocyst. The blastocyst wall is composed of a single layer of cells called the trophoblast, and within the cavity is an inner cell mass that is destined to form the embryo. After implantation of the blastocyst within the endometrium, the trophoblast proliferates over its entire surface and, by the eleventh day after ovulation, it consists of two distinct layers. The thicker outer layer consists of a multinucleated protoplasmic mass, the syncytiotrophoblast, from whose outer surface project numerous primary villi. Connective tissue containing fetal blood capillaries extends into the villi which are now termed secondary or chorionic villi. The inner layer of cells, the cytotrophoblast, is composed of cells with clearly defined cell boundaries. The growing chorionic villi destroy endometrial tissue in their locality, leaving intervillous spaces. With further enlargement of villi, the spaces become interconnecting and contain blood liberated by penetration of the maternal vessels by the trophoblast. After the tenth week of pregnancy, the cytotrophoblast progressively disappears until at parturition only isolated clumps of its cells remain.

The functional unit of the placenta concerned with exchange of materials between mother and fetus is the chorionic villus (Fig. 3.14). Passage of dissolved substances occurs between the maternal blood in the intervillous spaces and the fetal blood in the capillaries of the chorionic villi. The placental barrier is imposed by the syncytiotrophoblast, the discontinuous cytotrophoblast, the basal lamina of the trophoblast, loose connective tissue, the basal lamina of the fetal capillaries, and the capillary endothelium. Most sites of known mechanisms of placental transport are localized to the microvillous and basal plasma membranes of the syncytiotrophoblast.

3.3 Functional anatomy of the small and large intestine, liver and kidney

3.3.1 The small intestine

The small intestine (Fig. 3.15) is about 6 m in length and 3 cm in diameter in the adult human. It consists of three portions, starting with the duodenum, which is only about 30 cm long, and terminating at the ileocaecal valve. The jejunum accounts for the remaining two-fifths, and the ileum the remaining three-fifths.

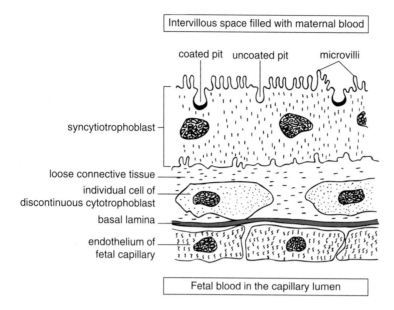

Intervillous space filled with maternal blood

coated pit   uncoated pit   microvilli

syncytiotrophoblast

loose connective tissue

individual cell of
discontinuous cytotrophoblast

basal lamina

endothelium of
fetal capillary

Fetal blood in the capillary lumen

Fig. 3.14 Diagram of part of the chorionic villus of the human placenta near term showing the cellular barrier between maternal and fetal blood. The chorionic villus consists of a core of connective tissue containing the fetal capillaries. The core is ensheathed by the two layers of the trophoblast, namely the outer syncytiotrophoblast and the inner cytotrophoblast. The syncytiotrophoblast is a multinuclear epithelial layer which is devoid of lateral cell boundaries; its microvillous surface is bathed by maternal blood circulating in the intervillous space, while its basal surface faces the fetal circulation. The microvillous surface of the syncytiotrophoblast presents a large area for nutrient absorption; also present are coated and uncoated pits that facilitate endocytosis of macromolecules. The cytotrophoblast consists of discrete cells that become progressively fewer in number. The basal laminae of the trophoblast and capillary endothelium are not shown.

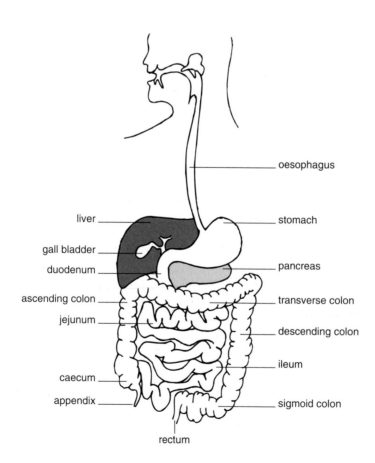

oesophagus

liver

stomach

gall bladder

duodenum

pancreas

ascending colon

transverse colon

jejunum

descending colon

ileum

caecum

appendix

sigmoid colon

rectum

Fig. 3.15 The gastrointestinal tract.

The intestinal wall comprises four principal layers as shown in Fig. 3.16. The outermost serosal layer is covered with peritoneum and contains blood vessels, lymphatics and nerve fibres which pass through it to the other layers. The next layer, the muscularis externa, consists of an inner band of circularly orientated and an outer band of longitudinally orientated smooth muscle fibres arranged in a spiral fashion. Contraction of these muscle fibres facilitates (1) segmentation, in which the gut contents are mixed by local contractions of small segments of gut wall and (2) peristalsis, which refers to propulsive movements stimulated by distension of the gut wall. The third layer, the submucosa, comprises coarse areolar connective tissue and contains plexuses of blood vessels and lymphatics. The innermost layer, the mucosa, consists of an epithelium, lubricated by mucus, resting upon a basal lamina. This, in turn, is supported by a layer of loose, areolar connective tissue termed the lamina propria, which is attached to a thin sheet of smooth muscle, the muscularis mucosa.

To allow a maximum efficiency of absorption, the intestinal mucosa shows specialization that increases its surface area to approximately 300 m². Firstly, the mucosa, with a core of submucosa, is thrown into permanent concentric folds called plicae circulares which protrude into the intestinal lumen. The folds are up to 1 cm in height and any one fold may extend two-thirds or more around the circumference of the intestine. Rarely do the folds completely encircle the lumen. The plicae circulares are found most frequently in the distal duodenum and proximal jejunum. Thereafter, they become less frequent and are rare in the distal ileum. As well as increasing the absorptive area, the plicae circulares retard the passage of chyme, allowing more time for effective digestion and absorption.

The absorptive area is greatly increased by the presence of tightly packed projections called villi, each about 1 mm long, giving the mucosal surface a velvet-like appearance. In the human, the villi are numerous in the duodenum and jejunum, but fewer in the ileum. In the proximal duodenum they are broad, ridge-like structures, changing to tall, leaf-like villi in the distal duodenum/proximal jejunum. Thereafter, they gradually transform into short finger-like processes in the distal jejunum and ileum.

The villus (Fig. 3.17) is the functional absorptive unit of the small intestine. Contained within the lamina propria core of each villus is a capillary network with a supplying arteriole and draining venule. A blind-ending lymphatic vessel (lacteal) in the centre of each villus drains into a plexus of collecting vesicles

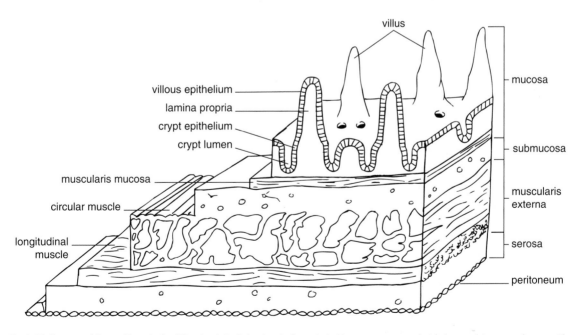

Fig. 3.16 Structure of the small intestinal wall (sectional view) showing the four principal layers: serosa, muscularis externa, submucosa and mucosa. The mucosa comprises the epithelium, lamina propria and muscularis mucosa.

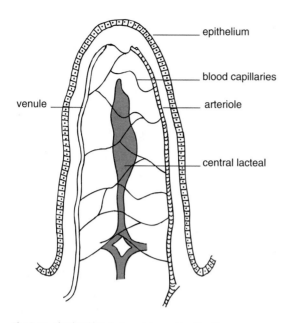

Fig. 3.17 Blood and lymphatic vessels supplying the villus.

in the submucosa. The lacteal is surrounded by smooth muscle elements that extend from the muscularis mucosa. During digestion the muscularis mucosa contracts, causing the villi to sway and contract intermittently. These movements and contractions may have the effect of 'milking' the lacteals, forcing the lymph and absorbed nutrients (fats) into the lymphatic vesicles. Each villus is covered by an epithelium composed of a single layer of columnar absorptive cells (enterocytes) interspersed occasionally with mucus-secreting goblet cells. Undifferentiated cells in the epithelium of the intestinal glands (crypts) proliferate and migrate upwards to replace enterocytes and other cells that are continuously being sloughed off from the tip of the villus into the intestinal lumen. During migration, the cells mature and the enzymes associated with the cells increase in activity. Complete cell renewal takes place every 5–6 days in the human small intestine.

The enterocyte constitutes the only anatomical barrier of physiological significance controlling the absorption of nutrients. As shown in Fig. 3.18, the apical membrane of the enterocyte (i.e. the membrane facing the intestinal lumen) is covered with microvilli, which are minute projections of the plasma membrane. The brush-like appearance of the apical membrane under the microscope gives rise to the alternative term 'brush-border membrane' for the

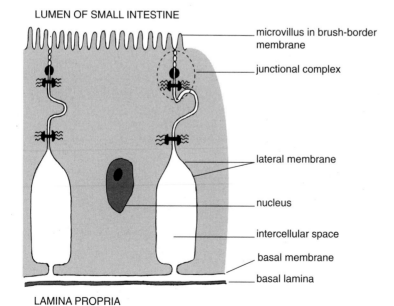

Fig. 3.18 Longitudinal section of an enterocyte.

apical membrane. The microvilli are packed at a density of 200 000 per mm² in the human jejunum. The basal membrane rests on a basal lamina composed of extracellular matrix proteins. The intercellular space between the lateral membranes only becomes dilated when nutrients and water are being absorbed. When absorption is not taking place, the intercellular space is collapsed and the lateral membranes are closely apposed.

3.3.2 The large intestine

Beginning at the ileocaecal valve, the greater part of the large intestine (Fig. 3.15) consists of the ascending, transverse, descending and sigmoid colon. The caecum is a cul-de-sac that projects from the proximal part of the ascending colon and is the major site of bacterial vitamin synthesis in the large intestine. The vermiform appendix, which extends from the caecum, is vestigial in the human. The length of the large intestine in the adult human is usually 1.5–1.8 m. The calibre is 7.5 cm at its commencement and diminishes gradually until it reaches a minimum of 2.5 cm at the rectosigmoid junction. The calibre then increases to form the rectal ampulla, which narrows abruptly at the tonically contracted anal canal.

The well-developed muscularis externa of the large intestine comprises an outer longitudinal and inner circular layer of smooth muscle. Most of the longitudinal muscle fibres aggregate into three equidistantly placed bundles known as taeniae. The combined contractions of the circular and longitudinal muscles cause the unstimulated portion of the large intestine to bulge outward into bag-like sacs called haustra. The mixing movements arising from haustral contractions gradually expose all the colonic contents to the intestinal epithelium. The slow but persistent haustral contractions gradually propel the fluid contents in the caecum and ascending colon anal-ward. From the beginning of the transverse colon to the sigmoid colon, the haustral contractions are taken over by peristalsis-like mass movements. The submucosa and muscularis mucosa of the large intestine are similar to those of the small intestine. The mucosa of the entire large intestine is devoid of villi. The intestinal glands are larger and more numerous than those in the small intestine, and contain a greater abundance of mucus-producing goblet cells.

3.3.3 The liver

The liver is divided into right and left lobes of approximately equal size and subdivided into a large number of lobules. It is covered by a fibroconnective tissue capsule from which thin septa enter the matrix. Each lobule (Fig. 3.19) contains an intralobular vein in its

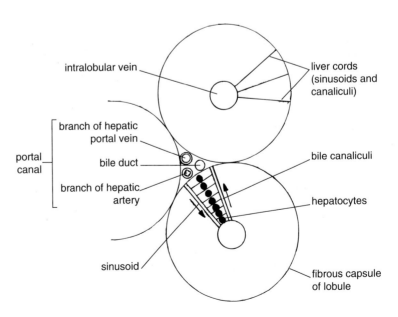

Fig. 3.19 Transverse section of liver showing the regular arrangement of lobules. (Arrows indicate fluid flow in sinusoids and canaliculi.)

centre and portal canals at its periphery. Portal canals are surrounded by small amounts of fibroconnective tissue and contain a branch of the hepatic artery, a branch of the portal vein, and a bile ductule. Lymphatic vessels within the portal canal produce lymph which passes indirectly into the lymphatic capillaries.

The matrix of the liver is composed of parenchymal cells (hepatocytes) arranged to form a sponge-like three-dimensional lattice in which the spaces (sinusoids) are filled with blood. At the surface adjacent to a sinusoidal blood space, the hepatocyte is separated from the sinusoidal lining by a narrow perisinusoidal space called the space of Disse (Fig. 3.20). This region serves as a lymphatic space containing proteoglycans and the microvilli of the hepatocytes. Bile produced by the hepatocytes passes into narrow channels (bile canaliculi), which are simply spaces between adjacent hepatocytes and lead to interlobular bile ductules.

In addition to its parenchymal cells, the liver contains various kinds of nonparenchymal cells; namely endothelial cells that line the sinusoidal spaces, Kupffer cells, pit cells and stellate cells. The endothelial cells are characterized by the presence of numerous circular openings (fenestrations) and by the absence of a supporting basal lamina. The fenestrations, along with spaces between adjacent endothelial cells, allow the plasma of the sinusoidal blood free access to the space of Disse, thus permitting easy exchange of metabolites between hepatocytes and the blood. Stellate cells are the major vitamin A-storing cells in the liver and comprise 5–15% of total liver cells; they are localized within the space of Disse between the hepatocytes and the endothelial cells.

Cirrhosis of the liver, common in chronic alcoholics, is caused by alcohol poisoning at such frequent intervals that the hepatocytes cannot recover fully between bouts of drinking. When this happens, fibroblasts grow in place of the hepatocytes and the liver becomes irreversibly clogged with connective tissue.

3.3.4   The kidney

The kidney facilitates the elimination of waste metabolic products in the urine and also subserves functions of fluid and salt balance by excreting these materials in varying quantities dependent upon need.

In histological section the kidney consists of an enormous number of tortuous and intertwined uriniferous tubules. Each tubule consists of two func-

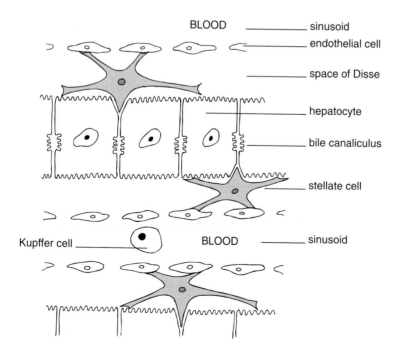

Fig. 3.20 Cellular structure of the liver showing the spatial relationship among endothelial, stellate and parenchymal cells (hepatocytes).

tional units: the nephron of 30–40 mm length and the collecting tubules of about 20 mm length. The nephron is responsible for urine production and the collecting tubule is the excretory duct leading eventually to the ureter.

As shown in Fig. 3.21, the first part of the nephron is the cup-shaped Bowman's capsule containing a tuft of blood capillaries called the glomerulus. The entire structure is known as the Malpighian corpuscle, where the process of filtration takes place. The glomerular pressure is sufficient to cause water and simple substances of low molecular weight to pass easily through the walls of the capillaries and Bowman's capsule into the lumen of the capsule. The glomerular filtration is discriminatory with regard to the size of macromolecules, and small proteins will traverse the glomerular barrier relatively easily. Filtration is not selective: both waste products and useful materials move from the blood into the nephron.

The selective reabsorption of essential constituents of the glomerular filtrate into the blood takes place in the proximal convoluted tubule – a region of the nephron which is composed of a single layer of epithelial cells with a brush border of microvilli at the luminal surface (Fig. 3.22). The tubules are enveloped by blood capillaries whose walls are highly permeable. The outer membrane of the tubule epithelial cell rests on a basal lamina and is invaginated to form a labyrinth of basal channels. Adjacent tubule cells are separated by intercellular spaces and fluid circulates through these spaces and basal channels. This fluid bathes the cells of the proximal convoluted tubule and the surrounding capillary network.

The basic mechanisms for transport through the tubule epithelial cell membranes are essentially the same as those discussed for transport in the intestine. An ATP-dependent sodium pump located in the basolateral membrane pumps sodium out of the epithelial cell (primary active transport). The removal of sodium from the cell creates an electrochemical gradient for sodium across the cell, which provides the energy for the carrier-mediated sodium-coupled transport of glucose, amino acids and certain water-soluble vitamins across the brush-border membrane into the cell (secondary active transport). Transport of glucose across the basolateral membrane of the tubule cell takes place by sodium-independent facilitated diffusion.

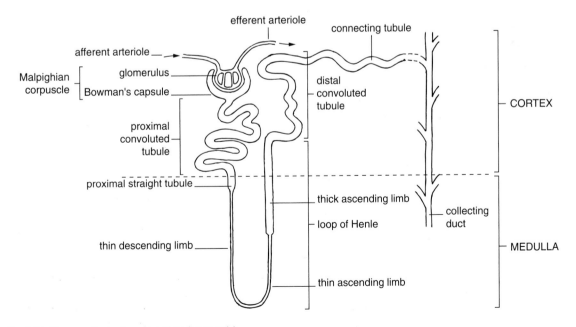

Fig. 3.21 Diagrammatic structure of a nephron (not to scale).

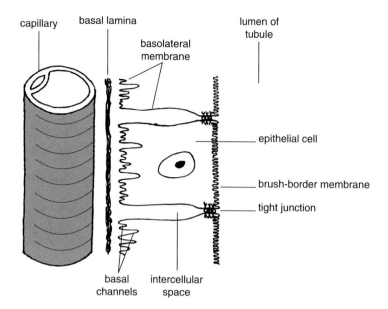

Fig. 3.22 Longitudinal section of an epithelial cell of the proximal convoluted tubule.

3.4   Digestion and absorption

3.4.1   General concepts

Digestion refers to the chemical and physical modifications which render ingested food constituents absorbable by the small intestine. Absorption is the process by which the products of digestion move from the lumen of the small intestine into the enterocytes and thence into the bloodstream or lymphatic system. A complex meal may be fully digested and absorbed in 3 hours.

After the digested food has passed through the wall of the small intestine, nutrients other than fats or fat-soluble substances enter the venules within the lamina propria. The venules eventually lead to the portal vein, which conveys nonlipid products of digestion from the intestine to the liver. Most of the absorbed non-lipid material passes through the liver, whose cells extract nutrients for storage or metabolic processing. The only exception to this portal route are the internal iliac veins which drain directly back into the systemic circulation (Granger *et al.*, 1987). The nutrient-enriched blood that has passed through the liver is then sent to the heart and thence to the lungs. The oxygenated blood returns to the heart for redistribution to all parts of the body. The nutrients pass from the blood capillaries into the extracellular fluid from which cells take up the nutrients they need.

Bile produced by the liver is secreted continuously into the gall bladder, which discharges it intermittently into the duodenum. Bile is necessary for the emulsification of ingested fats. Many vital micronutrients, including vitamin D, folate and vitamin B_{12}, are conserved through their excretion in bile and subsequent reabsorption by the small intestine (enterohepatic circulation). The liver also produces copious amounts of lymph to sustain the lymphatic system. Absorbed lipids and lipid-soluble substances in the form of chylomicrons are transported via the lymphatic system and thoracic ducts to the subclavian veins and into the systemic circulation, bypassing the liver.

Digestion commences as soon as the food enters the mouth. Chewing helps to break up large particles of food, whilst also mixing food with saliva, which acts as a lubricant and contains the enzymes salivary amylase and lingual lipase. Lingual lipase has only a minor role in digestion of dietary triglycerides; however, salivary amylase plays a major role in digestion of dietary starch. Most of the enzymatic activity of salivary amylase occurs in the stomach, where there is a much longer time for it to interact with the starch.

In the stomach, the churning action and the presence of hydrochloric acid and pepsin convert the food bolus into a liquid chyme. The stomach has three regions with regard to its glandular secretions: the fundus (in the proximal stomach), the body and the antrum (in the distal stomach). The folds of the stomach lining contain microscopic gastric pits into each of which drain four or five gastric glands. The mucosa of the body and fundus contains oxyntic glands whereas the mucosa of the antrum contains pyloric glands. Oxyntic glands are lined by parietal cells that secrete hydrochloric acid and intrinsic factor and by chief cells that secrete pepsinogen (the precursor of pepsin) and gastric lipase. The pyloric glands contain almost no parietal cells or chief cells but, rather, contain mucus-secreting cells and G cells, which produce the hormone gastrin.

Most absorption takes place and is completed in the small intestine. On arrival at the duodenum, the acidic chyme is buffered by the bicarbonate in pancreatic juice and bile. Brunner's glands in the duodenum produce an alkaline secretion containing mucus. The proteases, amylase, lipase and other enzymes of pancreatic origin are also secreted into the duodenum. The final stages of digestion take place on the luminal surface or within the epithelial cells lining the small intestine. When absorption has been accomplished, the jejunum and ileum are actively involved in the regulation of electrolyte and fluid balance. The various stages of digestion are co-ordinated by the action of the nervous system, endocrine system and circulatory system.

The principal functions of the colon are (1) absorption of water and inorganic salts (mainly sodium) from the chyme to form solid faeces and (2) storage of faecal matter until it can be expelled.

3.4.2 The luminal environment within the small intestine

The bulk luminal phase of the upper gastrointestinal tract is characterized by a wide range of pH values. Postprandial pH values in humans are within the following ranges: 1.8–3.4 in the stomach, 6.8–7.8 in the lower small intestine, and 3.5–7 in the duodenum and proximal jejunum.

Bulk contents of the intestinal lumen are mixed by segmentation and peristalsis, and water and solutes are brought to the surface of the mucosa by convection. However, the luminal environment immediately adjacent to the brush-border membrane is stationary and unaffected by gut motility. The lack of convective mixing in this region creates a series of thin layers,

each progressively more stirred, extending from the surface of the enterocyte to the bulk phase of the lumen. Together, these are the so-called 'unstirred layer', whose effective thickness in the human jejunum has been calculated to be 35 μm based on the rate of disaccharide hydrolysis at the brush border, rather than the 600-μm value derived from osmotic transient measurements (Levitt et al., 1992).

Solute movement within an unstirred layer takes place by diffusion, which is slow compared to the convective movement in the bulk luminal phase. The pH at the luminal surface is approximately two units lower than that of the bulk phase and varies less than ±0.5 units despite large pH variations in the intestinal chyme. It has been suggested that the formation of the low-pH microclimate is due to the presence of mucin which covers the entire surface of the epithelium (Nimmerfall & Rosenthaler, 1980; Shiau et al., 1985). Mucopolysaccharides possess a wide range of ionizable groups and hence mucin is an ampholyte. If the luminal chyme is of low pH, the ampholyte is positively charged and so it repels additional hydrogen ions entering the microclimate. If, on the other hand, the chyme is alkaline, the ampholyte becomes negatively charged and retains hydrogen ions within the microclimate. In this manner, the mucin layer functions as a restrictive barrier for hydrogen ions diffusing in and out of the microclimate.

3.4.3 Adaptive regulation of intestinal nutrient transport

Many patterns of adaptation fall into one or the other of two categories: (1) a non-specifically increased absorption of all nutrients, arising ultimately from an increase in the animal's overall nutrient requirements, and with an increase in absorptive surface area as the primary mechanism, and (2) phenomena involving the induction or repression of a specific transport mechanism, depending on the dietary availability or body store of the transported substrate.

Non-specific anatomical adaptation to changing metabolic requirements and food deprivation
Increases in metabolic requirements such as arise during pregnancy, lactation, growth, exercise and cold stress are met by an increased absorption of all available nutrients, mediated at least in part by an induced increase in food intake (hyperphagia). The increased

absorption is due to an increase in mucosal mass per unit length of intestine and a consequent increase in absorptive surface area. Not only is there an increase in the total number of cells (hyperplasia) but the villi become taller.

The mammalian intestine adapts to prolonged food deprivation by dramatically slowing the rate of epithelial cell production in the crypts in order to conserve proteins and biosynthetic energy. This effect on mitosis and enterocyte renewal leads to markedly shortened villi. Because cell migration along the crypt/villus axis is also slowed, more cells lining the villi are functionally mature. Therefore, food deprivation, by reducing mucosal mass and increasing the ratio of transporting to nontransporting cells, effectively increases solute transport per unit mass of intestine.

Dietary regulation of intestinal nutrient carriers
It is well established that certain intestinal nutrient carriers, including those transporting a number of sugars and amino acids, are adaptively regulated by their substrates. This type of regulation is transient and reversible. For example, the rate (V_{max}) of active glucose uptake doubles within 12 hours when mice fed a carbohydrate-free diet are switched to a high-carbohydrate diet (Diamond & Karasov, 1984). If the same mice were switched back to the carbohydrate-free diet, it would take up to 3 days for the glucose uptake to revert to the original rate. The sole mechanism responsible for these changes is a corresponding increase or decrease in the number of carriers at both the apical and basolateral membranes of the enterocytes. There is no effect on numerous variables of intestinal structure, such as length, circumference, weight, villus dimensions and density, and area at the villus level. The signal for regulation of brush-border glucose transport is the luminal concentration of sugars – not only glucose itself, but also nontransporting sugars. The signal for the basolateral glucose transport is yet to be established, but it involves signals from the plasma. The signals are perceived in the intestinal crypts, where the carrier proteins are synthesized within the developing enterocytes. The observed lag in response is attributed to the time taken for the cells to migrate from crypt to villus.

According to the adaptive regulation/modulation hypothesis (Karasov, 1992), a carrier should be repressed when its biosynthetic and maintenance costs

exceed the benefits it provides. The benefits can be provision of either metabolizable calories or an 'essential' nutrient, i.e. a nutrient such as an essential amino acid which cannot be synthesized in the body and must be obtained from the diet. Glucose carriers are up-regulated when the dietary supply of glucose is adequate or high because glucose provides valuable calories. The down-regulation of glucose carriers during a deficiency of glucose can be explained by the biosynthesis and maintenance costs outweighing the benefits of transporting this 'nonessential' nutrient.

One might expect carriers for water-soluble vitamins to be down-regulated by their substrates and up-regulated in deficiency of the vitamins. The rationale in this case is that carriers for these essential nutrients are most needed at low dietary substrate levels; at high levels the required amount of the vitamin could be extracted from the lumen by fewer carriers or even cross the enterocyte by simple diffusion. As vitamins do not provide metabolizable energy, there is nothing to gain from the cost of synthesizing and maintaining carriers when the vitamin supply is adequate or in excess.

The prediction of suppressed transport of vitamins at high dietary intakes has proved to be true for ascorbic acid, biotin and thiamin, but not for pantothenic acid, for which carrier activity is independent of dietary levels (Ferraris & Diamond, 1989). It appears that intestinal carriers are regulated only if they make the dominant contribution to uptake, as is the case for the three regulated vitamins. It can also be reasoned that carriers for ascorbic acid, biotin and thiamin would need to be regulated, because nutritional deficiencies of these vitamins can and do occur. In contrast, there is no need to regulate pantothenic acid carriers, because this vitamin is found naturally in almost all foods and cases of deficiency are extremely rare.

3.4.4 Alcoholism and its effect on intestinal transport

Chronic alcoholism is a complex disorder often characterized by malnutrition, vitamin deficiencies (particularly thiamin, vitamin B_6 and folate) and diarrhoea. Among the possible mechanisms for these disturbances are alterations in intestinal digestion, absorption and secretion. The following is based on a review by Wilson & Hoyumpa (1979) of the possible mechanisms by which ethanol directly affects intestinal transport.

Chronic ingestion of ethanol (1.09 M) results in shortening of the villi in the jejunum and degenerative changes in cellular ultrastructure of both jejunal and ileal villi. However, disturbances in intestinal function have been observed in the absence of such changes and so the changes cannot fully account for the impaired transport of nutrients.

The ethanol molecules (CH_3CH_2–OH) insert into the lipid bilayer of the plasma membrane with their hydrocarbon portions positioned between hydrophobic regions of membrane lipids and proteins. Ethanol causes a molecular rearrangement of membranes, which loosens the membrane and makes it more fluid. This effect of ethanol may increase the permeability of the gut wall and allow passive movement of large antigenic molecules, toxins and pathogenic organisms through the gut wall and into the bloodstream. It may also interfere with the conformational changes that carrier proteins need to make to effect solute transport. After chronic treatment with ethanol, cells adapt to this change in membrane fluidity by incorporating more rigid fatty acids into membrane phospholipids.

Ethanol inhibits the cell's sodium pump thereby interfering with sodium-coupled active transport of glucose, amino acids and certain water-soluble vitamins.

3.5 Glucose transport

Glucose transport has been well studied and the experimental techniques and postulated mechanisms help toward understanding the absorption of water-soluble vitamins.

3.5.1 Experimental approaches

Discussed here are a few selected *in vitro* studies which have contributed to a model for the intestinal absorption of glucose. Of course, any conclusions derived from *in vitro* experiments should be confirmed and extended using *in vivo* techniques in which the normal vascular channels are intact. This is particularly true for studies of regulation of transport function.

Everted intestinal sacs
The everted sac consists of a short length of isolated rat intestine turned inside out so that the epithelial brush border is on the outer surface. The sac is filled with a physiological solution, sufficient in volume to distend the wall, and an oxygen bubble is introduced. The sac is tied at both ends and suspended in an oxygenated incubation medium maintained at 37°C. The radioactively labelled solute under investigation is placed in the large volume of incubation medium and the solute taken up is measured both in the tissue and in the physiological solution within the sac. A number of adjacent portions of intestine from the same animal can be studied simultaneously.

The everted sac preparation allows both net absorption and tissue uptake of solutes to be studied under physiological conditions. Net absorption includes not only events at both boundaries of the enterocytes, but also possible contributions from interstitial connective tissue and several layers of serosal muscle. Experiments using everted intestinal sacs led Crane in 1960 to propose his sodium-gradient hypothesis for the active transport of glucose (Crane, 1962). The hypothesis stated that the energy necessary for glucose accumulation in intestinal tissue is provided by an inwardly directed sodium concentration gradient. Crane envisioned membrane carriers which have binding sites for Na+ as well as for glucose.

Short-circuit current technique
In a typical experiment, a segment of rabbit ileum is cut open to produce a sheet of tissue and the external muscle layers and submucosa are surgically removed. The remaining mucosal strip, consisting of the epithelial cell layer, the underlying lamina propria and the muscularis mucosa, is tightly mounted in the middle partition of an Ussing chamber, which separates solutions of identical composition and hydrostatic pressure. The bathing solutions are continuously oxygenated and circulated at the appropriate temperature during an experiment. In the open-circuited condition, in which no external current is applied to the system, the spontaneous electrical potential difference across the epithelium is continuously monitored using electrodes that are inserted into the chamber as close as possible to the surfaces of the mucosal strip.

In the short-circuited state, an external current just sufficient to abolish the transepithelial potential is passed across the tissue using another pair of electrodes connected to a variable electromotive force (Fig. 3.23). In this so-called 'voltage-clamped' preparation, there is no driving force for the net diffusional flows of ions across the tissue. Thus any

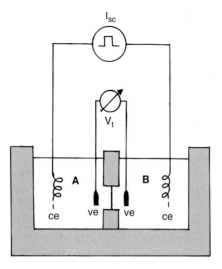

Fig. 3.23 Short-circuit current technique. The intestinal mucosal strip is represented by the vertical line between the voltage electrodes (ve) and separates compartments A and B. External current is applied across the tissue using the current electrodes (ce). The short-circuit current (I_{sc}) is the current needed to make the transepithelial potential difference (V_t) = 0. From Reuss (1997), in HANDBOOK OF PHYSIOLOGY, SECTION 14: CELL PHYSIOLOGY, edited by J Hoffmann & J Jamieson, copyright 1997 by the American Physiological Society. Used by permission of Oxford University Press, Inc.

net movements across the tissue must be the result of some form of active transport. Under these conditions the current necessary to abolish the transepithelial potential difference (referred to as the short-circuit current) is equal to the sum of the net transepithelial flows of all ions that are actively transported across the intestine. The practical importance of this relationship is that, by using radioisotopes to measure unidirectional mucosal-to-serosal and serosal-to-mucosal fluxes of individual ions under short-circuit conditions, one can identify those ions that are actively transported across the intestine. It was demonstrated that the only such ion was Na$^+$.

Using a tracer quantity of the ^{24}Na$^+$ isotope, Schultz & Zalusky (1964a,b) reported the following observations. The addition of glucose (11 mM) to the mucosal bathing solution results in a rapid increase in the transepithelial potential difference, the short-circuit current (I_{sc}) and the rate of active sodium transport from mucosa to serosa. These three effects are dependent upon the active transport of glucose and are independent of the metabolic fate of the sugar. Furthermore, they are inhibited by low concentrations of phloridzin (phlorizin) in the mucosa solution and by low concentrations of ouabain in the serosal solution. The increase in the short-circuit current (ΔI_{sc}) requires the presence of sodium in the perfusion medium and its magnitude is a linear function of the sodium concentration. On the other hand, ΔI_{sc} is a saturable function of the mucosal glucose concentration, which is consistent with Michaelis-Menten kinetics. These data were important in establishing the concept that glucose entry across the apical membrane promotes a simultaneous entry of Na$^+$, which is partially extruded at the basolateral membrane via the sodium pump. The unidirectional serosa-to-mucosa sodium flux, on the other hand, is attributed to simple ionic diffusion, there being no evidence for the presence of a carrier or the influence of solvent drag.

Isolated enterocytes

Isolated cells allow determination of initial rates of solute uptake and provide information on the intracellular accumulation and metabolic fate of the solute. If normally energized cells are used, the membrane potentials interfere with an accurate determination of the coupling ratio. To circumvent this problem, the membrane potential is experimentally maintained at or near zero using biochemical agents to deplete the cells of ATP and to confer a high K$^+$ permeability on the membrane.

Freshly isolated chicken enterocytes were used to establish that the true Na$^+$:glucose transport coupling ratio is 2:1 rather than 1:1 (Kimmich & Randles, 1980). They also provided data consistent with a model of brush-border sodium-glucose co-transport in which Na$^+$ binding to the Na$^+$-dependent glucose carrier at the luminal surface of the apical membrane and debinding at the cytoplasmic surface are both dependent on the membrane potential (Kimmich & Randles, 1988).

Membrane vesicles

Brush-border membrane vesicles can be prepared by homogenizing isolated enterocytes or mucosal scrapings and precipitating non-brush-border particulate matter with 10 mM Ca^{2+} or Mg^{2+}. The brush borders, because of their greater density of negative surface charges, are not precipitated and remain in the supernatant fluid. Centrifugation of this fluid provides a pellet of membrane vesicles, 95% of which have the same membrane orientation as in the intact enterocyte (i.e. they are 'the right side out'). Basolateral membrane vesicles can be obtained from a source of isolated enterocytes by differential centrifugation followed by separation on a density gradient. Vesicles of brush-border and basolateral membranes can be prepared simultaneously using the technique of free-flow electrophoresis to isolate them (Murer & Kinne, 1980).

Membrane vesicles allow solute transport properties to be investigated independently in brush-border and basolateral membranes without the complications of cellular metabolism or intracellular compartmentation. From such studies, the overall picture of intestinal glucose absorption has emerged. Three different membrane events have been identified: (1) entry of luminal glucose into the enterocyte by secondary active transport across the apical membrane via a sodium-glucose carrier, (2) facilitated diffusion of glucose out of the cell across the basolateral membrane via a sodium-independent carrier, and (3) primary active transport of sodium out of the cell via the sodium pump.

3.5.2 The GLUT family of facilitated-diffusion glucose transporters

The glucose transporters of the GLUT family are carrier proteins interwoven in the plasma membranes of many different cell types. Their function is to mediate facilitated diffusion of D-glucose across plasma membranes, either into or out of the cell. Five functional isoforms of GLUT, numbered 1 to 5, have been positively identified and characterized. Table 3.1 shows the tissue distribution of these isoforms. GLUT1 is widely distributed among many tissues and facilitates glucose transport across the blood–brain barrier. GLUT2 is preferably expressed in the liver. GLUT2 is also located in the basolateral membrane of small intestinal enterocytes, but is notably absent in the brush-border membrane. GLUT3 appears to be present in all tissues, with its largest expression in kidney, placenta, and neurons of the brain. Unlike the other GLUT proteins, which are constitutively expressed, GLUT4 is insulin-responsive and occurs primarily in intracellular vesicles in the cells of insulin-sensitive tissues. GLUT5 transports fructose far better than it does glucose, and facilitates fructose transport across the brush-border membrane of enterocytes.

Table 3.1 Human glucose transporters (GLUT) (compiled from Levin, 1999).

Isoform	Sugar transported	Major sites of expression
GLUT1	Glucose	Widely distributed, including heart, kidney, adipose cells, fibroblasts, placenta, retina, choroid plexus
GLUT2	Glucose, galactose, mannose, fructose	Sinusoidal membranes of liver, tubule cells of kidney, small intestinal enterocytes (basolateral membrane), insulin-secreting β cells of the pancreas
GLUT3	Glucose	Widely distributed. Highest expression in neurons of brain, kidney, placenta
GLUT4	Glucose	Insulin-sensitive tissues: brown and white adipocytes, skeletal muscle, cardiac muscle
GLUT5	Fructose, glucose (poor)	Jejunum (brush-border membranes), mature spermatozoa

3.5.3 Glucose absorption in the small intestine

Soon after eating a meal the high concentration of glucose in the intestinal lumen may allow uptake to take place by simple diffusion. After a while, the luminal concentration of glucose becomes lower than the concentration in the enterocyte or in the intercellular space, and therefore the glucose must be absorbed against a concentration gradient.

Fig. 3.24 shows how physiological amounts of glucose and fructose are absorbed by the small intestine. In the overall process, luminal glucose crosses the brush border and accumulates in the enterocyte by means of a sodium-dependent secondary active transport system located in the brush-border membrane. The immediate driving force for the sodium-coupled entry of glucose is the electrochemical gradient for sodium. This has two components – the sodium concentration gradient across the cell and the brush-border membrane potential. Fructose crosses the brush border by facilitated diffusion mediated by GLUT5. Exit of both glucose and fructose from the enterocyte to the serosa takes place by facilitated diffusion at the basolateral membrane and is mediated by GLUT2.

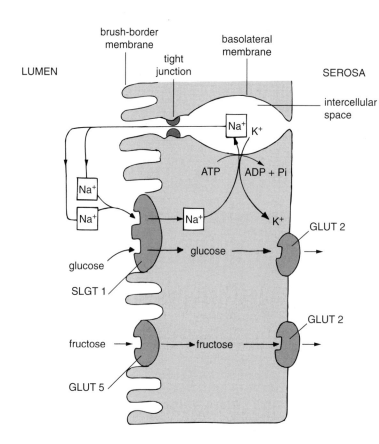

Fig. 3.24 Diagram showing the carrier-mediated transport of D-glucose and D-fructose across the apical membrane and basolateral membrane of an enterocyte. Na$^+$ extruded into the intercellular space by the basolateral Na$^+$-K$^+$-ATPase (sodium pump) is able to equilibrate with Na$^+$ on the luminal side of the enterocyte by permeation through the tight junction. ATP, adenosine triphosphate; ADP, adenosine diphosphate; P$_i$, inorganic phosphate.

The secondary active transport mechanism of glucose uptake at the apical membrane is mediated by a sodium-glucose co-transporting carrier (SGLT1), which requires four intact independent identical subunits in order to function. Each enterocyte contains an estimated 10^6–10^7 of such carriers. SGLT1 binds the substrates at a stoichiometric ratio of two sodium ions to a single glucose molecule. D-Galactose, having an almost identical structure to D-glucose, shares the same carrier site, but glucose has a greater affinity for the carrier and is transported at a greater rate. Sodium-glucose co-transport is specifically inhibited by phloridzin, a plant glycoside which competes with D-glucose for the binding site on the carrier but is not itself transported.

A model of sodium-glucose co-transport across the apical membrane is shown in Fig. 3.25. In this model the binding of sodium ions to and dissociation from the protein carrier (SGLT1) on opposing sides of the membrane are strongly influenced by changes in the membrane potential. Negatively charged residues residing in membrane-spanning domains of the protein might be involved in sodium binding. It has been proposed (Ugolev & Metel'skii, 1990) that the transporter has at least two channels – one for Na$^+$ and another for glucose.

Serosal transport of glucose acts to limit the gradient-forming capability of the brush-border transporting system, thereby maintaining a modest concentration of intracellular glucose. The carrier responsible for facilitated diffusion of glucose at the basolateral membrane is independent of sodium, has a low affinity for the sugar, and is competitively inhibited by cytochalasin B.

Fundamental to the understanding of sodium-coupled glucose absorption is the fact that carrier-mediated events at both brush-border and basolateral membranes are electrogenic, i.e. they result in a translocation of positive charge. At the brush-border membrane, the sodium-coupled entry of glucose results in a depolarization of the electrical potential difference across that barrier. In other words, the cell

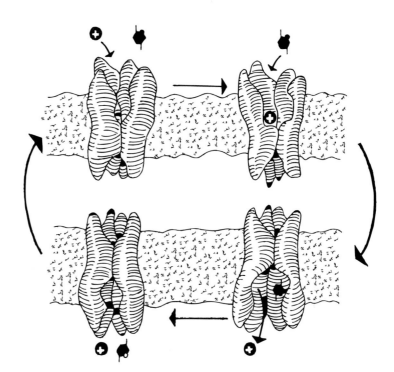

Fig. 3.25 Model of the membrane-bound arrangement of the intestinal brush-border Na⁺-glucose co-transporter. Two sodium ions (represented by the circle with a net positive charge) plus one glucose molecule (hexagon) are shown interacting with the co-transporter. At the extracellular surface Na⁺ binds to the co-transporter, which results in a conformational change that permits glucose to bind to the glucose-binding site. With both substrate species bound, the co-transporter undergoes a new conformational shift, placing Na⁺ and glucose near the inner surface of the membrane. Na⁺ and glucose are released to the cytoplasm, thereby triggering a co-transporter conformational shift to expose the binding sites once again to the extracellular surface of the membrane. The co-transporter thus again assumes the optimal conformation for binding extracellular Na⁺ and glucose. Reproduced, with permission, from Stevens *et al.* (1990), *Proceedings of the National Academy of Science U.S.A.* (©1990).

interior becomes less negative with respect to the luminal environment owing to the influx of sodium ions. The electrogenic nature of the sodium pump is due to more Na⁺ being extruded per unit time across the basolateral membrane than K⁺ accumulated.

The depolarization at the brush-border membrane seems to be self-defeating in that it markedly reduces the membrane potential. This component of the electrochemical driving force needs to be restored if the uptake process is to be perpetuated. The cellular model proposed by Schultz (1977) allows this to be achieved. This model takes into account the high conductivity of the intercellular tight junction, and the ease by which Na⁺ equilibrates between the extracellular media on the basolateral and luminal sides of the enterocyte. By virtue of this rapid paracellular pathway for the flow of Na⁺, the current generated at one of the limiting membranes can influence the potential difference across the other. This electrical coupling constitutes an electrochemical feedback between the co-transported entry of Na⁺ and Na⁺ extrusion at the opposite membranes. The circular movement of Na⁺ allows the co-transport of glucose to take place with minimal changes in the size of the intracellular sodium transport pool.

3.5.4   Paracellular movement – an alternative model for glucose absorption

Solvent drag, rather than active transport, has been proposed as the main mode of glucose absorption under physiological conditions (Madara & Pappenheimer, 1987). Pappenheimer suggested that a primary function of active transport is to transport glucose, together with sodium, at high concentration into the intercellular space, thus providing an osmotic force for the absorption of water into the space. The expansion of the intercellular spaces and an induced increase in tight junction permeability provide optimal conditions for the paracellular movement of glucose and other luminal nutrients in bulk by solvent drag. As nutrients are removed from the upper intestine, their concentrations decrease and active transport becomes a greater fraction of total uptake.

The Pappenheimer hypothesis of nutrient absorption is debatable because the presence of unstirred water layers in series with the epithelial cell membranes makes it difficult to calculate the magnitude of solvent drag. According to Ferraris *et al.* (1990), Pappenheimer's hypothesis is based on luminal glucose concentrations that are >10 times higher than those actually prevailing (Pappenheimer & Reiss, 1987). Using the recalculated lower glucose concentrations, Ferraris *et al.* (1990) reasoned that the contribution of solvent drag must be negligible, and carrier-mediated uptake rates are adequate to account for glucose absorption.

Fine *et al.* (1993) used a human intestinal perfusion technique to evaluate the Pappenheimer hypothesis. To assess the effect of D-glucose on intestinal permeability, the ratio of the diffusion rates of two passively absorbed solutes of different molecular size (urea/L-xylose and mannitol/L-xylose) was measured in the absence and presence of luminal D-glucose. If the effective radius through which the molecules diffuse were to increase, there would be a greater fractional change in the diffusion rate of the larger molecule than of the smaller molecule and the diffusion ratio (larger molecule/smaller molecule) would increase. No such increase was observed, which does not support the hypothesis that D-glucose increases the permeability of the human intestine. The fraction of total D-glucose absorption in the jejunum that could be attributed to a passive mechanism ranged from 2.8% to 8.4% (average 5%); there was no evidence of passive D-glucose absorption in the ileum. It was concluded that about 95% of the dietary D-glucose load is absorbed by stereospecific, carrier-mediated transport.

3.6   Digestion, absorption and transport of dietary fat

3.6.1   The plasma lipoproteins

The plasma lipoproteins are a family of globular proteins, each of which consists of a core of neutral lipid (predominantly triglyceride or cholesteryl ester) surrounded by a coat of phospholipid and protein. These particles can be divided into four broad categories: (1) chylomicrons, which primarily transport dietary triglyceride and cholesterol; (2) very-low-density lipoproteins (VLDL), which primarily transport triglycerides that have been synthesized in the liver;

and two lipoproteins that function primarily in the transport of endogenous cholesterol, namely (3) low-density lipoprotein (LDL) and (4) high-density lipoprotein (HDL). There is also an intermediate-density particle (IDL), having a density between that of VLDL and LDL. The IDL particles are very short-lived in the bloodstream, however, and seem to have little nutritional or physiological importance.

The protein components of the plasma lipoproteins are known as apolipoproteins. At least six different kinds of apolipoprotein have been identified in the intestinal lymph of humans: apoA, apoB (three different molecular sizes), apoC and apoE.

3.6.2   Digestion, absorption and transport

Absorption of the fat-soluble vitamins takes place mainly in the proximal jejunum and depends on the proper functioning of the digestion and absorption of dietary fat. The fat content of a typical Western diet is composed mainly of triglycerides accompanied by smaller amounts of phospholipids and sterols. The efficiency of absorption of fat-soluble vitamins parallels that of fat absorption and is affected by the nature of the lipid component of the diet.

The stomach is the major site for emulsification of dietary fat. The coarse lipid emulsion, on entering the duodenum, is emulsified into smaller globules by the detergent action of bile salts aided by the churning action of the intestine. The adsorption of bile salts on to the surface of the fat globules increases the lipolytic activity of pancreatic lipase, which hydrolyses triglycerides at the 1 and 3 positions and yields 2-monoglyceride and free fatty acids (Fig. 3.26). Secretion of bicarbonate from the pancreas and the biliary tract is needed to neutralize the pH to the optimal range for lipolysis. A cofactor called colipase is present in pancreatic juice and is required for lipase activity when bile salt is present. During their detergent action, bile salts exist in a monomolecular solution. Above a critical concentration of bile salts, the bile constituents (bile salts, phospholipid and cho-

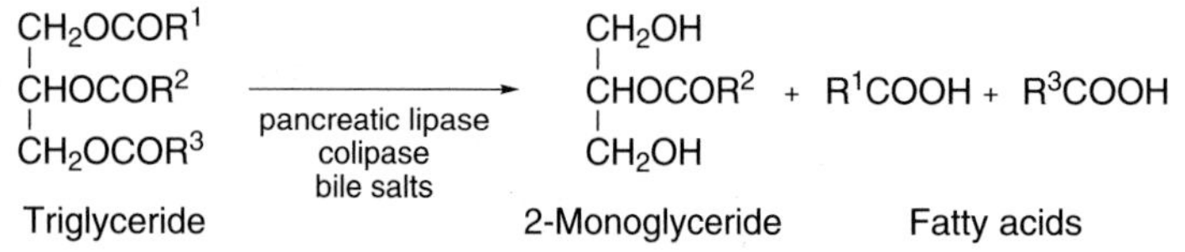

Fig. 3.26 Lipolysis of triglycerides in the small intestine.

lesterol) form aggregates called micelles, in which the polar ends of the molecules are orientated towards the surface and the nonpolar portions form the interior. The 2-monoglycerides and long-chain free fatty acids are sufficiently polar to combine with the micelles to form mixed micelles. These are stable water-soluble structures which can dissolve fat-soluble vitamins and other hydrophobic compounds in their oily interior.

The lipid components of the mixed micelles must be dissociated from these structures before they can be absorbed. Shiau & Levine (1980) showed that a low pH microclimate, representing the unstirred layer lining the luminal surface of the jejunum, facilitates micellar dissociation. Presumably, the fatty acid components of the mixed micelles become protonated when the mixed micelles enter the acidic microclimate of the unstirred layer. This protonation reduces fatty acid solubility in the mixed micelles, allowing release of the fatty acids together with other lipid constituents. Individual lipids, including fat-soluble vitamins, can then be absorbed across the brush-border membrane. The bile salts are left behind to be actively reabsorbed in the distal ileum, whence they return to the liver to be recycled via the gall bladder.

Triglycerides resynthesized within the enterocytes are packaged into chylomicrons (Fig. 3.27) in the endoplasmic reticulum together with free and esterified cholesterol, phospholipids, apolipoproteins, fat-soluble vitamins and carotenoids. The levels of lipids in chylomicrons are not strictly regulated, but depend on the dietary load. After processing through the Golgi apparatus, the chylomicrons are discharged from the enterocyte by exocytosis across the basolateral membrane, and enter the central lacteal of the villus. From there they pass into the larger lymphatic channels draining the intestine, into the thoracic duct, and ultimately into the systemic circulation.

3.6.3 Chylomicron metabolism

The chylomicrons are carried by the blood to all the tissues. Incorporated into the glycocalyx on the surface of capillary endothelia in most tissues is the enzyme lipoprotein lipase. Its extracellular action on the circulating chylomicrons releases free fatty acids and diglycerides which can then be absorbed by the tissue cells. The chylomicrons are thus converted into much smaller triglyceride-depleted particles known as chylomicron remnants. These particles contain apolipoprotein E (apoE) that they acquire from other circulating lipoproteins.

Uptake of chylomicron remnants by the liver and bone marrow

The liver has the capacity to rapidly remove chylomicron remnants from the circulation in all mammalian species studied. In the rabbit and nonhuman primate (marmoset), and probably also the human, the bone

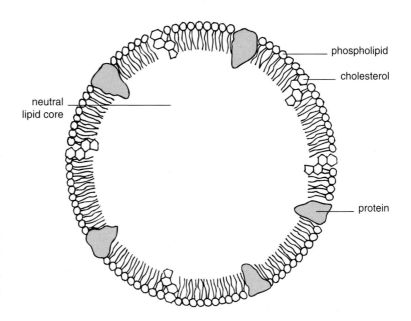

Fig. 3.27 Molecular structure of a chylomicron. The surface is mainly composed of a monomolecular layer of phospholipids with the polar head groups facing the outer aqueous environment. The phospholipids are interspersed with cholesterol molecules. Protruding from the surface are several different apolipoproteins, which are involved in the uptake and metabolism of chylomicron contents. The triglycerides within the oily centre make up about 90% of the weight of the particle. Also within the interior are cholesteryl esters, fat-soluble vitamins and traces of other lipids. The diameter of chylomicrons ranges from about 100 nm to about 500 nm.

phospholipid

cholesterol

neutral lipid core

protein

marrow also removes a significant amount of circulating chylomicrons and remnants.

Several overlapping mechanisms are involved in the hepatic uptake of chylomicron remnants (Cooper, 1997). The particles must first achieve a size that allows them to pass through the fenestrations of hepatic capillary endothelial cells and accumulate in the space of Disse. Sequestration of the remnants and further lipolysis by hepatic lipase precedes receptor-mediated uptake of the particles by the hepatocytes. The apoE on the remnants serves as the ligand for receptors present on hepatocyte surfaces facing the space of Disse.

The LDL receptor and the LDL receptor-related protein (LRP) facilitate uptake of the remnants by receptor-mediated endocytosis. The LDL receptor, whilst recognizing apoB-100 for the binding of LDL (Section 3.6.4), has a far higher affinity for particles containing several molecules of apoE than those containing a single molecule of apoB. Remnants can be taken up directly by LDL receptors but direct removal of remnants via the LRP seems to be limited. The remnants become enriched with apoE by taking up free apoE secreted into the space of Disse by the hepatocytes. apoE-enriched remnants bind avidly to the glycocalyx, specifically to heparan sulphate proteoglycans, on hepatocyte surfaces. This interaction appears to be required for the uptake of remnants by the LRP, as uptake can be inhibited by removal of heparan sulphate proteoglycans with heparinase. Ji *et al.* (1994) proposed that the remnants interacting with heparan sulphate proteoglycans may be transferred to the LRP, or the heparan sulphate proteoglycans may form a complex with the LRP and together mediate internalization.

In marmosets, uptake of chylomicrons and chylomicron remnants by the bone marrow is restricted to perisinusoidal macrophages, which protrude through the capillary endothelium into the marrow sinuses (Mahley & Hussain, 1991).

Formation of VLDL, HDL and LDL

In the liver, the constituent lipids of chylomicron remnants are repackaged into HDL and VLDL particles (mainly the latter), which are released into the circulation. There is no direct synthesis of LDL in the liver. VLDL contain high concentrations of triglycerides and moderate concentrations of cholesteryl esters and phospholipids. The triglycerides are removed from VLDL by the action of lipoprotein lipase located on the endothelial surface of blood vessels in extrahepatic tissues, enabling tissue uptake of free fatty acids. When much of the triglyceride has been removed, the VLDL become IDL. Newly released HDL contain a high concentration of protein (about 50 per cent), but very little cholesteryl ester. Circulating HDL take up the excess cholesterol released from cells into the plasma, converting it into cholesteryl esters by the action of lecithin:cholesterol acyltransferase. Much of the HDL cholesteryl ester is transferred to IDL which then become LDL. LDL is the major cholesterol-carrying lipoprotein and high levels of these particles in the circulation are associated with an increased risk of heart disease.

HDL participates in reverse cholesterol transport by acquiring cholesterol from tissues and other lipoproteins and transferring it to the liver for excretion. Elevated HDL levels in the circulation are associated with reduced risk of heart disease.

3.6.4   Role of plasma LDL in cholesterol transport

The LDL particle is composed of 75% lipid and 25% protein. The major lipid component is esterified cholesterol, which constitutes the bulk of the particle core. Surrounding this apolar core is a lipid coat composed of phospholipid and free cholesterol. The protein component apoB-100 consists of several subunits. The subunits form globules, of which a part is buried in the lipid core and a part is exposed at the water surface.

All growing cells need cholesterol for membrane synthesis. About 70% of the total plasma cholesterol is contained in LDL. Cells acquire cholesterol by taking up circulating LDL particles by the process of receptor-mediated endocytosis. apoB-100 is the ligand for the binding of LDL to the LDL receptor, a transmembrane glycoprotein. The internalized lipoproteins are conveyed to lysosomes where the cholesteryl esters are hydrolysed to free cholesterol. Most LDL receptors are expressed in the liver, where they facilitate the supply of cholesterol for secretion into bile, conversion to bile acids, and resecretion into the plasma in newly synthesized lipoproteins. LDL receptors are also present in high concentrations in the adrenal cortex and the ovarian corpus luteum, where they function to provide cholesterol for steroid hormone synthesis.

The intracellular concentration of cholesterol is subject to feedback control mediated by the LDL-derived cholesterol itself. The incoming cholesterol (1) suppresses the activity of 3-hydroxy-3-methylglutaryl coenzyme A reductase (HMG CoA reductase), which is the rate-controlling enzyme in cholesterol biosynthesis; (2) activates the cholesterol esterifying enzyme acyl-coenzyme A:cholesterol acyltransferase (ACAT), thereby sequestering excess cholesterol as cholesteryl esters; and (3) turns off the synthesis of the LDL receptor, thereby preventing further entry of LDL-cholesterol into the cell (Goldstein & Brown, 1977).

3.6.5 Absorption of the fat-soluble vitamins

Absorption of the individual fat-soluble vitamins is described in the relevant chapters. In summary, the vitamins are solubilized in mixed micelles to facilitate uptake by the intestinal epithelium. Inside the enterocytes the vitamins are incorporated into chylomicrons, which are released and transferred via the lymphatic system to the blood. The chylomicrons are attacked by lipoprotein lipase and the chylomicron remnants are taken up by the liver for storage, metabolism or subsequent release. Because of the existence of specific carrier proteins for vitamins A and D, transport of these vitamins from the liver to other tissues is not dependent on lipoproteins. No specific carrier proteins for vitamins E and K in plasma have been identified: plasma transport of these vitamins appears to be entirely mediated by lipoproteins.

3.7 Neural and endocrine communication systems

3.7.1 Introduction: the nervous, endocrine and neuroendocrine systems

Anatomically, the nervous system can be divided into the central nervous system (CNS) and the peripheral nervous system. The CNS is composed of the brain and spinal cord located in the cranium and vertebral canal; the peripheral nervous system includes all other nervous structures. The CNS receives all nervous impulses from the body (interoceptive) and all impulses following stimuli originating outside the body (exteroceptive). The peripheral nervous system serves to interconnect all other tissues and organs with the CNS.

Endocrine systems employ hormones as chemical messengers. Hormones are synthesized by the cells of endocrine glands and secreted from these glands directly into the bloodstream. They travel in the systemic circulation to the cells of distal target tissues where they initiate their biological response.

Neuroendocrine systems are those in which neurons secrete neurohormones that reach the systemic circulation and influence the function of cells at another location in the body.

3.7.2 The neuron

The functional unit of the nervous system is the neuron, which consists of a cell body and its thread-like processes – one or more dendrites and a single axon. The axon is commonly referred to as the nerve fibre and varies in length from a fraction of a millimetre to a metre or more. Most of the nerve cell bodies are located in or near the CNS. Their processes, which are capable of transmitting impulses, may lie totally within the CNS, may extend from the CNS system for great distances, or may lie entirely outside the CNS. The dendrites conduct impulses toward the cell body, and the axon conducts impulses away from the cell body. Nerve impulses are relayed from one neuron to another across synapses. At these meeting points the surface membranes of the two neurons are very close together, but there is never any cytoplasmic continuity. The width of the extracellular space separating the pre- and post-synaptic membranes, the synaptic cleft, is generally about 25 nm. Transmission of an impulse across a synapse is chemical rather than electrical. It depends on the release of a chemical transmitter from the presynaptic terminal, which then diffuses across the synaptic cleft and interacts with receptor sites on the postsynaptic membrane so as to cause a specific change in its ionic permeability.

An axon consists of a long cylinder of cytoplasm, the axoplasm, surrounded by an electrically excitable nerve membrane, the axolemma, which is continuous with the plasma membrane of the parent nerve cell body. Axons may be unmyelinated or myelinated. In myelinated nerves, the axon is surrounded by a tubular sheath composed of multiple layers of tightly packed concentric membranes formed by and continuous with the plasma membrane of Schwann cells. This myelin sheath contains the lipid sphingomyelin, which is an excellent electrical insulator. The myelin

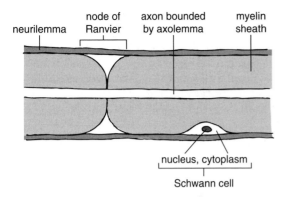

Fig. 3.28 Diagram of a myelinated nerve fibre. The myelin sheath is an insulating layer derived from Schwann cell plasma membranes spiralling concentrically to form a wrapping around the axon. The outer layer of the myelin, the neurilemma, is a basal lamina beneath which lie the flattened nuclei of Schwann cells.

sheath is interrupted at intervals by the nodes of Ranvier. The structure of a typical myelinated axon of the peripheral nervous system is shown in Fig. 3.28.

3.7.3   Propagation of a nerve impulse

It is possible to place microelectrodes on the surface of a myelinated axon at a node of Ranvier and record spike-like electrical currents that are associated with changes in potential difference taking place across the axonal membrane. A nerve impulse is propagated in the form of an action potential and depends upon rapid changes in membrane ion permeability. During the initial phase of the action potential a rapid influx of sodium ions through voltage-gated sodium channels causes rapid depolarization of the membrane, i.e. the inside surface of the membrane becomes less negative relative to the outside of the membrane. The more a membrane is depolarized, the greater the number of sodium channels that will be opened. The entry of Na^+ does not continue indefinitely: it is halted partly because the membrane potential soon reaches the sodium ion equilibrium potential, where the net inward driving force acting on sodium ions becomes zero, and partly because the rise in sodium permeability decays inexorably with time from the moment when it is first triggered. After the peak of the spike has been reached, therefore, the sodium permeability is rapidly reduced. At the same time, the opening of potassium channels and chloride channels allow K^+

efflux and Cl^- influx, thereby increasing the degree of intracellular negativity. This hyperpolarization inhibits the neuron because the membrane potential is now further away than ever from the –45 mV threshold for excitation. The fact that potassium channels are 50 times more numerous than sodium channels (Hille, 1970) ensures that hyperpolarization is rapid. The membrane then adjusts to its normal resting potential of –65 mV in readiness for another action potential.

In myelinated fibres, the sodium channels are concentrated at the nodes of Ranvier. The function of the myelin sheath is to restrict the inward and outward passage of local circuit current to the nodes of Ranvier, so causing the nerve impulse to be propagated along myelinated fibres from node to node in a series of jumps (saltatory conduction). The generation of an action potential at each node results in the depolarization of the next node and subsequently the generation of an action potential with an internode delay of only about 20 μs.

3.7.4   Hormones and cell signalling

General principles

There are three general classes of hormones: (1) peptide hormones, e.g. thyroid-stimulating hormone and adrenocorticotropic hormone; (2) steroid hormones, e.g. oestrogens, testosterone and cortisol; and (3) derivatives of the amino acid tyrosine, e.g. thyroxine and adrenaline (epinephrine). Peptide and amine hormones are stored in secretory vesicles until needed. Steroid hormones are not stored: they are synthesized from intracellular stores of cholesteryl esters after a stimulus.

Hormone action is initiated by the binding of hormone to receptors in the cells of target tissues. Hormonal receptors are large proteins which have both high affinity and high specificity for their hormonal ligands. Each cell within a target tissue contains some 2000 to 100 000 receptors. The target tissues for a particular hormone are those whose cells contain receptors for that hormone: cells that lack such receptors do not respond. Thus receptors provide the first level of specificity for hormone action. Formation of the hormone–receptor complex triggers a cascade of reactions in the target cell, with each stage becoming more powerfully activated, so that very low concentrations of circulating hormone can elicit a robust biological response.

The receptors for peptide hormones and catecholamines are located in or on the surface of the cell membrane. These hormones, being hydrophilic, cannot cross the lipid bilayer of the cell's plasma membrane and so many of them recruit a 'second messenger' to mediate their intracellular action. (The hormone is the 'first messenger'.) The best-known second messenger is cyclic AMP; others include diacylglycerol and inositol triphosphate (these are products of membrane phospholipid breakdown) and calcium ions.

The receptors for the steroid hormones reside within the cell. The steroid hormones, being hydrophobic, are able to cross the plasma membrane and bind to their specific receptors. The liganded receptors interact with specific sites on the DNA and directly regulate gene transcription. The newly formed proteins become the controllers of new or increased cellular function.

Regulation of hormonal activity

Hormonal activity can be regulated at both the endocrine gland and the target tissue. Positive or negative feedback to the endocrine gland may regulate any step during the synthesis, processing or release of the hormone. Positive feedback results in additional secretion of the hormone, while negative feedback has the opposite effect. Most hormones are controlled through negative feedback in order to prevent overactivity of the target tissues and to allow responses to subsequent signals. The controlled variable is often the degree of activity of the target tissue. Above a certain level of activity, feedback signals to the endocrine gland become powerful enough to shut down hormone production or prevent secretion.

Formation of the hormone–receptor complex may cause the number of active receptors to decrease, either because of inactivation or destruction or because of decreased production by the cell's protein-manufacturing capacity. This down-regulation of receptors leads to a decreased response of the target tissue to the hormone. Some hormones can cause up-regulation of receptors by inducing synthesis of the receptors. When this occurs, the target tissue becomes progressively more sensitive to the stimulating effects of the hormone.

3.7.5 G proteins

The signal from most peptide hormones (but not from insulin) is relayed from the activated (i.e. hormone-bound) membrane receptor across the plasma membrane and into the cytosol by means of a guanosine triphosphate (GTP)-binding protein (G protein). Translocation of the G protein from the lipid environment of the membrane to the aqueous environment of the cytosol and back again is made possible by the detachment and re-attachment of a lipophilic palmitate group.

G proteins are a family of heterotrimeric proteins composed of three subunits, designated α, β and γ in order of decreasing molecular weight. The α-subunit of the G protein (with GTP bound) binds to and activates the effector, which may be a membrane-bound enzyme or an ion channel. Activation of an enzyme effector results in the formation of the second messengers cyclic AMP and diacylglycerol/inositol triphosphate; activation of calcium channels causes an influx of Ca^{2+} second messenger into the cell.

G protein-coupled receptors comprise the largest superfamily of proteins in the body with more than 1000 having been identified. Their common structural feature is the presence of seven helical membrane-spanning domains with an extracellular amino terminus and an intracellular carboxyl terminus. In addition to peptide hormones, ligands for G protein-coupled receptors include biogenic amines, glycoproteins, lipids, nucleotides, ions and proteases. Moreover, the sensation of exogenous stimuli, such as light, odours and taste, is mediated via these receptors.

One member of the family of G proteins, G_s, transmits signals from a wide variety of G protein-coupled receptors to adenylyl cyclase (formerly called adenylate cyclase), an enzyme which catalyses the formation of cyclic AMP from ATP within cells. Wedegaertner & Bourne (1994) proposed a model (Fig. 3.29) for the role of the G protein in relaying the signal across the plasma membrane. In the inactive state, G_s exists as a heterotrimeric complex with GDP bound to the α-subunit. The inactive complex is tightly associated with the inner leaflet of the plasma membrane by virtue of a lipophilic palmitate group attached to the α-subunit. Upon binding of hormone to the G protein-coupled receptor, the activated receptor interacts with the α-subunit of the G_s protein to promote the replacement of GDP with GTP. GTP binding changes the conformation of $G_s\alpha$, leading to its dissociation from the stable $\beta\gamma$ dimer. The α and $\beta\gamma$ subunits remain associated with the plasma membrane by virtue of their respective palmitate and isoprenyl attachments. Palmitate is

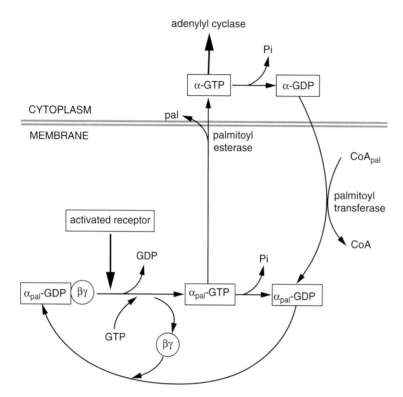

Fig. 3.29 Model of Gα$_s$ palmitoylation and depalmitoylation as a means for reversible translocation of the subunit between the plasma membrane and the cytoplasm. Reprinted from *Cell*, Vol. 77, Wedegaertner, P. B. and Bourne, H. R. Activation and depalmitoylation of G$_s$α, pp. 1063–70, ©1994, with permission from Elsevier Science.

rapidly cleaved from GTP-bound G$_s$α by a palmitoyl esterase and some or all of the depalmitoylated α-subunit is released from the membrane into the cytoplasm. The active GTP-bound G$_s$α stimulates adenylyl cyclase to catalyse the conversion of ATP to cyclic AMP. The latter then activates cyclic AMP-dependent protein kinase, which phosphorylates specific proteins in the cell, triggering biochemical reactions that ultimately lead to the cell's response to the hormone. A GTPase intrinsic to the α-subunit converts the active GTP-bound subunits in both membrane and cytoplasm into the inactive GDP-bound forms. Re-attachment of palmitate to the cytoplasmic subunit by a palmitoyl transferase facilitates the return of the GDP-bound G$_s$α to the plasma membrane.

3.7.6   Second messengers

Cyclic AMP and cyclic GMP

The main components of the cyclic AMP signalling system are shown in Fig. 3.30. A similar alternative second messenger, cyclic guanosine monophosphate (cyclic GMP), can be formed from GTP by guanylyl cyclase in response to a few peptide hormones.

Amplification of the hormonal signal is achieved as follows. The binding of a single molecule of hormone to one receptor molecule activates many G-protein molecules, each of which activates a molecule of adenylyl cyclase. Each molecule of adenylyl cyclase catalyses the formation of multiple cyclic AMP molecules, each of which activates one molecule of cyclic AMP-dependent protein kinase (protein kinase A). This kinase then initiates a cascade of enzymes by activating a second kinase, which activates a third kinase, and so forth. Such a multistep system has the potential for additional regulation, allowing fine-tuning of the signal and the ability to override a given stimulus under appropriate circumstances.

A given hormone can bind to several different receptors, each of which is coupled to a different G protein. This allows the same hormone to either stimulate or inhibit a particular action. For example, adrenaline can bind to both α- and β-adrenergic receptors. The β$_2$-adrenergic receptor is coupled to G$_s$, and therefore the binding of adrenaline leads to an increase in cyclic AMP levels. The α$_2$-adrenergic receptor is coupled to an inhibitory G protein, G$_i$, so that adrenaline binding leads to a decrease in cyclic AMP levels.

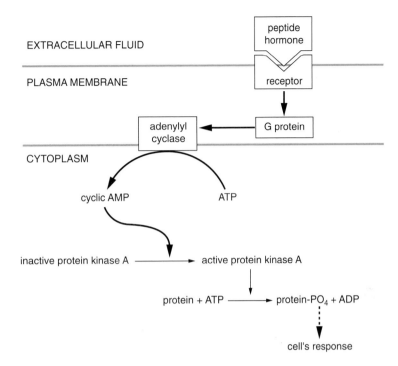

Fig. 3.30 The adenylyl cyclase-cyclic AMP second messenger system.

The specific action that occurs in response to increases or decreases of cyclic AMP in each type of target cell depends on the nature of the intracellular machinery – some cells having one set of enzymes, and other cells having other enzymes. Therefore, different functions are elicited in different target cells – such functions as alterations in cell membrane permeability, muscle contraction or relaxation, secretion of substances by the cell and synthesis of intracellular chemicals. The cyclic AMP signalling system is also able to control transcription of specific genes. Protein kinase A-mediated phosphorylation of the cyclic AMP response element-binding protein (CREB) enhances the binding of this protein to a specific site on the gene termed the cyclic AMP response element (CRE). This protein–DNA interaction initiates transcription, leading to synthesis of new protein.

Diacylglycerol and inositol triphosphate

Diacylglycerol acts as a second messenger in the transduction of extracellular signals initiated by peptide hormones, neurotransmitters (e.g. acetylcholine), antigens and some growth factors (e.g. platelet-derived growth factor and epidermal growth factor). The main components of the diacylglycerol second messenger system are shown in Fig. 3.31. Phosphatidylinositol, a phospholipid constituent of the plasma membrane, can be doubly phosphorylated to form phosphatidylinositol biphosphate. Activation of phospholipase C in response to appropriate ligand binding of the cell-surface receptor results in the hydrolysis of phosphatidylinositol biphosphate and the formation of diacylglycerol and inositol triphosphate. Both of these hydrolysis products act as intracellular second messengers. Diacylglycerol and calcium ions together activate protein kinase C, which catalyses the covalent addition of a phosphate group to serine and threonine residues of various proteins, thereby altering their activity. Inositol triphosphate causes the release of Ca^{2+} from storage compartments in mitochondria and the endoplasmic reticulum, thereby triggering the activation of a variety of calcium-dependent enzymes and hormonal responses. Protein kinase C activation and Ca^{2+} mobilization act synergistically to cause a variety of cellular responses.

Signalling is desensitized in response to chronic activation by dephosphorylation of the protein kinase C effected by a membrane-associated heterotrimeric type 2A phosphatase (Hansra et al., 1996). This event is followed by increased proteolysis of the kinase. These two independent desensitization processes are triggered by the membrane-associated activation of protein kinase C itself.

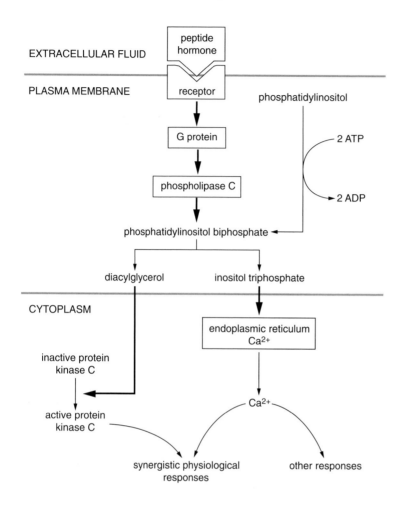

Fig. 3.31 The diacylglycerol second messenger system.

Calcium ions

Another second messenger system operates in response to the entry of Ca^{2+} into cells or to the release of Ca^{2+} from intracellular pools through the action of inositol triphosphate. The Ca^{2+} entry may be initiated (1) by changes in membrane potential that open membrane calcium channels or (2) by a hormone interacting with membrane receptors that open calcium channels. The increased intracellular Ca^{2+} binds with high affinity to the protein calmodulin, which has four Ca^{2+}-binding sites. When three or four of these sites have bound with Ca^{2+}, the calmodulin molecule undergoes a conformational change, thereby exposing hydrophobic regions that are involved in interaction with more than twenty target enzymes, including several protein kinases. Activation of calmodulin-dependent protein kinases causes, via phosphorylation, activation or inhibition of proteins involved in the

cell's response to a hormone. The kinases include the multifunctional calmodulin-dependent multiprotein kinase and dedicated kinases such as myosin light chain kinase, phosphorylase kinase and elongation factor 2 kinase that regulate muscle contraction, glycogenolysis and protein synthesis, respectively (Cohen, 1992). Other calmodulin-dependent enzymes include adenylyl cyclase, nitric oxide synthase, calmodulin-dependent protein phosphatase (calcineurin), cyclic 3′,5′-nucleotide phosphodiesterase and Ca^{2+}-Mg^{2+}-ATPase.

3.7.7 Protein tyrosine kinases

Not all extracellular signals mediate their responses through G protein-coupled generation of intracellular second messengers. Some membrane receptors bypass the G proteins and second messengers and directly initiate the final common pathway that transduces the extracellular signals. Receptors for insulin and other growth factors possess intrinsic tyrosine kinase activity and are referred to as protein tyrosine kinases. These receptors straddle the plasma membrane; their extracellular domain contains the ligand binding site and the intracellular domain contains the tyrosine kinase. The receptors are activated upon binding of ligand and respond by phosphorylating themselves at specific multiple tyrosine residues, using phosphate derived from ATP. Autophosphorylation of the receptors allows them to phosphorylate many intracellular proteins, which then mediate the appropriate cellular response.

3.7.8 Regulation of signal transduction

The hormonal stimulus can be blunted or shut off at several levels of the signal transduction system. (1) The stimulus can be diminished by decreasing the number of receptors at the cell surface. This can be achieved by decreased production of the receptors by the protein-manufacturing mechanism of the cell. Alternatively, the receptor proteins themselves are inactivated or destroyed during the course of their function, one example being endocytosis of the receptor prior to intracellular destruction of the ligand. In any event, this down-regulation of the receptor decreases the responsiveness of the target tissue to the hormone. (2) The G_s protein is inactivated by an intrinsic GTPase activity that hydrolyses the bound GTP to GDP. This GTPase activity allows the G_s protein to act as a molecular switch: it rapidly turns the hormonal signal on or off by binding or hydrolysing GTP, respectively. (3) The inhibitory G protein, G_i, when activated by other receptors, leads to direct inhibition of adenylyl cyclase and thus cessation of cyclic AMP production. (4) The ability to hydrolyse cyclic AMP by phosphodiesterase allows the cell to respond transiently to a given signal.

An additional mechanism of regulating signal transduction, known as desensitization, allows a receptor to be rapidly inactivated and then reactivated despite the continued presence of a stimulus of constant intensity. Persistent or excessive stimulation of a G protein-coupled receptor leads to activation of a G protein-coupled receptor kinase (GRK) that phosphorylates the receptor. The receptor then binds an arrestin protein which sterically prevents signalling to

the G protein (Lefkowitz, 1998). The family of GRKs includes at least six members (GRKs 1–6) of which the most thoroughly investigated are rhodopsin kinase (GRK1) and β-adrenergic receptor kinase (GRK2). GRKs recognize only the liganded or stimulus-modified forms of the receptors that they phosphorylate (Lorenz et al., 1991). Desensitization of rhodopsin, the photoreceptor in the rod cells of the retina, occurs in less than one second following light stimulation, thereby preventing a brief flash of light from being perceived as continuous illumination.

3.7.9 Role of protein kinase C in stimulus–response coupling

The role of protein kinase C in stimulus–response coupling was first demonstrated for the release of serotonin from platelets. The enzyme has since been shown to be involved in the release of certain hormones and neurotransmitters, the secretion of certain enzymes, smooth muscle contraction and relaxation, activation of T and B lymphocytes, inhibition of gap junctions, modulation of ion conductance, interaction and down-regulation of receptors, cell proliferation, expression of certain genes, steroidogenesis, lipogenesis and glucose metabolism. When intracellular Ca^{2+} concentrations become too high, protein kinase C activates the Ca^{2+}-transport ATPase (calcium pump) and the Na^+/Ca^{2+} exchange protein, both of which remove Ca^{2+} from the cell (Nishizuka, 1986).

Protein kinase C is synthesized as an unphosphorylated and catalytically inactive protein of 74 kDa that is bound to the plasma membrane of the cell. The protein is converted into an active form of 77 kDa and then into an 80 kDa form by at least two phosphorylation steps. The first phosphorylation is initiated by an as yet unidentified kinase ('protein kinase C kinase'). This phosphorylation step takes place on the activation loop of the newly synthesized protein and renders it catalytically competent. The membrane-bound enzyme, when stimulated by phosphatidylserine, then phosphorylates itself at the carboxy terminus. This autophosphorylation decreases the enzyme's affinity for the membrane so that it partitions into the cytosol (Dutil et al., 1994). The doubly phosphorylated enzyme is allosteric, i.e. regulatable. Binding of the activator (diacylglycerol) to the allosteric site of the enzyme causes a conformational change, thereby exposing the catalytic site that is normally blocked by the so-called pseudosubstrate region.

There are several subtypes of protein kinase C, each the product of a separate gene; these are identified by a Greek letter, the α-subtype being the most ubiquitous. Isoforms of the β-subtype (β1 and β2) are generated post-translationally by the alternative splicing of the primary mRNA transcript. The eleven subspecies of protein kinase C (PKC) so far identified have been divided into three groups: the conventional (cPKC) group comprises α, β1, β2 and γ; the new (nPKC) group comprises δ, ε, η, θ and μ; and the atypical (aPKC) group comprises ζ and λ(ι) (Nishizuka, 1995). The ability of the individual subspecies to elicit different physiological responses is presumably due to their localization in different tissues and subcellular sites.

In the absence of diacylglycerol, protein kinase C resides in the cytosol. When diacylglycerol is generated, it recruits the kinase from the cytosol to the plasma membrane. Diacylglycerol, aided by *cis*-unsaturated fatty acids, also increases the affinity of protein kinase C for Ca^{2+}, thereby causing full enzyme activity when Ca^{2+} concentrations are basal (Nishizuka, 1995). A proportion of the activated enzyme is targeted to the nucleus where the phosphorylation of nuclear regulatory proteins (transcription factors) could provide a mechanism for the direct regulation of gene expression, leading to changes in cell proliferation and differentiation (Olson *et al.*, 1993).

The diacylglycerol produced by receptor-mediated hydrolysis of phosphatidylinositol biphosphate is short-lived, either being re-incorporated into phosphoinositides or hydrolysed to arachidonic acid, the precursor of prostaglandins and thromboxane. Long-term cellular responses, such as cell proliferation and

activation of T lymphocytes, requires sustained activation of protein kinase C through other pathways. For example, hydrolysis of membrane phosphatidylcholine by phospholipase D produces phosphatidic acid and choline. Phosphatidic acid is converted to diacylglycerol by the action of a phosphomonoesterase, thereby indirectly activating protein kinase C. Phosphatidic acid may also activate protein kinase C directly (Nishizuka, 1995).

Protein kinase C exerts negative feedback control over various steps of its activation pathway, including down-regulation of the cell-surface receptor. In addition, protein kinase C exerts negative feedback control at the level of the receptors for various growth factors, such as epidermal growth factor.

Protein kinase C is a target for phorbol esters, such as 12-*O*-tetradecanoylphorbol-13-acetate (TPA), and probably serves as a receptor for these compounds. A number of phorbol esters are well known as potent tumour promoters. Extremely low concentrations of phorbol esters are able to substitute for diacylglycerol and activate protein kinase C. Unlike diacylglycerol, however, phorbol esters are metabolically stable; moreover, their entry into the cell is not susceptible to feedback control. Phorbol esters are therefore able to activate protein kinase C in a sustained rather than transient manner. Prolonged treatment of cells with phorbol esters leads to disappearance of protein kinase C owing to an increased rate of proteolysis (Young *et al.*, 1987). Depletion of protein kinase C would remove the negative feedback control that the kinase exerts over growth factor receptors, leading to uncontrolled cell proliferation in the presence of a mitogenic stimulus. This possible effect of phorbol esters on protein kinase C is shown in Fig. 3.32.

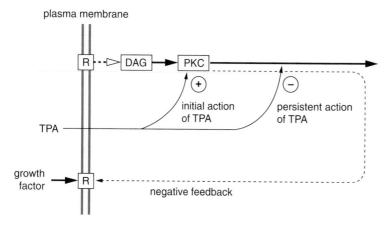

Fig. 3.32 Effect of phorbol ester on protein kinase C. Initially, TPA (12-*O*-tetradecanoylphorbol-13-acetate) mimics diacylglycerol (DAG) and activates protein kinase C (PKC), but a secondary persistent action of TPA leads to degradation of PKC thereby removing the negative feedback control of growth factor receptors exerted by PKC. R, receptors in plasma membrane. Reprinted with permission from Nishizuka (1988), *Nature*, Vol. 334, pp. 661–5, © 1988, Macmillan Magazines Limited.

The microbial product calphostin C is a highly potent and specific inhibitor of protein kinase C in cell cultures (Kobayashi *et al.*, 1989). The potent cytotoxic activity and antitumour activity of calphostin C might be due to the inhibition of protein kinase C.

3.8 Structure of bone and its growth and development

Bone, or osseous tissue, is a dynamic living tissue with a well developed vascular and nerve supply. Histologically, bone is a rigid form of connective tissue that consists of cells and an intercellular matrix. In order to maintain its required toughness, bone is constantly being destroyed and renewed by a process known as remodelling.

3.8.1 Composition of bone matrix

The bone matrix consists of an organic component, largely type I collagen, called the osteoid, and a mineral component comprising mainly calcium phosphate in the form of hydroxyapatite $[Ca_{10}(PO_4)_6(OH)_2]$. Hydroxyapatite comprises 90% of bone, with collagen making up 90% of the remaining organic matrix. Individual collagen molecules become interconnected by the formation of pyridinoline cross-links, which are unique to bone. The hydroxyapatite crystals are regularly distributed along the length of the collagen fibres and take the form of needles, thin plates or leaves. The surface ions of hydroxyapatite are hydrated, allowing the exchange of ions between the crystals and the surrounding fluid. The collagen fibres and crystals are embedded in an amorphous ground substance containing phosphoproteins, glycoproteins and γ-carboxyglutamic acid-containing proteins. These components all play a role in calcification (mineralization). They are acidic in nature and possess high aggregation tendencies and calcium-binding properties. The association of hydroxyapatite with collagen fibres accounts for the hardness and resistance of the bone structure. Matrix synthesis determines the volume of bone but not its density. Calcification of the matrix increases the density of bone by displacing water, but does not alter its volume.

3.8.2 Bone cells

There are three types of functional cells in bone tissue: osteoblasts, osteocytes and osteoclasts (Fig. 3.33).

Osteoblasts

Osteoblasts arise from mesenchymal stem cells present in the stroma (framework) of the bone marrow. These cells have the potential to differentiate into a variety of mesenchymal tissues, such as bone, cartilage, tendon, muscle, marrow, fat and dermis. The stem cells proliferate and then commit themselves to a particular pathway of lineage progression, differentiation and

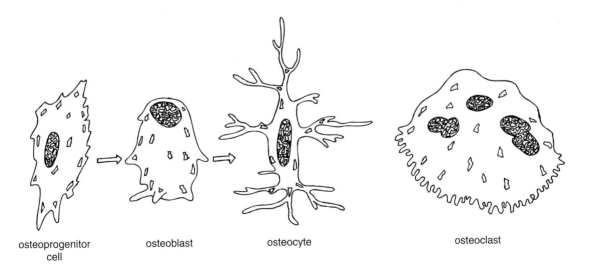

osteoprogenitor   osteoblast   osteocyte   osteoclast
cell

Fig. 3.33 Types of cells in bone tissue.

maturation (Bruder *et al.*, 1994). The commitment event and lineage progression involve the action of locally generated cytokines and growth factors, many of which are controlled by circulating hormones. Mesenchymal stem cells committed to bone formation are referred to as osteoprogenitor cells. These cells give rise to pre-osteoblasts which differentiate into secretory osteoblasts.

Osteoblasts synthesize and secrete type I collagen and a number of noncollagenous proteins. The latter include osteocalcin, which functions to limit bone formation, and osteonectin, which appears to play a role in the survival of bone cells. The osteoblasts also secrete large quantities of alkaline phosphatase, providing the inorganic phosphate component of bone. Osteoblasts initiate bone resorption by producing proteases which remove surface osteoid. The presence of cell-surface receptors for most chemical mediators of bone metabolism is evidence of the role of osteoblasts in the regulation of bone turnover. A subpopulation of osteoblasts, known as lining cells, lie as nonsynthesizing, flattened cells along trabecular surfaces.

Osteocytes

Calcification induces morphological and metabolic changes in the osteoblast, converting this bone cell into an osteocyte. Osteocytes are surrounded by newly synthesized bone matrix. They are mature bone cells and have no mitotic potential or secretory activity. In developing bone, their cytoplasmic processes extend for considerable distances in narrow channels called canaliculi and make contact with processes of neighbouring osteocytes via gap junctions. The network thus formed allows molecules to be passed from cell to cell. In mature bone the processes are almost completely withdrawn, but the canaliculi remain to provide an avenue for the exchange of nutrients and waste products between the blood and the imprisoned osteocytes.

Osteoclasts

Osteoclasts are multinucleated giant cells that are solely responsible for the resorption (destruction) of bone matrix – both mineral and organic components. Their progenitors are mononucleate haematopoietic cells of the monocyte/macrophage lineage which, when stimulated, fuse together to become mature osteoclasts. Resorption is important in the development, growth, maintenance and repair of bone. The

cells are found in or near cavities called Howship's lacunae on bone surfaces. Osteoclasts express on their surfaces many receptors for calcitonin, which is a potent inhibitor of the cell's resorptive activity. The surface of the osteoclast facing the bone matrix is termed the ruffled border, owing to extensive infoldings. Adjacent to the ruffled border in the cell's interior is a so-called clear zone that is rich in actin filaments but devoid of organelles. The clear zone is a site of adhesion of the osteoclast to the bone matrix and creates a microenvironment of low pH and lysosomal enzymes for bone resorption. Osteoclasts secrete acid, collagenase and other proteolytic enzymes that dissolve the bone matrix. The ruffled border is essential for the activity of the osteoclast. In osteopetrosis, a genetic disease characterized by dense heavy bone, the osteocytes lack ruffled borders and bone resorption is defective.

3.8.3   Architecture of bone

There are two types of bone tissue: woven or primary bone and lamellar or mature bone. All of the bone in the newborn baby is woven and this bone type occurs also in localized regions of the growing skeleton and in repairing fractures. Woven bone is characterized by a random orientation of its collagen fibres and a low mineral content relative to that of lamellar bone. Except in a very few locations, such as tooth sockets, woven bone is replaced in infants over one year old by lamellar bone, so-called because the collagen fibres are orientated in parallel arrays. The bone tissue described in the following is lamellar bone.

There are two types of lamellar bone: cortical bone and cancellous or trabecular bone. Cortical bone is a dense solid mass which forms the external layer of all bones of the body and predominates in the shafts of long bones. Cancellous bone takes the form of an irregular latticework of rods, plates and arches individually known as trabeculae. Cancellous bone makes up most of the bone tissue of short, flat and irregularly shaped bones such as the vertebrae, pelvis and shoulder blade; it is also found in the bulbous ends of long bones. In early life, the spaces between the trabeculae of all cancellous bones are filled with haemopoietic (blood-producing) red bone marrow, but later the red marrow is confined to the cancellous bones of the trunk. The spaces in other cancellous bones are filled with yellow bone marrow, which consists mostly of fat.

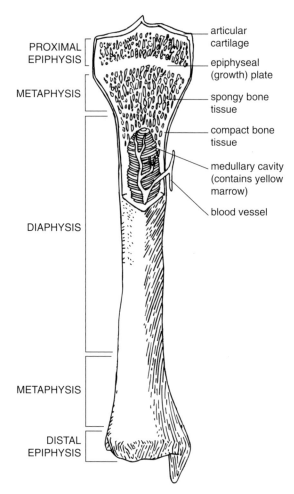

PROXIMAL
EPIPHYSIS

articular
cartilage

epiphyseal
(growth) plate

METAPHYSIS

spongy bone
tissue

compact bone
tissue

medullary cavity
(contains yellow
marrow)

blood vessel

DIAPHYSIS

METAPHYSIS

DISTAL
EPIPHYSIS

Fig. 3.34 Gross anatomy of a typical long bone with interior partially exposed.

periosteum consists of dense fibrous connective tissue and contains a network of blood vessels. The inner layer is composed of more loosely arranged connective tissue and numerous osteoprogenitor cells. Some component collagenous fibres of the periosteum penetrate the bone matrix as Sharpey's fibres. Inside the bone, the medullary cavity and the cavities of cancellous bone are lined by the endosteum. This membrane is composed of a single layer of osteoprogenitor cells and a very small amount of connective tissue. The principal functions of the periosteum and endosteum are nutrition of the osseous tissue and the provision of new osteoblasts for bone repair.

Cortical bone

In cortical bone, the calcified bone matrix is formed of layers called lamellae arranged in a manner determined by the distribution of blood vessels. The lamellae are organized into osteons (Haversian systems) in which four to twenty lamellae are concentrically arranged around a central Haversian canal containing the blood vessels and nerves. A segment of an Haversian system is shown diagrammatically in Fig. 3.35. Between, and occasionally within, the lamellae there are small cavities called lacunae which contain osteocytes. Radiating from each lacuna are the canaliculi. These channels penetrate adjacent lamellae to unite with canaliculi of neighbouring lacunae and eventually open to extracellular fluid at bone surfaces.

Each osteon is a long often bifurcated cylinder which in long bones is orientated mainly in the long

In a typical long bone (Fig. 3.34) the shaft (diaphysis) is composed almost entirely of cortical bone with a small component of cancellous bone surrounding the medullary cavity. In the adult, the medullary cavity contains yellow bone marrow. The bulbous ends (epiphyses) and the metaphyses consist of cancellous bone covered by a shell of cortical bone. In the growing animal, the epiphysis is separated from the metaphysis by a thick plate of hyaline cartilage known as the epiphyseal plate; it is in this region that bone elongation occurs. In the adult, the cartilaginous plate has been replaced by cancellous bone.

The outer surfaces of most bones, but not the articular surfaces of joints, are covered by a bilayered sheath called the periosteum. The outer layer of the

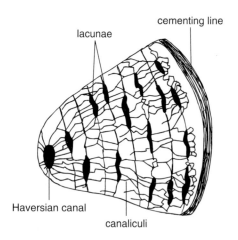

cementing line

lacunae

Haversian canal

canaliculi

Fig. 3.35 Diagram of a segment of an osteon (Haversian system) in cross-section.

axis of the diaphysis. The Haversian canals communicate with the periosteum bone marrow cavity and each other through transverse or oblique Volkmann's canals, which perforate the lamellae. The intervals between osteons are occupied by interstitial lamellae, which are the remnants of osteons partly destroyed during the internal reconstruction of the bone.

Cancellous bone

Each trabecula consists of a mosaic of angular segments formed by parallel sheets of lamellae. These segments of lamellar bone are called trabecular packets and are functionally analogous to the osteons of compact bone. The latticework of the trabeculae is orientated along lines of stress.

Within the trabeculae are osteocytes that lie in lacunae. Most trabeculae are less than 0.2 mm in thickness and the entrapped osteocytes are nourished by diffusion through canaliculi extending to the surface. A few trabeculae are thicker than 0.2 mm and their central portion generally contains concentric lamellae surrounding a blood vessel.

3.8.4 Mineralization

Although a continuous process, mineralization has been divided into primary and secondary phases. Primary mineralization lasts several days and is responsible for 70% of total mineralization, while secondary mineralization occurs over several following months and completes the total process. The primary phase is under the control of chondrocytes and osteoblasts, whereas the secondary phase is most likely governed by the chemical composition of the fluid surrounding the matrix.

Mineral crystals appear to be formed initially in extracellular matrix vesicles, which have been found at sites of rapid calcification, namely embryonic bone, calcifying epiphyseal growth cartilage and healing fractures. The vesicles are formed by budding from the plasma membranes of chondrocytes and osteoblasts, and are active at the commencement of primary mineralization. The newly released matrix vesicles undergo maturation, exhibiting increased alkaline phosphatase and phospholipase A_2 activities, and increasing in diameter as discrete hydroxyapatite crystals form on the inner leaflet of the vesicle membrane. Rupture of the membrane releases the crystals which adhere to each other and serve as foci for continued crystal deposition in the extracellular matrix. The vesicles also release proteases which facilitate matrix calcification by degrading surrounding proteoglycan aggregates.

3.8.5 Bone formation: ossification

Ossification begins around the sixth or seventh week of embryonic life and continues throughout adulthood. There are two types of ossification, which differ by the initial material on which the bone is formed. Intramembranous ossification refers to the formation of bone directly within mesenchymal connective tissue. Endochondral ossification refers to the replacement of cartilage by bone in a miniature cartilage 'model'. In both types of ossification, woven bone is formed initially.

Intramembranous ossification

The frontal and parietal bones of the skull are examples of bones that develop by intramembranous ossification. This process also contributes to the growth of short bones and the thickening of long bones.

During the eighth week of life in the human fetus, an area of mesenchyme becomes richly vascularized. This prompts mesenchymal cells to differentiate into a variety of cell types, including osteoblasts. The osteoblasts secrete the osteoid and when they are completely surrounded by it, they become osteocytes. Within a few days, minute crystals of calcium salts are deposited in an orderly fashion upon collagen fibrils, and the matrix calcifies. Lacunae and canaliculi are formed around the osteocytes and their cytoplasmic processes. As the bone matrix forms, it develops into trabeculae that fuse with one another to create the open latticework appearance of cancellous bone. The spaces between trabeculae fill with vascularized connective tissue which differentiates into red bone marrow. The mesenchyme located near the endosteal surface transforms into the endosteum and the remaining envelope of connective tissue at the periosteal surface develops into the periosteum. Eventually, most surface layers of the cancellous bone are replaced by cortical bone, but cancellous bone remains in the centre of the bone.

Endochondral ossification

Most bones of the body are formed by endochondral ossification. This is a slow process which is not achieved until the bone has reached its full size and growth has ceased. The process is best observed in a long bone.

At the site where the bone is going to form, mesenchymal cells cluster together in the shape of the future bone. The mesenchymal cells differentiate into chondroblasts that produce the cartilage model. In addition, a membrane called the perichondrium develops around the cartilage model. The cartilage model grows in length by continual cell division of chondrocytes accompanied by further secretion of cartilage matrix by the daughter cells. This pattern of growth from within is called interstitial growth. The increase in thickness of the cartilage model is due mainly to appositional growth. This refers to the addition of more matrix to its periphery by new chondroblasts that develop from the perichondrium.

As the cartilage model continues to grow, chondrocytes in its mid-region hypertrophy, probably because they accumulate glycogen for ATP production. Some hypertrophied cells burst, releasing their contents, and changing the pH of the matrix. The resultant chemical changes trigger calcification. Once the cartilage becomes calcified, other chondrocytes die because nutrients no longer diffuse quickly enough through the matrix. The lacunae of the cells that have died are now empty, and the thin partitions between them break down forming small cavities.

In the meantime, a nutrient artery penetrates the perichondrium and then the developing bone through a hole in the mid-region of the model. This stimulates osteoprogenitor cells in the perichondrium to differentiate into osteoblasts. The cells lay down a thin sheet of cortical bone under the perichondrium called the periosteal bone collar. Once the perichondium starts to form bone, it is known as the periosteum.

Near the mid-region of the model, the periosteum sends out osteogenic buds into the disintegrating calcified cartilage through holes made by osteoclasts in the bone collar. The buds, containing blood capillaries and osteoprogenitor cells, enter the spaces left by the dead and degenerating chondrocytes. The invading osteoprogenitor cells proliferate and develop into osteoblasts, which begin to deposit bone matrix over the remnants of calcified cartilage, forming cancellous bone. This region of bone deposition is called the primary ossification centre, in which ossification proceeds inward from the external surface of the model. As the ossification centre expands towards the ends of the model, osteoclasts break down the newly formed

cancellous bone. This bone-resorbing activity leaves a hollow cavity, the medullary cavity, in the core of the diaphysis along its length. The cavity then fills with red bone marrow. The longitudinal expansion of the primary ossification centre is accompanied by a widening of the periosteal bone collar in the same direction. The bone collar also thickens, providing support to the central zone of resorbing cartilage prior to its replacement by bone.

At about the time of birth, epiphyseal arteries enter the epiphyses and secondary ossification centres develop. Osteoprogenitor cells invade the area via vascular osteogenic buds originating from the diaphysis. Cartilage removal and bone matrix deposition follow. Bone formation is similar to that in the primary ossification centre. One difference, however, is that no medullary cavities are formed in the epiphyses. Secondary ossification proceeds outward in all directions from the centre of the epiphysis until there is almost complete replacement of cartilage by cancellous bone. Two regions at each epiphysis, the articular surface and the epiphyseal plate, do not undergo secondary ossification. Articular cartilage persists throughout adult life and, in the absence of a perichondrium, no equivalent of a bone collar is formed here. The epiphyseal plate is converted to cancellous bone much later in life, when growth of the long bone is complete.

3.8.6   Bone growth and remodelling

Growth

As a child grows, long bones lengthen by addition of bone material at the cartilaginous epiphyseal plate. In this process, chondrocytes are produced mitotically on the epiphyseal side of the plate. The chondrocytes then die and the cartilage is replaced by bone on the diaphyseal side. In this way, the thickness of the plate remains almost constant, but the bone on the diaphyseal side increases in length. Eventually, chondrocytes stop dividing and bone replaces the cartilage in the epiphyseal plate. The newly formed bony structure is called the epiphyseal line and, with its appearance, bone stops growing in length but continues to thicken. In the thickening of long bones, bone lining the medullary cavity is first destroyed by osteoclasts in the endosteum so that the cavity increases in diameter. At the same time, osteoblasts from the periosteum add new bone tissue to the outer surface. During the growth spurt, there is a rapid increase in bone mineral density, followed by a slower increase until peak bone mass is achieved sometime in young adulthood. Exercise and sports activity in children and young adults increases peak bone mass, particularly if the sport is weight-bearing.

Before puberty, bone growth is stimulated mainly by growth hormone. Oestrogens and testosterone, the sex hormones produced at puberty, are responsible for the acceleration in growth of the long bones during the teenage years. The sex hormones also promote morphological changes in the skeleton that are typical of males and females.

Remodelling

The mineral component of bone, although nonliving, is capable of being continuously resorbed and reformed. This turning over of bony material is called remodelling and is a natural process of renewal and repair. Remodelling occurs at discrete foci called basic multicellular units (BMUs) and involves a sequence of highly co-ordinated cellular events.

Cancellous bone remodelling starts on the bone surface, which is covered by a single layer of flat lining cells. These cells respond to stimuli such as parathyroid hormone or mechanical stress, which initiate the remodelling cycle. Firstly, the lining cells retract and the underlying layer of osteoid is digested, possibly by enzymes secreted by osteoblasts. Osteoclast progenitor cells are recruited to the site by chemotaxis and, stimulated by contact with mineralized bone matrix, are transformed to osteoclasts. The osteoclasts then begin to excavate resorption pits in the bone matrix. After removing a suitable volume of bone, osteoclasts undergo apoptosis and dissolve away. Osteoblasts then move in and begin to replace the resorbed bone with new bone. When this renewal process is finished at a particular site, osteoblasts remaining at the surface become quiescent and transform into lining cells, effectively sealing the new bone surface. Osteoblasts imprisoned within the bone become osteocytes.

The remodelling of cortical bone is triggered by signals which may originate in cells lining the Haversian canals or in osteocytes. Osteoclasts excavate a cone-shaped tunnel which is refilled by the products of activated osteoblasts.

During bone turnover in healthy young adults, the amount of bone removed by osteoclasts is quantitatively replaced by osteoblasts. This phenomenon, known as coupling, is achieved by a complex chemical communication network between osteoblasts and osteoclasts. An imbalance in bone remodelling leads to a progressive decrease in bone density (osteopenia) and a breakdown of bone architecture which, in combination, results ultimately in osteoporosis. Remodelling imbalance may be due to increased osteoclastic activity, creating resorption pits which are too deep for normal osteoblasts to fill; alternatively, or in addition, osteoclastic activity may be normal but the ability of osteoblasts to fill the resorption pits is impaired.

The sex hormones (oestrogens, androgens and progestins) are essential in maintaining proper coupling during bone remodelling. Oestradiol and oestrone are the predominant circulating sex hormones in premenopausal women, while testosterone predominates in men. However, androgens and oestrogens circulate in both men and women and there is evidence that these hormones affect bone homeostasis in both sexes. In women, when oestrogen levels fall following menopause, circulating androgens may have significant influences on bone metabolism (Oursler et al., 1996).

3.8.7   Osteoporosis

Elderly women during their lifetime lose about a third of cortical bone mass and half of cancellous bone mass from the skeleton (Riggs & Melton, 1986). Osteoporosis is a disease in which reduced bone mass and deterioration of bony microarchitecture render the bones so fragile that they fracture after only minor trauma, such as falling from a standing height. We are concerned with involutional osteoporosis, of which there are two types, I and II (Kassem et al., 1996).

Type I osteoporosis

This syndrome manifests in women typically between 50 to 75 years of age, and results from an acceleration of cancellous bone loss after the menopause. About one in five postmenopausal women will develop type I osteoporosis unless treated. Within the first 1 to 5 years after the onset of menopause, the rate of cancellous bone loss is two to six times the pre-menopausal rate of about 1% per year, but it gradually returns to the pre-menopausal rate about the 10th year after onset of menopause (Krall & Dawson-Hughes, 1999). There is only a slight corresponding increase in cortical bone loss. Fractures occur most commonly in the distal radius (forearm) and the spinal vertebrae. The vertebral fractures are of the crush or collapse type, causing a >25% reduction of vertebral height, and may be acutely painful.

Osteoporosis in post-menopausal women is due to the dramatic decrease in oestrogen production that accompanies menopause; this is evident by the well-established efficacy of hormone replacement therapy (Lindsay, 1993). The accelerated phase of bone loss is associated with increased osteoclastic resorption and oestrogen exerts its protective effect against bone loss mainly by inhibiting resorption. Inhibition is due to both decreased osteoclastogenesis and diminished resorptive activity of mature osteoclasts. Oestrogen receptors have been found in both osteoblasts and osteoclasts. Oestrogen could therefore directly modulate the secretion of local regulatory factors by these cells or modulate the cells' response to regulatory factors. Oestrogen could also act indirectly by modulating the production of factors involved in bone resorption (Pacifici, 1996). For example, the cytokines interleukin-1 (IL-1) and tumour necrosis factor (TNF), which stimulate bone resorption, activate osteoclasts indirectly via a primary effect on osteoblasts. In addition, these two cytokines stimulate osteoclast progenitor cell proliferation and fusion. Furthermore, they act synergistically to increase the secretion of other bone-resorbing cytokines such as macrophage-colony stimulating factor (M-CSF) and IL-6. The finding of increased expression of IL-1 and TNF in the bone cells of women with post-menopausal osteoporosis is consistent with the suppressive effect of oestrogen (when present) upon the production and activity of these cytokines. Oestrogen can also act positively by increasing the production of transforming growth factor β (TGFβ), a cytokine which decreases both recruitment and activity of osteoclasts.

Type II osteoporosis
Type II osteoporosis is a purely age-related syndrome, which affects men and women over 70 and is twice as common in women as in men. Bone loss increases gradually with aging, unlike the accelerated loss seen in type I osteoporosis. In both sexes, cancellous bone loss begins at about age 40 and continues into old age. Cortical bone loss commences five to ten years later but slows or ceases later in life (Riggs & Melton, 1986). In elderly women, type I and type II osteoporosis overlap and result in a disproportionate loss of cancellous bone. Type II osteoporotic fractures occur most commonly in the proximal femur (hip) and the spinal vertebrae. The vertebral fractures are of the compression type causing the normally cube-shaped vertebrae to become wedge-shaped. A severe consequence of vertebral compression fractures is kyphosis, known as 'dowager's hump'.

A number of age-related factors are implicated in the aetiology of type II osteoporosis (Kassem et al., 1996). Two important factors are (1) impaired bone formation at the cellular level, where osteoblasts fail to refill the resorption pits created by osteoclasts during bone remodelling, and (2) secondary hyperparathyroidism, which leads to increased bone turnover. Impaired bone formation may be due to a decreased production of osteoblasts or to their decreased responsiveness to regulatory factors. Secondary hyperparathyroidism could arise from an age-related impairment of 25-hydroxyvitamin D conversion to 1,25-dihydroxyvitamin D in the kidneys. This would lead to a decrease in the intestinal absorption of calcium and the lowered blood calcium level would trigger the release of parathyroid hormone. In the presence of defective osteoblastic bone formation, the parathyroid hormone-mediated increase in bone turnover will result in a net increase in bone loss. Obviously, a nutritional deficiency of vitamin D will have a similar outcome.

Impaired γ-carboxylation of osteocalcin is associated with increased risk of hip fracture, which suggests that vitamin K deficiency contributes to the development of type II osteoporosis. The role of vitamin K in bone metabolism is discussed in Section 10.5.5.

Measurement of bone mineral density and rate of bone loss
Bone mineral density is measured noninvasively by dual energy X-ray absorptiometry (DXA) performed on the forearm, lumbar spine and proximal femur. Rates of bone loss can be predicted by measuring serum or urinary biochemical markers of remodelling. Serum markers of bone formation include osteocalcin and bone specific alkaline phosphatase (BSAP). Urinary markers of bone resorption are based on the pyridinoline cross-links of collagen, specifically the amino terminal telopeptide and lysyl and hydroxylysyl pyridinoline (Kleerekoper, 1996).

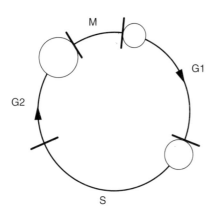

Fig. 3.36 The cell cycle. See text for explanation of phases. The enlarging circles represent an idealized proliferative cell growing to an optimum size for cell division.

3.9   Cell proliferation

3.9.1   The cell cycle

The cell cycle (Fig. 3.36) is the sequence of events whereby a proliferative cell divides into two. The newly-born cell increases its volume and mass during a post-mitotic interphase (G1 phase), doubles its complement of chromosomes during a DNA synthesis phase (S phase), increases further in volume and mass during a post-synthetic interphase (G2 phase) and then divides by mitosis and cytokinesis (M phase). During the G1 phase (and for some cell types also during the G2 phase), the cell may exit the cycle and enter a quiescent state, the G0 phase. Whether it does or not is determined by intrinsic signals or signals from neighbouring cells.

The time required to complete a eukaryotic cell cycle depends on the cell type. Embryonic cells do not need to grow between divisions and can complete a cell cycle in 8 min. The most rapidly dividing somatic cells have cycling times of 10–24 hours; liver cells divide about once a year and mature neurons never divide.

3.9.2   Control of cell proliferation

Genetic influences

Regulation of the cell cycle is a balance between gene products that promote cell replication and those that deter cell replication. Genes that can cause resting cells to divide are classified as proto-oncogenes, while genes that can prevent a cell from dividing are called tumour suppressor genes. The protein products of tumour suppressor genes serve as transducers of anti-proliferative signals.

Cell signalling

Two major cell surface receptor mechanisms mediate the effects of extracellular messengers on intracellular processes. Many hormones, including glucagon, ACTH and adrenaline, interact with plasma membrane-bound receptors to activate adenylyl cyclase to increase the production of cyclic AMP. Numerous other agents, including peptide hormones and growth factors, interact with receptors to induce a rapid turnover of phosphatidylinositol in the plasma membrane of target cells to produce diacylglycerol. Diacylglycerol can markedly stimulate calcium-dependent protein kinase C, which catalyses the phosphorylation of pre-existing proteins. Phosphorylation is an important mechanism for controlling the activities of enzymes involved in cell proliferation and many other cellular systems. Cyclic AMP inhibits receptor-mediated phosphatidylinositol turnover, thereby decreasing diacylglycerol production and preventing the activation of protein kinase C (Anderson *et al.*, 1985).

Extracellular growth factors

The mitotic proliferation of animal cells is initiated and regulated by a variety of extracellular polypeptide growth factors, which exert control over individual cells. These factors stimulate intracellular messengers, which in turn induce the expression of a set of primary response genes. Induction is both rapid and transient: protein synthesis is not required and gene expression is greatly diminished within a few hours. The levels of gene products are very low in quiescent or unstimulated cells; stimulation by various agents results in a rapid and transient increase in mRNA and protein. Primary response genes encode proteins that either activate or repress the transcription of other genes, resulting in biological responses specific to the stimulating growth factor. The encoded proteins include members of the Fos and Jun families.

Intercellular communication

Certain cells seem to produce signal molecules which regulate the growth of cell populations. These putative molecules are transmitted to neighbouring cells by diffusion through gap junction channels and never leave the intercellular space. Many studies have shown that intercellular communication is necessary for normal growth regulation and that cell proliferation occurs when intercellular communication is decreased. Inhibiting the gap-junctional flow of growth-controlling factors leads to neoplastic transformation of cells and the formation of cancerous tumours. The specific implication of intercellular communication in growth control has been demonstrated by experiments in which an exogenous gene for the gap junctional protein connexin43 was incorporated into communication-deficient cancer cells in culture. Expression of that gene led to the formation of functional gap junctions and concomitant increase in intercellular communication, and to inhibition of growth of these cancer cells (Mehta *et al.*, 1991). Furthermore, injection of exogenous connexin-expressing cells into mice suppressed tumour formation (Rose *et al.*, 1993).

Lowenstein's group (Mehta *et al.*, 1986) reported that the growth of cultured cancer cells was arrested when they were in contact with normal cells. This growth inhibition was dependent on the presence of gap junctional communication between the two types of cell. This finding supports the hypothesis that the gap junctional channels transmit growth-regulating molecules and that blocking of these channels causes deregulation. The results are compatible with such molecules being either inhibitory or stimulatory signals. The authors suggested two models to accommodate these alternatives.

In the model operating with inhibitory signals, the normal (growth-arrested) cell population is the signal source. The growth-inhibiting signals are transmitted via the gap junctions to adjacent cancer cells, and from there are disseminated by the junctional channels throughout the cancer cell population. In the model operating with stimulatory signals, the cancer cells are the signal source. Transmittance of stimulatory signal to the normal cells reduces the concentration of signal at source to below threshold level with the result that the cancerous cells are no longer stimulated to grow by an excess of their own signals. In either model the crucial link in the growth inhibition of cancer cells is the gap junctional communication between the cancer cells and normal cells.

3.9.3 Apoptosis

Apoptosis is a genetically controlled process of cell death. Regulation of cell death is essential for normal development and is an important defence against viral infection and the emergence of cancer. Excessive cell death can lead to impaired development and degenerative diseases, whereas too little cell death can lead to cancer and persistent and sustained viral infection. The process of apoptosis is controlled through the expression of specific genes. Some gene products are activators of apoptosis, whereas others are inhibitors. NGFI-B, among other primary response gene products, is an essential mediator of apoptosis (Liu *et al.*, 1994; Woronicz *et al.*, 1994).

3.9.4 Cancer

Cancer is the result of unregulated cell proliferation and manifests as malignant tumours, which are either haematological or solid. Cancer cells have the property of no longer recognizing appropriate territorial behaviour and relationships with neighbouring cells. Cancer can result from the activation of proto-oncogenes to oncogenes (cancer genes), whose altered protein products cannot be properly controlled by the cell. Activation can be induced by point mutations (altered triplet codon) and frameshift mutations (insertions or deletions of a single nucleotide or a segment of DNA); a proto-oncogene can fuse with another cellular gene; and a normal proto-oncogene product can be over-expressed. One common feature of oncogenes is their dominance: only one of the two copies needs to be altered to induce tumour formation. Furthermore, the biochemical activity of the oncoprotein is usually more active than the normal gene product. Examples of proto-oncogenes are *c-jun* and *c-fos*, whose protein products are components of the dimeric transcription factor AP-1.

Cancer can also result from inactivation of tumour suppression genes, allowing the unconstrained growth of the cancer cell. Deletions or elimination of the gene itself occur frequently among tumour suppression genes. These genes are recessive and both copies must become defective for tumour formation to occur. Tumour suppression genes are responsible for many, if not all, of the inherited cancer syndromes.

Examples of this class of genes are *p53*, which induces apoptosis, and *rb-1*, which regulates the cell cycle.

The induction of cancer by chemicals can be divided into three stages: initiation, promotion and progression. Initiation refers to the damage to DNA by a chemical or its metabolite in a linear, dose-related manner that does not possess a clearly defined threshold. Proliferation of initiated cells allows the genetic damage to be passed on to daughter cells, after which event initiation becomes irreversible. Promotion involves the induction of proliferation of initiated cells that allows for the 'locking in' of the initiation damage as well as facilitating an environment for further mutational events in the preneoplastic initiated cells. Promotion is dose-dependent, exhibits a threshold and is reversible. The third stage, progression, is the least defined and involves the irreversible transition from preneoplastic to neoplastic cells. The combined sequence of events is referred to as neoplastic transformation.

Chemical carcinogens may be either genotoxic or nongenotoxic: both stimulate DNA synthesis and cell proliferation in target tissues. Genotoxic compounds function in the initiation stage of cancer; they damage nuclear DNA through mutation and chromosome changes. The mode of action of nongenotoxic carcinogens has not been established, but they are capable of inhibiting intercellular communication. Tumour-promoting phorbol esters are nongenotoxic compounds which bind to and activate protein kinase C, apparently by substituting for diacylglycerol as an activator of this enzyme. One common cellular effect of phorbol esters and other nongenotoxic carcinogens is the inhibition of intercellular communication through gap junctions.

Further reading

Gabbay, R. A. & Flier, J. S. (1999) Transmembrane signaling: a tutorial. In: *Modern Nutrition in Health and Disease*, 9th edn. (Ed. M. E. Shils, J. A. Olson, M. Shike & A. C. Ross), pp. 585–94. Lippincott, Williams & Wilkins, Philadelphia.

Gether, U. (2000) Uncovering molecular mechanisms involved in activation of G protein-coupled receptors. *Endocrine Reviews*, **21**, 90–113.

Krupnick, J. G. & Benovic, J. L. (1998) The role of receptor kinases and arrestins in G protein-coupled receptor regulation. *Annual Review of Pharmacology and Toxicology*, **38**, 289–319.

Manolagas S. C. (2000) Birth and death of bone cells: basic regulatory mechanisms and implications for the pathogenesis and treatment of osteoporosis. *Endocrine Reviews*, **21**, 115–37.

Martin, T. J. & Ng, K. W. (1994) Mechanisms by which cells of the osteoblast lineage control osteoclast formation and activity. *Journal of Cellular Biochemistry*, **56**, 357–66.

Newton, A. C. (1995) Protein kinase C: structure, function, and regulation. *Journal of Biological Chemistry*, **270**(48), 28495–8.

Spector, R. (1986) Nucleoside and vitamin homeostasis in the mammalian central nervous system. *Annals of the New York Academy of Sciences*, **481**, 221–30.

References

Anderson, R. G. W. (1993) Potocytosis of small molecules and ions by caveolae. *Trends in Cell Biology*, **3**, 69–72.

Anderson, R. G. W. & Orci, L. (1988) A view of acidic intracellular compartments. *Journal of Cell Biology*, **106**, 539–43.

Anderson, R. G. W., Kamen, B. A., Rothberg, K. G. & Lacey, S. W. (1992) Potocytosis: sequestration and transport of small molecules by caveolae. *Science*, **255**, 410–11.

Anderson, W. B., Estival, A., Tapiovaara, H. & Gopalakrishna, R. (1985) Altered subcellular distribution of protein kinase C (a phorbol ester receptor). Possible role in tumor promotion and the regulation of cell growth: relationship to changes in adenylate cyclase activity. *Advances in Cyclic Nucleotide and Protein Phosphorylation Research*, **19**, 287–306.

Avers, C. J. (1986) Membrane structure and function. In: *Molecular Cell Biology*, pp. 141–81. Addison-Wesley Publishing Company, Reading, Massachusetts.

Ballard, S. T., Hunter, J. H. & Taylor, A. E. (1995) Regulation of tight-junction permeability during nutrient absorption across the intestinal epithelium. *Annual Review of Nutrition*, **15**, 35–55.

Bowman, E. J., Siebers, A. & Altendorf, K. (1988) Bafilomycins: a class of inhibitors of membrane ATPases from microorganisms, animal cells, and plant cells. *Proceedings of the National Academy of Sciences of the U.S.A.*, **85**, 7972–6.

Bruder, S. P., Fink, D. J. & Caplan, A. I. (1994) Mesenchymal stem cells in bone development, bone repair, and skeletal regeneration therapy. *Journal of Cellular Biochemistry*, **56**, 283–94.

Cereijido, M., Robbins, E. S., Dolan, W. J., Rotunno, C. A. & Sabatini, D. D. (1978) Polarized monolayers formed by epithelial cells on a permeable and translucent support. *Journal of Cell Biology*, **77**, 853–80.

Cohen, P. (1992) Signal integration at the level of protein kinases, protein phosphatases and their substrates. *Trends in Biochemical Sciences*, **17**, 408–13.

Cooper, A. D. (1997) Hepatic uptake of chylomicron remnants. *Journal of Lipid Research*, **38**, 2173–92.

Crane, R. K. (1962) Hypothesis for mechanism of intestinal transport of sugars. *Federation Proceedings*, **21**, 891–5.

Diamond, J. M. & Karasov, W. H. (1984) Effect of dietary carbohydrate on monosaccharide uptake by mouse small intestine *in vitro*. *Journal of Physiology*, **349**, 419–40.

Duffey, M. E., Hainau, B., Ho, S. & Bentzel, C. J. (1981) Regulation of epithelial tight junction permeability by cyclic AMP. *Nature*, **294**, 451–3.

Dutil, E. M., Keranen, L. M., DePaoli-Roach, A. A. & Newton, A. C. (1994) *In vivo* regulation of protein kinase C by trans-phosphorylation followed by autophosphorylation. *Journal of Biological Chemistry*, **269**(47), 29359–62.

Ferraris, R. P. & Diamond, J. M. (1989) Specific regulation of intestinal nutrient transporters by their dietary substrates. *Annual Review of Physiology*, **51**, 125–41.

Ferraris, R. P., Yasharpour, S., Lloyd, K. C. K., Mirzayan, R. & Diamond, J. M. (1990) Luminal glucose concentrations in the gut under normal conditions. *American Journal of Physiology*, **259**, G822–37.

Fine, K. D., Santa Ana, C. A., Porter, J. L. & Fordtran, J. S. (1993) Effect of D-glucose on intestinal permeability and its passive absorption in human small intestine in vivo. *Gastroenterology*, **105**, 1117–25.

Frizzell, R. A. & Schultz, S. G. (1972) Ionic conductances of extracellular shunt pathway in rabbit ileum. Influence of shunt on transmural sodium transport and electrical potential differences. *Journal of General Physiology*, **59**, 318–46.

Goldstein, J. L. & Brown, M. S. (1977) The low-density lipoprotein pathway and its relation to atherosclerosis. *Annual Review of Biochemistry*, **46**, 897–930.

Granger, D. N., Kvietys, P. R., Perry, M. A. & Barrowman, J. A. (1987) The microcirculation and intestinal transport. In: *Physiology of the Gastrointestinal Tract*, 2nd edn. (Ed. by L. R. Johnson), pp. 1671–97. Raven Press, New York.

Hansra, G., Bornancin, F., Whelan, R., Hemmings, B. A. & Parker, P. J. (1996) 12-*O*-Tetradecanoylphorbol-13-acetate-induced dephosphorylation of protein kinase Cα correlates with the presence of a membrane-associated protein phosphatase 2A heterotrimer. *Journal of Biological Chemistry*, **271**(51), 32785–8.

Hille, B. (1970) Ionic channels in nerve membranes. *Progress in Biophysics and Molecular Biology*, **21**, 1–32.

Ji, Z.-S., Fazio, S., Lee, Y.-L. & Mahley, R. W. (1994) Secretion-capture role for apolipoprotein E in remnant lipoprotein metabolism involving cell surface heparan sulfate proteoglycans. *Journal of Biological Chemistry*, **269**(4), 2764–72.

Karasov, W. H. (1992) Tests of the adaptive modulation hypothesis for dietary control of intestinal nutrient transport. *American Journal of Physiology*, **263**, R496–R502.

Kassem, M., Melton, L. J. III & Riggs, B. L. (1996) The type I/type II model for involutional osteoporosis. In: *Osteoporosis*. (Ed. R. Marcus, D. Feldman & J. Kelsey), pp. 691–702. Academic Press, San Diego.

Kimmich, G. A. (1981) Intestinal absorption of sugar. In: *Physiology of the Gastrointestinal Tract*, Vol. 2. (Ed. L. R. Johnson), pp. 1035–61. Raven Press, New York.

Kimmich, G. A. & Randles, J. (1980) Evidence for an intestinal Na$^+$: sugar transport coupling stoichiometry of 2:0. *Biochimica et Biophysica Acta*, **596**, 439–44.

Kimmich, G. A. & Randles, J. (1988) Na$^+$-coupled sugar transport: membrane potential-dependent K_m and K_i for Na$^+$. *American Journal of Physiology*, **255**, C486–94.

Klaunig, J. E. & Ruch, R. J. (1990) Role of inhibition of intercellular communication in carcinogenesis. *Laboratory Investigation*, **62**, 135–46.

Kleerekoper, M. (1996) The evaluation of patients with osteoporosis. In: *Osteoporosis*. (Ed. R. Marcus, D. Feldman & J. Kelsey), pp. 1011–18. Academic Press, San Diego.

Kobayashi, E., Nakano, H., Morimoto, M. & Tamaoki, T. (1989) Calphostin C (UCN-1028C), a novel microbial compound, is a highly potent and specific inhibitor of protein kinase C. *Biochemical and Biophysical Research Communications*, **159**, 548–53.

Krall, E. A. & Dawson-Hughes, B. (1999) Osteoporosis. In: *Modern Nutrition in Health and Disease*, 9th edn. (Ed. M. E. Shils, J. A. Olson, M. Shike & A. C. Ross), pp. 1353–64. Lippincott, Williams & Wilkins, Philadelphia.

Lefkowitz, R. J. (1998) G protein-coupled receptors. III. New roles for receptor kinases and β-arrestins in receptor signaling and desensitization. *Journal of Biological Chemistry*, **273**(30), 18677–80.

Levin, R. J. (1999) Carbohydrates. In: *Modern Nutrition in Health and Disease*, 9th edn. (Ed. M. E. Shils, J. A. Olson, M. Shike & A. C.

Ross), pp. 49–65. Lippincott, Williams & Wilkins, Philadelphia.

Levitt, M. D., Strocchi, A. & Levitt, D. G. (1992) Human jejunal unstirred layer: evidence for extremely efficient luminal stirring. *American Journal of Physiology*, **262**, G593–6.

Lindsay, R. (1993) Hormone replacement therapy for prevention and treatment of osteoporosis. *American Journal of Medicine*, **95**, 37S–9S.

Liu, Z.-G., Smith, S. W., McLaughlin, K. A., Schwartz, L. M. & Osborne, B. A. (1994) Apoptotic signals delivered through the T-cell receptor of a T-cell hybrid require the immediate-early gene *nur77*. *Nature*, **367**, 281–4.

Lorenz, W., Inglese, J., Palczewski, K., Onorato, J. J., Caron, M. G. & Lefkowitz, R. J. (1991) The receptor kinase family: primary structure of rhodopsin kinase reveals similarities to the β-adrenergic receptor kinase. *Proceedings of the National Academy of Sciences of the U.S.A.*, **88**, 8715–9.

Madara, J. L. & Pappenheimer, J. R. (1987) Structural basis for physiological regulation of paracellular pathways in intestinal epithelia. *Journal of Membrane Biology*, **100**, 149–64.

Mahley, R. W. & Hussain, M. M. (1991) Chylomicron and chylomicron remnant catabolism. *Current Opinion in Lipidology*, **2**, 170–6.

Mehta, P. P., Bertram, J. S. & Loewenstein, W. R. (1986) Growth inhibition of transformed cells correlates with their junctional communication with normal cells. *Cell*, **44**, 187–96.

Mehta, P. P., Hotz-Wagenblatt, A., Rose, B., Shalloway, D. & Loewenstein, W. R. (1991) Incorporation of the gene for a cell-to-cell channel protein into transformed cells leads to normalization of growth. *Journal of Membrane Biology*, **124**, 207–25.

Mellman, I., Fuchs, R. & Helenius, A. (1986) Acidification of the endocytic and exocytic pathways. *Annual Review of Biochemistry*, **55**, 663–700.

Murur, H. & Kinne, R. (1980) The use of isolated membrane vesicles to study epithelial transport processes. *Journal of Membrane Biology*, **55**, 81–95.

Musil, L. S. & Goodenough, D. A. (1991) Biochemical analysis of connexin43 intracellular transport, phosphorylation, and assembly into gap junctional plaques. *Journal of Cell Biology*, **115**, 1357–74.

Nimmerfall, F. & Rosenthaler, J. (1980) Significance of the goblet-cell mucin layer, the outermost luminal barrier to passage through the gut wall. *Biochemical and Biophysical Research Communications*, **94**, 960–6.

Nishizuka, Y. (1986) Studies and perspectives of protein kinase C. *Science*, **233**, 305–12.

Nishizuka, Y. (1988) The molecular heterogeneity of protein kinase C and its implications for cellular regulation. *Nature*, **334**, 661–5.

Nishizuka, Y. (1995) Protein kinase C and lipid signaling for sustained cellular responses. *FASEB Journal*, **9**, 484–96.

Olson, E. N., Burgess, R. & Staudinger, J. (1993) Protein kinase C as a transducer of nuclear signals. *Cell Growth & Differentiation*, **4**, 699–705.

Oursler, M. J., Kassem, M., Turner, R., Riggs, B. L. & Spelsberg, T. C. (1996) Regulation of bone cell function by gonadal steroids. In: *Osteoporosis*. (Ed. R. Marcus, D. Feldman & J. Kelsey), pp. 237–60. Academic Press, San Diego.

Pacifici, R. (1996) Postmenopausal osteoporosis. How the hormonal changes of menopause cause bone loss. In: *Osteoporosis*. (Ed. R. Marcus, D. Feldman & J. Kelsey), pp. 727–43. Academic Press, San Diego.

Pappenheimer, J. R. & Reiss, K. Z. (1987) Contribution of solvent drag through intercellular junctions to absorption of nutrients by the small intestine of the rat. *Journal of Membrane Biology*, **100**, 123–36.

Peracchia, C. & Bernardini, G. (1984) Gap junction structure and cell-to-cell coupling regulation: is there a calmodulin involvement? *Federation Proceedings*, **43**, 2681–91.

Reuss, L. (1997) Epithelial transport. In: *Handbook of Physiology. Section 14: Cell Physiology*. (Ed. J. F. Hoffman & J. D. Jamieson), pp. 309–88. Oxford University Press, New York.

Riggs, L. & Melton, L. J. III (1986) Involutional osteoporosis. *New England Journal of Medicine*, **314**, 1676–86.

Rodman, J. S., Mercer, R. W., & Stahl, P. D. (1990) Endocytosis and transcytosis. *Current Opinion in Cell Biology*, **2**, 664–72.

Rose, B., Mehta, P. P. & Loewenstein, W. R. (1993) Gap-junction protein gene suppresses tumorigenicity. *Carcinogenesis*, **14**, 1073–5.

Rose, R. C. & Schultz, S. G. (1971) Studies on the electrical potential profile across rabbit ileum. Effects of sugars and amino acids on transmural and transmucosal electrical potential differences. *Journal of General Physiology*, **57**, 639–63.

Rowland, L. P., Fink, M. E. & Rubin, L. (1991) Cerebrospinal fluid: blood–brain barrier, brain edema, and hydrocephalus. In: *Principles of Neural Science*, 3rd edn. (Ed. E. R. Kandel, J. H. Schwartz & T. M. Jessell), pp. 1050–60. Prentice-Hall International, Englewood Cliffs, New Jersey.

Schultz, S. G. (1977) Sodium-coupled solute transport by small intestine: a status report. *American Journal of Physiology*, **233**, E249–54.

Schultz, S. G. & Zalusky, R. (1964a) Ion transport in isolated rabbit ileum. I. Short-circuit current and Na fluxes. *Journal of General Physiology*, **47**, 567–84.

Schultz, S. G. & Zalusky, R. (1964b) Ion transport in isolated rabbit ileum. II. The interaction between active sodium and active sugar transport. *Journal of General Physiology*, **47**, 1043–59.

Shiau, Y.-F. & Levine, G. M. (1980) pH dependence of micellar diffusion and dissociation. *American Journal of Physiology*, **239**, G177–82.

Shiau, Y.-F., Fernandez, P., Jackson, M. J. & McMonagle, S. (1985) Mechanisms maintaining a low-pH microclimate in the intestine. *American Journal of Physiology*, **248**, G608–17.

Smart, E. J., Ying, Y.-S. & Anderson, R. G. W. (1995) Hormonal regulation of caveolae internalization. *Journal of Cell Biology*, **131**, 929–38.

Spector, R. (1989) Micronutrient homeostasis in mammalian brain and cerebrospinal fluid. *Journal of Neurochemistry*, **53**, 1667–74.

Spector, R. & Johanson, C. E. (1989) The mammalian choroid plexus. *Scientific American*, **261**(5), 48–53.

Stevens, B. R., Fernandez, A., Hirayama, B., Wright, E. M. & Kempner, E. S. (1990) Intestinal brush border membrane Na$^+$/glucose cotransporter functions *in situ* as a homotetramer. *Proceedings of the National Academy of Sciences of the U.S.A.*, **87**, 1456–60.

Ugolev, A. M. & Metel'skii, S. T. (1990) Two-channel transporter versus a single-channel Na$^+$-dependent transporter for glucose and amino acids in rat and turtle. *Biomedical Science*, **1**, 578–84.

Wedegaertner, P. B. & Bourne, H. R. (1994) Activation and depalmitoylation of G$_s\alpha$. *Cell*, **77**, 1063–70.

Wilson, F. A. & Hoyumpa, A. M. Jr. (1979) Ethanol and small intestinal transport. *Gastroenterology*, **76**, 388–403.

Woronicz, J. D., Calnan, B., Ngo, V. & Winoto, A. (1994) Requirement for the orphan steroid receptor Nurr77 in apoptosis of T-cell hybridomas. *Nature*, **367**, 277–81.

Xie, X.-S., Crider, B. P. & Stone, D. K. (1989) Isolation and reconstitution of the chloride transporter of clathrin-coated vesicles. *Journal of Biological Chemistry*, **264**(32), 18870–3.

Young, S., Parker, P. J., Ullrich, A. & Stabel, S. (1987) Down-regulation of protein kinase C is due to an increased rate of degradation. *Biochemical Journal*, **244**, 775–9.

4
Background Biochemistry

Key discussion topics

- Cellular biochemical processes convert the chemical energy locked within ingested foodstuffs to useful metabolic energy.
- Amino acids can be used to build proteins or they can be metabolized to carbohydrate intermediates of the tricarboxylic acid cycle.

- Free radicals and other harmful reactive species are kept at bay by the provision of metal-binding proteins, enzymes and antioxidants.
- Atherosclerosis is initiated by the oxidative modification of low-density lipoprotein.

4.1   Major degradation pathways in which B-group vitamins are involved as coenzymes

Many of the enzymes involved in cellular metabolism consist of a protein (apoenzyme) and an organic coenzyme, which is either a derivative of a B-group vitamin or the vitamin itself. The entire enzyme (apoenzyme plus coenzyme) is referred to as the holoenzyme. Coenzymes of these metabolic enzymes and their parent vitamins are listed in Table 4.1. The coenzymes participate in the overall reaction by acting as a donor of a particular chemical group (e.g. acyl, amino, one-carbon fragments) or electrons.

4.1.1   The role of ATP in energy storage

The cell derives its energy from chemical reactions arising from the catabolism of dietary carbohydrates, fats and proteins. The reactions occur sequentially as the nutrients are systematically oxidized through a pathway of intermediates, ultimately to carbon dioxide and water. All the reactions are enzyme catalysed and each exhibits a free energy change. Within a given catalytic pathway, some reactions may be energy-consuming. However, energy-producing reactions will prevail so there is a net gain in energy.

The energy produced through the catabolism of nutrient molecules is used to form the high-energy anhydride bonds connecting the β- and γ-phosphates (terminal phosphates) of adenosine triphosphate (ATP) and these bonds can in turn be hydrolysed to release the energy when needed. The released energy is free energy (G) which can be used to drive the various energy-requiring processes and anabolic reactions. ATP, as the reservoir of cellular energy, is the major link between energy-releasing and energy-demanding reactions. In nearly all cases, the energy is released by enzymatic hydrolysis of the terminal anhydride bond. The products of this hydrolysis are adenosine diphosphate (ADP) and a free phosphate group. The latter can be transferred to various phosphate acceptors, thereby activating the acceptors to a higher energy level.

4.1.2   Catabolism of polysaccharides, lipids and proteins

The dietary macronutrients – polysaccharides, lipids and proteins – are degraded in a three-stage process to produce cellular energy (Fig. 4.1).

Stage 1 is digestion, during which the macronutrients are hydrolysed into their component substituents: polysaccharides to glucose and other monosaccharides, lipids to glycerol and fatty acids, and proteins to amino acids. The energy released from these hydrolytic processes is made available to the body as heat.

In Stage 2, glucose is oxidized anaerobically to pyruvate in the cell cytoplasm by the process of glycolysis. Glycolysis produces a net gain of two molecules of ATP for each molecule of glucose degraded. This ATP is used for energy-consuming processes by the cells carrying out the anaerobic degradation of glucose. Skeletal muscle, with its poor oxygen supply, is ideally designed for carrying out glycolysis. If the oxygen supply to the tissue is adequate, pyruvate is oxidized to acetyl coenzyme A (acetyl-CoA) after entering the mitochondria. Long-chain fatty acids are broken down to acetyl-CoA by mitochondrial enzymes of the β-oxidation system, while the glycerol takes part in the glycolytic pathway. The carbon skeletons of the amino acids yield either an intermediate of the tricarboxylic acid (TCA) cycle or acetyl-CoA.

Acetyl-CoA is oxidized in Stage 3 by means of the TCA cycle. The enzymes catalysing the TCA cycle, in contrast to those of glycolysis, are located in the mitochondria. Three steps in the TCA cycle produce reduced nicotinamide adenine dinucleotide (NADH), while one step produces reduced flavin adenine dinucleotide ($FADH_2$).

Table 4.1   Coenzymes derived from B-group vitamins.

Coenzyme	Parent vitamin
Thiamin pyrophosphate (TPP)	Thiamin
Flavin adenine dinucleotide (FAD) and flavin mononucleotide (FMN)	Riboflavin
Nicotinamide adenine dinucleotide (NAD^+) and nicotinamide adenine dinucleotide phosphate ($NADP^+$)	Niacin
Pyridoxal phosphate (PLP)	Vitamin B_6
Coenzyme A (CoA)	Pantothenic acid
Biotin	Biotin
Tetrahydrofolate (THF)	Folate
Methylcobalamin and adenosylcobalamin	Vitamin B_{12}

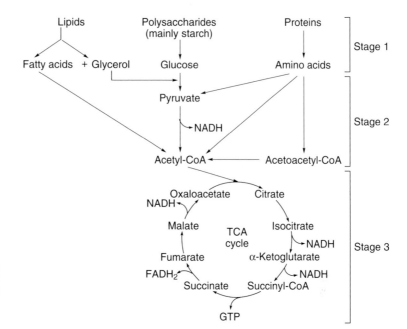

Fig. 4.1 Main stages in the catabolism of lipids, polysaccharides and proteins. Amino acids can also be converted to certain intermediates of the tricarboxylic acid (TCA) cycle (not shown). GTP, guanosine triphosphate.

4.1.3 Electron transport and oxidative phosphorylation

NADH and FADH$_2$ are reoxidized in the mitochondria by the electron transport chain, in which a series of electron acceptors are alternately reduced and oxidized. The electron acceptors are an integral part of the inner membrane of the mitochondrion. The electron transport chain has been divided into four complexes (I, II, III and IV), each of which represents a portion of the chain. Fig. 4.2 is a simplified scheme in which intermediate iron sulphide proteins are omitted and the complexes are not shown.

It is fundamental in biochemistry that (1) the hydrogen atom is composed of a proton (H$^+$) and an electron, and (2) all oxidation-reduction reactions involve the reversible transfer of electrons, with electrons being lost from a compound undergoing oxidation and gained by a compound undergoing reduction. The electron carriers are arranged in order of increasing tendency to undergo oxidation so that each electron transfer can proceed spontaneously. The process begins

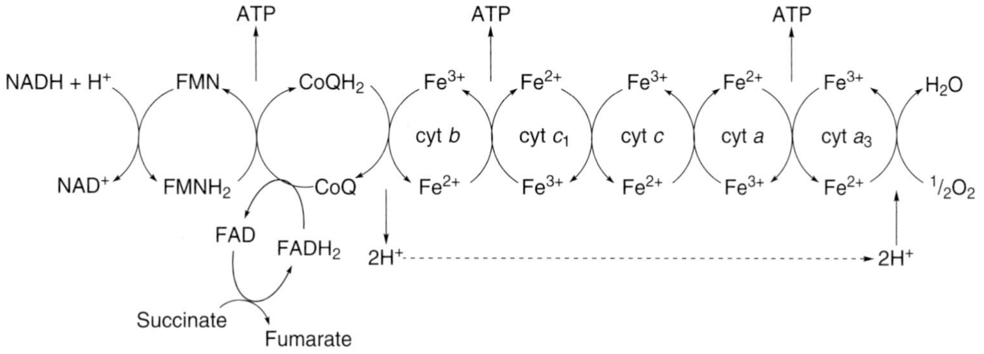

Fig. 4.2 Electron transport chain (simplified) showing the coupled formation of ATP. NADH enters the chain at FMN and FADH$_2$ enters at CoQ. The cytochromes b, c_1, c, a and a_3 transfer electrons through a valency change of the iron (Fe) cofactor.

with a transfer of electrons from NADH to FMN to yield NAD$^+$ and FMNH$_2$. The electrons are then passed on to coenzyme Q (CoQ, also known as ubiquinone), and from there they go through a specific sequence of cytochromes. The hydrogens of reduced CoQ are released as protons, and thereafter no hydrogen transfer takes place within the cytochrome sequence. The final carrier, cytochrome a_3, transfers electrons to elemental oxygen to form ionic oxygen, which then combines with the protons liberated at the interaction between CoQ and cytochrome b to form water.

The downhill flow of electrons generates sufficient energy to effect the phosphorylation of ADP to ATP (oxidative phosphorylation) at specific sites along the chain. There are three phosphorylation sites if NADH is being reoxidized (Fig. 4.2) and two if FADH$_2$ is being reoxidized. The energy yield is three molecules of ATP for each of the three molecules of NADH produced by the TCA cycle and two ATP for the FADH$_2$, giving a total of eleven molecules of ATP. The guanosine triphosphate (GTP) produced in the TCA cycle makes a total of twelve energy-rich phosphate bonds for each molecule of acetyl-CoA oxidized. The oxidation of pyruvate to acetyl-CoA in the mitochondria generates an additional NADH which, when reoxidized in the electron transport chain, will produce an additional three molecules of ATP; this gives a total of fifteen energy-rich bonds per molecule of pyruvate.

4.1.4   The hexose monophosphate shunt

The hexose monophosphate shunt (also known as the pentose phosphate pathway) has two main purposes:

(1) to generate pentose phosphates, necessary for the synthesis of nucleotides and nucleic acids (RNA and DNA), and (2) to produce NADPH, used for important metabolic functions, such as the synthesis of fatty acids. NADPH is a reduction product of the two dehydrogenase reactions involved in the conversion of glucose-6-phosphate to ribulose-5-phosphate (Fig. 4.3). Tissues that are active in the synthesis of fatty acids, such as the mammary gland, adipose tissue, the adrenal cortex and the liver, have a particularly high demand for NADPH. These tissues predictably engage the entire pathway, recycling pentose phosphates back to glucose-6-phosphate to perpetuate the cycle and to assure an ample supply of NADPH. The reversibility of the transketolase and transaldolase reactions allows the direct conversion of hexose phosphates into pentose phosphates, bypassing the oxidative (dehydrogenase) reactions. Cells with a high proliferation rate have a corresponding demand for nucleic acid synthesis and can produce pentose phosphates in this manner.

4.1.5   Gluconeogenesis

Although most tissues can utilize energy sources other than glucose, the brain and red blood cells are wholly reliant on glucose as their metabolic fuel. When the demand for glucose is high, as in diabetes, starvation or lactation, the liver can produce glucose by the separate processes of glycogenolysis and gluconeogenesis.

Gluconeogenesis is essentially a reversal of glycolysis. Most of the cytoplasmic enzymes involved in the conversion of glucose to pyruvate catalyse their reac-

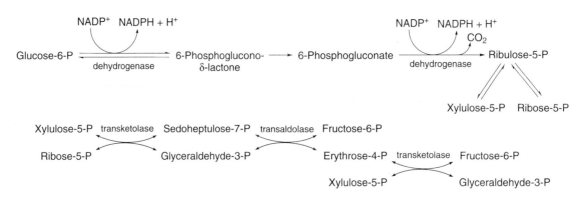

Fig. 4.3 The hexose monophosphate shunt. The cycle can be completed by reversible isomerization of fructose-6-phosphate to glucose-6-phosphate. P, phosphate.

tions reversibly and therefore provide the means for also converting pyruvate to glucose. There are, however, three reactions in glycolysis that are not reversible: (1) hexokinase, catalysing the conversion of glucose to glucose-6-phosphate; (2) phosphofructokinase, catalysing the conversion of fructose-6-phosphate to fructose-1,6-biphosphate; and (3) pyruvate kinase, catalysing the conversion of phosphoenolpyruvate (PEP) to pyruvate. The irreversibility of the first two reactions is overcome by the alternative use of specific phosphatases that remove phosphate groups by hydrolysis.

Bypassing the pyruvate kinase system is a greater problem because there is no alternative enzyme for converting pyruvate directly to PEP. Thus the pyruvate kinase system must be circumvented. The cell achieves this by involving oxaloacetate as an intermediate (Fig. 4.4). The enzyme that converts pyruvate to oxaloacetate, pyruvate carboxylase, is located solely in the mitochondrion. Thus it is mitochondrial pyruvate that is converted to oxaloacetate. The enzyme that converts oxaloacetate to PEP, PEP carboxykinase, is solely cytoplasmic, and so oxaloacetate needs to pass back to the cytoplasm. However, the mitochondrial membrane is impermeable to oxaloacetate, necessitating its conversion to malate, which can freely pass out of the mitochondrion. In the cytoplasm, the malate is converted back to oxaloacetate, which in turn is converted to PEP. Two of the enzymes involved in the bypass, pyruvate carboxylase and PEP carboxykinase, are unique to gluconeogenesis. The reactions of the bypass also allow the carbon skeletons of certain amino acids to enter the gluconeogenic pathway and lead to a net synthesis of glucose. Such amino acids are accordingly described as glucogenic (Section 4.2.4).

4.2 Amino acid utilization

4.2.1 The amino acid pool

Dietary protein of plant or animal origin is hydrolysed to constituent amino acids by enzymes in the gastrointestinal tract. A portion of the absorbed amino acids is retained by the intestinal cells for synthesizing digestive enzymes and other compounds. The remaining amino acids enter the bloodstream and are transported to the liver. Here, a portion of them is used to synthesize several plasma proteins and another portion is conveyed to extrahepatic tissues for the purpose of protein synthesis. The liver also metabolizes amino acids, converting the nitrogen atoms into urea and the carbon skeleton into intermediates utilized in the metabolism of carbohydrates and fats. In addition to the hydrolysis of dietary protein, most of the tissue

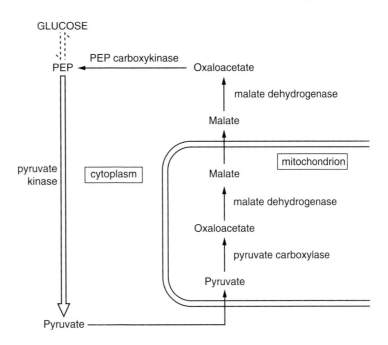

Fig. 4.4 The bypass of the unidirectional pyruvate kinase reaction in gluconeogenesis.

proteins, both structural and functional, are continually undergoing hydrolysis. The amino acids released likewise enter the circulation and become part of the general amino acid pool. This pool has no anatomical reality, but represents an availability of amino acids for utilization by the body. The pool is constantly undergoing depletion and repletion. This amino acid turnover is greatest in intestinal mucosa, followed by kidney, liver, brain and muscle, in that order.

Depletion of the amino acid pool is largely due to removal of the amino groups from the amino acids. The ammonia (NH_3) split off is (1) converted into and excreted as urea, or (2) used to aminate various keto acids to form other amino acids, or (3) indirectly excreted as ammonium ions (NH_4^+) in the urine.

4.2.2   The essentiality of amino acids

The protein content of the body is made up of 20 amino acids (Table 4.2), which are selected for protein

Table 4.2 The 20 amino acids incorporated into mammalian protein.

Amino acid	Standard abbreviation
Essential	
Isoleucine	Ile
Leucine	Leu
Lysine	Lys
Methionine	Met
Phenylalanine	Phe
Threonine	Thr
Tryptophan	Trp
Valine	Val
Histidine[a]	His
Nonessential	
Alanine	Ala
Arginine	Arg
Aspartic acid	Asp
Asparagine	Asn
Glutamic acid	Glu
Glutamine	Gln
Glycine	Gly
Proline	Pro
Serine	Ser
Conditionally essential	
Cysteine	Cys
Tyrosine	Tyr

[a] The essentiality for histidine has only been shown for infants, but probably small amounts are needed for adults as well (Laidlaw & Kopple, 1987).

synthesis by binding with transfer RNA. Some of these amino acids are synthesized *de novo* in the body from other amino acids or simple precursors; they are referred to as nonessential and are dispensable from the diet. However, several amino acids have no synthetic pathways in humans and are therefore essential or indispensable to the diet. Some nonessential amino acids may become conditionally essential under conditions when the supply of precursors becomes inadequate.

The terms 'essential' and 'nonessential' apply only to the diet. Within the body, the so-called nonessential amino acids are just as important metabolically as the essential ones. If they are not present in the diet they must be synthesized from other nitrogenous compounds.

Besides the 20 amino acids that are incorporated into protein, other metabolically important amino acids are present in the body. For example, ornithine and citrulline are linked to arginine through the urea cycle.

Most mammalian enzymes recognize only the L form of amino acids, although some reactions will operate with lower efficiency when presented with the D form.

4.2.3   Amino acid metabolism

The first step in the metabolism of most amino acids, once they have reached the liver, is removal of the α-amino group by transamination or deamination.

Transamination

Transamination reactions involve the transfer of an amino group from an amino acid to an α-keto acid. The keto acid that gains the amino group becomes an amino acid and the amino acid that loses its amino group becomes an α-keto acid. Transamination reactions are reversible and catalysed by aminotransferases, which all have a coenzyme form of vitamin B_6 as the prosthetic group. In many transamination reactions, α-ketoglutarate is the amino group acceptor, forming glutamic acid and another keto acid (Fig. 4.5). The effect of transamination reactions is to collect the amino groups from many different amino acids in the form of glutamate. The glutamate then functions as an amino group donor, the amino group being used for biosynthetic pathways or excretion pathways that lead to the elimination of nitrogenous waste products.

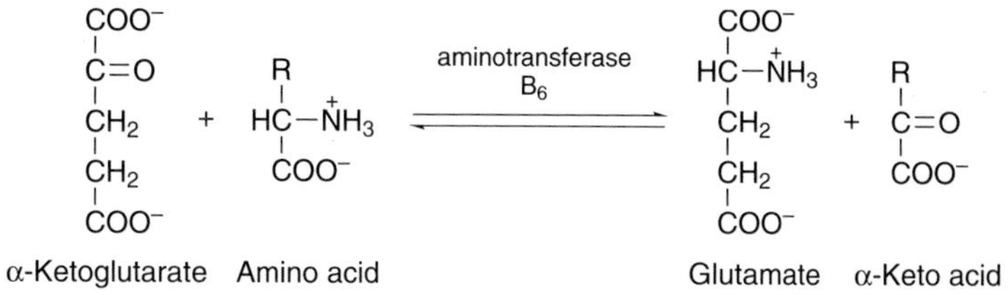

Fig. 4.5 A transamination reaction.

α-Ketoglutarate   Amino acid   Glutamate α-Keto acid

Deamination

Deamination reactions involve the removal of an amino group with no direct transfer to another compound. Figure 4.6 shows the oxidative deamination of glutamate catalysed by glutamate dehydrogenase, which takes place in the liver. The α-ketoglutarate formed from glutamate deamination can be used in the TCA cycle for the production of energy. The coupled action of an aminotransferase and glutamate dehydrogenase (Fig. 4.7) is referred to as transdeamination. Glutamic acid formed by the reaction between an amino acid and α-ketoglutarate is transported to liver mitochondria where glutamate dehydrogenase liberates the amino group as the ammonium ion. The toxic ammonium ion enters the ornithine cycle to be converted into urea. The urea passes into the bloodstream and thence to the kidneys where it is excreted into the urine.

4.2.4 Fate of amino acid carbon skeletons (α-keto acids)

Once an amino group has been removed from an amino acid, the remaining molecule, the α-keto acid, is referred to as a carbon skeleton. The amino acids from which the carbon skeletons are derived are described as either glucogenic or ketogenic, according to the metabolic fate of the skeletons. Those amino acids whose skeletons give rise to pyruvate or TCA cycle intermediates (α-ketoglutarate, succinyl-CoA, fumarate and oxaloacetate) are glucogenic, while those whose skeletons give rise to acetyl-CoA or acetoacetyl-CoA are ketogenic. As shown in Table 4.3, some amino acids are both glucogenic and ketogenic.

The points of entry of amino acid carbon skeletons into central metabolic pathways are shown in Fig. 4.8.

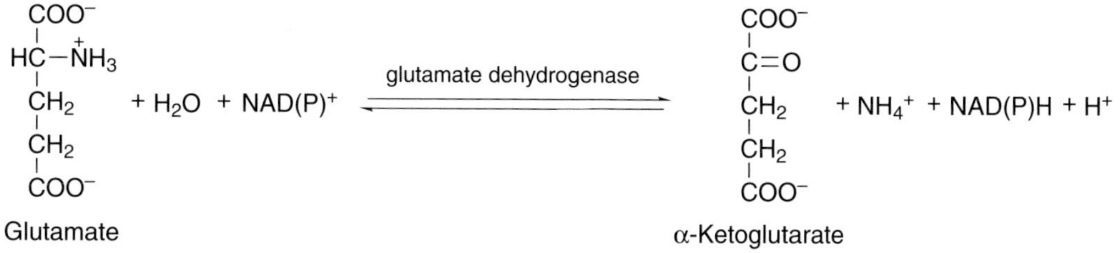

Fig. 4.6 A deamination reaction.

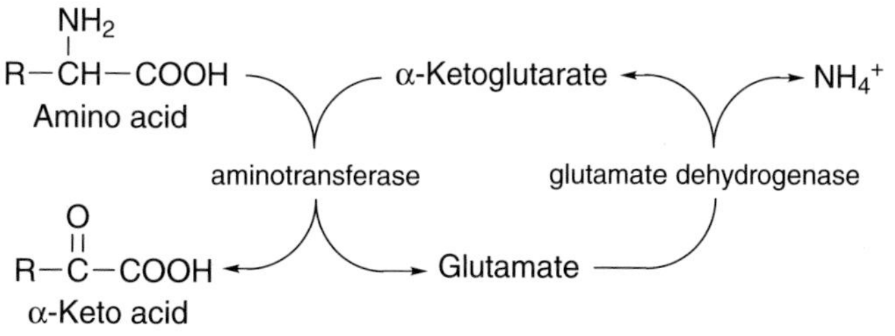

Fig. 4.7 The coupled action of an aminotransferase and glutamate dehydrogenase.

Table 4.3 End products of amino acid degradation. According to Nelson & Cox (2000).

Amino acid[a]	End product
Glucogenic	
Alanine, glycine, serine, cysteine	Pyruvate
Arginine, histidine, proline, glutamic acid, glutamine	α-Ketoglutarate
Valine, methionine, threonine	Succinyl-CoA
Aspartic acid, asparagine	Oxaloacetate
Ketogenic	
Leucine	Acetyl-CoA, acetoacetyl-CoA
Lysine	Acetoacetyl-CoA
Both glucogenic and ketogenic	
Phenylalanine, tyrosine	Fumarate, acetoacetyl-CoA
Isoleucine	Succinyl-CoA, acetyl-CoA
Tryptophan	Pyruvate, acetyl-CoA, acetoacetyl-CoA

[a]For an amino acid to be considered glucogenic, its catabolism must yield pyruvate or selected intermediates of the TCA cycle. Catabolism of a ketogenic amino acid must generate acetyl-CoA or acetoacetyl-CoA. Also see Fig. 4.8.

The glucogenic amino acids, by increasing the supply of TCA cycle intermediates, permit the utilization of oxaloacetate for gluconeogenesis without the danger of impairing TCA cycle activity. Those amino acids that give rise to pyruvate also increase the mitochondrial pool of oxaloacetate through the reaction catalysed by pyruvate carboxylase. The acetyl-CoA produced by ketogenic amino acids can enter the TCA cycle directly or be used for fatty acid synthesis. It can also be converted, as can acetoacetyl-CoA, to ketone bodies (acetoacetate and β-hydroxybutyrate) which are exported to extrahepatic tissues for use as an energy source (especially in muscle, but not in brain) if glucose supply is deficient. Since acetoacetyl-CoA can be cleaved to acetyl-CoA, the carbon skeletons of all 20 amino acids can ultimately be oxidized via the TCA cycle. The purely ketogenic amino acids (leucine and lysine) cannot be used for the synthesis of glucose. However, these amino acids are important under conditions of starvation because they allow sparing of whatever glucose is available for use by the brain. Thus the manner in which all of the amino acids are utilized depends on the nutritional state of the body.

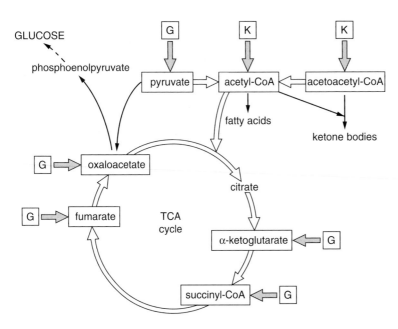

Fig. 4.8 The fate of amino acid carbon skeletons derived from glucogenic (G) and ketogenic (K) amino acids. See Table 4.3 for details.

4.3 Defences against free radicals and other reactive species

4.3.1 Reactive oxygen/nitrogen species

Reactive oxygen species (ROS) and reactive nitrogen species (RNS) of biological importance are listed in Table 4.4. ROS comprise oxygen-centred free radicals and non-radical derivatives of oxygen. These species can be generated within the body by a variety of processes and, if not adequately removed, can subject the body to oxidative stress. Severe oxidative stress produces harmful effects such as (1) physical damage to biological membranes and lipoproteins through lipid peroxidation; (2) modification of proteins, manifested by an inactivation of certain enzymes; and (3) damage to DNA with the potential for causing mutations. The accumulated damage may form the basis of age-dependent diseases such as atherosclerosis, arthritis, neurodegenerative disorders and cancer.

Animals have evolved mechanisms to deplete ROS, to limit their formation or to repair the damage caused by them. Many of these mechanisms arise through the direct activation of oxidative stress-inducible genes and the resultant synthesis of antioxidant enzymes, DNA repair enzymes and a host of other beneficial proteins (Storz *et al.*, 1990).

Free radicals

The electrons in an atom revolve in orbitals around the nucleus. Each orbital can hold a maximum of two electrons paired with antiparallel spin, resulting in no net spin. A free radical can be defined as an atom or molecule capable of independent existence that contains one or more unpaired electron(s). The unpaired electron is found alone in the outer orbital and is denoted by a superscript dot next to the element. The simplest free radical is an atom of hydrogen ($H^{\bullet}$), with one proton and a single electron. Reduction of oxygen by the transfer to it of a single electron will produce the superoxide anion radical ('superoxide'), usually represented by $O_2^{\bullet-}$. The oxygen molecule itself is a free radical because it has two unpaired electrons in different orbitals. Owing to their unstable electronic configuration, free radicals are much more reactive than non-radicals. They readily extract electrons from other molecules with which they collide, and these molecules in turn become free radicals. Thus a chain reaction is propagated.

Free radicals are generally produced by electron transfer reactions catalysed either enzymatically or non-enzymatically through the redox chemistry of transition metal ions. There are many ways of generating free radicals. Examples include phagocytosis during infection; metabolic processing of foreign compounds (e.g. constituents of tobacco smoke, drugs, pesticides, solvents and pollutants); ultraviolet irradiation of the skin; and ionizing radiation. A major source of superoxide is electron 'leakage' from the mitochondrial electron transport chain to molecular oxygen. Another source of superoxide is the metal-catalysed autoxidation of certain compounds including catecholamines, ascorbic acid, thiols (e.g. glutathione, cysteine), tetrahydrofolate and reduced flavins. Physical exercise leads to a greater production of free radicals relative to the greater oxygen consumption (Giuliani & Cestaro, 1997).

Free radicals range from very oxidizing to very reducing and their reduction potentials can be used to predict a hierarchy for free radical reactions (Buettner, 1993). The most oxidizing free radical is the hydroxyl radical ($^{\bullet}OH$) which, with a half-life of only 1 nanosecond at $37^{\circ}C$, is so reactive that there is no time for any molecule or radical to remove it before damage is done. Damage to DNA and proteins is therefore unavoidable and must be dealt with by repair enzymes.

Singlet oxygen

Singlet oxygen ($^{1}O_2$) is an exceptionally reactive and destructive form of oxygen, which has been implicated in the inactivation of enzymes, the peroxidation of lipids in membranes and lipoproteins, and in DNA strand breakage. It is produced when a molecule of ground-state triplet oxygen is excited by absorbing

Table 4.4 Examples of reactive oxygen species (ROS) and reactive nitrogen species (RNS).

	Free radicals	Non-radicals
ROS	Superoxide anion ($O_2^{\bullet-}$)	Singlet oxygen ($^{1}O_2$)
	Hydroxyl radical ($^{\bullet}OH$)	Hydrogen peroxide (H_2O_2)
	Nonlipid alkoxyl radical ($RO^{\bullet}$)	Hypochlorous acid ($HOCl$)
	Lipid alkoxyl radical ($LO^{\bullet}$)	
	Nonlipid peroxyl radical ($ROO^{\bullet}$)	
	Lipid peroxyl radical ($LOO^{\bullet}$)	
RNS	Nitric oxide ($NO^{\bullet}$)	Peroxynitrite anion ($ONOO^{-}$)
	Nitrogen dioxide ($NO_2^{\bullet}$)	

energy from a photochemical reaction. Excitation can be achieved when biological pigments such as retinaldehyde, flavins and porphyrins are illuminated in the presence of oxygen. The pigment absorbs light, enters a higher electronic state and transfers energy to the oxygen molecule. The result is a movement of one of the unpaired electrons in a way that alleviates the spin restriction. As there are no unpaired electrons, singlet oxygen does not qualify as a radical. Certain biological antioxidants, particularly carotenoids, are able to inactivate singlet oxygen by quenching, as discussed in Chapter 7.

Hydrogen peroxide

Hydrogen peroxide is produced by several oxidase enzymes and can also be formed enzymatically from the superoxide radical. Hydrogen peroxide is important in free radical biochemistry because it is a potential source of the highly reactive hydroxyl radical in the presence of free transition metal ions. It is relatively stable and its high diffusibility, both within and between cells, extends the range of free radical reactions.

Hypochlorous acid

Hypochlorous acid is an oxidizing and chlorinating agent produced by certain phagocytes (Section 5.2.3).

4.3.2   Defence systems

Transition metal ions in the free state promote free radical reactions and so the body ensures as far as possible that iron and copper ions, at least, are safely bound in storage or transport proteins. There is three times as much transferrin iron-binding capacity in plasma as iron needing to be transported (Halliwell, 1991). Iron ions bound to transferrin cannot stimulate lipid peroxidation or formation of hydroxyl free radicals. The same is true of copper ions bound to the plasma protein caeruloplasmin or albumin. The binding of iron to proteins depends on the plasma or tissue pH values being normal. A slight displacement of pH towards acidosis (as occurs in cases of ischaemia, trauma, inflammatory states and tumours) is sufficient to allow detachment of the metal and the initiation of radical-forming reactions (Cestaro et al., 1997).

The body's next line of defence is the removal of reactive oxygen species or their precursors by certain enzymes. For example, most of the superoxide generated in the body undergoes a dismutation reaction, forming hydrogen peroxide and oxygen (reaction 4.1). This reaction can take place spontaneously (albeit rather slowly) or can be catalysed by either of two superoxide dismutases, one a cytosolic copper–zinc enzyme and the other a mitochondrial manganese-centred enzyme.

$$2O_2^{\bullet-} + 2H^+ \rightarrow H_2O_2 + O_2 \tag{4.1}$$

Two enzymes remove hydrogen peroxide in mammalian cells: catalase (reaction 4.2) and selenium-dependent glutathione peroxidase (reaction 4.3). The latter enzyme is the more important of the two: catalase is probably limited to destroying hydrogen peroxide generated by oxidase enzymes located within peroxisomes.

$$2H_2O_2 \rightarrow 2H_2O + O_2 \tag{4.2}$$

$$H_2O_2 + 2GSH \rightarrow GSSG + 2H_2O \tag{4.3}$$

Oxidized glutathione is then converted back to GSH by an NADPH-dependent enzyme, glutathione reductase.

Enzymes do not completely prevent the formation of free radicals, and the body must now rely on antioxidants that 'scavenge' free radicals and convert them to harmless stable derivatives. Among naturally occurring antioxidants, vitamin E, vitamin C and carotenoids are the most important. Vitamin E is the major chain-breaking antioxidant in membrane lipids and lipoproteins. Vitamin C is an effective scavenger of several reactive oxygen species in the aqueous environment of the cytosol and extracellular fluids. Carotenoids have an important role in inactivating singlet oxygen. The ways in which each of these antioxidants function are discussed in the relevant chapters.

4.4   Haemostasis

4.4.1   Overview

Immediately after a blood vessel has been severed or ruptured, bleeding is stemmed by local vasoconstriction resulting from nervous reflexes, vascular spasm, and humoral factors released from the traumatized tissues and blood platelets. The damaged vessel is then sealed temporarily with a plug of aggregated platelets. Localized blood coagulation leads to subsequent formation of a blood clot composed of a three-dimensional meshwork of fibrin fibres entrapping blood cells, platelets and plasma. A large amount of plasminogen is also trapped in the clot along with other plasma proteins. The clot begins to develop in 15–20 s if the trauma to the vascular wall has been severe and in 1–2 min if the trauma has been minor. Within 3–6 min after rupture of a vessel (if the opening is not too large), the entire opening or broken end of the vessel is filled with clot. After 20 min to 1 hour, the clot retracts, closing the vessel still further. Clot retraction is effected by entrapped platelets which activate themselves to contract, thereby pulling attached fibrin fibres towards them and compressing the fibrin meshwork into a smaller mass. Within a few hours after clot formation, the clot is invaded by fibroblasts and the deposition of fibrous connective tissue throughout the clot seals the vessel permanently. A day or so after the clot has stopped the bleeding, the injured tissues and vascular endothelium very slowly release tissue plasminogen activator. This activator converts the plasminogen within the clot to plasmin, which dissolves the clot. After 1 or 2 weeks, the clot has been replaced by connective tissue.

4.4.2   Formation of the platelet plug

Platelets are colourless, round or oval discs of diameter 1–4 μm (cf. erythrocytes with a mean diameter of 7.8 μm). They arise by fragmentation of megakaryocytes within the bone marrow or soon after the megakaryocytes enter the blood. Although platelets have no nuclei and cannot reproduce, they have many functional characteristics of whole cells. The presence of contractile proteins in their cytoplasm enables them to contract; they have the capacity to synthesize various enzymes, generate ADP and ATP, and store large quantities of calcium ions; and they can synthesize prostaglandins, fibrin-stabilizing factor and a growth factor that stimulates the proliferation of vascular endothelial and smooth muscle cells. On the platelet surface is a coat of glycoproteins (the glycocalyx) that repulses adherence to normal endothelium and yet causes adherence to injured areas of the vessel wall. Adherence is mediated by von Willebrand factor, a multimeric plasma adhesive protein that binds to a specific receptor, glycoprotein 1b, on the platelet membrane.

When platelets come in contact with a damaged vascular surface, such as the collagen fibres in the vessel wall, the platelets themselves undergo an immediate and drastic change, an event known as activation. They swell to a spherical form and extend long pseudopodia; their contractile proteins contract forcefully and cause the release of granules that contain multiple active factors; they become sticky so that they adhere to exposed collagen in damaged vessels and tissues; and they secrete large quantities of ADP. The ADP in turn acts on nearby platelets to activate them as well, and the stickiness of these additional platelets causes them to adhere to the originally activated platelets. Activated platelets also release thromboxane A_2, which is both a vasoconstrictor and an aggregating agent (Marcus, 1978). The recruitment of platelets to the damaged site in this manner leads to the formation of a platelet plug.

An increase in the cytosolic Ca^{2+} concentration is a major signal underlying platelet activation. Physiological agonists such as collagen, thrombin, ADP, platelet-activating factor and thromboxane A_2 mobilize Ca^{2+} by stimulating its release from intracellular stores in the endoplasmic reticulum and also its entry into the cell across the plasma membrane. After stimulation, the cytosolic Ca^{2+} concentration is restored to the resting level by sequestration of the ion into the endoplasmic reticulum and extrusion out of the cell. These movements of Ca^{2+} are carried out by Ca^{2+}-ATPases (calcium pumps).

4.4.3   Blood coagulation

The complexity of the blood coagulation system ensures that it only becomes active when necessary. Each component is inactive and must be activated to participate in clot formation.

Initiation of coagulation: formation of prothrombin activator

There are two pathways leading to the formation of prothrombin activator: the extrinsic pathway (Fig. 4.9) and the intrinsic pathway (Fig. 4.10). In both of these pathways, a series of plasma proteins, the blood-clotting factors, create a cascade which enormously amplifies the original stimulus for clotting. Most of the blood-clotting factors circulate as inactive precursors (zymogens) of proteolytic enzymes. Each factor

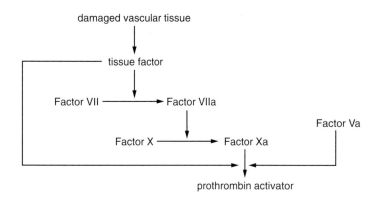

Fig. 4.9 Extrinsic pathway for initiating blood coagulation.

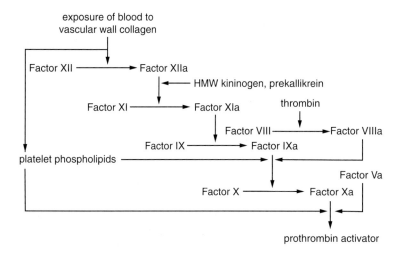

Fig. 4.10 Intrinsic pathway for initiating blood coagulation.

is activated by partial proteolysis, and then in turn activates the next factor. Most of the clotting factors (Table 4.5) are designated by Roman numerals. In the pathways described below, a small letter 'a' after the Roman numeral denotes the activated form of the factor.

Extrinsic pathway

This pathway is triggered by injury to the tissues and is initiated by a glycoprotein known as tissue factor (also called tissue thromboplastin). Tissue factor is an integral membrane protein found on the surface of non-vascular cells in close association with phospholipids. When injury occurs, tissue factor is exposed to blood and forms a one-to-one complex with circulating Factor VII in the presence of calcium ions. Formation of this complex facilitates the conversion of Factor VII to its active protease form (Factor VIIa) by minor pro-

Table 4.5 Components of the blood coagulation cascade.

Factor	Identity	Function
Factor I	Fibrinogen	Structural
Factor II	Prothrombin	Protease zymogen
Factor III	Tissue factor (thromboplastin)	Cofactor/initiator
Factor IV	Calcium	Cofactor
Factor V	See text	Cofactor
Factor VII	See text	Protease zymogen
Factor VIII	See text	Cofactor
Factor IX	See text	Protease zymogen
Factor X	See text	Protease zymogen
Factor XI	See text	Protease zymogen
Factor XII	See text	Protease zymogen
Factor XIII	See text	Protease zymogen
Protein C	See text	Protease zymogen
Protein S	See text	Cofactor
von Willebrand factor	See text	Adhesion

teolysis. The Factor VIIa–tissue factor complex then converts Factor X to another protease (Factor Xa) by the cleavage of a single peptide bond. Factor Xa combines immediately with the tissue factor as well as with Factor Va and phospholipids provided by activated platelets to form the complex prothrombin activator.

Intrinsic pathway

This pathway begins in the blood itself. Exposure of the blood to vascular wall collagen following damage to blood vessels causes circulating Factor XII to change its molecular configuration, converting it into a proteolytic enzyme (Factor XIIa). Simultaneously, platelets are stimulated to release phospholipids. Factor XIIa activates Factor XI, a reaction which also requires HMW (high-molecular-weight) kininogen and is accelerated by prekallikrein. Activated Factor XI then activates Factor IX. Activated Factor IX, acting in concert with activated Factor VIII and with the platelet phospholipids, activates Factor X. The last step in the intrinsic pathway is the same as that in the extrinsic pathway. That is, activated Factor X combines with Factor Va and platelet or tissue phospholipids to form prothrombin activator.

Factor VIII is the factor that is missing in a person who has classic haemophilia. The bleeding disease called thrombocytopenia is caused by a deficiency of platelets.

Conversion of prothrombin to thrombin and clot formation

A scheme of these events is given in Fig. 4.11. Pro-thrombin activator, in the presence of sufficient amounts of calcium ions and phospholipids provided by activated platelets, causes conversion of prothrombin to thrombin. Once generated, thrombin exerts positive feedback upon its formation by activating Factor V. Prothrombin is a plasma protein that is formed continually in the liver; it splits easily into smaller compounds, one of which is thrombin. Much of the prothrombin first formed attaches to pro-thrombin receptors on the platelets that have already stuck to the damaged tissue. This binding stimulates the formation of still more thrombin in the localized area of damage.

Fibrinogen is a soluble plasma protein of high molecular weight (MW = 340 000), which is formed in the liver. Thrombin, a weakly proteolytic enzyme, selectively removes four peptides from each molecule of fibrinogen to form a molecule of fibrin monomer. Many fibrin monomer molecules then spontaneously polymerize into long fibres of insoluble fibrin that constitute the reticulum of the clot. The formation of fibrin accelerates the conversion of fibrin-stabilizing factor (Factor XIII) to an enzyme (Factor XIIIa) by thrombin in the presence of calcium ions. Fibrin-stabilizing factor is a plasma protein, but is also released from platelets entrapped in the clot. Factor XIIIa causes covalent bonding between fibrin monomer molecules as well as multiple cross-linking between adjacent fibrin fibres; it also causes cross-linking of other plasma proteins to fibrin, so incorporating them into the clot. The result is a greatly strengthened reticulum.

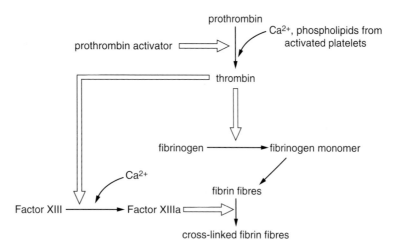

Fig. 4.11 Scheme for conversion of prothrombin to thrombin and conversion of fibrinogen to cross-linked fibrin fibres.

Regulation of the coagulation cascade

Many plasma proteins are involved in the regulation of coagulation. Among them, antithrombin III is a plasma protease inhibitor that scavenges any of the blood-clotting enzymes that move away from the growing clot. Protein C inactivates the active cofactor forms of Factors V and VIII, thus rapidly slowing blood clotting. Protein C is converted to its active enzyme form on endothelial cell membranes by a complex of two proteins, thrombomodulin and thrombin. Activated protein C, anchored to the membrane through binding to membrane-bound protein S, converts the Factors Va and VIIIa to their inactive forms by limited proteolysis. Tissue-factor-pathway inhibitor binds to Factor Xa, and this complex in turn binds to the tissue-factor–Factor VII complex, thus inactivating the extrinsic pathway.

Lysis of blood clots

Circulating in the bloodstream is a protein called plasminogen that, when activated, becomes a proteolytic enzyme called plasmin. Whenever plasmin is formed, it causes lysis of the clot by destroying fibrin fibres as well as fibrinogen, prothrombin, and Factors V, VIII and XII. During clot formation, plasminogen is trapped within the clot along with other plasma proteins. The injured tissues and vascular endothelium very slowly release a potent substance called tissue plasminogen activator that, after the clot has stopped the bleeding, eventually converts plasminogen to plasmin. Plasmin plays an important role in removing minute clots from millions of tiny peripheral vessels that otherwise would become occluded.

4.5   Atherosclerosis

Atherosclerosis is a degenerative disease of large- and medium-sized arteries with a predisposition for critical arterial beds such as the coronaries, which supply heart muscle with nutritive, oxygenated blood. The disease is characterized by the progressive formation of an atheromatous plaque upon the innermost layer of the arterial wall. This build-up of fatty material reduces the bore of the artery whilst also causing hardening and loss of elasticity of the arterial wall. Plaque formation is preceded by a reduced ability of the arterial smooth muscle to relax. Atherosclerosis is the principal cause of cardiovascular and cerebro-vascular disease, leading to heart attacks and strokes, respectively.

The causal relationship between high blood cholesterol levels and atherosclerosis is well established (Levine et al., 1995). Hypercholesterolaemia may be thought of as any plasma cholesterol level above 160 mg/100 mL. Cholesterol-lowering therapy is effective in both the primary prevention of coronary artery disease and the secondary prevention of subsequent cardiac events in patients with established coronary disease.

4.5.1   Association between high blood cholesterol and atherosclerosis

An early demonstration of the link between hypercholesterolaemia and atherosclerosis took place in 1913 when Anitschkow in Russia observed that feeding pure cholesterol to rabbits produced elevated blood cholesterol levels as well as atherosclerosis in the aorta and coronary arteries.

The causal relationship between high blood cholesterol levels and atherosclerosis is demonstrated unequivocally by the genetic disorder familial hypercholesterolaemia (FH). This disorder is an example of an inborn error of metabolism and is due to impaired production of the LDL receptor. There are two forms of FH: a heterozygous form and a more severe homozygous form. FH heterozygotes inherit one mutant gene and number about one in 500 people in most ethnic groups. The cells of these individuals produce approximately half the normal number of LDL receptors. As a result, LDL is removed from the circulation at half the normal rate, the lipoprotein accumulates in blood to levels twofold above normal, and heart attacks occur typically in the fourth and fifth decades of life. If two heterozygotes of the opposite sex have a child, that child has a one in four chance of inheriting two copies of the mutant gene, one from each parent. Such FH homozygotes (about one in a million people) have plasma LDL levels 6–10-fold above normal. Heart attacks can occur at the age of two and are almost inevitable by the age of 20 (Goldstein & Brown, 1987).

4.5.2   The lesions of atherosclerosis

The wall of a typical artery is composed of three coats. The innermost coat, the tunica intima, consists of an inner endothelium, a subendothelial layer of delicate fibroelastic connective tissue and an external band of elastic fibres, which may be absent in many vessels. The middle coat, the tunica media, consists chiefly of circularly arranged smooth muscle cells. The outer coat, the tunica adventitia, is composed principally of connective tissue, most of the elements of which run parallel to the long axis of the vessel. The structure and relative thickness of each coat vary according to the type and size of the vessel.

The lesions of atherosclerosis represent a continuum from the early fatty streak to the intermediate fibrofatty lesion to the mature fibrous plaque. Early lesions are commonly found at intimal sites where changes in blood flow occur at branches and curves in the arterial system. Changes in the mature lesion involve all three coats of the arterial wall. Not all fatty streaks progress to fibrous plaques; some remain stable or regress and disappear.

The fatty streak

The fatty streak is composed mainly of an aggregation of lipid-filled macrophages and smooth muscle cells known as foam cells within the intima. The overlying endothelium is frequently thinned and distorted by the subjacent foam cells. Blood monocytes are continuously recruited to the evolving fatty streak where they differentiate into macrophages.

The fibrofatty lesion

This intermediate lesion is characterized by necrosis of the foam cells with the release of foam cell lipids to the interstitium. There is mitogen-stimulated proliferation of smooth muscle cells and subsequent synthesis of collagen, elastin and proteoglycans. Monocyte recruitment continues and the endothelium begins to fragment.

The fibrous plaque

The fibrous plaque comprises a dense cap of fibrous connective tissue containing multiple layers of smooth muscle cells that occupy slit-like spaces. Foam cells accumulate at the shoulders of the plaque. Beneath the fibrous cap is a region rich in macrophages, T lymphocytes and smooth muscle cells, and beneath that is a core of extracellular lipid, cholesterol crystals, necrotic debris and calcification. Microvascular channels ramify throughout the thickened lesion, presumably to provide nutrients and oxygen to the cells.

Although there may be severe atherosclerotic narrowing of arteries, atherosclerosis alone rarely results in occlusion, defined as complete obliteration of the arterial lumen. However, rheological forces may cause the plaque to rupture or fissure, resulting in haemorrhage into the plaque, thrombosis and occlusion. This happening is a major cause of myocardial infarction.

4.5.3   The LDL oxidation hypothesis

It was recognized in the 1950s that an elevation of plasma LDL is strongly associated with atherosclerosis. Goldstein et al. (1979) discovered that cultured mouse peritoneal macrophages were converted into foam cells in the presence of chemically modified LDL, but not native LDL. Oxidized LDL (oxLDL) emerged as a candidate modified form when a newly discovered receptor named 'scavenger receptor' was shown to mediate rapid uptake of oxLDL, but not native LDL, by macrophages. Unlike the LDL receptor, the scavenger receptor was not down-regulated when the cholesterol content of the cell increased, thus scavenger receptor could allow cholesterol to accumulate in macrophages and lead to foam cell formation. The transformation of native LDL to a form (modified LDL) which is more rapidly endocytosed by macrophages almost certainly involves oxidation, but not all oxidative treatments necessarily lead to the formation of modified LDL (Bedwell et al., 1989).

Immunological evidence exists for a role of oxLDL in the development of atherosclerosis. Human and rabbit atherosclerotic lesions contain an immunoglobulin (IgG) that recognizes epitopes present in oxLDL but not in native LDL (Ylä-Herttuala et al., 1994). The titres of antibodies that recognize epitopes of oxLDL increase with the progression of atherosclerosis in mice (Palinski et al., 1995) and humans (Salonen et al., 1992).

It seems likely that oxidative modification of LDL is confined to microdomains within the arterial intima where LDL would be isolated from the many antioxidants present in extracellular fluid. It has been shown in vitro that LDL can be oxidatively modified to cytotoxic oxLDL by all the major cell types in the arterial wall, namely endothelial cells, smooth muscle cells and macrophages. These cells generate reactive substances which are then transferred to the LDL.

Cell-mediated stimulation of LDL modification is prevented by antioxidants and is dependent on redox-active metals in the medium (Steinbrecher *et al.*, 1984). This suggests that the oxidative modification of LDL involves the peroxidation of constituent polyunsaturated fatty acids. During modification, there is extensive degradation of lecithin (phosphatidylcholine) to lysolecithin catalysed by phospholipase A_2 present in the apoB-100 moiety of LDL (Parthasarathy & Barnett, 1990). The removal of lysolecithin from the surface of the particle aids the peroxidation of core lipids. There is also fragmentation of apoB-100 by direct oxidative scission. Extensive oxidation of LDL leads to aggregation of the LDL particles.

4.5.4 Lipid peroxidation

The polyunsaturated fatty acids (PUFAs) incorporated into the phospholipids of cell plasma membranes, the membranes of subcellular organelles (e.g. mitochondria) and plasma lipoproteins are susceptible to attack by certain free radicals such as $^•OH$, $LOO^•$ and $LO^•$. These free radicals initiate chain reactions that, if not stopped by chain-breaking antioxidants, result in the accumulation of toxic products. The process of lipid peroxidation can be conveniently divided into three stages: initiation, propagation and termination.

Initiation

$$LH + {^•OH} \rightarrow L^• + H_2O \qquad (4.4)$$

Propagation

$$L^• + O_2 \rightarrow LOO^• \qquad (4.5)$$

$$LOO^• + L'H \rightarrow LOOH + L'^• \qquad (4.6)$$

Termination

$$LOO^• + LOO^• \rightarrow \text{molecular products} \qquad (4.7)$$

Transition metals can decompose lipid hydroperoxides into peroxyl and alkoxyl radicals that bring about a dramatic intensification of the propagative stage.

$$LOOH + Fe^{2+} \text{ (or } Cu^+) \rightarrow \\ LO^• + OH^- + Fe^{3+} \text{ (or } Cu^{2+}) \qquad (4.8)$$

$$LOOH + Fe^{3+} \text{ (or } Cu^{2+}) \rightarrow \\ LOO^• + H^+ + Fe^{2+} \text{ (or } Cu^+) \qquad (4.9)$$

In reactions 4.4 to 4.9, LH represents a PUFA side chain of a phospholipid; $L^•$, a carbon-centred lipid radical; $LOO^•$, a lipid peroxyl radical; $LO^•$, a lipid alkoxyl radical; and LOOH, a lipid hydroperoxide. Reactions 4.4 to 4.6 are illustrated in Fig. 4.12.

Initiation involves removal of a hydrogen atom $(H^•)$ from a methylene $(–CH_2–)$ carbon in the PUFA molecule by any chemical species that is sufficiently reactive. Reaction 4.4 shows initiation by a hydroxyl radical. Removal of the hydrogen atom leaves behind an unpaired electron on the methylene carbon atom, $(–C^•H–)$. The presence of a double bond in the fatty acid weakens the C–H bonds on the carbon atom adjacent to the double bond and so makes $H^•$ removal easier. Thus the greater the number of double bonds in a PUFA, the more susceptible is the PUFA to peroxidation.

The lipid radical $L^•$ undergoes a molecular rearrangement to form a conjugated diene that reacts with molecular oxygen to give $LOO^•$. The peroxyl radical then attacks an adjacent PUFA side chain of a phospholipid ($L'H$), removing a hydrogen atom and converting itself into a lipid hydroperoxide. The new $L'^•$ reacts with oxygen to yield another peroxyl radical and thus a chain reaction is propagated. In this manner, a single initiation can result in hundreds of PUFA side chains being converted into lipid hydroperoxides. The length of the propagation chain depends on the lipid–protein ratio in a membrane, the fatty acid composition, the oxygen concentration, and the presence or absence within the membrane of chain-breaking antioxidants. In the absence of a chain-breaking antioxidant, the propagation chain (reactions 4.5 and 4.6) is eventually broken when two peroxyl radicals react together to give molecular products (reaction 4.7).

In the body, lipid hydroperoxides are cleaved by phospholipase A_2, releasing the peroxidized fatty acid from the phospholipid. The peroxidized free fatty acid can now be reduced to a harmless hydroxy fatty acid by the action of glutathione peroxidase (reaction 4.10). The reducing equivalents for this reaction are provided by the tripeptide glutathione (reduced form, GSH; oxidized form, GSSG).

$$PUFA\text{-}OOH + 2GSH \rightarrow \\ PUFA\text{-}OH + H_2O + GSSG \qquad (4.10)$$

Alternatively, a phospholipid hydroperoxide glutathione peroxidase can convert lipid hydroperoxides directly to a hydroxy acid (Buettner, 1993). Both of

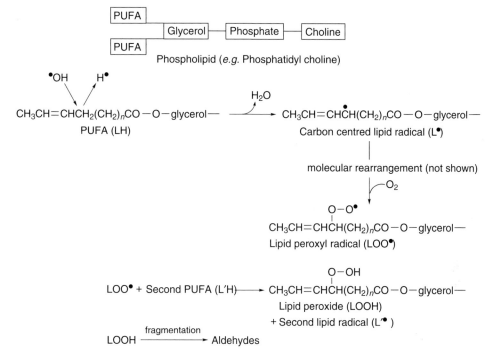

Fig. 4.12 Initiation and propagation stages of lipid peroxidation.

these peroxidase enzymes uniquely require the trace element selenium as a cofactor. [Note: A non-selenium-dependent glutathione peroxidase exists which reduces hydrogen peroxide, but has no activity against organic hydroperoxides (Lawrence & Burk, 1976)].

The PUFAs in LDL are protected from peroxidation by the presence of several indigenous lipid-soluble antioxidants. By far the major antioxidant is α-tocopherol (vitamin E): on average about six molecules of this antioxidant are present in each LDL molecule. Vitamin E is a very efficient free radical scavenger and terminates chains almost as soon as they are initiated. In doing so, vitamin E and other antioxidants are gradually used up. When the LDL is finally depleted of its antioxidants, the chain reaction will proceed unchallenged until all LDL PUFAs are converted into lipid hydroperoxides. At termination the lipid hydroperoxides break down to a wide range of products, including aldehydes, hydrocarbons, epoxides and alcohols. Some of these breakdown products are diffusible toxins which irritate endothelial cells and may contribute to disruption of endothelial integrity.

The aldehydes arising from lipid hydroperoxide decomposition are particularly important in atherogenesis. Malondialdehyde, 4-hydroxynonenal and probably other aldehydes bind covalently to the ε amino group of lysine residues on the apoB protein moiety of LDL particles, causing a progressive decrease in the positive charge and a conformational change. This modification results in a loss of recognition by the LDL receptor and the creation of new epitopes of apoB that are recognized by the macrophage scavenger receptor. Evidence for the involvement of aldehydes is the observation by Picard *et al.* (1992) that aminoguanidine, a compound with high binding affinity for aldehydes, prevents apoB lysine modification, thereby inhibiting the oxidatively induced uptake of LDL by macrophages.

4.5.5   Possible mechanisms of cell-mediated LDL oxidation

Several biochemical systems have been shown to promote LDL oxidation *in vitro*; these systems involve thiols, lipoxygenase, myeloperoxidase, superoxide and peroxynitrite radical (Berliner & Heinecke, 1996). Physiologically relevant mechanisms underlying LDL oxidation *in vivo* are largely a matter of speculation.

Superoxide

Superoxide has been proposed as a primary cell-derived oxidant with a role in LDL oxidation on the basis that superoxide dismutase inhibits rapid uptake of LDL by macrophages. However, Jessup *et al.* (1993) showed that the use of superoxide dismutase is inappropriate as a test for the involvement of superoxide because it has metal-chelating properties. These authors found that superoxide generated in a cell-free system could not modify LDL. Similarly, LDL modification by macrophages was not accelerated when extracellular superoxide generation was increased 5–10-fold by stimulation of NADPH oxidase. Thus there is no secure evidence for the direct involvement of superoxide in cell-mediated oxidative modification of LDL.

To account for the apparent toxicity of superoxide, the secondary production of the far more reactive hydroxyl radical by the iron-catalysed Haber–Weiss reaction (reactions 4.11–4.13) has been frequently proposed.

$$2O_2^{\bullet -} + 2H^+ \rightarrow H_2O_2 + O_2 \tag{4.11}$$

$$O_2^{\bullet -} + Fe^{3+} \rightarrow O_2 + Fe^{2+} \tag{4.12}$$

$$Fe^{2+} + H_2O_2 \rightarrow {}^{\bullet}OH + OH^- + Fe^{3+} \tag{4.13}$$

The contribution of superoxide to hydroxyl radical formation by the Haber–Weiss reaction may not be significant *in vivo*, as ascorbate and other reducing agents compete with superoxide in reducing iron.

Peroxynitrite anion

Superoxide and nitric oxide (a modulator of vascular tone; Section 4.5.6) are generated in excess by the endothelium of hypercholesterolaemic arteries (Minor *et al.*, 1990; Ohara *et al.*, 1993) and can react together to produce peroxynitrite anion. This reaction is faster than both the superoxide dismutase-catalysed and spontaneous dismutation of superoxide to hydrogen peroxide (Huie & Padmaja, 1993). At physiological pH, the reaction product, peroxynitrite radical (ONOO⁻), is protonated to peroxynitrous acid (ONOOH), which decomposes spontaneously to yield nitrogen dioxide ($NO_2^{\bullet}$) and hydroxyl radical (Beckman *et al.*, 1990). Both ${}^{\bullet}OH$ and $NO_2^{\bullet}$ can separately initiate lipid peroxidation. This way of producing hydroxyl radical is not dependent on transition metal ions.

$$NO^{\bullet} + O_2^{\bullet -} \rightarrow ONOO^- \tag{4.14}$$

$$ONOO^- + H^+ \rightarrow ONOOH \tag{4.15}$$

$$ONOOH \rightarrow {}^{\bullet}OH + NO_2^{\bullet} \tag{4.16}$$

Radi *et al.* (1991) synthesized peroxynitrite and showed that it induced lipid peroxidation in phosphatidylcholine (lecithin) liposomes. Peroxynitrous acid and/or its decomposition products (i.e. ${}^{\bullet}OH$ and $NO_2^{\bullet}$) served as the oxidizing species. Darley-Usmar *et al.* (1992) showed that a system which simultaneously generated superoxide and nitric oxide was capable of initiating lipid peroxidation in human LDL, whereas a system which generated only nitric oxide was unable to do so. Graham *et al.* (1993) reported that chemically synthesized peroxynitrite converted LDL to a form recognized by the macrophage scavenger receptor. These results are consistent with the hypothesis that the reaction of superoxide with nitric oxide contributes to the pathogenesis of atherosclerosis by yielding a potent mediator of LDL oxidation without the requirement for transition metal ions (White *et al.*, 1994).

4.5.6   Atherogenic properties of oxLDL

OxLDL may be atherogenic by numerous mechanisms, some of which are listed below.

- The lysolecithin present in oxLDL increases vascular superoxide production resulting in a self-perpetuating cycle of LDL oxidation (Ohara *et al.*, 1994).
- OxLDL, by virtue of its lysolecithin content, exhibits chemotactic activity for circulating monocytes (Quinn *et al.*, 1988) and T lymphocytes (McMurray *et al.*, 1993).
- OxLDL induces monocyte chemotactic protein-1 (MCP-1) synthesis in endothelial cells and smooth muscle cells (Cushing *et al.*, 1990).
- Both oxLDL (Cominacini *et al.*, 1997) and lysolecithin (Kume *et al.*, 1992) can induce the expression of the endothelial adhesion molecules ICAM-1 and VCAM-1.
- Monocytes/macrophages exposed to oxLDL release cytokines which stimulate endothelial cells to synthesize cell adhesion molecules (Frostegård *et al.*, 1993).

- OxLDL inhibits the motility of resident macrophages in the subendothelial space, thereby favouring macrophage accumulation in developing lesions (Quinn *et al.*, 1985).
- OxLDL induces endothelial cells to synthesize macrophage colony-stimulating factor (MCSF), which can induce differentiation of monocytes into macrophages, including an increased expression of scavenger receptor (Rajavashisth *et al.*, 1990).
- OxLDL stimulates proliferation of macrophages (Yui *et al.*, 1993) and aortic smooth muscle cells (Chatterjee & Ghosh, 1996) in culture.
- Lysolecithin present in oxLDL induces migration of smooth muscle cells in human coronary arteries (Kohno *et al.*, 1998).
- OxLDL enhances lipopolysaccharide-induced tissue factor expression in human adherent monocytes (Brand *et al.*, 1994). Normally, tissue factor is not expressed within the vasculature; however, its expression can be induced in monocytes and endothelial cells by a variety of agonists, including lipopolysaccharide. Activation of the blood coagulation cascade by aberrant expression of tissue factor on the surface of monocytes or endothelial cells could lead to thrombus formation in ruptured plaques.
- OxLDL stimulates platelet aggregation (Katzman *et al.*, 1994).
- Endothelial cells chronically exposed to oxLDL have a severely impaired capacity to release prostacyclin, a potent cytoprotective agent, which inhibits cell proliferation, platelet adhesion and aggregation, and monocyte adhesion (Thorin *et al.*, 1994).
- Lysolecithin in oxLDL decreases the responsiveness of isolated rabbit aorta to endothelium-dependent relaxants (Mangin *et al.* 1993).
- OxLDL decreases the expression of nitric oxide synthase, the enzyme responsible for producing the epithelium-derived relaxing factor, nitric oxide (Liao *et al.*, 1995).
- OxLDL enhances agonist-induced vasoconstrictions by a direct effect on the vascular smooth muscle (Galle *et al.*, 1990).

Cytotoxicity

Oxidative modifications of LDL by lipid peroxidation renders the oxLDL toxic to cells *in vitro* (Morel *et al.*, 1983). Cytotoxicity of oxLDL to endothelial cells, smooth muscle cells, fibroblasts, monocytes, neutrophils and macrophages in culture has been demonstrated (Henriksen *et al.*, 1979; Hessler *et al.*, 1979, 1983; Cathcart *et al.*, 1985; Reid & Mitchinson, 1993). The capacity of oxLDL to injure or kill cells may contribute to endothelial damage and may account for the necrotic debris found in the core regions of atherosclerotic plaques. Electron microscopic examination of mouse peritoneal macrophages exposed to oxLDL revealed the following ultrastructural changes: chromatin condensation, reduction in cell volume, cell break-up into membrane-bound bodies and blebbing of the plasma membrane. These changes are more characteristic of apoptosis than necrosis. In contrast, cells exposed to native LDL exhibited no such changes (Reid *et al.*, 1993).

The presence during lipoprotein preparation of general free radical scavengers (vitamin E, butylated hydroxytoluene) or the divalent cation chelator EDTA prevented the formation of cytotoxic oxLDL. However, the toxic action of oxLDL could not be prevented by the addition of any of these agents during incubation of the oxLDL with cells (Morel *et al.*, 1983). These observations indicate that an oxidized lipid is responsible for cytotoxicity rather than free radicals generated in culture by the action of oxLDL. Hughes *et al.* (1994) extracted the toxic components from lipid extracts of oxLDL and identified them as the oxysterols 7-ketocholesterol and 7-hydroxycholesterol. When the two toxins were added to native LDL at concentrations equivalent to those present in oxLDL, the resultant LDL was not rendered cytotoxic. This suggests that the oxysterols are released more rapidly from oxLDL than from native LDL because of the severe disruption of the lipoprotein's lipid environment during oxidative modification. The mechanism(s) by which oxysterols exert their cytotoxicity has not been established.

4.5.7 Development of the atherosclerotic lesion

Initiation

Plasma LDL enters the subendothelial space of the arterial intima where it is trapped in microenvironments secluded from plasma antioxidants. LDL lipid is mildly oxidized to minimally oxidized LDL through the action of resident vascular cells. The modified lipoprotein induces local vascular cells to produce

MCP-1, which attracts circulating monocytes, and M-CSF, which stimulates monocyte differentiation to macrophages in the subendothelium. Monocyte recruitment also requires highly organized interactions between signalling and adhesion molecules (McEver, 1992). Adhesion of leucocytes to endothelial cells is mediated through selective cell surface adhesion molecules expressed by both types of cell. Adhesion molecules expressed by endothelial cells include ICAM-1, VCAM-1 and E-selectin. ICAM-1 is constitutively expressed, but its expression can be augmented by the cytokines IL-1β, IFN-γ and TNF-α. VCAM-1 and E-selectin are not constitutively expressed, but expression of the former is induced by TNF-α and that of the latter by IL-1β and TNF-α. Adhesion molecules expressed by leucocytes are known as integrins; they include LFA-1, VLA-4α and MAC-1.

ICAM-1 and VCAM-1 may mediate monocyte adherence to the developing atherosclerotic lesion. Both are up-regulated in endothelium adjacent to fatty streaks in the aorta of rabbits fed a hypercholesterolaemic diet and in the LDL-receptor deficient Watanabe heritable hyperlipidaemic rabbit (Cybulsky & Gimbrone, 1991). ICAM-1 is a receptor for the LFA-1 and MAC-1 integrins and mediates the adhesion of monocytes, lymphocytes and neutrophils to the endothelium. VCAM-1, by binding to VLA-4 integrin, mediates the adhesion of lymphocytes and monocytes to the activated endothelium (Meydani, 1998). The endothelial adhesion molecules may have distinct functions in the recruitment of leucocytes. E-selectin and VCAM-1 may mediate rapid but transient adhesion of circulating leucocytes to endothelium, whereas ICAM-1 may mediate subsequent leucocyte transendothelial migration (Collins, 1993).

Foam cell formation

The macrophages within the subendothelial space produce reactive oxygen species that further modify minimally oxidized LDL to completely oxidized LDL (oxLDL). Macrophages and smooth muscle cells take up the oxLDL by endocytosis, mediated by scavenger receptors on the macrophage surface. Circulating monocytes do not express the scavenger receptor; the receptor is induced when the monocytes differentiate into macrophages. There is evidence (Hoff et al., 1992) that, because of LDL particle aggregation, the mode of oxLDL uptake by macrophages changes with increasing degrees of LDL oxidation from one involv-

ing the scavenger receptor to an alternative one in which aggregates are phagocytosed. The macrophages become so bloated with accumulated cholesterol that they transform into foam cells. Scavenger receptors increase in number in response to macrophage colony-stimulating factor and other cytokines, which are induced in endothelial cells by oxLDL (Berliner & Heinecke, 1996). Oxidation of LDL and its uptake by macrophages is increased by factors released from activated platelets (Aviram, 1995).

Aggregation of oxLDL occurs in the aortic intima and macrophages can ingest such aggregates by phagocytosis. Macrophages are also able to phagocytose oxLDL–antibody aggregates via the antibody-binding Fc receptor (Khoo et al., 1992).

Advanced stages

Foam cell formation stimulates the local synthesis of proteoglycans and lipoprotein lipase, which promote further LDL retention and aggregation in the subendothelium. Endothelial cells and smooth muscle cells are capable of elaborating all of the elements of connective tissue. The deposition of connective tissue advances the fatty streak to the intermediate fibrofatty lesion. Activation of the resident macrophages and T lymphocytes promotes the formation of molecules that stimulate the transformation of local smooth muscle cells from the contractile to the proliferative state. Migration and proliferation of smooth muscle cells significantly enlarge the lesion. The necrotic mass at the base of advanced plaques is mainly due to the accumulation of the remnants of dead macrophage-derived foam cells (Aqel et al., 1985).

4.5.8 Arterial calcification

Calcification is a common pathological finding in the aging human arteries and heart valves. There are two distinct types of arterial calcification, designated according to their site in the arterial wall. Intimal calcification refers to the atherosclerotic plaque calcification that develops in the tunica intima. Calcification develops at the fatty streak stage as small scattered deposits of calcium hydroxyapatite crystals, which form in matrix vesicles similar to those of developing bone. Medial calcification, known as Monckeberg's sclerosis, is confined to the tunica media. It proceeds in a linear fashion and is not necessarily associated with plaque formation. It often progresses to ossification characterized by the formation of bone trabeculae and the presence of osteocytes and bone marrow within the vessel wall. Medial calcification occurs at a much earlier age in lower-limb arteries of diabetics.

It was once thought that plaque calcification was a passive process resulting from the accumulation of calcium released from dying cells within necrotic regions of the plaque. However, recent evidence suggests that this process is active and regulatable, with remarkable similarities to organized bone formation (osteogenesis). The mineral within calcified atherosclerotic plaques is hydroxyapatite, the same mineral as found in bone. Bone matrix proteins, such as osteopontin, osteonectin, osteocalcin and matrix Gla protein (MGP), have been demonstrated in atherosclerotic plaques, as have bone morphogenetic proteins (Shanahan et al., 1998).

The question arises: what cells are responsible for producing the mineralized matrix in arterial calcification? In cultured bovine aortic smooth muscle cells grown slightly beyond confluency, multicellular nodules formed and these nodules subsequently calcified. Cells cloned from these nodules were termed calcifying vascular cells (CVCs). These cells were capable of producing bone matrix proteins and in this respect behaved like osteoblasts. CVC cells were subsequently found among artery wall cells in calcified human atherosclerotic lesions (Watson, 2000). In answer to the question, it can be postulated that, in response to some stimulus associated with atherosclerosis, smooth muscle cells in the vessel media migrate into the intima where they proliferate and differentiate into osteoblast-like cells. The stimulus that activates the normally quiescent vascular smooth muscle cells is likely to be endothelial damage, which would expose the underlying smooth muscle cells to cytokines released by platelets and circulating blood cells.

4.5.9 Endothelial dysfunction

Vasomotor control

The blood flow to a particular tissue is regulated at the minimal level that will supply the tissue's requirements. This ensures that the tissues are always adequately supplied, whilst keeping the workload on the heart to a minimum. Acute control of local blood flow is achieved within seconds to minutes by changes in local vasodilator/vasoconstriction of the arterioles and small arteries effected through

relaxation/contraction of the vascular smooth muscle. The state of contraction of the vascular smooth muscle is referred to as vascular tone. The arteries are normally maintained in a partial state of contraction (vasomotor tone) by the continual firing of nervous impulses from the vasomotor centre.

The vascular endothelium lining the lumen can modulate vascular tone by the synthesis and release of potent vasorelaxant and vasoconstrictor substances. Release of these substances is usually balanced in favour of vasodilators, notably epithelium-derived relaxing factor, prostacyclin and endothelium-derived hyperpolarizing factor. Epithelium-derived relaxing factor has been identified as the nitric oxide radical (NO•) (Palmer et al., 1987; Ignarro et al., 1987), which is formed within endothelial cells by the oxidative deamination of L-arginine (Palmer et al., 1988). The enzyme responsible, endothelial constitutive nitric oxide synthase, requires tetrahydrobiopterin as a cofactor and is regulated by protein kinase C. Inhibition of protein kinase C increases the expression of the synthase, resulting in an increased synthesis of nitric oxide (Ohara et al., 1995). The synthesis/release of nitric oxide is mediated directly by shear stress on the endothelial cells caused by the viscous drag that results from an increase in blood flow. There is a constant basal release under the stimulus of pulsatile blood flow. Nitric oxide is also synthesized and released in response to a large number of agents which activate endothelial surface receptors. These agents include local mediators (e.g. bradykinin, histamine and substance P), ADP released by aggregating platelets, and thrombin formed after activation of the coagulation cascade. The hormone noradrenaline, acting via endothelial α_2 adrenergic receptors, can also cause the release of nitric oxide. The calcium ionophore A23187 is an endothelium-dependent vasodilator that acts independently of a membrane receptor. With some agents, relaxation may be limited to certain animal species (Furchgott & Vanhoutte, 1989).

The nitric oxide generated in the endothelium diffuses to the underlying smooth muscle where it stimulates guanylyl cyclase to produce cyclic guanosine monophosphate (cyclic GMP). Relaxation of the smooth muscle may be effected through a cyclic GMP-dependent protein kinase which controls the phosphorylation and dephosphorylation of myosin light chains (Lüscher, 1991). Nitric oxide and prostacyclin act synergistically to cause relaxation because two different second messengers, cyclic GMP and cyclic AMP, are involved. Endothelium-derived hyperpolarizing factor may facilitate relaxation and attenuate the responsiveness of the smooth muscle to certain vasoconstrictor hormones (Lüscher, 1990). A simplified scheme of nitric oxide-mediated vascular relaxation in normal blood vessels is shown in Fig. 4.13.

Treatment of isolated segments of rabbit artery with pharmacological concentrations of acetylcholine causes nitric oxide-mediated vasodilation through the activation of muscarinic receptors on the endothelial cells. If the endothelial layer is removed from the segments, thereby removing the source of nitric oxide, the normal vasodilator response to acetylcholine is replaced by vasoconstriction resulting from the direct effect of this agent on the smooth muscle (Furchgott & Zawadski, 1980). This discovery has been regarded as an indication of a pathological mechanism rather than a physiological one because acetylcholine, as a neurotransmitter released from the periarterial nerves, is unlikely to diffuse all the way through the medial muscle coat before acting on endothelial cells. However, Burnstock (1987) demonstrated ultrastructural localization of choline acetyltransferase in endothelial cells in rabbit cerebral, femoral and mesenteric arteries, indicating that endothelial cells can synthesize acetylcholine and store it.

Hypercholesterolaemia and atherosclerosis profoundly impair endothelium-dependent arterial relaxation as demonstrated, for example, in the aortas of rabbits (Habib *et al.*, 1986; Verbeuren *et al.*, 1986), the iliac arteries of monkeys (Freiman *et al.*, 1986) and the coronary arteries of pigs (Shimokawa & Vanhoutte, 1989) and humans (Ludmer *et al.*, 1986; Bossaller *et al.*, 1987; Förstermann *et al.*, 1988a). Depletion of tetrahydrobiopterin, an essential cofactor for nitric oxide synthase, causes impaired nitric oxide generation (Schmidt *et al.*, 1992). Stroes *et al.* (1997) speculated that decreased nitric oxide-dependent vasodilation in hypercholesterolaemia could be related to a relative deficiency of tetrahydrobiopterin, resulting in impaired nitric oxide synthase activity. They then showed that tetrahydrobiopterin did indeed restore the disturbed nitric oxide-dependent vasodilation in patients with familial hypercholesterolaemia, at a stage when macrovascular disease had not yet occurred.

Ludmer *et al.* (1986) showed that the hypercontractility of diseased coronary arteries might be attributable to an abnormal vascular response to acetylcholine. Graded concentrations of acetylcholine and, for comparison, the endothelial-independent vasodilator glyceryl trinitrite were infused into a coronary artery of eight patients with advanced coronary stenoses (>50% narrowing), six patients with mild coronary atherosclerosis (<20% narrowing), and four control subjects with angiographically normal coronary arteries. Acetylcholine produced dilation in each of the normal coronary arteries. In contrast, all eight of the arteries with advanced stenosis and five of the six vessels with minimal disease showed dose-dependent

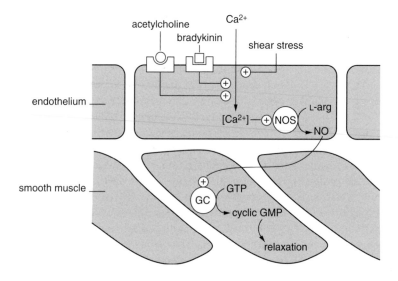

Fig. 4.13 Vascular relaxation mediated by nitric oxide. Shear stress or receptor activation of vascular endothelium by an agent such as bradykinin or acetylcholine results in an influx of calcium ions. The consequent increase in intracellular calcium stimulates the constitutive nitric oxide synthase (NOS). The nitric oxide (NO) formed from L-arginine (L-arg) by this enzyme diffuses to underlying smooth muscle cells, in which it stimulates the soluble guanylyl cyclase (GC), resulting in enhanced synthesis of cyclic GMP from guanosine triphosphate (GTP). This increase in cyclic GMP in the smooth muscle cells leads to their relaxation. Plus signs indicate stimulation. Reproduced from Moncada & Higgs (1993), copyright ©1993 Massachusetts Medical Society. All rights reserved.

constriction. All vessels dilated in response to glyceryl trinitrite.

Förstermann *et al.* (1988a) used isometric tension recording to study the effects of several vasodilators upon atherosclerotic coronary arteries excised from the hearts of cardiac transplantation patients. In most of the arteries, acetylcholine was a direct vasoconstrictor. Nitric oxide-mediated relaxations in response to substance P, bradykinin and Ca^{2+}-ionophore A23187 were significantly attenuated but not abolished. In de-endothelialized tissues these compounds had no effect. In contrast, endothelium-independent relaxation induced by isoprenaline was not affected by atherosclerosis. These observations suggest that the impaired relaxation in response to acetylcholine was specific for relaxation mediated by muscarinic receptors, as the activators of other receptor types still caused some degree of relaxation in atherosclerotic arteries.

Oxidized LDL causes impaired vasodilation by inhibiting the ability of arterial endothelial cells to release nitric oxide (Kugiyama *et al.*, 1990) and inactivating nitric oxide that is released (Chin *et al.* 1992). Oxidized LDL also stimulates the expression and release of the vasoconstrictor, endothelin, from vascular endothelium (Boulanger *et al.*, 1992). Ohgushi *et al.* (1993) showed that inhibition of protein kinase C activity with staurosporine or calphostin C prevented impairment of endothelial dysfunction by oxLDL, thereby implicating the kinase in the impairment. Ohgushi *et al.* (1993) further showed that lysolecithin was capable of activating protein kinase C. It can be concluded from these experiments that lysolecithin, formed and released during the oxidative modification of LDL, is transferred to the vascular endothelium where it activates protein kinase C. This enzyme in turn inhibits the release of nitric oxide, resulting in impaired relaxation of vascular smooth muscle in response to chemical mediators and shear stress.

Atherosclerotic arteries generate excessive amounts of oxygen-derived free radicals (Hennig & Chow, 1988) and these radicals likely contribute to endothelial dysfunction (Mügge *et al.*, 1991a,b). Nitric oxide is rapidly destroyed by superoxide anions (Gryglewski *et al.*, 1986) and the release of nitric oxide from endothelial cells depends on the activity of endothelial superoxide dismutase, the enzyme which converts superoxide to hydrogen peroxide and oxygen. Pre-treatment of rabbit aorta with an inhibitor of the dismutase, but not with inhibitors of other antioxidant defence mechanisms, markedly reduced endothelium-dependent relaxation in response to acetylcholine (Mügge *et al.*, 1991a). This finding suggests that inactivation of nitric oxide by intracellularly produced superoxide is normally prevented by intrinsic superoxide dismutase activity. It was further shown (Mügge *et al.*, 1991b) that treatment of cholesterol-fed rabbits with an assimilatable form of superoxide dismutase improved the impaired endothelium-dependent vasorelaxation in response to acetylcholine.

Interactions between platelets and the vascular endothelium

The vascular endothelium plays an important role in maintaining the normal fluidity of the blood. Among other mechanisms, this is achieved by the synthesis and release of anticoagulants (e.g. thrombomodulin), fibrinolytic (e.g. tissue plasminogen activator) and platelet inhibitory (e.g. nitric oxide, prostacyclin) substances.

Platelet aggregation is an essential process in preventing blood loss in the event of vascular injury, but it is equally important for platelets to circulate freely at other times. Platelets are easily activated so there is a potential danger of inappropriate aggregation. This is prevented by the action of nitric oxide and prostacyclin continuously released by the endothelial cells into the lumen of the blood vessel. The nitric oxide diffuses into the platelets and increases the concentration of cyclic GMP through activation of guanylyl cyclase. The cyclic GMP initiates a number of protein phosphorylation steps that finally lead to suppression of Ca^{2+} release from intracellular storage sites (Bassenge, 1991). The consequent inhibition of Ca^{2+} signalling limits platelet activity. Prostacyclin acts in a parallel manner to nitric oxide, except that the second messenger is cyclic AMP rather than cyclic GMP. Because their actions are mediated by different second messengers, there is synergism between nitric oxide and prostacyclin in inhibiting platelet aggregation. Thus, even when the concentrations of each are subthreshold, they are effective in combination. Unlike prostacyclin, nitric oxide also inhibits platelet adhesion.

At sites of injury, ADP released by aggregating platelets and thrombin formed during blood clotting stimulate the release of endothelial nitric oxide and prostacyclin, which act synergistically to cause relaxation of the vascular smooth muscle. Aggregating platelets also release vasoconstrictors such as serotonin, thromboxane A_2 and prostaglandin E_2. However, the endothelial nitric oxide produced in response to aggregating platelets normally overrides the direct vasoconstrictor effects of the platelet products and so the net effect is vasodilation (Förstermann *et al.*, 1988b). This effect of platelet aggregation and blood clotting upon the vascular endothelium constitutes a protective mechanism against vasospasm, which is associated with angina (Schroeder *et al.*, 1977). The release of endothelial inhibitors of platelet aggregation (nitric oxide and prostacyclin) in response to platelet aggregation controls adhesion and aggregation in the manner of negative feedback.

Shimokawa & Vanhoutte (1989) showed that endothelium-dependent relaxation in response to aggregating platelets is severely impaired in atherosclerosis and moderately impaired in hypercholesterolaemia. Thus endothelial damage or dysfunction shifts the balance of vasoactive compounds toward vasoconstriction, a state conducive to vasospasm. Under clinical conditions, the spasms can be complicated by thrombosis leading to vessel occlusion and myocardial infarction.

4.5.10 Protective effects of HDL

Epidemiological studies have generally shown a strong inverse correlation between plasma HDL concentration and incidence of coronary heart disease. The role of HDL in reverse-cholesterol transport is well established and many other protective effects against development of atherosclerosis have been reported (Barter & Rye, 1996). For example, HDL inhibits the oxidative modification of LDL; inhibits the transmigration of monocytes induced by oxLDL; blocks the induction by oxLDL of monocyte adhesion to the endothelium; prevents oxLDL-induced cytotoxicity in vascular smooth muscle cells and endothelial cells; removes cholesterol from cells in the arterial intima, thereby preventing the formation of foam cells; ameliorates the abnormal vasoconstriction that is a feature of early atherosclerosis; and stimulates prostacyclin synthesis and prolongs its half-life by binding to it.

Further reading

Diaz, M. N., Frei, B., Vita, J. A. & Keaney, J. F. Jr. (1997) Antioxidants and atherosclerotic heart disease. *New England Journal of Medicine*, **337**, 408–16.

Esterbauer, H., Gebicki, J., Puhl, H. & Jürgens, G. (1992) The role of lipid peroxidation and antioxidants in oxidative modification of LDL. *Free Radical Biology and Medicine*, **13**, 341–90.

Halliwell, B., Gutteridge, J. M. C. & Cross, C. E. (1992) Free radicals, antioxidants, and human disease: where are we now? *Journal of Laboratory and Clinical Medicine*, **119**, 598–620.

Loft, S. & Poulsen, H. E. (1996) Cancer risk and oxidative DNA damage in man. *Journal of Molecular Medicine*, **74**, 297–312.

Parthasarathy, S. & Rankin, S. M. (1992) Role of oxidized low density lipoprotein in atherogenesis. *Progress in Lipid Research*, **31**, 127–43.

Reaven, P. D. & Witztum, J. L. (1996) Oxidized low density lipoproteins in atherogenesis: role of dietary modification. *Annual Review of Nutrition*, **16**, 51–71.

Rubanyi, G. M. (1991) Endothelium-derived relaxing and contracting factors. *Journal of Cellular Biochemistry*, **46**, 27–36.

Schwartz, C. J., Valente, A. J., Sprague, E. A., Kelley, J. L. & Nerem, R. M. (1991) The pathogenesis of atherosclerosis: an overview. *Clinical Cardiology*, **14**, 1–16.

Steinberg, D. (1997) Oxidative modification of LDL and atherogenesis. *Circulation*, **95**, 1062–71.

Yu, B. P. (1994) Cellular defenses against damage from reactive oxygen species. *Physiological Reviews*, **74**, 139–62.

References

Aqel, N. M., Ball, R. Y., Waldmann, H. & Mitchinson, M. J. (1985) Identification of macrophages and smooth muscle cells in human atherosclerosis using monoclonal antibodies. *Journal of Pathology*, **146**, 197–204.

Aviram, M. (1995) LDL-platelet interaction under oxidative stress induces macrophage foam cell formation. *Thrombosis and Haemostasis*, **74**, 560–4.

Barter, P. J. & Rye, K.-A. (1996) High density lipoproteins and coronary heart disease. *Atherosclerosis*, **121**, 1–12.

Bassenge, E. (1991) Antiplatelet effects of endothelium-derived relaxing factor and nitric oxide donors. *European Heart Journal*, **12** (Supplement E), 12–15.

Beckman, J. S., Beckman, T. W., Chen, J., Marshall, P. A. & Freeman, B. A. (1990) Apparent hydroxyl radical production by peroxynitrite; implications for endothelial injury from nitric oxide and superoxide. *Proceedings of the National Academy of Sciences of the U.S.A.*, **87**, 1620–4.

Bedwell, S., Dean, R. T. & Jessup, W. (1989) The action of defined oxygen-centred free radicals on human low-density lipoprotein. *Biochemical Journal*, **262**, 707–12.

Berliner, J. A. & Heinecke, J. W. (1996) The role of oxidized lipoproteins in atherogenesis. *Free Radical Biology & Medicine*, **20**, 707–27.

Bossaller, C., Habib, G. B., Yamamoto, H., Williams, C., Wells, S. & Henry, P. D. (1987) Impaired muscarinic endothelium-dependent relaxation and cyclic guanosine 5′-monophosphate formation in atherosclerotic human coronary artery and rabbit aorta. *Journal of Clinical Investigation*, **79**, 170–4.

Boulanger, C. M., Tanner, F. C., Béa, M.-L., Hahn, A. W. A., Werner, A. & Lüscher, T. F. (1992) Oxidized low density lipoproteins induce mRNA expression and release of endothelin from human and porcine endothelium. *Circulation Research*, **70**, 1191–7.

Brand, K., Banka, C. L., Mackman, N., Terkeltaub, R. A., Fan, S.-T. & Curtiss, L. K. (1994) Oxidized LDL enhances lipopolysaccharide-induced tissue factor expression in human adherent monocytes. *Arteriosclerosis and Thrombosis*, **14**, 790–7.

Buettner, G. R. (1993) The pecking order of free radicals and antioxidants: lipid peroxidation, α-tocopherol, and ascorbate. *Archives of Biochemistry and Biophysics*, **300**, 535–43.

Burnstock, G. (1987) Mechanisms of interaction of peptide and nonpeptide vascular neurotransmitter systems. *Journal of Cardiovascular Pharmacology*, **10** (Suppl. 12), S74–S81.

Cathcart, M. K., Morel, D. W. & Chisholm, G. M. III (1985) Monocytes and neutrophils oxidize low density lipoprotein making it cytotoxic. *Journal of Leukocyte Biology*, **38**, 341–50.

Cestaro, B., Giuliani, A., Fabris, F. & Scarafiotti, C. (1997) Free radicals, atherosclerosis, ageing and related dysmetabolic pathologies: biochemical and molecular aspects. *European Journal of Cancer Prevention*, **6** (Suppl. 1), S25–S30.

Chatterjee, S. & Ghosh, N. (1996) Oxidized low density lipoprotein stimulates aortic smooth muscle cell proliferation. *Glycobiology*, **6**, 303–11.

Chin, J. H., Azhar, S. & Hoffman, B. B. (1992) Inactivation of endothelial derived relaxing factor by oxidized lipoprotein. *Journal of Clinical Investigation*, **89**, 10–18.

Collins, T. (1993) Endothelial nuclear factor-κβ and the initiation of the atherosclerotic lesion. *Laboratory Investigation*, **68**, 499–508.

Cominacini, L., Garbin, U., Pasini, A. F., Davoli, A., Campagnola, M., Contessi, G. B., Pastorino, A. M. & Cascio, V. L. (1997) Antioxidants inhibit the expression of intercellular cell adhesion molecule-1 and vascular cell adhesion molecule-1 induced by oxidized LDL on human umbilical vein endothelial cells. *Free Radical Biology and Medicine*, **22**, 117–27.

Cushing, S. D., Berliner, J. A., Valente, A. J., Territo, M. C., Navab, M., Parhami, F., Gerrity, R., Schwartz, C. J. & Fogelman, A. M. (1990) Minimally modified low density lipoprotein induces monocyte chemotactic protein 1 in human endothelial cells and smooth muscle cells. *Proceedings of the National Academy of Sciences of the U.S.A.*, **87**, 5134–8.

Cybulsky, M. I. & Gimbrone, M. A. Jr. (1991) Endothelial expression of a mononuclear leukocyte adhesion molecule during atherosclerosis. *Science*, **251**, 788–91.

Darley-Usmar, V. M., Hogg, N., O'Leary, V. J., Wilson, M. T. & Moncada, S. (1992) The simultaneous generation of superoxide and nitric oxide can initiate lipid peroxidation in human low density lipoprotein. *Free Radical Research Communications*, **17**, 9–20.

Förstermann, U., Mügge, A., Alheid, U., Haverich, A. & Frölich, J. C. (1988a) Selective attenuation of endothelium-mediated vasodilation in atherosclerotic human coronary arteries. *Circulation Research*, **62**, 185–90.

Förstermann, U., Mügge, A., Bode, S. M. & Frölich, J. C. (1988b) Response of human coronary arteries to aggregating platelets: importance of endothelium-derived relaxing factor and prostanoids. *Circulation Research*, **63**, 306–12.

Freiman, P. C., Mitchell, G. C., Heistad, D. D., Armstrong, M. L. & Harrison, D. G. (1986) Atherosclerosis impairs endothelium-dependent vascular relaxation to acetylcholine and thrombin in primates. *Circulation Research*, **58**, 783–9.

Frostegård, J., Wu, R., Haegerstrand, A., Patarroyo, M., Lefvert, A.-K. & Nilsson, J. (1993) Mononuclear leukocytes exposed to oxidized low density lipoprotein secrete a factor that stimulates endothelial cells to express adhesion molecules. *Atherosclerosis*, **103**, 213–19.

Furchgott, R. F. & Vanhoutte, P. M. (1989) Endothelium-derived relaxing and contracting factors. *FASEB Journal*, **3**, 2007–18.

Furchgott, R. F. & Zawadzki, J. V. (1980) The obligatory role of endothelial cells in the relaxation of arterial smooth muscle by acetylcholine. *Nature*, **288**, 373–6.

Galle, J., Bassenge, E. & Busse, R. (1990) Oxidized low density lipoproteins potentiate vasoconstrictions to various agonists by direct interaction with vascular smooth muscle. *Circulation Research*, **66**, 1287–93.

Giuliani, A. & Cestaro, B. (1997) Exercise, free radical generation and vitamins. *European Journal of Cancer Prevention*, **6** (Suppl. 1), S55–S67.

Goldstein, J. L. & Brown, M. S. (1987) Regulation of low-density lipoprotein receptors: implications for pathogenesis and therapy of hypercholesterolemia and atherosclerosis. *Circulation*, **76**, 504–7.

Goldstein, J. L., Ho, Y. K., Basu, S. K. & Brown, M. S. (1979) Binding site on macrophages that mediates uptake and degradation of acetylated low density lipoprotein, producing massive cholesterol deposition. *Proceedings of the National Academy of Sciences of the U.S.A.*, **76**, 333–7.

Graham, A., Hogg, N., Kalyanaraman, B., O'Leary, V., Darley-Usmar, V. & Moncada, S. (1993) Peroxynitrite modification of low-density lipoprotein leads to recognition by the macrophage scavenger receptor. *FEBS Letters*, **330**, 181–5.

Gryglewski, R. J., Palmer, R. M. J. & Moncada, S. (1986) Superoxide anion is involved in the breakdown of endothelial-derived vascular relaxing factor. *Nature*, **320**, 454–6.

Habib, J. B., Bossaller, C., Wells, S., Williams, C., Morrisett, J. D. & Henry, P. D. (1986) Preservation of endothelium-dependent vascular relaxation in cholesterol-fed rabbit by treatment with the calcium blocker PN 200110. *Circulation Research*, **58**, 305–9.

Halliwell, B. (1991) Reactive oxygen species in living systems: source, biochemistry, and role in human disease. *American Journal of Medicine*, **91** (Suppl. 3C), 14S–22S.

Hennig, B. & Chow, C. K. (1988) Lipid peroxidation and endothelial cell injury: implications in atherosclerosis. *Free Radical Biology & Medicine*, **4**, 99–106.

Henriksen, T., Evensen, S. A. & Carlander, B. (1979) Injury to human endothelial cells in culture induced by low density lipoproteins. *Scandinavian Journal of Clinical & Laboratory Investigation*, **39**, 361–8.

Hessler, J. R., Morel, D. W., Lewis, L. J. & Chisholm, G. M. (1983) Lipoprotein oxidation and lipoprotein-induced cytotoxicity. *Arteriosclerosis*, **3**, 215–22.

Hessler, J. R., Robertson, A. L. Jr. & Chisholm, G. M. III (1979) LDL-induced cytotoxicity and its inhibition by HDL in human vascular smooth muscle and endothelial cells in culture. *Atherosclerosis*, **32**, 213–29.

Hoff, H. F., Whitaker, T. E. & O'Neil, J. (1992) Oxidation of low density lipoprotein leads to particle aggregation and altered macrophage recognition. *Journal of Biological Chemistry*, **267**(1), 602–9.

Hughes, H., Mathews, B., Lenz, M. L. & Guyton, J. R. (1994) Cytotoxicity of oxidized LDL to porcine aortic smooth muscle cells is associated with the oxysterols 7-ketocholesterol and 7-hydroxycholesterol. *Arteriosclerosis and Thrombosis*, **14**, 1177–85.

Huie, R. E. & Padmaja, S. (1993) The reaction of NO with superoxide. *Free Radical Research Communications*, **18**, 195–9.

Ignarro, L. J., Buga, G. M., Wood, K. S., Byrns, R. E. & Chaudhuri, G. (1987) Endothelium-derived relaxing factor produced and released from artery and vein is nitric oxide. *Proceedings of the National Academy of Sciences of the U.S.A.*, **84**, 9265–9.

Jessup, W., Simpson, J. A. & Dean, R. T. (1993) Does superoxide radical have a role in macrophage-mediated oxidative modification of LDL? *Atherosclerosis*, **99**, 107–20.

Katzman, P. L., Bose, R., Henry, S., McLean, D. L., Walker, S., Fyfe, C., Perry, Y., Mymin, D. & Bolli, P. (1994) Serum lipid profile determines platelet reactivity to native and modified LDL-cholesterol in humans. *Thrombosis and Haemostasis*, **71**, 627–32.

Khoo, J. C., Miller, E., Pio, F., Steinberg, D. & Witztum, J. L. (1992)

Monoclonal antibodies against LDL further enhance macrophage uptake of LDL aggregates. *Arteriosclerosis and Thrombosis*, **12**, 1258–66.

Kohno, M., Yokokawa, K., Yasunari, K., Minami, M., Kano, H., Hanehira, T. & Yoshikawa, J. (1998) Induction by lysophosphatidylcholine, a major phospholipid component of atherogenic lipoproteins, of human coronary artery smooth muscle cell migration. *Circulation*, **98**, 353–9.

Kugiyama, K., Kerns, S. A., Morrisett, J. D., Roberts, R. & Henry, P. D. (1990) Impairment of endothelium-dependent arterial relaxation by lysolecithin in modified low-density lipoproteins. *Nature*, **344**, 160–2.

Kume, N., Cybulsky, M. I. & Gimbrone, M. A. Jr. (1992) Lysophosphatidylcholine, a component of atherogenic lipoproteins, induces mononuclear leukocyte adhesion molecules in cultured human and rabbit arterial endothelial cells. *Journal of Clinical Investigation*, **90**, 1138–44.

Laidlaw, S. A. & Kopple, J. D. (1987) Newer concepts of the indispensable amino acids. *American Journal of Clinical Nutrition*, **46**, 593–605.

Lawrence, R. A. & Burk, R. F. (1976) Glutathione peroxidase activity in selenium-deficient rat liver. *Biochemical and Biophysical Research Communications*, **71**, 952–8.

Levine, G. N., Keaney, J. F. Jr. & Vita, J. A. (1995) Cholesterol reduction in cardiovascular disease. *New England Journal of Medicine*, **332**, 512–21.

Liao, J. K., Shin, W. S., Lee, W. Y. & Clark, S. L. (1995) Oxidized low-density lipoprotein decreases the expression of endothelial nitric oxide synthase. *Journal of Biological Chemistry*, **270**(1), 319–24.

Ludmer, P. L., Selwyn, A. P., Shook, T. L., Wayne, R. R., Mudge, G. H., Alexander, R. W. & Ganz, P. (1986) Paradoxical vasoconstriction induced by acetylcholine in atherosclerotic coronary arteries. *New England Journal of Medicine*, **315**, 1046–51.

Lüscher, T. F. (1990) Imbalance of endothelium-derived relaxing and contracting factors. A new concept in hypertension? *American Journal of Hypertension*, **3**, 317–30.

Lüscher, T. F. (1991) Endothelium-derived nitric oxide: the endogenous nitrovasodilator in the human cardiovascular system. *European Heart Journal*, **12** (Suppl. E), 2–11.

McEver, R. P. (1992) Leukocyte–endothelial cell interactions. *Current Opinion in Cell Biology*, **4**, 840–9.

McMurray, H. F., Parthasarathy, S. & Steinberg, D. (1993) Oxidatively modified low density lipoprotein is a chemoattractant for human T lymphocytes. *Journal of Clinical Investigation*, **92**, 1004–8.

Mangin, E. L. Jr., Kugiyama, K., Nguy, J. H., Kerns, S. A. & Henry, P. D. (1993) Effects of lysolipids and oxidatively modified low density lipoprotein on endothelium-dependent relaxation of rabbit aorta. *Circulation Research*, **72**, 161–6.

Marcus, A. J. (1978) The role of lipids in platelet function: with particular reference to the arachidonic acid pathway. *Journal of Lipid Research*, **19**, 793–826.

Meydani, M. (1998) Nutrition, immune cells, and atherosclerosis. *Nutrition Reviews*, **56**, S177–82.

Minor, R. L. Jr., Myers, P. R., Guerra, R. Jr., Bates, J. N. & Harrison, D. G. (1990) Diet-induced atherosclerosis increases the release of nitrogen oxides from rabbit aorta. *Journal of Clinical Investigation*, **86**, 2109–16.

Moncada, S. & Higgs, A. (1993) The L-arginine–nitric oxide pathway. *New England Journal of Medicine*, **329**, 2002–12.

Morel, D. W., Hessler, J. R. & Chisolm, G. M. (1983) Low density lipoprotein cytotoxicity induced by free radical peroxidation of lipid. *Journal of Lipid Research*, **24**, 1070–6.

Mügge, A., Elwell, J. H., Peterson, T. E. & Harrison, D. G. (1991a)

Release of intact endothelium-derived relaxing factor depends on endothelial superoxide dismutase activity. *American Journal of Physiology*, **260**, C219–25.

Mügge, A., Elwell, J. H., Peterson, T. E., Hofmeyer, T. G., Heistad, D. D. & Harrison, D. G. (1991b) Chronic treatment with polyethylene-glycolated superoxide dismutase partially restores endothelium-dependent vascular relaxations in cholesterol-fed rabbits. *Circulation Research*, **69**, 1293–300.

Nelson, D. L. & Cox, M. M. (2000) *Lehninger. Principles of Biochemistry*, 3rd edn. Worth Publishers, New York.

Ohara, Y., Peterson, T. E. & Harrison, D. G. (1993) Hypercholesterolemia increases endothelial superoxide anion production. *Journal of Clinical Investigation*, **91**, 2546–51.

Ohara, Y., Peterson, T. E., Zheng, B., Kuo, J. F. & Harrison, D. G. (1994) Lysophosphatidylcholine increases vascular superoxide anion production via protein kinase C activation. *Arteriosclerosis and Thrombosis*, **14**, 1007–13.

Ohara, Y., Sayegh, H. S., Yamin, J. J. & Harrison, D. G. (1995) Regulation of endothelial constitutive nitric oxide synthase by protein kinase C. *Hypertension*, **25**, 415–20.

Ohgushi, M., Kugiyama, K., Fukunaga, K., Murohara, T., Sugiyama, S., Miyamoto, E. & Yasue, H. (1993) Protein kinase C inhibitors prevent impairment of endothelium-dependent relaxation by oxidatively modified LDL. *Arteriosclerosis and Thrombosis*, **13**, 1525–32.

Palinski, W., Tangirala, R. K., Miller, E., Young, S. G. & Witztum, J. L. (1995) Increased autoantibody titers against epitopes of oxidized LDL in LDL receptor-deficient mice with increased atherosclerosis. *Arteriosclerosis, Thrombosis, and Vascular Biology*, **15**, 1569–76.

Palmer, R. M. J., Ferrige, A. G. & Moncada, S. (1987) Nitric oxide release accounts for the biological activity of endothelium-derived relaxing factor. *Nature*, **327**, 524–6.

Palmer, R. M. J., Ashton, D. S. & Moncada, S. (1988) Vascular endothelial cells synthesize nitric oxide from L-arginine. *Nature*, **333**, 664–6.

Parthasarathy, S. & Barnett, J. (1990) Phospholipase A_2 activity of low density lipoprotein: evidence for an intrinsic phospholipase A_2 activity of apoprotein B-100. *Proceedings of the National Academy of Sciences of the U.S.A.*, **87**, 9741–5.

Picard, S., Parthasarathy, S., Fruebis, J. & Witztum, J. L. (1992) Aminoguanidine inhibits oxidative modification of low density lipoprotein and the subsequent increase in uptake by macrophage scavenger receptors. *Proceedings of the National Academy of Sciences of the U.S.A.*, **89**, 6876–80.

Quinn, M. T., Parthasarathy, S. & Steinberg, D. (1985) Endothelial cell-derived chemotactic activity for mouse peritoneal macrophages and the effects of modified forms of low density lipoprotein. *Proceedings of the National Academy of Sciences of the U.S.A.*, **82**, 5949–53.

Quinn, M. T., Parthasarathy, S. & Steinberg, D. (1988) Lysophosphatidylcholine: a chemotactic factor for human monocytes and its potential role in atherosclerosis. *Proceedings of the National Academy of Sciences of the U.S.A.*, **85**, 2805–9.

Radi, R., Beckman, J. S., Bush, K. M. & Freeman, B. A. (1991) Peroxynitrite-induced membrane lipid peroxidation; the cytotoxic potential of superoxide and nitric oxide. *Archives of Biochemistry and Biophysics*, **288**, 481–7.

Rajavashisth, T. B., Andalibi, A., Territo, M. C., Berliner, J. A., Navab, M., Fogelman, A. M. & Lusis, A. J. (1990) Induction of endothelial cell expression of granulocyte and macrophage colony-stimulating factors by modified low-density lipoproteins. *Nature*, **344**, 254–7.

Reid, V. C. & Mitchinson, M. J. (1993) Toxicity of oxidized low density lipoprotein towards mouse peritoneal macrophages in vitro.

Atherosclerosis, **98**, 17–24.

Reid, V. C., Mitchinson, M. J. & Skepper, J. N. (1993) Cytotoxicity of oxidized low-density lipoprotein to mouse peritoneal macrophages: an ultrastructural study. *Journal of Pathology*, **171**, 321–8.

Salonen, J. T., Ylä-Herttuala, S., Yamamoto, R., Butler, S., Korpela, H., Salonen, R., Nyyssönen, K., Palinski, W. & Witztum, J. L. (1992) Autoantibody against oxidized LDL and progression of carotid atherosclerosis. *Lancet*, **339**, 883–7.

Schmidt, K., Werner, E. R., Mayer, B., Wachter, H. & Kukovetz, W. R. (1992) Tetrahydrobiopterin-dependent formation of endothelium-derived relaxing factor (nitric oxide) in aortic endothelial cells. *Biochemical Journal*, **281**, 297–300.

Schroeder, J. S., Bolen, J. L., Quint, R. A., Clark, D. A., Hayden, W. G., Higgins, C. B. & Wexler, L. (1977) Provocation of coronary spasm with ergonovine maleate. *American Journal of Cardiology*, **40**, 487–91.

Shanahan, C. M., Proudfoot, D., Farzaneh-Far, A. & Weissberg, P. L. (1998) The role of Gla proteins in vascular calcification. *Critical Reviews in Eukaryotic Gene Expression*, **8**, 357–75.

Shimokawa, H. & Vanhoutte, P. M. (1989) Impaired endothelium-dependent relaxation to aggregating platelets and related vasoactive substances in porcine coronary arteries in hypercholesterolemia and atherosclerosis. *Circulation Research*, **64**, 900–14.

Steinbrecher, U. P., Parthasarathy, S., Leake, D. S., Witztum, J. L. & Steinberg, D. (1984) Modification of low density lipoprotein by endothelial cells involves lipid peroxidation and degradation of low density lipoprotein phospholipids. *Proceedings of the National Academy of Sciences of the U.S.A.*, **81**, 3883–7.

Storz, G., Tartaglia, L. A. & Ames, B. N. (1990) Transcriptional regulator of oxidative stress-inducible genes: direct activation by oxidation. *Science*, **248**, 189–94.

Stroes, E., Kastelein, J., Cosentino, F., Erkelens, W., Wever, R., Koomans, H., Lüscher, T. & Rabelink, T. (1997) Tetrahydrobiopterin restores endothelial function in hypercholesterolemia. *Journal of Clinical Investigation*, **99**, 41–6.

Thorin, E., Hamilton, C. A., Dominiczak, M. H. & Reid, J. L. (1994) Chronic exposure of cultured bovine endothelial cells to oxidized LDL abolishes prostacyclin release. *Arteriosclerosis and Thrombosis*, **14**, 453–9.

Verbeuren, T. J., Jordaens, F. H., Zonnekeyn, L. L., Van Hove, C. E., Coene, M.-C. & Herman, A. G. (1986) Effect of hypercholesterolemia on vascular reactivity in the rabbit. I. Endothelium-dependent and endothelium-independent contractions and relaxations in isolated arteries of control and hypercholesterolemic rabbits. *Circulation Research*, **58**, 552–64.

Watson, K. E. (2000) Pathophysiology of coronary calcification. *Journal of Cardiovascular Risk*, **7**, 93–7.

White, C. R., Brock, T. A., Chang, L.-Y., Crapo, J., Briscoe, P., Ku, D., Bradley, W. A., Gianturco, S. H, Gore, J., Freeman, B. A. & Tarpey, M. M. (1994) Superoxide and peroxynitrite in atherosclerosis. *Proceedings of the National Academy of Sciences of the U.S.A.*, **91**, 1044–8.

Ylä-Herttuala, S., Palinski, W., Butler, S. W., Picard, S., Steinberg, D. & Witztum, J. L. (1994) Rabbit and human atherosclerotic lesions contain IgG that recognizes epitopes of oxidized LDL. *Arteriosclerosis and Thrombosis*, **14**, 32–40.

Yui, S., Sasaki, T., Miyazaki, A., Horiuchi, S. & Yamazaki, M. (1993) Induction of murine macrophage growth by modified LDLs. *Arteriosclerosis and Thrombosis*, **13**, 331–7.

5
Background Immunology

Key discussion topics

- The human immune system has two components: a ready-made innate immunity that relies largely on phagocytosis of pathogenic microorganisms, and a longer-term, more specific acquired immunity that has a 'memory'.
- Phagocytic leucocytes (e.g. neutrophils, monocytes and macrophages) internalize pathogenic microorganisms and kill them by the release of toxic products into cytoplasmic vacuoles.
- The acquired immune response is mediated by two main types of lymphocyte; cytotoxic T lymphocytes combat intracellular viruses and other pathogens; antibody-producing B lymphocytes combat pathogens occurring freely in the body fluids.
- Antibody molecules (immunoglobulins) attach to pathogens and recruit effector cells to destroy the pathogens.
- The protein components of the complement system mediate several effector mechanisms of the immune response.
- Cytokines are short-acting signalling molecules that affect the function of cells of the immune system and other systems of the body.

5.1 General features of the immune system

Immunity refers to the body's resistance to invasive pathogens (viruses, bacteria, fungi, protozoa and multicellular parasites) or their toxic products, to allergens (pollen, animal hair, chemicals, etc.) and to unwanted cells or cell products arising within the body from cancer or autoimmune diseases. The immune system comprises (1) cellular defence mechanisms mediated by several types of leucocytes and (2) humoral defence mechanisms mediated by soluble proteins, so-called because they are dissolved in the body fluids rather than being primarily associated with cells. Any immune response involves, firstly, recognition of the pathogen or other foreign material and, secondly, elimination of these invaders. When an immune response occurs in an exaggerated or inappropriate form, the term 'hypersensitivity' is applied. The fundamental concept underlying the function of the immune system is the ability to distinguish, at the molecular level, 'self' from 'non-self' (foreign) materials.

All cells of the immune system originate from just one cell type in the bone marrow of adult mammals, the haemopoietic stem cell. These pluripotent cells give rise to two main lineages: (1) the lymphoid lineage produces lymphocytes and (2) the myeloid lineage produces mononuclear and polymorphonuclear phagocytes, megakaryocytes (precursors of platelets) and mast cells. The precise origin of natural killer cells and dendritic cells is uncertain, although they do develop ultimately from haemopoietic stem cells.

With regard to pathogens, the immune response depends on the site of infection and the nature of the pathogen. All viruses, some bacteria and some protozoan parasites replicate inside host cells, whereas many bacteria and larger parasites replicate in extracellular spaces and body fluids. To clear an intracellular infection, it is necessary to destroy the infected host cells. Extracellular pathogens are selectively destroyed and their toxic products neutralized.

Immune responses may be either innate (natural) or acquired (adaptive). Innate immunity, being genetically determined, is present from birth and is in full readiness for an attack by invading pathogens. The innate defence mechanisms act non-specifically against a wide range of microorganisms and foreign material and can be mobilized at the site of infection within hours. The main characteristics and components of innate immunity occur in the inflammatory response. There is no immunological memory; that is, the response is not dependent upon prior exposure to a particular infectious agent.

Acquired immunity is not immediately ready to combat a foreign invader that has never previously entered the body; it develops over a long period only after invasion by a novel intruder. However, once an acquired immune response has occurred, the body acquires the capacity to recognize and destroy that particular invader very rapidly the next time it is encountered, and the individual is now said to be immune to

it. Not only is there an immunological memory, but the response to the particular invader on subsequent occasions is much more vigorous and effective than the response to the first encounter.

It is well documented that a decline in immune function takes place with advancing age (Walford, 1980).

5.2   Innate immunity

Innate immunity is conferred by the physical barriers of the skin and mucous membranes and by cellular and humoral defence mechanisms.

5.2.1   Barriers imposed by the skin and mucous membranes

Intact skin is a resistant barrier because the outer horny layer of keratin is impenetrable to most microorganisms. The skin is further protected by sebaceous secretions and sweat which contain bactericidal and fungicidal fatty acids. In the respiratory tract, mucus containing entrapped particles is constantly being swept by the action of cilia towards the oropharynx where it is swallowed. The acidic pH of the stomach contents destroys most microorganisms.

5.2.2   Cells of the innate immune system

The cell types involved in the innate immune system include phagocytes, natural killer cells, mast cells and platelets.

Phagocytes
Phagocytic leucocytes are classified into two main types, according to the shape of their nuclei. Mononuclear phagocytes have a simple-shaped nucleus and polymorphonuclear phagocytes or granulocytes have a bi- or multi-lobed nucleus. Phagocytes engulf foreign particles such as bacteria, internalize them and destroy them in a two-stage process. Firstly, the phagocyte is stimulated to generate lethal reactive oxidants in a biochemical process known as the respiratory burst; secondly, the phagocyte releases a large number of enzymes and other bioactive molecules from intracellular storage granules called lysosomes. This release of lysosomal products is known as degranulation. The lysosomal products are responsible for digesting the bacteria which have been killed by the reactive oxidants.

Mononuclear phagocytes

These cell types include macrophages and their precursors, monocytes. Monocytes circulate in the blood but in time they migrate to the tissues where they differentiate into macrophages.

Polymorphonuclear phagocytes

These cell types are subdivided into neutrophils, basophils and eosinophils on the basis of the affinity of their granules for the acidic and basic dyes used in histology. Neutrophils [commonly referred to in the literature as PMN (polymorphonuclear leucocytes)] outnumber by far all other types of phagocyte in human peripheral blood. Eosinophils are particularly effective against extracellular parasites. Basophils are not obviously phagocytic, their main function being secretion of soluble molecules that mediate inflammatory responses.

Macrophages

These cells are able to carry out a remarkable array of different functions and are an important link between the innate and acquired immune systems. In the absence of a stimulus, macrophages remain relatively quiescent at a particular site and in this state they are known as resident macrophages. Resident macrophages line the body cavities and blood capillaries where they can make early contact with invading pathogens. They acquire characteristic morphologies and specialized functions depending on where they are localized. Examples of resident macrophages are Kupffer cells (liver), osteoclasts (bone), microglia (brain), mesangial cells (kidney), alveolar macrophages (lung) and peritoneal macrophages (lining the peritoneal cavity). Resident macrophages possess a variety of cell surface receptors which allow them to respond to specific stimuli very rapidly. A variety of inflammatory agents stimulate the resident macrophages to develop into inflammatory macrophages, which express a greater number of receptors and secrete in copious amounts a variety of products involved in the inflammation process. Among these products are protein components of the complement system, various coagulation factors and proteolytic enzymes. Both resident and inflammatory macrophages can be stimulated during acquired immune responses to become activated macrophages, now with a greatly enhanced ability to destroy certain pathogens and some types of tumour cells.

Natural killer cells

Found in blood, liver and spleen, these large non-phagocytic cells kill virally infected host cells and tumour cells extracellularly by the spontaneous release of various cytotoxic molecules. Perforins and cytolysins insert themselves into the plasma membrane of target cells where they polymerize to form transmembrane pores. The passage of ions through these pores disturbs the osmotic equilibrium and water rapidly enters the cell, causing the cell to swell and eventually burst. Other molecules enter the target cell and cause apoptosis by enhanced fragmentation of its nuclear DNA. Recognition of target cells is aided by receptors to glycoproteins which appear on the target cell membrane following viral infection or oncogenic transformation.

Mast cells

The cytoplasm of these cells is full of membrane-bound granules containing a variety of preformed mediators that produce inflammation in surrounding tissues. It is mainly the mast cells that release vasoactive amines (e.g. histamine and bradykinin) during acute inflammation. Mast cells are often situated next to arterioles, so that the amines can immediately cause vasodilation when released in response to injury or infection.

Platelets

These are fragments of megakaryocytes, which pass from the bone marrow into the bloodstream. Platelets contribute to the inflammatory response through the release of vasoactive amines and various cytokines. The role of platelets in haemostasis is discussed in Section 4.4.2.

5.2.3   Phagocytosis

Circulating phagocytes are directed to the site of infection by chemotaxis and attach to the surface of the particle to be engulfed. They recognize a particle as being foreign usually because the particle has been coated (opsonized) with an opsonin, which binds to a specific receptor on the surface of the phagocyte. The C3b fragment of the C3 complement protein is such an opsonin (Section 5.2.6). The edges of the plasma membrane around the points of attachment extend outward to engulf the particle, finally enclosing it within a vacuole called the phagosome. The energy required for particle engulfment is derived from glycolysis (Selvaraj & Sbarra, 1966). Actin and other contractile fibrils in the cytoplasm surround the phagosome around its outer edge, pushing it to the interior. When the phagocyte is activated by any one of a number of signal molecules, an unusual enzyme, NADPH oxidase, comes into play. This enzyme, which is bound to the phagosome membrane and to the plasma membrane, begins to generate superoxide – a precursor of several microbicidal oxidants. Almost simultaneously, the membrane of the phagosome fuses with the unit membrane of adjacent lysosomes, the fused membranes rupture, and the lysosomal contents are discharged into the enlarged vacuole, now called a phagolysosome. Lysosomal contents also leak into the extracellular fluid, with the potential for damage to local host cells.

The selective discharge of lysosomal enzymes (but not cytoplasmic enzymes) from human neutrophils in response to immunological stimuli is regulated by the opposing actions of intracellular cyclic GMP and cyclic AMP (Ignarro & George, 1974). Cyclic GMP, in the presence of calcium, mediates the discharge of lysosomal enzymes, whereas cyclic AMP inhibits the discharge. Many cellular functions are similarly regulated by the opposing effects of these two cyclic nucleotides. Cellular concentrations of cyclic GMP and cyclic AMP, and thus cellular functions, can be influenced by hormones and neurotransmitters. For example, acetylcholine promotes the accumulation of cyclic GMP and thus enhances lysosomal enzyme discharge, while adrenaline and histamine promote the accumulation of cyclic AMP and inhibit enzyme discharge.

The respiratory burst

The toxic reactive oxidants produced by phagocytes fall into two classes: oxidizing radicals, such as the hydroxyl radical ($^\bullet$OH), and oxidized halogens, such as hypochlorous acid (HOCl). The oxidants are generated ultimately from oxygen, which is converted to superoxide ($O_2^{\bullet-}$) through a metabolic pathway aptly called the respiratory burst. As far as is known, this pathway is unique to phagocytes. Activation of NADPH oxidase reduces molecular oxygen to superoxide by electron transfer from NADPH. The increased oxygen consumption is due to the oxidation of glucose-6-phosphate via the hexose monophosphate shunt to produce the required NADPH.

$$2O_2 + NADPH \rightarrow 2O_2^{\bullet-} + NADP^+ + H^+ \quad (5.1)$$

The phagocytes are stimulated to initiate the respiratory burst by many agents, including opsonized particles, the complement fragment C5a, leukotriene B_4 (produced by stimulated phagocytes) and N-formylated oligopeptides of bacterial origin that are actively secreted or are released by lysis of dead organisms (Babior, 1984).

The superoxide dismutates to hydrogen peroxide which, being relatively stable, diffuses to more distant sites and extends the range of antimicrobial action. Superoxide and hydrogen peroxide are only moderately reactive and the cellular damage resulting from the respiratory burst is due to the conversion of either products to more highly reactive oxidants. For example, hydrogen peroxide breaks down in the presence of free transition metal ions (e.g. Fe^{2+}) to produce the highly reactive hydroxyl radical; this is lethal to many pathogens, including large parasites that the phagocytes cannot engulf.

Lysozyme

Lysozyme, one of the lysosomal enzymes released by phagocytes, lyses bacteria by splitting sugars off the peptidoglycan component of the bacterial cell wall. Gram-positive bacteria (e.g. *Staphylococcus aureus*) are easily lysed by lysozyme, as their cell wall is composed almost exclusively of peptidoglycan. Pure cultures of Gram-negative bacteria (e.g. *Escherichia coli*), on the other hand, are resistant to lysis because their surface layers of lipopolysaccharides, proteins and lipids make the underlying peptidoglycan inaccessible to the lysozyme. Nevertheless, Gram-negative bacteria are killed by phagocytes. Studies by Miller (1969) suggest that reactive oxidants generated by the respiratory burst during phagocytosis disrupt the integrity of the outermost layer of Gram-negative bacteria, allowing lysozyme to reach its substrate. The reactive oxidants cause bacterial death and the effects of lysozyme permit subsequent digestion of the dead bacterium.

The myeloperoxidase–hydrogen peroxide–halide system

The lysosomes of most phagocytes, with the notable exception of macrophages, contain peroxidases that catalyse the formation of hypochlorous acid (HOCl) from hydrogen peroxide produced by dismutation of superoxide during the oxidative burst of phagocytosis.

$$H_2O_2 + H^+ + Cl^- \rightarrow HOCl + H_2O \qquad (5.2)$$

Theoretically, any of the halides (Cl^-, Br^-, I^-) and the pseudohalide (SCN^-) can participate in reaction 5.2. Chloride is most probably used at most sites in the body because its plasma concentration is more than a thousand times that of the other halides.

In the case of neutrophils and monocytes, the enzyme is myeloperoxidase, whereas in eosinophils it is eosinophil peroxidase; macrophages contain neither of these peroxides. The hypochlorous acid damages invading catalase-negative microorganisms by oxidizing a wide range of biomolecules (e.g. thiols and amino compounds), destroying the biological activity of nucleotides such as ATP, and inactivating certain redox enzymes (e.g. haem-containing enzymes). Catalase-positive microorganisms are able to prevent the formation of hypochlorous acid and thus are not susceptible to attack by this oxidant.

Chloramines

Hypochlorous acid reacts rapidly and spontaneously with primary or secondary amines that are either released from the neutrophil itself or are present in the surrounding medium, thus generating a family of chloramines. In general, chloramines are less powerful oxidants than hypochlorous acid itself, but they are able to chlorinate or oxidize a wide range of target molecules (Weiss, 1989).

$$R'RNH + HOCl \rightarrow R'RNCl + H_2O \qquad (5.3)$$

Nitric oxide

Phagocytes, including macrophages, can produce nitric oxide, which is toxic to bacteria and tumour cells. Cytotoxicity is attributable to the nitric oxide combining with iron-containing moieties in enzymes concerned with DNA synthesis and essential metabolic processes in the target cells.

5.2.4   Self-protection of phagocytes

The phagocytes themselves are susceptible to attack by the reactive oxidants that they produce. However, they are able to defend themselves against self-destruction, at least to a limited extent. The antioxidant systems of the phagocytes include superoxide dismutase, which converts superoxide to oxygen and hydrogen peroxide; catalase and glutathione peroxidase, both of which reduce hydrogen peroxide to water; and other antioxidants, such as α-tocopherol and ascorbic acid. These systems protect neutrophils long enough for them to deliver their lethal cocktail of toxins to extracellular and phagocytosed pathogens, but after phagocytosis the neutrophils die. Macrophages live much longer than neutrophils and can phagocytose during their whole life span by resynthesis of lysosomal enzymes. Macrophages are therefore better protected against self-destruction, possibly by their ascorbic acid content, which is about twice as high as that of neutrophils and monocytes (Schmidt & Moser, 1985).

5.2.5   Defects of phagocytic cell function

Chronic granulomatous disease

The importance of the respiratory burst as a means of destroying pathogens is underlined by the appearance of chronic granulomatous disease (CGD). This disease is caused by a genetic defect of NADPH oxidase in phagocytes and consequent failure to generate superoxide. The disease manifests as excessive susceptibility to pathogenic organisms positive for catalase. Catalase-negative organisms are not a problem because they cannot detoxify the hydrogen peroxide they produce during growth; therefore, these organisms are quickly eliminated. Patients with CGD typically develop serious infections with *Staphylococcus aureus*, Gram-negative bacilli and fungi, but not with routine upper respiratory bacterial pathogens or usual childhood viral pathogens (Wolf & Keusch, 1999).

Chediak–Higashi syndrome

Patients with the Chediak–Higashi syndrome suffer frequent and severe pus-forming infections that are secondary to impaired microbicidal activity of neutrophils. This impairment appears to be related to delayed delivery of lysosomal contents into phagosomes and may arise from abnormal assembly of microtubules. The diminished chemotaxis observed in the syndrome may also be caused by impaired microtubular function (Boxer *et al.*, 1976). There is experimental evidence suggesting a functional link between chemotactic activation as well as degranulation of phagocytes and post-translational fixation of tyrosine into the alpha-chain of tubulin catalysed by tyrosine ligase (Schmidt & Moser, 1985).

5.2.6 Humoral defence mechanisms

Among the many substances in extracellular fluids which destroy microorganisms, complement, interferons and acute phase proteins are produced in response to infection.

Complement

Complement is a collective term for at least 25 proteins that indirectly elicit various biological effects upon the immune system. These complement components are produced primarily in the liver and circulate in the blood and extracellular fluid, normally in low concentration. The circulating components are present in their inactive, precursor forms. There are two pathways of complement activation, the classical and the alternative. Although both pathways share some common components, they differ in the ways in which they are initiated. The classical pathway requires antigen–antibody complexes for initiation, and therefore defends the body against a specific invader. The alternative pathway is initiated by various substances, including the cell walls of some bacteria; it therefore has a non-specific defensive role.

The protein components of the classical pathway of activation are each assigned a number and react in the order: C1q, C1r, C1s, C4, C2, C3, C5, C6, C7, C8 and C9. Binding of antigen to antibody unmasks a specific reactive site on the antibody, which in turn binds directly with the first component, C1q. This sets into motion a cascade reaction, with each component sequentially acting on others. A number of the proteins involved are split into two fragments, designated a and b fragments, by the product of the previous step. The early components of the alternative pathway are known as factors and are identified by single letters. C3 participates in both pathways and is cleaved by separate convertases to C3a and C3b (Fig. 5.1). The binding of C3b to the surfaces of microorganisms and antigen–antibody complexes stimulates the cleavage of more C3 by positive feedback, resulting in the rapid deposition of many molecules of C3b. The binding of C3b to a surface is the key step in the distinction of self from non-self by complement. Self cell surfaces are protected by molecules that effectively limit C3b deposition; non-self surfaces lack such proteins.

In the later stages of activation, the alternative pathway uses identical components to the classical pathway, i.e. components C5 through to C9. The terminal reaction sequence is non-enzymatic and produces a complex comprising components C5b and C6–C9 (designated C5b6789). This end-product, known as the membrane-attack complex, has a direct effect of lysing the cell membranes of a variety of bacteria and viruses. The binding of C7 to C5b6 during complex assembly marks the transition of the complex from a hydrophilic to a hydrophobic state. This allows C5b67 to be inserted into the membrane lipid bilayer at the focus of complement activation. Formation of the pore-forming macromolecule is completed by the binding of C8, followed by a stepwise addition of up to 14 C9 monomers.

Specific stages of the complement activation cascade are controlled by regulatory molecules. In addition, a number of proteins present in body fluids prevent lysis of healthy cells by binding to fluid phase

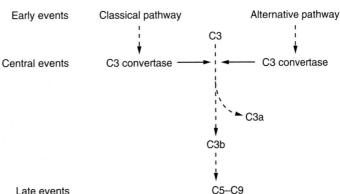

Fig. 5.1 The two pathways for complement activation.

C5b67. The cells of the host's immune system can endocytose and exocytose portions of membrane containing membrane-attack complex and are thus relatively resistant to lysis.

The membrane-attack complex is effective in lysing most, but not all, Gram-negative bacteria. Gram-positive bacteria are generally resistant because the thick peptidoglycan layer in their cell wall prevents insertion of the membrane-attack complex into the lipid bilayer. Viruses, being enveloped in a membrane that is largely derived from the plasma membrane of the infected host cell, are susceptible to complement-mediated lysis.

In addition to producing cell lysis, activation of the complement system yields fragments of components that possess various important biological activities. The amplification that occurs with C3 activation results in a coating of C3b on antigens (e.g. bacteria) and on antigen–antibody complexes. Phagocytic cells carry receptors for C3b and are therefore able to recognize and bind the coated particles (Fig. 5.2). Thus the coating of foreign particles by fragments of complement proteins results in the particles being phagocytosed more readily and ultimately destroyed. This process – enhancement of phagocytosis by the deposition of an opsonin (e.g. C3b) on the antigen – is known as opsonization. Phagocytosis is further aided by adherence of the coated particles to the endothelium of blood vessels. Encapsulated bacteria such as *Streptococcus pneumoniae* evade phagocytosis because the capsule prevents interaction between C3b deposited on the cell membrane and the CR1 receptor on phagocytic cells.

Two small fragments of complement proteins, C3a and C5a, bind to receptors on mast cells and induce degranulation. The release of histamine and other vasoactive mediators from the granules contributes to the inflammatory response. Fragment C5a also causes chemotactic migration of neutrophils and macrophages toward the site of complement activation.

Interferons

Interferons are included among the cytokines – soluble proteins that act as signalling molecules between different types of cells (Section 5.5). Interferons (specifically IFN-α and -β) induce a state of antiviral resistance in uninfected tissue cells. When a cell is infected with a virus, it secretes interferon which then binds to receptors on uninfected neighbouring cells. This binding of interferon induces the synthesis of enzymes that inhibit translation and destroy mRNA, therefore the virus cannot replicate. The virally infected cell is thus isolated from healthy cells and the virus is unable to spread.

Acute phase proteins

Acute phase proteins are so-called because their normally low concentrations in serum can rise over 1000-fold during an infection. They are processed in the liver in response to stimulation by cytokines such as interleukin-1. Interleukin-1 in turn is produced by macrophages in response to stimulation by microbial products such as lipopolysaccharide (endotoxin). One important acute phase protein is C-reactive protein which binds to the phosphorocholine residues in the

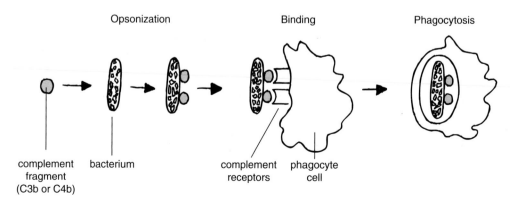

Fig. 5.2 Steps in the uptake of a particle such as a bacterium opsonized by a fragment of complement protein.

cell wall of certain microorganisms and is very efficient at activating the classical complement pathway.

5.3 Inflammation

Inflammation is the manifestation of the body's response to tissue injury, whether caused by infection, physical trauma, chemicals or heat. It is often considered in terms of acute inflammation and chronic inflammation. The inflammatory response is immensely complex and no attempt is made here to describe it in full. We will focus instead upon the physiological actions of selected inflammatory mediators that have relevance to the immunogenic properties of certain vitamins (vitamins A, D, E, B_6 and C; see relevant chapters).

5.3.1 The inflammatory response

The purpose of an inflammatory response is to bring fluid, proteins and cells from the blood into the damaged tissues, where they effect host defence and repair. The main events that facilitate this are dilation of the arterioles to increase blood flow to the affected area; increased permeability of venules, which allows plasma fluid to pass through the endothelium; and migration of leucocytes across venular endothelium to the site of injury. The classical signs of inflammation – redness, heat, swelling and pain – are a direct result of these events.

The acute vascular response to infection takes place within seconds of the initial stimulus, and lasts for some minutes. Mast cells are stimulated to release preformed molecules from storage granules. Some of these molecules (e.g. histamine) are vasoactive, while others are chemotactic. Platelets also release vasoactive amines, as well as coagulation factors which lead to localized fibrin deposition.

The acute cellular response takes place over the next few hours. The first of the phagocytic cells to act are the resident macrophages already present in the affected area. When stimulated by products from the inflamed tissue, these cells enlarge and break away from their attachments, once again becoming mobile macrophages with phagocytic activity. Polymorphonuclear phagocytes (mainly neutrophils) from the bloodstream arrive on the scene by the controlled process of migration. In this process, capillary endothelial cells close to

inflammation sites are induced to produce adhesion molecules on their luminal surface. The phagocytes passing through the capillaries also have adhesion molecules on their surface. Interaction between the respective adhesion molecules causes the phagocytes to stick to the endothelium. The phagocytes are then activated to squeeze between the endothelial cells and to secrete collagenases and other enzymes in order to 'digest' their way through the basal lamina. Having now reached the tissue, the phagocytes are guided to the inflammation zone by chemotactic molecules. Cells of inflamed tissues increase their synthesis of heat shock proteins in response to the thermal stress, despite a decrease in total protein synthesis.

If the infection is sufficiently severe, a chronic cellular response may follow over the next few days. Circulating monocytes arrive and enlarge to become macrophages. More leucocytes are made available through mobilization of bone marrow stores. Finally, after days or weeks, in-growth of fibrous tissue helps in the healing process.

If the inflammatory response is unable to destroy the infectious agent or to completely remove all of the accumulated products, the affected area is walled off from the surrounding healthy tissue by granulomatous tissue. A ball of cells known as a granuloma is formed when macrophages and lymphocytes, and later epithelioid cells and giant cells, surround the affected area.

Inflammatory diseases such as rheumatoid arthritis arise because the host's immune system fails in some way to regulate the inflammatory response.

5.3.2 Mediators of the inflammatory response

The inflammatory response is mediated by chemicals released from cells of the tissue and from cells of the immune system. An important early phase mediator is histamine, which is released from the storage granules of mast cells and also by platelets within seconds of initiation. Later, about 6–12 hours after initiation, vascular events are mediated by prostaglandins and leukotrienes, which are products of arachidonic acid metabolism. These molecules are newly synthesized and secreted by a wide variety of cell types in response to an appropriate stimulus. Cytokines (Section 5.5) are important in signalling between cells as inflammatory reactions develop.

Histamine

Histamine induces relaxation of the smooth muscle walls of pre-capillary arterioles, causing the vessels to dilate and thereby increasing blood flow; this produces the redness and heat. Histamine also causes retraction of endothelial cells in post-capillary venules, forming intracellular gaps; the resultant increase in permeability leads to oedema (leakage of plasma into the interstitial space) and produces the swelling and, in part, pain. These effects on the blood vessels are mediated through stimulation of histamine type 1 (H1) receptors.

Histamine also participates in immune suppression through stimulation of histamine type 2 (H2) receptors on neutrophils and suppressor T cells (Section 5.6). Thus histamine may have either an amplifying or an inhibiting effect on the inflammatory response, depending upon the stage of inflammation and whether H1 or H2 receptors are stimulated.

Excess histamine leads to hypersensitivity and antihistamine therapy is well known for alleviating conditions such as hay fever and inflammatory skin disorders.

Prostaglandins

The prostaglandins are a family of lipids that are synthesized from arachidonic acid, a 20-carbon unsaturated fatty acid component of cell membrane phospholipids. They are produced in every tissue in the body and act as local hormones in the immediate area of their production and release. Prostaglandins do not exist free in tissues, but have to be synthesized and released in response to an appropriate stimulus. Their biological activity is incredibly diverse and, as far as immunoregulation is concerned, some are stimulatory and some are inhibitory. One particular prostaglandin, PGE_2, increases the vasoactive and chemotactic properties of several other mediators of the inflammatory response.

The biosynthesis of prostaglandins involves several sequential steps as shown in Fig. 5.3. The first step is the hormone-induced release of arachidonic acid from membrane phospholipids. In many cells, most of the arachidonic acid is generated directly through the hydrolytic action of phospholipase A_2; alternative, indirect pathways involve phospholipases C and D (Smith, 1992). The arachidonic acid undergoes a cyclooxygenation to form a peroxide, PGG_2, and this in turn is reduced to a transient hydroxyendoperoxide, PGH_2, by peroxidation. These two reactions are catalysed by dual cyclooxygenase (COX) and peroxidase functions of prostaglandin H synthase (PGHS). PGH_2 is converted to one of a series of possible prostanoid products, including prostaglandins. COX is the rate-limiting enzyme in prostaglandin biosynthesis and requires hydroperoxide as an activator. In general, this process is cell-specific with differentiated cells producing only one of the major prostanoids in abundance. PGE_2, for

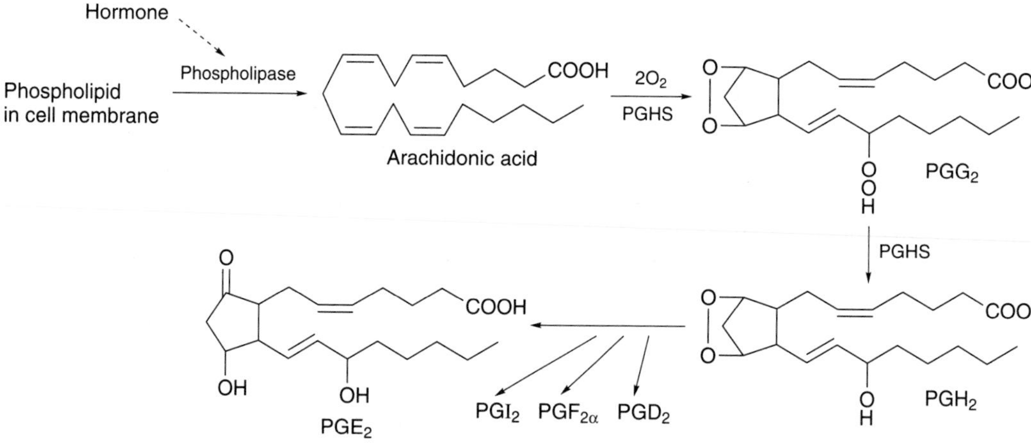

Fig. 5.3 Biosynthesis of prostaglandin E_2. PGHS, prostaglandin H synthase.

example, is formed by simple molecular rearrangement (isomerization).

Leukotrienes

One of this family of mediators, LTB4, induces degranulation of mast cells (releasing histamine), and causes the chemotaxis and/or chemokinesis of a number of cell types, including neutrophils.

Cytokines

The cytokines interleukin-1, interleukin-6 and tumour necrosis factors have overlapping biological activities and mediate multi-functional inflammatory effects. In combination, they trigger the synthesis of the acute phase proteins.

5.4 Acquired immunity

Acquired immune responses are directed specifically against antigenic determinants or epitopes. An antigenic determinant is a constituent part of an antigen, an antigen being any material that is recognized as foreign by the acquired immune system. Epitopes are characteristic three-dimensional chemical groups on the surfaces of microorganisms and foreign material.

The acquired immune response takes two forms: (1) cell-mediated responses result from the actions of different types of cells and (2) humoral responses are mediated in part by circulating antibodies.

5.4.1 Cell-mediated responses

Lymphocytes

The predominant cell type in the acquired immune system is the lymphocyte – a non-phagocytic, motile cell which is found mainly in the lymphoid tissues. Unlike cells of the innate immune system, which have non-specific recognition systems, lymphocytes have unique antigen-recognizing receptors inserted into their plasma membranes, enabling the lymphocytes to recognize specific pathogens. Therefore, before exposure to antigen, there exists in an individual vast numbers of lymphocytes, each with a different antigen-binding specificity governed by the molecular conformation of its receptor.

In the absence of an immune response, lymphocytes are in an inactive or 'resting state'. When an immune response is triggered, for example during a virus in-fection, lymphocytes that can respond to the virus become activated to carry out their specific functions. After they have been activated, the lymphocytes proliferate and become much larger cells called lymphoblasts. Activation signals that trigger this event (blastogenesis) are delivered by immunostimulatory cells, particularly dendritic cells. Once the immune response has ceased (for example, because the virus has been successfully eliminated) the lymphoblasts are transformed back to inactive lymphocytes. However, some of them form part of a population of 'memory' cells which constantly recirculate through the blood and lymph. Memory cells are specific for the particular virus; they are able to mount a vigorous and effective secondary response should the same virus be encountered in the future.

There are two functionally distinct types of lymphocytes – B lymphocytes (B cells for short) and T lymphocytes (T cells). In adult mammals, B cells develop in the bone marrow before they enter the blood as mature cells. T cells, however, develop only partly in the bone marrow: T cell precursors leave the marrow and travel via the blood to the thymus where they complete their development. The bone marrow and thymus are called primary lymphoid tissues because mature lymphocytes are actually produced at these sites. The mature B and T cells then enter the bloodstream and travel to secondary lymphoid tissues, which include the spleen and lymph nodes.

B lymphocytes

Different B cells are genetically programmed to encode an antibody for a particular antigen. The antibody is found as a transmembrane protein on the B-cell surface where it acts as the antigen-recognizing receptor. When the B cell interacts with its specific antigen, it multiplies and differentiates into a plasma cell, which then produces and secretes antibody in a soluble form. The soluble antibody has the same molecular structure as the B-cell receptor, except for the extreme carbon-terminal end. The soluble antibody circulates in the blood and other body fluids and recognizes native (i.e. unmodified) antigenic determinants on bacteria or foreign materials occurring freely in the body fluids.

T lymphocytes

T cells are divided into major subsets which have effector and regulatory functions. These subsets are cytotoxic T cells, helper T cells and suppressor T cells.

Cytotoxic T cells are effector cells that bind to host tissue cells infected by viruses and other intracellular pathogens, and then perforate their cell membranes by secretion of hole-forming perforins and cytolysins. In addition, the cytotoxic T cells release cytotoxic substances directly into the attacked cell. Almost immediately, the cell becomes greatly swollen, and it usually dissolves shortly thereafter.

Various regulatory helper T cells are stimulated by B cells, dendritic cells and macrophages to produce cytokines, which act upon all immune cells to regulate their function. For example, one group of helper cells helps resting cytotoxic T cells to become cytotoxic; another group helps resting B cells to divide, differentiate into plasma cells and make antibody; and a third group helps mononuclear phagocytes to destroy pathogens they have taken up.

Suppressor T cells are those T cells that release soluble inhibitors of the immune system, such as transforming growth factor-β.

Antigen presentation

Because viruses and other intracellular pathogens are enveloped within the cells of host tissues, the cell needs to be able to display antigens on the plasma membrane where they can be recognized by T cell receptors. The host cells accomplish this by antigen presentation (Fig. 5.4). Inside the infected cell, protein antigens are degraded to small peptides which then become bound to a self molecule called an MHC molecule. MHC molecules are encoded in a set of genes known as the major histocompatibility complex located within one chromosome of the tissue cell or phagocytic cell. The peptide–MHC complex is transported to the cell surface where it is specifically recognized by T cell receptors. This method of recognizing cell-associated antigens – MHC-restricted antigen recognition – is unique to T cells. Antigen presentation is also carried out by so-called accessory cells of the immune system, particularly by macrophages and dendritic cells.

Approximately 90–95% of circulating T cells are of the αβ type, in which the antigen receptor is a heterodimer of two polypeptides (α and β). Most of the αβ cells contain either CD4 or CD8 co-receptor molecules in addition to a common CD3 co-receptor. Cells which carry the CD4 co-receptor (CD4+ T cells) are mainly helper T cells, while those which carry the CD8 co-receptor (CD8+ T cells) are predominantly

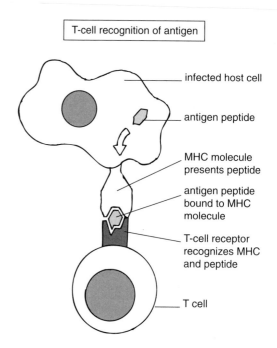

T-cell recognition of antigen

- infected host cell
- antigen peptide
- MHC molecule presents peptide
- antigen peptide bound to MHC molecule
- T-cell receptor recognizes MHC and peptide
- T cell

Fig. 5.4 Activation of T lymphocytes by antigen presentation. See text for details.

cytotoxic. CD4+ and CD8+ T cells recognize antigens in association with different classes of MHC molecules (class II and class I, respectively). CD4+ T cells are further divided into Th1 and Th2 subsets on the basis of their patterns of cytokine secretion. Th1 cells mediate several functions associated with cytotoxicity and are thus important for dealing with intracellular pathogens. Th2 cells are more effective at stimulating B cells to proliferate and produce antibodies; they therefore function primarily to protect against free-living microorganisms. Prostaglandin E_2 plays a regulatory role in maintaining the balance in activity between the Th1 and Th2 subsets (Phipps et al., 1991).

The LFA-1/ICAM-1 adhesion system

For a T cell to enter an inflamed or infected tissue, it must first adhere to the endothelium of a blood vessel at that site, and cross the vessel wall by extravasation. Adhesion and extravasation are mediated by the interaction of adhesion molecules expressed on the endothelial cells with cell surface receptors (integrins) on the T cells. An important endothelial adhesion molecule is the intercellular adhesion molecule-1 (ICAM-1), a cell-surface glycoprotein and member of the immunoglobulin gene superfamily. Although weakly expressed in non-stimulated cells, ICAM-1 expression is strongly increased by pro-inflammatory cytokines such as IL-1β, IFN-γ and TNF-α, as well as by bacterial lipopolysaccharides and phorbol esters. ICAM-1 interacts with lymphocyte-function-associated antigen-1 (LFA-1), a member of the β$_2$ subfamily of integrins, which is constitutively expressed by lymphocytes and other cells of the immune system. In addition to its role in adhesion and extravasation of T cells, the LFA-1/ICAM-1 adhesion system is important for antigen presentation (Altmann *et al.*, 1989).

5.4.2   *Humoral responses*

Structure and function of antibodies

Soluble antibodies are Y-shaped glycoproteins of the immunoglobulin (Ig) family synthesized and secreted by plasma cells in response to antigenic stimulation of naive B cells. Occurring freely in the blood and lymph, antibodies act as flexible adapters, allowing various mediators of the immune system to recognize specific pathogens and their products and to exert their action. The body can make several million different antibodies, each one able to recognize a specific infectious agent.

All antibody molecules consist of four polypeptide chains – two identical heavy chains and two identical light chains. Each of the arms of the Y-shaped molecule represents a Fab region, which binds to antigen; the stem represents the Fc region, which interacts with immune system mediators. The terminal half of each of the Y arms is highly variable in its amino acid sequence from one antibody to the next, the remainder of the molecule being relatively constant. These differences give rise to the terms 'variable' and 'constant' regions. Immunoglobulins are classified on the basis of structural differences in the heavy chains. The most important classes are IgG, IgA, IgM, IgD and IgE. The constant regions of the heavy chains, and consequently the class of the antibody, can change during the course of an immune response, although the antigen specificity of the antibody is unchanged. This process is known as antibody class switching and as a result the effector functions performed by the antibody will also change.

Phagocytes and natural killer cells, among other cells, have Fc receptors on their surfaces, allowing these cells to bind and destroy antibody-coated bacteria and tumour cells. Antibodies can also bind to the first component (C1q) of the complement system, thereby activating the complement cascade.

The primary function of an antibody is to bind antigens. In a few cases this has a direct effect; for example, neutralization of toxins by blocking active sites and inhibition of viral attachment to the target cell or penetration of the cell. In other cases, including precipitation of soluble antigen, agglutination of particulate antigen and activation of the complement system, secondary effector functions come into play. These secondary functions result from the formation of immune complexes between multivalent antigens and divalent antibody.

The variable region of a particular antibody may represent a unique structure that has appeared for the first time within a certain individual. Consequently, an immune response may be directed against epitopes on the variable domains. Each of these epitopes is known as an idiotope and the sum of all the idiotopes determines the antibody's idiotype. An immune response that is elicited by the host's own antibody molecules is called an auto-anti-idiotype response and the 'anti-antibodies' that are produced are termed auto-anti-idiotype antibodies. It has been postulated (Jerne, 1984) that idiotype and anti-idiotype antibodies can interact to form a network that can influence the outcome of an immune response.

Antibody responses to different types of antigen

In general, B cell responses to complex protein antigens require helper T cells; these responses and the antigens that elicit them are described as T-dependent (TD). TD responses fall into two categories, primary and secondary antibody responses. B cells can also respond to other types of antigen in the absence of T helper cells, in which case the responses and antigens are described as T-independent (TI). TI responses are usually unable to elicit a secondary response. TI and TD antigens can be distinguished according to whether or not, respectively, they can stimulate antibody production in the athymic mouse (mutants without a functional thymus).

T-dependent (TD) responses

An animal's first exposure to a TD antigen elicits a primary response, during which selected B cells undergo differentiation and clonal expansion to become antibody-secreting plasma cells. At the same time, other B cells (and T cells) differentiate and proliferate to become memory cells. The primary response is characterized by a lag phase and the production of mainly the IgM class of antibody. IgM is particularly effective in activating the complement cascade (15 times more so than IgG). If the antigenic determinant is present on a pathogenic microorganism, complement may either kill the organism directly or stimulate phagocytosis via complement receptors on phagocytes. After a plateau of antibody production, the response declines.

Once primed during the primary response, an animal can produce a more vigorous secondary response when subsequently challenged by the same antigen. This is partly due to the fact that the memory cells produced during the primary response are more readily activated by antigen than are resting cells. The lag phase is much shorter, and antibody production is higher and more persistent compared with the primary response. B cells expressing receptors with a higher affinity for antigen are selected for clonal expansion as the secondary response progresses, a phenomenon known as affinity maturation. The switching of antibody class from IgM to other classes brings other effector functions into play.

T-independent (TI) responses

TI antigens can be divided into type 1 and type 2 antigens according to whether or not, respectively, they elicit antibody production in neonatal and xid mice. The latter mice have a particular X-linked immunodeficiency gene called *xid* which makes them unable to respond to certain types of antigen.

Type 1 antigens are immunogenic early in life. An example is the lipopolysaccharide component of bacterial cell walls. Type 2 antigens are immunogenic in later life because they have more stringent requirements for mature B cells and cytokines. Examples are polysaccharide capsules of bacteria such as *Streptococcus pneumoniae* and synthetic polysaccharides like dextran and Ficoll. *In vivo*, type 2 antigens localize selectively on marginal zone macrophages in the spleen.

5.5   Cytokines

Cytokines are short-acting signalling molecules which affect the function of cells of the immune system and other systems of the body. They are proteins whose action is mediated by binding to specific receptors on target cells. Cytokines are not stored preformed within their cells of origin; rather they are synthesized by a cell in response to a specific stimulus and immediately secreted. Cytokines exhibit pleiotropism; that is, a given cytokine can act on many different cell types. They also display functional redundancy in the sense that many particular responses are elicited by a number of different cytokines. This can be explained by several cytokines sharing at least one chain of a common multichain receptor.

Cytokines play a crucial role in the amplification of the immune response because their release from just a few stimulated cells results in the activation of multiple cell types, which are not necessarily located in the immediate area. Different cytokines can either enhance or inhibit a given immune response. One cell may synthesize many different cytokines; moreover, one cell may be the target of many cytokines, each binding to its own cell-surface receptor. Cytokines often influence the synthesis of and affect the actions of other cytokines. An immune response can be fine-tuned not only by varying the type and amount of cytokine production, but also by regulating the density and affinity of cytokine receptors.

Cytokines are involved in both innate and acquired immune responses and exhibit a great diversity of action. The various cytokines include interleukins (IL-1 to IL-17), interferons (IFN-α, -β and -γ), transforming growth factor-β (TGF-β), tumour necrosis factors (TNF-α and -β) and colony-stimulating factors (CSFs). Interleukins are produced largely by T helper cells and many are involved in directing cells of the immune system to proliferate and differentiate. The overall effect of interferons is to inhibit viral replication and activate host defence mechanisms. Transforming growth factor-β is a family of three closely related molecules that stimulate connective tissue growth and collagen formation, but are inhibitory to virtually all immune and haemopoietic functions. The tumour necrosis factors are involved in the acute phase response to infection and injury, as well as regulation of cell proliferation and differentiation. TNF-α (cachetin) has multiple effects upon leucocytes and endothelial cells. TNF-β (lymphotoxin) is cytotoxic and may play an important role in immunoregulation. Both TNF-α and TNF-β have potent antiviral effects, which in part may be related to their ability to

Table 5.1   Examples of some cytokines and some of their functions.

Cytokine	Produced by	Functions
Interleukin-1 (IL-1)	Macrophages Epithelial cells	Potentiates IL-2 release from activated Th1 cells. Stimulates synthesis of acute phase proteins.
Interleukin-2 (IL-2)	Th1 cells	Stimulates Th1 and B cell proliferation. Induces secretion of other cytokines from activated T cells.
Interleukin-4 (IL-4)	Th2 cells Mast cells	Stimulates Th2 and B cell proliferation. Inhibits proliferation of Th1 cells. IL-4 activates resting B cells and directs antibody class switching to IgG1 and IgE.
Interleukin-5 (IL-5)	Th2 cells	Induces growth and differentiation of eosinophils.
Interleukin-6 (IL-6)	Th2 cells	Causes a generalized increase in Ig synthesis by activated B cells. Promotes the secretion of IgM and IgG by mitogen-stimulated B cells.
Interleukin-8 (IL-8)	Macrophages Other cell types	Chemotactic for neutrophils.
Interleukin-10 (IL-10)	Th2 cells	Inhibits cytokine synthesis by Th1 cells.
Interleukin-12 (IL-12)	B cells Macrophages	Activates natural killer cells. Stimulates differentiation of Th1 cells.
Interferon-α and -β (IFN-α, -β)	Many types of leucocyte	Antiviral effect. Increases cellular expression of MHC class I molecules.
Interferon-γ (IFN-γ)	Th1 cells Natural killer cells	Activates macrophages and natural killer cells. Increases cellular expression of MHC class II molecules. Inhibits IL-4-induced proliferation of Th2 cells. Inhibits IL-4-induced activation and proliferation of B cells. Inhibits IL-4-induced Ig class switching.
Tumour necrosis factor (TNF-α)	Activated macrophages Other cell types	Augments the capacity of macrophages to release IL-1 and PGE_2. Increases adhesion of lymphocytes and neutrophils to endothelial cells. Enhances proliferation of activated B cells. Increases antibody production in presence of IL-2.

Th1 and Th2 cells are subsets of CD4$^+$ (helper) T cells.
MHC class I molecules participate in antigen presentation to CD8$^+$ (cytotoxic) T cells.
MHC class II molecules participate in antigen presentation to CD4$^+$ (helper) T cells.

induce IFN-γ. Colony-stimulating factors direct the maturation of haemopoietic stem cells in the bone marrow. Examples of some cytokines and some of their functions are presented in Table 5.1.

5.6   Hypersensitivity

Hypersensitivity is the result of an immune response that occurs inappropriately or to an exaggerated degree. The immune response can be directed towards the body's own tissues (autoimmunity) and towards transplanted organs. Four main types of hypersensitivity have been defined: types I, II, III, which are antibody-mediated, and type IV. Type IV, known as delayed-type hypersensitivity, results from the action of cytokines that are produced by activated T helper cells. The helper cells respond to antigen and MHC class II molecules on antigen-presenting cells by releasing cytokines that recruit inflammatory cells to the site where the antigen is localized. The cytokines include IFN-γ, which activates macrophages and natural killer cells. The response is manifested as tissue swelling and local cellular proliferation. Type IV hypersensitivity is thought to occur during transplantation reactions.

5.7   Immune suppression

Immune responses can be suppressed by a variety of mechanisms, and some examples follow.

1   Oxidant secretory products of phagocytic leucocytes suppress the functional activity of lymphocytes (both B and T cells) and natural killer cells (El-Hag *et al.*, 1986).
2   Suppressor T cells release inhibitory cytokines, such as TGF-β.
3   IL-2 regulates the expression of its own receptors on T lymphocytes.
4   High concentrations of soluble antibody block the antigen-recognizing receptors (membrane-bound antibody) on B lymphocytes. The consequent inability of the B cells to recognize their specific antigen renders them unable to differentiate and produce soluble antibody.
5   Antibodies may be regulated by idiotype–anti-idiotype interactions.
6   Macrophages can produce prostaglandins, which non-specifically inhibit lymphocyte responses.
7   Cortisol inhibits the proliferation of lymphocytes and induces the production of TGF-β.

Histamine, after first mediating the immune response, helps to suppress it by activating suppressor T cells that have H2 receptors (Griswold *et al.*, 1984, 1986). In neutrophils, stimulation of H2 receptors by histamine promotes an increase in intracellular levels of cyclic AMP, which lowers chemotactic responsiveness (Anderson *et al.*, 1977) and inhibits release of lysosomal enzymes (Busse & Sosman, 1976).

5.8   Neuroendocrine modulation of immune responses

It has long been known that stressful conditions can suppress immune functions, reducing the ability of an individual to recover from infection. This can be explained by the fact that the neuroendocrine and immune systems are interconnected, forming an integrated system with common mediators and receptors. Cells of the immune system have receptors for many hormones, hormone-releasing factors and neurotransmitters – evidence that these molecules regulate immune responses. Moreover, immune cells themselves produce hormones and endorphins.

The interplay between the neuroendocrine and immune systems is bi-directional, as exemplified by the control of cortisol release from the adrenal glands during stress. Cortisol has well-known anti-inflammatory properties and it also suppresses the immune system. The signal for the release of cortisol originates in the brain. Electrical signals generated in the brain, and also IL-1 and IL-6 synthesized in brain cells, stimulate the hypothalamus to produce corticotrophin-releasing hormone (CRH), which induces the anterior lobe of the pituitary gland to release adrenocorticotrophic hormone (ACTH). CRH can also induce lymphocytes to produce their own ACTH. The ACTH is released into the bloodstream and, on reaching the target organ (adrenal glands), stimulates the adrenal cells to secrete cortisol. At excessive concentrations, ACTH inhibits the release of CRH and ACTH by negative feedback to the hypothalamus and anterior pituitary gland.

Further reading

Arai, K., Lee, F., Miyajima, A., Miyatake, S., Arai, N. & Yokota, T. (1990) Cytokines: coordinators of immune and inflammatory responses. *Annual Review of Biochemistry*, **59**, 783–836.

References

Altmann, D. M., Hogg, N., Trowsdale, J. & Wilkinson, D. (1989) Cotransfection of ICAM-1 and HLA-DR reconstitutes human antigen-presenting cell function in mouse L cells. *Nature*, **338**, 512–14.
Anderson, R., Glover, A. & Rabson, A. R. (1977) The *in vitro* effects of histamine and metiamide on neutrophil motility and their relationship to intracellular cyclic nucleotide levels. *Journal of Immunology*, **118**, 1690–6.
Babior, B. M. (1984) Oxidants from phagocytes: agents of defense and destruction. *Blood*, **64**, 959–66.
Boxer, L. A., Watanabe, A. M., Rister, M., Besch, H. R. Jr., Allen, J. & Baehner, R. L. (1976) Correction of leukocyte function in Chediak-Higashi syndrome by ascorbate. *New England Journal of Medicine*, **295**, 1041–5.
Busse, W. W. & Sosman, J. (1976) Histamine inhibition of neutrophil lysosomal enzyme release: an H2 histamine receptor response. *Science*, **194**, 737–8.
El-Hag, A., Lipsky, P. E., Bennett, M. & Clark, R. A. (1986) Immunomodulation by neutrophil myeloperoxidase and hydrogen peroxide: differential susceptibility of human lymphocyte functions. *Journal of Immunology*, **136**, 3420–6.
Griswold, D. E., Alessi, S., Badger, A. M., Poste, G. & Hanna, N. (1984) Inhibition of T suppressor cell expression by histamine type 2 [H$_2$] receptor antagonists. *Journal of Immunology*, **132**, 3054–7.
Griswold, D. E., Alessi, S., Badger, A. M., Poste, G. & Hanna, N. (1986) Differential sensitivity of T suppressor cell expression to

inhibition by histamine type 2 receptor antagonists. *Journal of Immunology*, **137**, 1811–15.

Ignarro, L. J. & George, W. J. (1974) Mediation of immunologic discharge of lysosomal enzymes from human neutrophils by guanosine 3′,5′-monophosphate. *Journal of Experimental Medicine*, **140**, 225–38.

Jerne, N. K. (1984) Idiotype networks and other preconceived ideas. *Immunological Reviews*, **79**, 5–24.

Miller, T. E. (1969) Killing and lysis of gram-negative bacteria through the synergistic effect of hydrogen peroxide, ascorbic acid, and lysozyme. *Journal of Bacteriology*, **98**, 949–55.

Phipps, R. P., Stein, S. H. & Roper, R. L. (1991) A new view of prostaglandin E regulation of the immune response. *Immunology Today*, **12**, 349–52.

Schmidt, K. & Moser, U. (1985) Vitamin C – a modulator of host defense mechanism. *International Journal for Vitamin and Nutrition Research*, Suppl. No. 27, 363–79.

Selvaraj, R. J. & Sbarra, A. J. (1966) Relationship of glycolytic and oxidative metabolism to particle entry and destruction in phagocytosing cells. *Nature*, **211**, 1272–6.

Smith, W. L. (1992) Prostanoid biosynthesis and mechanisms of action. *American Journal of Physiology*, **263**, F181–91.

Walford, R. L. (1980) Immunology and aging. *American Journal of Clinical Pathology*, **74**, 247–53.

Weiss, S. J. (1989) Tissue destruction by neutrophils. *New England Journal of Medicine*, **320**, 365–76.

Wolf, L. & Keusch, G. T. (1999) Nutrition and infection. In: *Modern Nutrition in Health and Disease*, 9th edn. (Ed. M. E. Shils, J. A. Olson, M. Shike & A. C. Ross), pp. 1569–88. Lippincott, Williams & Wilkins, Philadelphia.

6
The Genetic Control of Protein Synthesis and its Regulation by Nuclear Hormone Receptors

Key discussion topics

- Chromatin structure and modification have major controlling roles in transcriptional regulation.
- Regulated transcription requires the participation of a multitude of regulatory proteins working under combinatorial control.
- Signal transduction pathways convert transient cell-surface stimuli into a long-term transcriptional response.
- Hormone response elements on the DNA act as enhancers to increase the transcriptional activity of an adjacent promoter.

6.1 Functional structure of DNA

6.1.1 Base pairing and the genetic code

The DNA molecule is made up of two polynucleotide strands twisted together into a double helix. Each nucleotide residue consists of a five-carbon sugar molecule (deoxyribose) to which is attached one of four organic bases and a phosphate group (Fig. 6.1). The names of the bases – adenine, thymine, cytosine and guanine – are abbreviated to A, T, C and G, respectively. The respective nucleotides are named deoxyadenosine monophosphate (dAMP),

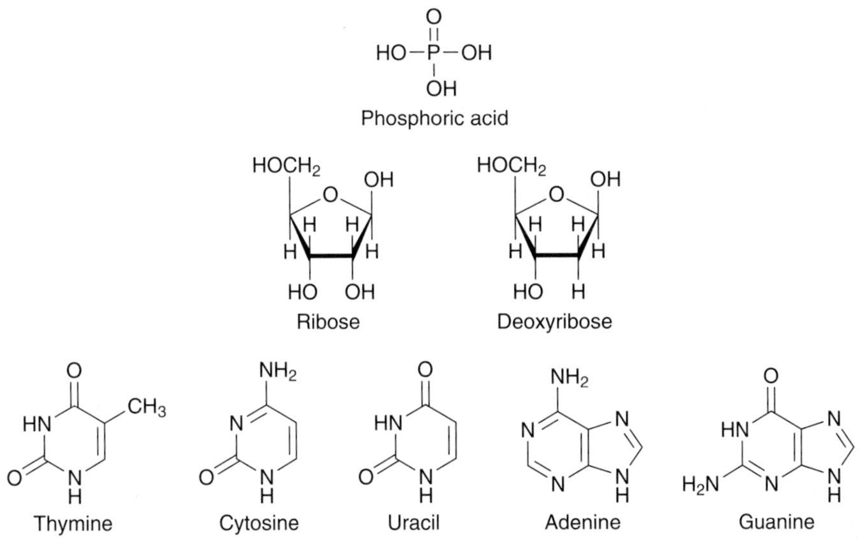

Fig. 6.1 The structural components of the nucleic acids. In DNA, the sugar is deoxyribose and the bases are adenine, guanine, cytosine and thymine. In RNA, the sugar is ribose and the bases are adenine, guanine, cytosine and uracil.

deoxythymidine monophosphate (dTMP), deoxycytidine monophosphate (dCMP) and deoxyguanosine monophosphate (dGMP). Each strand of the DNA is a chain composed of alternating sugar and phosphate residues resulting from the formation of 3′→5′ phosphodiester bonds between nucleotide residues (Fig. 6.2). The paired strands are juxtaposed in opposite directions so that the 5′ end of one strand is aligned with the 3′ end of the other. The two strands are held together by hydrogen bonds between specific pairs of bases. The two glycosidic bonds that attach a base pair to its sugar residues do not lie directly opposite each other. This results in the grooves that form between the two sugar–phosphate backbones of the double helix being of unequal sizes, creating a major groove and a minor groove. The bases are always paired in the same way: A bonds only to T and G bonds only to C. The two strands are therefore complementary; given the sequence of bases in one strand, the sequence in the other is completely defined.

The amino acid sequence of the polypeptide chain of the protein to be synthesized is determined by the sequence of bases in the DNA – the genetic code. The genetic code consists of successive triplets of bases, with more than one arrangement of triplets specifying a given amino acid. For example, GGC, AGA and CTT are among the triplets responsible for the respec-

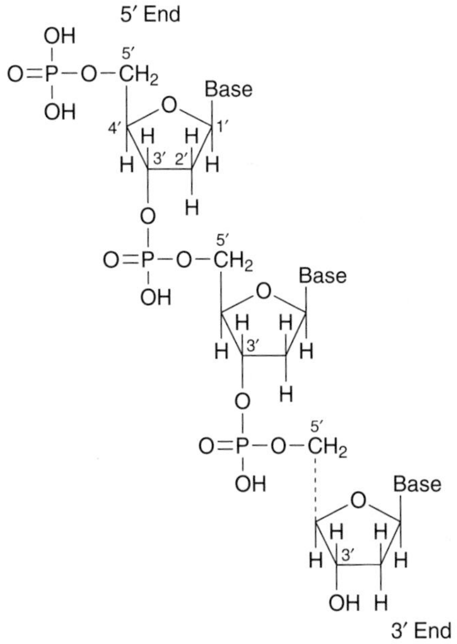

Fig. 6.2 Structure of the polynucleotide chain of DNA resulting from the formation of 3′ → 5′ phosphodiester bonds between nucleotide residues.

tive placement of proline, serine and glutamic acid in a polypeptide.

DNA

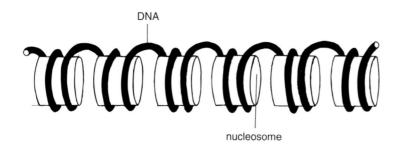

nucleosome

Fig. 6.3 Model for the beads-on-a-string structure of chromatin. Reproduced, with permission, from Brown (1999), *Genomes*, ©1999, BIOS Scientific Publishers Ltd.

6.1.2   Nucleosomal DNA

In the human nucleus each of the 23 chromosomes contains a single molecule of DNA double helix comprising 10^7 to 10^8 base pairs; this equates to an average length of about 5 cm. How can such a long molecule fit into a nucleus of 10 μm diameter? The answer is that naked DNA does not exist in nuclei – the DNA is compacted into chromatin by winding around specific DNA-binding proteins called histones. The histones bind to DNA largely through ionic bonds between the negatively charged phosphate groups of DNA and positively charged amino acid residues (arginine and lysine) exposed on the histone surfaces. The fundamental repeating unit of chromatin is the nucleosome, which appears in electron micrographs as beads on a string (see Fig. 6.3 for a model). Each nucleosome consists of core histones (H2A, H2B, H3 and H4), linker histones (H1 or variants thereof) and variable lengths of linker DNA. Two molecules each of the core histones form a barrel-shaped nucleosome core particle, around which 146 base pairs of DNA are wrapped in nearly two complete turns. Models of the octamer of core histones and the nucleosome core particle are shown in Fig. 6.4. The H3 and H4 histones form a central tetramer that is flanked by two H2A/H2B heterodimers. The linker histone acts as a clamp, preventing the unwinding of DNA from the octameric complex. Each of the four types of core histone comprises a globular, hydrophobic carboxy terminus and an extended hydrophilic amino-terminal tail containing a number of positively charged amino acid residues. The tails lie on the outside of the nucleosome, where they can interact ionically with the negatively charged phosphates of the DNA backbone. Linker histones are very elongated, with both C and N terminal arms extending from a more globular central body. During interphase (the period between cell divisions) the chromatin filaments form higher order structures by winding into a solenoid containing six nucleosomes per turn.

As will become evident, histones and other packaging proteins are not simply inert structures around which the DNA is wound, but instead are active participants in the processes that determine which genes are expressed in an individual cell.

A.

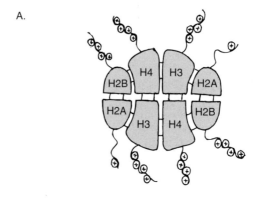

B.

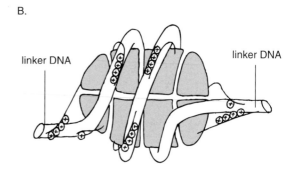

linker DNA   linker DNA

Fig. 6.4 Models for (A) the octamer of core histones and (B) the nucleosome core particle with linker DNA. Reproduced with permission, from Csordas, A., 1990, *Biochemical Journal*, Vol. 265, pp. 23–8. © the Biochemical Society.

6.2   Role of RNA in protein synthesis

Most people know that a gene is a unit of heredity in a chromosome, controlling a particular inherited characteristic of an individual. However, it is not widely appreciated that genes control cell function by determining what proteins will be synthesized within the cell. By far the majority of the proteins are enzymes; the remaining proteins play important roles in cellular structure and regulation of cellular activities.

The overall process of protein synthesis is depicted in Fig. 6.5. Note that the assembly of amino acids into proteins takes place in the cytoplasm. Both the transfer and the utilization of information are mediated by ribonucleic acid (RNA) – a single-stranded nucleic acid which is similar in structure to DNA but has the base uracil in place of thymine, and the sugar

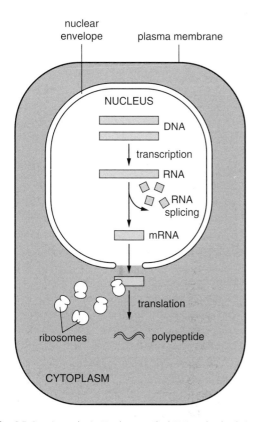

Fig. 6.5 Protein synthesis. Newly transcribed RNA molecules (primary transcripts) are extensively processed (spliced) to become mRNA molecules. These are transported out of the nucleus into the cytoplasm, where they are translated into protein by ribosomes. Reproduced, with permission, from Brown (1999), *Genomes*, ©1999, BIOS Scientific Publishers Ltd.

ribose instead of deoxyribose (see Fig. 6.1). The uracil nucleotide is named deoxyuridine monophosphate (dUMP). There are three different types of RNA molecules present in the cell, each of which plays a key role in the biosynthesis of proteins: these are messenger RNA, transfer RNA and ribosomal RNA.

Messenger RNA (mRNA) carries the genetic message between the DNA in the nucleus and the site of protein synthesis on the ribosomes. The codon (the unit that codes for a given amino acid) consists of a triplet of bases in mRNA that are exactly complementary to the code triplets of the DNA. There are 64 codons; 60 correspond to the 20 amino acids (many amino acids have several codons), one is a start codon and the remaining three are stop codons.

The mRNA itself is synthesized from DNA by the aptly named process of transcription (copying). Before this can take place, the DNA at the site of transcription must be accessible to proteins required to initiate and regulate this process. That is, the chromatin in this localized region must be 'unpackaged' as opposed to compact. Within the unpackaged region, the nucleosomes are repositioned so as to expose a short stretch of naked DNA.

Detailed aspects of transcription are discussed later in this chapter, but the basic process is given here as an introduction. The mechanism of transcription is depicted in Fig. 6.6. Transcription is catalysed by the enzyme RNA polymerase II, which combines with a host of protein transcription factors and regulatory proteins to form a pre-initiation complex at a precise site on the DNA called the promoter. The polymerase moves along the DNA, temporarily unwinding and separating the two strands at each stage of its movement. As it moves along, RNA is formed by the linking of ribonucleotides under the influence of the polymerase and using one of the DNA strands as a template. The ribonucleotides originate from free ribonucleoside triphosphates. Release of two of the three phosphate radicals from each ribonucleoside triphosphate liberates large amounts of energy from the broken high-energy phosphate bonds. This energy is used to cause covalent linkage of the remaining phosphate on the ribonucleoside (now a ribonucleotide) with the ribose on the end of the growing RNA molecule. Hydrogen bonds are created between the successive bases of the DNA strand and the bases of the ribonucleotides. Base pairing is the same as that found in the DNA molecule, except that the uracil

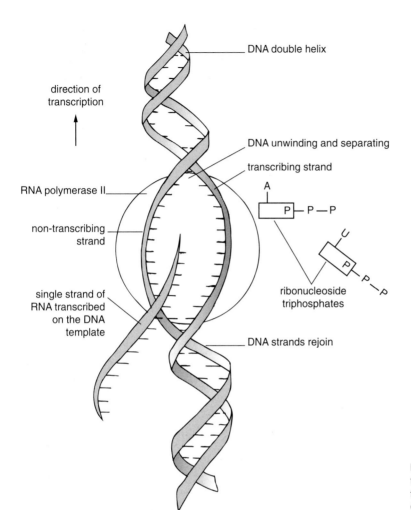

direction of
transcription

DNA double helix

DNA unwinding and separating

transcribing strand

RNA polymerase II

non-transcribing
strand

single strand of
RNA transcribed
on the DNA
template

ribonucleoside
triphosphates

DNA strands rejoin

Fig. 6.6 Diagram showing the mechanism of transcription. Reproduced, with permission, from Green *et al.* (1990), *Biological Science*, © Cambridge University Press.

of RNA is paired with the adenine of DNA. As the synthesis of the RNA strand proceeds, its hydrogen bonds with the DNA template break because the other strand of DNA has a higher energy of bonding. The two DNA strands are reunited and the new RNA strand is released into the nucleoplasm.

The newly transcribed RNA, the primary transcript, contains many unwanted nucleotide sequences, constituting more than 90 per cent of the total strand. A series of nuclear enzymes carries out RNA processing, which usually entails modification of the ends of the primary transcript and excision of unwanted sequences called introns. Accompanying the excision of introns is a rejoining of the coding segments (exons) to form a shortened RNA molecule, now mRNA. These excision and rejoining events are called RNA

splicing. Often a cell can splice the primary transcript in different ways. This process of alternative RNA splicing allows different proteins to be produced from a single gene. The newly made mRNA diffuses from the nucleus into the cytoplasm through pores in the nuclear membrane.

Transfer RNA (tRNA) is found in the cytoplasm. Its function is to pick up amino acids and to carry them to the ribosomes, so that they can be joined together into polypeptides. There are at least 20 different tRNA molecules, one for each amino acid. They all have a similar structure (Fig. 6.7) in which the single strand of RNA is folded back upon itself in a clover-leaf arrangement due to pairing between complementary bases. One unpaired end of each tRNA molecule contains a triplet of exposed nucleotides, known as

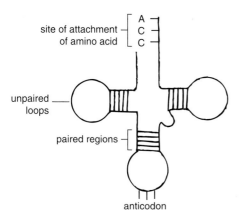

Fig. 6.7 Simplified diagram of the structure of transfer RNA (tRNA). Each tRNA molecule is characterized by having its own anticodon and a site of attachment for a specific amino acid. Reproduced, with permission, from Green *et al.* (1990), *Biological Science*, © Cambridge University Press.

the anticodon, while another unpaired end has a site for attachment to a specific amino acid. Each tRNA therefore picks up its own particular amino acid and, by matching of its anticodon with the complementary codon in mRNA, the amino acids can be assembled in the correct sequence.

Ribosomal RNA (rRNA) is a component of the ribosomes. These are composed of two spherical subunits of unequal size, each of which is made up of about equal parts of RNA and of protein. By attachment of the smaller subunit of the ribosome to mRNA, the latter is held in such a way that its codons can be recognized and paired with the complementary anticodons in the tRNA. As shown in Fig. 6.8, a ribosome can accommodate two tRNAs at any one time, allowing their amino acids to be peptide-linked. As the

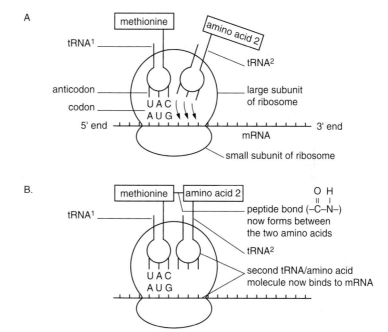

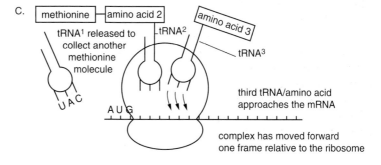

Fig. 6.8 Translation. (A) and (B) Consecutive stages in the attachment of tRNA/amino acid complexes by their anticodons to the codons on mRNA and the formation of a peptide bond between adjacent amino acids. (C) The relative movements of mRNA and ribosome exposing a new triplet (frame) for the attachment of the tRNA/amino acid complex. The initial tRNA molecule is now released from the ribosome and cycles back into the cytoplasm to be reactivated by enzymes to form a new tRNA/amino acid complex. Reproduced, with permission, from Green *et al.* (1990), *Biological Science*, © Cambridge University Press.

peptide bond is formed, the ribosome simultaneously moves one codon further along the mRNA molecule. The tRNA on the left is then released, to be used again, and the next one moves in from the right to pair with the newly positioned codon and to add another amino acid to the growing polypeptide chain. The process by which the transcribed information carried in the base sequence of mRNA is used to produce a sequence of amino acids in a polypeptide chain is known as translation. The sequence is completed when the ribosome comes to one of the three stop codons on the mRNA.

Once the polypeptide is synthesized, it dissociates from the ribosome and is released into the cytoplasm. There it undergoes some post-translational modification, such as folding or associating with other polypeptides, to form a functional protein.

6.3   Gene expression

A gene is a segment of double-stranded nuclear DNA. The transfer of genetic information from DNA into protein constitutes gene expression. Apart from housekeeping genes, which are expressed in all tissues, genes are expressed in a highly controlled manner so that only those proteins needed by a specific cell for a specific purpose are synthesized. Each step in the pathway of protein synthesis may be regulated. Controlled processes include transcription, RNA processing, RNA transport to the cytoplasm, mRNA stability, selection of mRNAs for translation, and post-translational modification of the protein product. Most genes are regulated in part at the transcriptional level.

In adult mammalian cells, the majority of the DNA is methylated, specifically at the cytosines of CpG dinucleotides. DNA methylation is associated with repression of gene expression (see Section 6.6.5 for the mechanism) and is retained after cell division. Most tissue-specific genes are methylated (and thus repressed) in every cell type, except those that actually express the gene. Housekeeping genes have a non-methylated CpG island tightly associated with their promoter and are thought not to be regulated by DNA methylation (Laird & Jaenisch, 1994).

The pattern of gene expression is determined to a large extent by the conditions of the extracellular environment. Growth factors, cytokines and other extracellular agents stimulate cell-surface receptors, which initiate a complicated biochemical pathway of signal transduction to the nucleus. Steroid hormone receptors can enter the nucleus directly. The transduced signals can cause gene expression to be either enhanced or suppressed. In this manner, a transient external stimulus can be converted into a long-term biological response.

6.4   Mutation and polymorphism

The nuclei of diploid organisms contain homologous pairs of chromosomes, each chromosome consisting of a molecule of DNA and associated proteins. Each genetic locus is occupied by two alleles, one on each chromosome of the pair. An allele is one of a series of alternative genes that can potentially occupy a particular locus. A heterozygote is a person whose alleles at a particular locus are different; in a homozygote the alleles are identical.

A perfectly healthy person may carry a particular single allele which produces an abnormal protein that can potentially create an hereditary disease. The fact that the disease is not manifested means that the person is a heterozygote and the allele is recessive. In this situation, the allele on the other chromosome produces sufficient normal protein to override the effect of the abnormal protein. If the allele were dominant rather than recessive in the heterozygote, the abnormal protein would exert its effect even in the presence of the normal protein and the disease would be manifested. If heterozygous parents each carry the recessive allele, there is a chance that both copies of the allele will be passed to a child and the child, a homozygote, will suffer from the disease. This is illustrated in Fig. 6.9.

The common allele is called the normal or wild-type. If the variant allele is very rare it is called a mutant. Mutation is a change in the sequence of base pairs along the double-stranded DNA molecule. The change may be simple, such as the substitution of one pair of bases for a different pair, or more complex, such as the deletion or addition of base pairs. The change in the DNA base pair will alter the genetic code, resulting in a change in the codon in the mRNA. The new codon will combine with a tRNA bearing a different amino acid, and so a different amino acid will be incorporated into the polypeptide chain during protein synthesis. Shorthand for the wild-type homozygote is +/+, for the wild-type/mutant het-

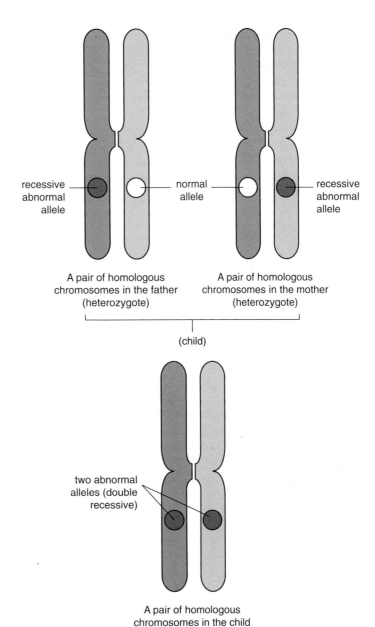

recessive abnormal allele — normal allele — recessive abnormal allele

A pair of homologous chromosomes in the father (heterozygote)

A pair of homologous chromosomes in the mother (heterozygote)

(child)

two abnormal alleles (double recessive)

A pair of homologous chromosomes in the child (homozygote)

Fig. 6.9 The inheritance of an hereditary disease from parents who are both heterozygous for a locus with a recessive allele.

erozygote is +/m, and for the mutant homozygote is m/m. If the mutant is dominant to normal its symbol is capitalized, i.e. +/M.

Although an individual person has only two alleles at a particular locus, human populations can have many different alleles of that locus. When the occurrence of a variant allele is too high to be explained by recurrent mutation (conventionally 1% or more), it is called a polymorphism. Specific loci of populations that exhibit multiple alleles are therefore said to be polymorphic. Any specific allele constitutes a fraction of all alleles in the population, that fraction being called its allele frequency (also called gene frequency). Allele frequencies change over time owing to the combined processes of mutation and natural selection, among others.

6.5   Basal transcription

Basal or minimal transcription is defined as transcription in the absence of activators. The step-wise assembly of protein transcription factors described below can take place *in vitro* with purified factors, but is unlikely to occur *in vivo* where a host of regulatory proteins will be present. Nevertheless, knowledge of the protein–protein interactions involved in basal transcription is fundamental to understanding how transcription is regulated in the cell.

6.5.1   The core promoter

The core promoter refers to a group of control modules that are clustered around the transcriptional start site on the DNA. Positions in promoters are given as distances in base pairs from the start site at +1. A positive sign denotes a downstream position, in the direction of transcription; a negative sign denotes an upstream position. There is no position 0. There are two core promoter elements, the TATA box around −30 and the initiator at the start site. Together these elements fix the exact start site of transcription. The TATA box acts as a recognition and binding site for TFIID – the first of several protein factors that assemble to eventually form the pre-initiation complex. The initiator interacts later with a component of the pre-initiation complex, probably with RNA polymerase II, and determines the exact start site of transcription (Kollmar & Farnham, 1993). All promoters examined to date contain either one or both of the core elements, and either element can support basal transcription.

6.5.2   General transcription factors

In addition to RNA polymerase II, at least seven different general transcription factors (GTFs) are involved in the initiation of basal transcription via the TATA box. RNA polymerase II plus the GTFs are referred to as the basal transcription machinery. The GTFs, designated TFIIA, TFIIB, TFIID, TFIIE, TFIIF, TFIIH and TFIIJ, assemble stepwise into a basal pre-initiation complex in a definite (but non-alphabetical) order. There is a remarkable conservation, based on polypeptide sequences, of the GTFs from yeast to humans. Proposed functions of GTFs IIA to IIH are listed in Table 6.1. There is as yet no clearly defined role for TFIIJ.

Most of the GTFs are complex molecules composed of two or more polypeptide subunits (Table 6.1). Among these, TFIID contains TBP (TATA-binding protein) and multiple, tightly-bound TBP-associated factors (TAFs); only the TBP subunit is required for basal transcription. TFIIH possesses kinase, helicase and ATPase activities, all of which play essential roles in transcription.

Table 6.1   Functions of general transcription factors from human cells.

Factor	Number of subunits	MW (kDa) (of subunits)	Function
TFIID — TBP	1	38	Recognition of the TATA box; recruitment of TFIIB
TFIID — TAFs	12	15–250	Recognition of the core promoter in the absence of a TATA box; positive and negative regulatory functions
TFIIA	3	12, 19, 35	Stabilization of TBP binding and TAF–DNA interactions; anti-repression function
TFIIB	1	35	Recruitment of RNA polymerase II–TFIIF complex; influences selection of transcription start site
TFIIF	2	30, 74	Promoter targeting of RNA polymerase II; destabilization of non-specific polymerase–DNA interactions
RNA polymerase II	12	10–220	Catalysis of RNA polymerization from ribonucleotides; recruitment of TFIIE
TFIIE	2	34, 57	Recruitment of TFIIH and regulation of its enzyme activities
TFIIH	9	35–89	Conversion of closed initiation complex to an open complex using helicase and ATPase activities; promoter clearance by CTD kinase activity

From Roeder, *et al.* (1996).
Abbreviation: CTD, carboxy-terminal domain of largest subunit of RNA polymerase II.

6.5.3 Formation of the pre-initiation complex and subsequent events

The process of transcription can be divided into discrete stages: pre-initiation complex assembly, initiation, promoter clearance, transcript elongation and termination. Initiation is defined by the formation of the first phosphodiester bond. The following events (also see Fig. 6.10) are based largely on evidence reviewed by Roeder (1996).

The first step in the formation of the pre-initiation complex is nucleation whereby TBP binds specifically

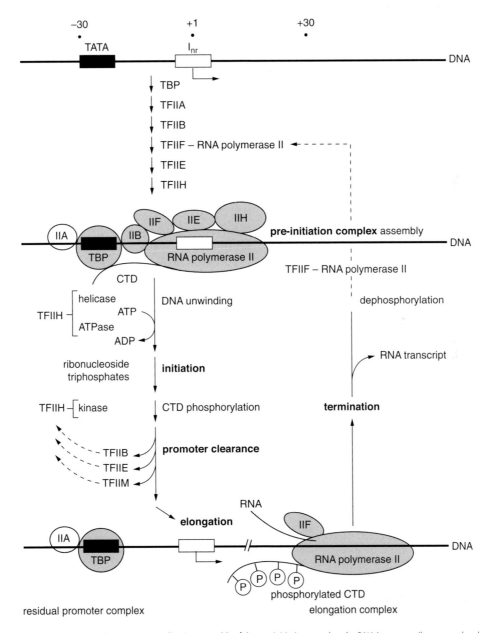

Fig. 6.10 Scheme of events in basal transcription. Following assembly of the pre-initiation complex, the DNA is temporarily unwound and separated in a localized region. The presence of ribonucleoside triphosphates results in initiation, which is followed by promoter clearance, elongation and termination as described in the text. Inr, initiator; CTD, carboxy-terminal domain of RNA polymerase II. Reprinted from *Trends in Biochemical Science*, Vol. 21, Roeder, R. G., The role of general initiation factors in transcription by RNA polymerase II, pp. 327–35, © 1996, with permission from Elsevier.

to the TATA box to form an initial committed complex. TBP is a molecular saddle whose concave underside binds to DNA in the minor groove, leaving the convex surface free to bind to other proteins. The binding of TBP has a dramatic effect upon the DNA, causing kinking and bending. This distortion brings sequences upstream and downstream of the TATA box into close apposition. The next factor to arrive is TFIIA, whose anti-repressive function is to displace TBP-bound negative cofactors (NC1 and NC2) and thus allow TFIIB to bind to TBP. TFIIA also stabilizes the committed complex under physiological conditions. Next to arrive is TFIIB, which binds through direct interactions with TBP and with DNA sequences both upstream and downstream of the TATA box. TFIIB further stabilizes the assembling complex and recruits a pre-formed TFIIF–RNA polymerase II complex through interactions with both components. The role of TFIIF is to direct the polymerase to the correct site on the promoter. The next factors, TFIIE and TFIIH, bind co-operatively. The binding of TFIIJ completes the assembly of the pre-initiation complex.

Initiation commences with the temporary unwinding of about two turns of the DNA double helix and separation of the two strands. DNA unwinding is effected by the helicase activity of TFIIH, aided by the ATPase, which releases the required energy from ATP. The formation of an open pre-initiation complex allows the RNA molecule to be synthesized from free ribonucleoside triphosphates using one of the DNA strands as a template. The RNA polymerase II within the complex is then phosphorylated in its carboxy-terminal domain by the kinase activity of TFIIH. The resultant disruption of contacts between GTFs and the polymerase leads to promoter clearance in which the polymerase, with TFIIF still attached, moves down the DNA to establish an elongation complex. The remaining GTFs are released, except for TBP which remains attached to the TATA box. TFIIB is re-associated with the promoter-bound TBP, enabling recruitment of RNA polymerase II and the GTFs for subsequent rounds of initiation.

6.6   Regulated transcription

The formation of a multiprotein pre-initiation complex allows for multiple points of regulation. Regulated transcription requires the participation of a multitude of regulatory DNA elements and proteins acting to either enhance or repress transcription, and working under combinatorial control.

6.6.1   Enhancers and silencers

Enhancers and silencers are DNA binding sites for a variety of transcriptional activator and repressor proteins, respectively. The function of an enhancer is to increase the recruitment rate of transcription factors and RNA polymerase II molecules at the promoter, while that of a silencer is to suppress transcription. The majority of enhancers are located upstream of the transcriptional start site, often many kilobases away, but some are located downstream and a few occur within the promoter region (Fig. 6.11). A particular enhancer functions preferably or exclusively in certain cell types and so enhancers provide tissue-specific gene expression. Distant upstream or downstream enhancers and silencers can make contact with the promoter region by looping of the intervening DNA.

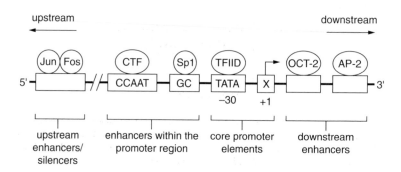

Fig. 6.11 Features of the transcriptional control region for a mammalian, protein-coding gene. Cis-acting elements are denoted by rectangles; trans-acting factors are denoted by circles. X indicates the transcription start site.

6.6.2   Activators and coactivators

Transcription of protein-coding genes can be stimulated above the basal rate by combinations of various protein activators, which bind to specific enhancer sequences and act synergistically. An activator molecule has two important domains: a DNA-binding domain, which anchors the protein to its enhancer, and a transcription activation domain, which interacts with a coactivator. Coactivators are another class of regulatory proteins, which are essential for activated transcription. At least some of the TAFs associated with the TFIID complex are coactivators. Coactivators do not bind to DNA, but function as adaptors, forming molecular bridges connecting the upstream DNA-bound activator to the core promoter.

The versatility of some activators is illustrated by VP16, which has the ability to interact with TBP, TFIIB and TFIIH. The effect of VP16 upon TBP is to stimulate nucleation, while interactions with TFIIB and TFIIH stimulate RNA polymerase II recruitment and promoter clearance, respectively. The regulated coupling of polymerase entry and exit from the promoter is essential to ensure multiple initiation cycles in an efficient manner.

Roberts & Green (1994) proposed a model for the effect of VP16 on TFIIB (Fig. 6.12). TFIIB possesses two functional domains: an amino-terminal portion that interacts with TFIIF and a carboxy-terminal portion that interacts with RNA polymerase II, TBP and VP16. The unstimulated TFIIB molecule exists in a closed conformation owing to interaction between the amino and carboxy terminals. In such a conformation, TFIIB is relatively inaccessible to TBP, RNA polymerase II and TFIIF. VP16 induces a conformational change in TFIIB, opening up the molecule and making it more accessible to the above factors. The implication is that activators, by changing the conformation of TFIIB, facilitate protein–protein interactions between TFIIB and TBP and also between TFIIB and the TFIIF–RNA polymerase II complex. Coactivators and other TAFs provide additional protein surfaces to

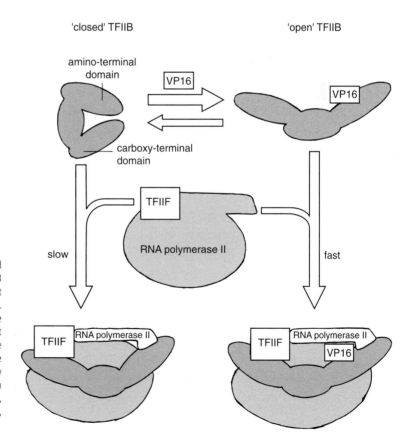

Fig. 6.12 Model for the VP16-induced conformational change in TFIIB. Native TFIIB exists in a closed conformation, making it inaccessible to other transcription factors. Opening of the TFIIB molecule in the presence of VP16 (activator) stimulates TFIIB recruitment to the promoter, which in turn stimulates the recruitment of TFIIF–RNA polymerase II. In the absence of VP16, the opening of TFIIB is likely to be much slower. Reprinted from Sheldon & Reinberg (1995), *Current Biology*, Vol. 5, Tuning-up transcription, pp. 43–6, © 1995, with permission from Elsevier.

accommodate multiple protein–protein interactions with a diverse assortment of activators. The stimulation of TFIIB recruitment to the promoter and the stimulated recruitment of the polymerase and general transcription factors increase the proportion of DNA templates on which a functional pre-initiation complex is assembled, rather than increasing the rate of complex assembly.

Regulation of CREB

The regulation of one particular activator, cyclic AMP response element-binding protein (CREB), is fairly well understood. In non-stimulated cells, CREB binds constitutively to specific cyclic AMP response elements (CREs) on the DNA, but fails to activate transcription. Under certain circumstances, inactive CREB may act as a repressor and block the action of upstream enhancer-binding transcription factors. Upon stimulation of cell-surface receptors that positively regulate adenylyl cyclase, intracellular cyclic AMP levels rise and activation of protein kinase A (PKA) ensues. The catalytic subunit of PKA then translocates to the nucleus, where it phosphorylates CRE-bound CREB on serine 133, located in a critical position within its activation domain. The resultant increase in CREB transcriptional activity leads to activation of CRE-containing promoters.

One possible way through which phosphorylation at Ser133 may stimulate CREB activity is by allowing it to bind to another protein, CBP (CREB-binding protein). CBP functions as a coactivator, linking CREB to the basal transcription machinery. Following dissociation of ligand or receptor down-modulation, cyclic AMP levels drop and the catalytic subunit of PKA is inactivated through binding to the enzyme's regulatory subunit. This drop in PKA activity results in a net increase in phosphatase activity, leading to dephosphorylation of CREB and its inactivation.

6.6.3   *The RNA polymerase II holoenzyme*

In intact cells, about 20% of RNA polymerase II and GTFs other than TFIID and TFIIA form a megadalton-sized conglomerate known as the RNA polymerase II holoenzyme. In addition to the polymerase itself (the core polymerase) and general transcription factors, the holoenzyme also contains Srb proteins and (debatably) Swi/Snf proteins, as well as other known and unknown proteins. A multisubunit complex containing the nine known Srb proteins and TFIIF among other proteins can be dissociated from a preparation of the holoenzyme. This complex, known as the Srb/mediator, participates in the promoter's response to transcriptional activators.

Several lines of evidence indicate that the holoenzyme is the form of RNA polymerase II that initiates transcription at most, if not all, promoters *in vivo* (Koleske & Young, 1995). Biochemical data support a model in which the assembled holoenzyme is recruited to promoters at which TFIID is already bound.

6.6.4   *Chromatin remodelling*

The organization of chromatin into nucleosomes is an essential feature in the regulation of transcription. Nucleosomes are transcriptional repressors because they impede access of the basal transcription machinery to the core promoter. Of particular significance, nucleosomes virtually prevent the binding of TBP to the TATA box *in vitro*, and TBP does not associate with the core promoter *in vivo* in the absence of a functional activator. The inability of TBP to bind nucleosomal DNA means that recruitment of the basal transcription machinery is excluded. On the other hand, nucleosomes have only a modest inhibitory effect on the binding of activator proteins to their upstream enhancers. The repressive action of nucleosomes is important in closing off those parts of the genome that need to be transcriptionally silenced. When it becomes necessary for a gene to be expressed, changes in cell physiology elicit a remodelling of chromatin, which allows binding of transcription factors at promoters. Two important chromatin remodelling systems have been studied. In one system, the changes in chromatin structure are mediated by ATP-driven Swi/Snf proteins; the other system involves the post-translational modification of core histones by acetylation. Both systems disrupt histone–DNA interactions in a transient and reversible manner.

Swi/Snf remodelling proteins

Members of the Swi/Snf family of chromatin remodelling proteins comprise highly conserved multisubunit complexes of ~2 MDa – huge proteins about half the size of a ribosome. In yeast Swi/Snf, the Swi2/Snf2 subunit is an ATPase that contains sequence motifs closely related to those found in DNA helicases. Although Swi/Snf does not catalyse DNA unwinding, it may function in a manner similar to helicase. That is, it may move along a nucleosome in a wave-like manner using the energy derived from the hydrolysis of ATP (Pazin & Kadonaga, 1997). This movement is accompanied by a partial and localized alteration of chromatin structure in a manner that permits the binding of site-specific transcription factors. Although the mechanism by which Swi/Snf functions has not yet been elucidated, it appears that these remodelling proteins increase accessibility of transcription factors to DNA without displacing histones. Swi/Snf could either perturb but not fully disrupt the structure of nucleosome core particles or they could influence the spacing of nucleosome arrays. With regard to the latter possibility, the twisting of DNA at the edges of the nucleosome may cause the nucleosome to slide along the DNA (Varga-Weisz & Becker, 1998). The accessible chromatin reverts to an inaccessible form unless a transcription factor binds to the DNA.

Acetylation

Nuclear histone acetyltransferases (HATs) catalyse the transfer of an acetyl group from acetyl coenzyme A onto the ε-amino group of specific lysine residues present exclusively in the amino-terminal tails of each of the core histones. Neutralization of the positively charged lysines reduces the net positive charge of the histone tails and weakens their association with DNA. The displacement of the flexible tails (Fig. 6.13) permits subtle changes in nucleosomal structure and a partial unwinding or loosening of the core DNA. Acetylation may also inhibit formation of higher-order chromatin. The overall result is an increase in accessibility of transcription factors to their DNA-binding sites. Acetylation does not occur randomly; multiple HATs have specificities for different lysines in the histone tails. A steady-state equilibrium is maintained by the opposing activity of histone deacetylases (Fig. 6.14).

The connection between histone acetylation and transcriptional activation was established beyond doubt when the HAT activity of the yeast protein Gcn5, a known coactivator, was shown to be critical for activation of target genes *in vivo* (Kuo *et al.*, 1998; Wang *et al.*, 1998). Gcn5 does not act alone to mediate transcriptional activation: it functions within a

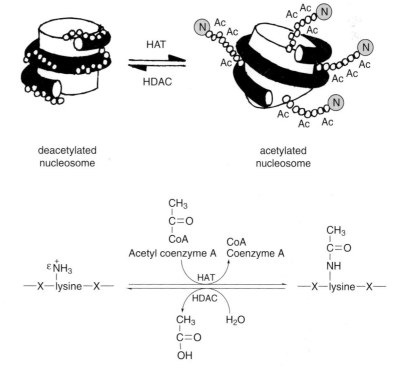

Fig. 6.13 Effects of histone acetylation on nucleosome structure. In the deacetylated repressive nucleosome, the positively charged amino-terminal tails of the core histones are closely associated with the core DNA. Acetylation of specific lysines in the histone tails neutralizes their positive charges thereby releasing the tails from contact with the DNA. The consequent loosening of the nucleosomal structure permits access of the transcription machinery. Ac, acetyl group. Reproduced, with permission, from *Cellular and Molecular Life Sciences*, Vol. 54, pp. 6–20, © 1998, Birkhäuser Verlag AG.

deacetylated nucleosome

acetylated nucleosome

Fig. 6.14 The enzyme-catalysed acetylation and deacetylation of lysine residues in histone amino-terminal tails. X, other amino acids.

large complex called SAGA that includes Spt and Ada proteins. Three constituent proteins of SAGA (Spt3, Spt20 and Ada2) interact with TBP. Also, Ada2 and/or Gcn5 interact with activators such as VP16 (Roberts & Winston, 1997). Thus the catalytic activity of Gcn5 is potentially targeted to a promoter through any one of a number of protein–protein interactions.

Cosma *et al.* (1999) measured the association of five transcriptional regulators with promoter sequences of the yeast *HO* gene. They concluded that Swi/Snf altered nucleosomes in a manner that permitted their association with SAGA. Both chromatin remodelling and histone acetylation steps were obligatory for binding of SBF (a transcription factor) to take place. Although the changes in nucleosome structure induced by Swi/Snf are quite stable *in vitro*, it is likely that histone acetylation is needed *in vivo* to stabilize these changes.

The presence of HAT activity in TAF$_{II}$250 suggests a possible means for TBP to bind to the TATA box in nucleosomal DNA. As both TAF$_{II}$250 and TBP are components of the TFIID complex, the TFIID itself comes equipped to modify the core histones and facilitate access of TBP.

Since the discovery that yeast Gcn5 exhibits HAT activity *in vitro* (Brownell *et al.*, 1996), many previously isolated coactivators have subsequently been shown to be HATs. Such HATs include CBP and its functional homologue p300, PCAF, SRC-1 and ACTR. Table 6.2 shows that HATs interact and appear to vary in their histone substrate preference. CBP/p300 stands out as an integrator of activation signals from diverse regulatory proteins. The sum total of acetylation in a given cell may be shared by multiple, partially redundant HAT activities.

6.6.5   Repressors and co-repressors

Histone deacetylases (HDACs) counter the effects of HATs by restoring the nucleosomes to their transcriptionally repressive configurations. The best described HDACs are yeast Rpd3 and the related HDAC1 of human origin. HDACs form a complex with a co-repressor such as Sin3. Neither the HDAC nor the co-repressor bind directly to DNA. However, the co-repressor interacts not only with the HDAC but also with a DNA-binding repressor such as Ume6, which tethers the complex to upstream silencer elements. Thus the co-repressor bridges the gene-specific repressor to the HDAC, whose activity at the core promoter is necessary to achieve full repression.

As previously mentioned, DNA methylation is associated with repression of gene expression. The mediator responsible is MeCP (methyl-CpG binding protein), a chromosomal protein which recruits the HDAC–co-repressor complex to methylated sites on the DNA via interaction with the co-repressor (Ng & Bird, 1999). Thus, DNA methylation strengthens transcriptional silencing by histone deacetylation.

6.6.6   Interaction of regulatory transcription factors

In the overall scheme, chromatin structure is reversibly altered to allow or prevent access of the basal transcription machinery by targeting HATs or HDACs to the core promoter and thereby activating or repressing transcription, respectively. It is now clear that transcriptional activators such as VP16 function by recruiting coactivators such as CBP/p300 whose HAT activity disrupts the repressive chromatin structure. Similarly, repressors such as Ume6 do not directly

Table 6.2   Histone acetyltransferases (HATs).

	Histone substrate	Origin	Remarks
Gcn5	Free H3, H4	Yeast, mammalian	Component of SAGA which interacts with TBP through Spt3, Spt20 and Ada2
PCAF	Free H3, H4, nucleosomal H3	Mammalian	Associates with CBP/p300, SRC-1, ACTR
CBP/p300	Free and nucleosomal H2A, H2B, H3, H4	Mammalian	Associates with nuclear hormone receptors, P/CAF, SRC-1, ACTR, CREB, AP-1 and other regulatory proteins
TAF$_{II}$250	Free H3, H4	Yeast, mammalian	Component of TFIID
SRC-1	Free and nucleosomal H3, H4	Yeast, mammalian	Associates with nuclear hormone receptors, P/CAF, CBP/p300
ACTR	Free and nucleosomal H3, H4	Yeast	Associates with nuclear hormone receptors, P/CAF, CBP/p300

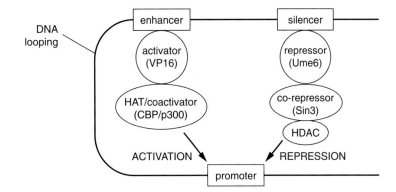

Fig. 6.15 Arrangement of regulatory proteins involved in transcriptional activation and repression. Coactivators harbour intrinsic HAT activity while co-repressors interact with a complex containing HDAC.

inhibit transcription, but rather recruit HDACs via a bridging co-repressor such as Sin3. The activators and repressors bind to upstream regulatory elements and the indirect contacts with the promoter are facilitated by looping of the intervening stretches of DNA (Fig. 6.15).

6.7   Jun, Fos and the AP-1 complex

AP-1 is the collective name for a variety of dimers composed of members of the Jun and Fos protein families (Angel & Karin, 1991). Among these proteins, c-Jun is the major component of the dimeric complex and c-Fos is its best-known partner. AP-1 is a transcriptional activator that binds to promoter elements in genes that are required for cell proliferation. Typical genes are those that encode collagenase, stromelysin and osteocalcin. The response element that is recognized by AP-1 (the AP-1 binding site) functions as an inducible enhancer (Angel *et al.*, 1987). Its consensus DNA sequence is a palindromic 5′-TGA(G/C)TCA-3′. Jun and Fos proteins are described as bZIP proteins because of their conserved basic regions and leucine zipper motifs that are required for DNA binding and dimerization, respectively. Their activation domains, which contain high densities of specific amino acids, are envisioned to interact directly or indirectly with other regulatory proteins and with the basal transcription machinery.

AP-1 is an example of a transcription factor that responds to extracellular signals. The occupancy of specific cell-surface receptors by growth factors and cytokines triggers tightly coordinated multistep signal transduction cascades to the nucleus. In this cascade AP-1 is the terminal acceptor responsible for converting the transient stimulation at the cell surface into a long-term transcriptional response.

The functional forms of AP-1 are Jun/Fos heterodimers and Jun homodimers; Fos proteins do not form homodimers. Dimerization is a prerequisite for DNA binding. The various heterodimers differ not only in their direct effects on transcription, but also in their interactions with other transcription factors, thereby increasing the combinatorial possibilities for gene regulation. There is also evidence that Jun family members can modulate each other's action.

c-Jun and c-Fos are the respective products of the genes c-*jun* and c-*fos*, whose own transcription is induced by growth factors, cytokines, tumour promoters and various other stimuli which trigger signal transduction pathways to the nucleus via protein kinase C. c-*jun* and c-*fos* are primary response genes, whose transcription is activated independently of concomitant protein synthesis within a few minutes of cell stimulation. Induction of c-*jun* is long lasting, varying from a few hours to several days in a manner that is dependent on cell type and stimulus. It is noteworthy that c-*jun* transcription is stimulated by its own protein product. This positive autoregulation serves an important role in amplifying the initial transient stimulus to produce the long-term response. In contrast to c-*jun*, c-*fos* induction is rapid and highly transient, resulting in appearance of the c-Fos protein within 1 hour of the initial stimulus. Induction of c-*fos* transcription depends on another transcription factor, serum response factor, and is inhibited by its own product. Thus c-*fos* acts as a genetic switch, being rapidly induced, then quickly shut off again.

AP-1 activity is regulated by post-translational modification of both pre-existing and newly synthesized AP-1 proteins, as well as through induction of *jun* and *fos* genes. Protein phosphorylation is the post-translational modification of choice when rapid modulation of protein activity in response to changes in environmental conditions is required. c-Jun is phosphorylated at five regulatory sites bearing threonine or serine residues. Three sites (Thr231, Ser243 and Ser249) are clustered within the carboxy-terminal DNA-binding domain and the other two sites (Ser63 and Ser73) are located in the amino-terminal activation domain. Phosphorylation of c-Jun at the carboxy-terminal sites inhibits DNA binding by c-Jun homodimers, but has no measurable effect on c-Jun/c-Fos heterodimers (Karin, 1994). Dephosphorylation of these sites through activation of protein kinase C removes this inhibition, allowing DNA binding and contributing to increased AP-1 activity (Boyle *et al.*, 1991). Phosphorylation of the amino-terminal sites stimulates the transcriptional activity of c-Jun, without affecting its DNA-binding activity; this stimulation also takes place when c-Jun is heterodimerized with c-Fos (Karin, 1994). In this case, the phosphorylation, which is mediated by c-Jun N-terminal kinase (JNK) (Hibi *et al.*, 1993), is required to recruit the transcriptional coactivator, CBP (Arias *et al.*, 1994).

A third mechanism to regulate AP-1 activity is physical interaction with nuclear receptors. In contrast to the interaction between AP-1 and steroid hormone receptors, which is nonmutual and can be either negative or positive (Shemshedini *et al.*, 1991), the interaction between AP-1 and the retinoid receptors is mutual and solely inhibitory.

In addition to repression by protein–protein interactions, AP-1 activity is also negatively regulated at the level of c-*jun* and c-*fos* transcription. This negative regulation is important for normal cellular function. Because of its ability to positively autoregulate its own transcription, c-*jun* is at the risk of being permanently transcribed. Over-expression of c-*jun* is dangerous because it can lead to uncontrolled cell proliferation and tumour formation.

Another property of Jun and Fos is their ability to induce DNA bending in opposite orientations (Kerppola & Curran, 1991). The bending is caused at least in part by charge interactions. Contact between proteins bound to separated sites on DNA requires looping of the intervening DNA. Although long DNA fragments of several hundred to thousands of base pairs are flexible, short DNA fragments of ten to a few hundred base pairs have the characteristics of stiff rods. Therefore, interaction between proteins separated by short distances is constrained by the unfavourable free energy of DNA looping. The bending of DNA by Jun and Fos reduces this thermodynamic barrier and facilitates protein–protein interactions.

6.8 Nuclear hormone receptors as regulators of protein synthesis

6.8.1 Steroid hormones

Steroid hormones include the male sex hormones (collectively called androgens), the female sex hormones (oestrogens and progestins) and the hormones secreted by the cortex of the adrenal glands (the corticosteroids). The hormones circulate in the blood both free and in combination with carrier proteins. The free steroids diffuse in and out of cells but are retained only in target cells through binding to specific receptor proteins, which are constitutively present. It was initially thought that, in the absence of hormone, the receptors were located in the cytoplasm and, after binding hormone, were rapidly translocated into the nucleus. It is now known that the unoccupied receptors are actively transported from the cytoplasm to the nucleus, but then diffuse back into the cytoplasm. This constant movement between nucleus and cytoplasm is known as nucleocytoplasmic shuttling.

The binding of steroid hormones to their intracellular receptors causes the receptors to bind as homodimers to specific hormone response elements on the DNA. These elements can be regarded as enhancers and the receptors as ligand-inducible activator proteins. In the absence of ligand, steroid receptors exist in the form of large complexes with various heat shock proteins, and it is logical to suppose that these proteins sterically hinder DNA binding. The binding of ligand induces a conformational change in the steroid receptor, which allows it to dissociate from the heat shock proteins and also to pair up with a similar receptor to form a homodimer. Ligand activation and dimeric DNA binding of the receptor stimulates regulated transcription, after which the hormone and receptor dissociate from one another and from the DNA. The hormone is metabolized and excreted from the cell, while the free receptor is recycled to await binding by another hormone molecule.

6.8.2   Classification of nuclear hormone receptors into types I and II

Vitamin A (as retinoic acid) and vitamin D (as 1,25-dihydroxyvitamin D_3) also induce the synthesis of specific proteins through receptor-mediated regulation of gene transcription. Receptors for vitamins A and D share certain structural and functional properties with steroid hormone receptors, and all may be considered as members of a nuclear hormone receptor superfamily. The superfamily can be conveniently divided into two types based on functionally distinct properties. Type I comprise receptors (R) for the classic steroid hormones such as (o)estrogen (ER), progesterone (PR), androgen (AR), glucocorticoid (GR) and mineralocorticoid (MR). Type II comprise receptors for thyroid hormone (TR), retinoic acid (RAR and RXR), vitamin D_3 (VDR) and prostanoids (PPAR). Also included in the superfamily are orphan receptors whose cognate ligands (if any exist) are as yet unidentified.

There are several important functional differences between the type I and type II receptors. Type I receptors are unable to bind DNA in the absence of ligand, whereas type II receptors are able to do so. Type I receptors bind to their DNA response elements as homodimers, whereas type II receptors are able to form stable heterodimers with the retinoid X receptor (RXR) *in vitro*. It is this constitutive dimerization that facilitates DNA binding in the absence of ligand. RAR and TR possess a silencing function, the CoR (co-repressor) box, which, in the absence of ligand, interacts with a co-repressor protein. Type I receptors do not have a CoR box but, unlike type II receptors, associate with heat shock proteins in the absence of ligand.

6.8.3   Hormone response elements

The hormone response elements on the DNA are binding sites for nuclear receptors and act as enhancers to increase the transcriptional activity of an adjacent promoter. The response elements are composed of two half-sites or core recognition motifs, each with six base pairs, separated by base pair spacers. The dyad symmetry of these elements permits receptor–ligand complexes to bind as dimers, with each monomer recognizing one of the half-sites.

Three main features determine the specificity of receptor binding to hormone response elements: (1) the precise nucleotide sequence of the half-site, (2) the orientation of half-sites with respect to each other and (3) the spacing between half-sites. There are only two consensus half-site sequences. The sequence 5′-AGAACA is recognized by the GR, MR, AR and PR; the sequence 5′-AGGTCA is recognized by the ER, RAR, VDR and TR, as well as virtually all other known members of the nuclear receptor superfamily. The orientation of half-sites can be as inverted repeats, everted repeats or direct repeats, as illustrated in Fig. 6.16. Table 6.3 shows the features of response

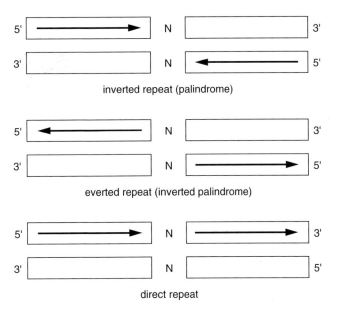

inverted repeat (palindrome)

everted repeat (inverted palindrome)

direct repeat

Fig. 6.16 Half-site orientations of hormone response elements. Arrows indicate the 5′ to 3′ direction. N, nucleotide spacer(s).

Hexanucleotide sequences	Type of response element	Receptor dimers
Inverted repeat sequences		
5′-AGAACAnnnTGTTCT-3′ 3′-TCTTGTnnnACAAAGA-5′	IR3	GR/GR, MR/MR, AR/AR, PR/PR
5′-AGGTCAnnnTGACCT-3′ 3′-TCCAGTnnnACTGGA-5′	IR3	ER/ER
Direct repeat sequences		
5′-AGGTCAnAGGTCA-3′ 3′-TCCAGTnTCCAGT-5′	DR1	RXR/RXR, RAR/RXR, PPAR/RXR
5′-AGGTCAnnAGGTCA-3′ 3′-TCCAGTnnTCCAGT-5′	DR2	RAR/RXR
5′-AGGTCAnnnAGGTCA-3′ 3′-TCCAGTnnnTCCAGT-5′	DR3	VDR/VDR
5′-AGGTCAnnnnAGGTCA-3′ 3′-TCCAGTnnnnTCCAGT-5′	DR4	TR/RXR
5′-AGGTCAnnnnnAGGTCA-3′ 3′-TCCAGTnnnnnTCCAGT-5′	DR5	RAR/RXR

Table 6.3 Features of hormone response elements preferentially recognized by nuclear receptors.

Base pairs: adenine (A); thymine (T); cytosine (C); guanine (G).
IR3, inverted repeat with three nucleotide spacers (n). DR1, DR2, DR3, etc., direct repeats with one, two, three, etc. nucleotide spacers.
Receptors (R) for: GR, glucocorticoid; MR, mineralocorticoid; AR, androgen; PR, progesterone; ER, (o)estrogen; RXR, retinoid X; RAR, retinoic acid; PPAR peroxisome proliferator-activated; VDR, vitamin D_3; TR, thyroid hormone.

elements recognized by the principal nuclear receptors. Those elements recognized by type I steroid receptors are designated IR3 elements because the half-sites are arranged exclusively as inverted repeats separated by three nucleotides. Specificity between GR, MR and PR is determined by differences in the individual nucleotides of the spacer.

In contrast to the strict palindromic organization of steroid hormone response elements, the highest affinity binding sites for type II receptors are arranged as direct repeats, with AGGTCA as the consensus core recognition motif. The preferred spacing between the direct repeats (DR) is three nucleotides (DR3) for VDR/RXR, four nucleotides (DR4) for TR/RXR, and five nucleotides (DR5) for RAR/RXR. RAR/RXR is also capable of binding to DR1 and DR2 elements, but with somewhat lower affinity than to the DR5 element. DR1 is also a response element for an RXR homodimer and for a PPAR/RXR heterodimer. The orphan receptor COUP-TF in dimeric partnership with RXR recognizes DRs with 0 to 5 spacers, although the binding is most avid with DR1 elements.

6.8.4 Classification of steroid-responsive genes

Genes regulated by steroid hormones may be divided into three categories: primary response genes, delayed primary response genes and secondary response genes (Dean & Sanders, 1996). This classification is based principally on whether or not the gene directly binds the hormone-bound nuclear receptor. In the case of primary response genes, the hormone–receptor complex acts as a transcription factor and directly binds, or binds through tethering, to a specific hormone response element within the target gene. The liganded receptor is only involved in one signal transduction pathway to affect transcription. Increases in mRNA steady-state levels occur within 15 min of steroid hormone administration. This rapid response has given rise to the term 'early genes'. The protein product of a primary response gene is the steroid responsive protein; there is no attendant synthesis of protein and therefore cycloheximide does not inhibit the hormonal response.

Secondary response genes, by definition, do not bind the hormone–receptor complex. Transcription of these genes is regulated by the action of an intermediary protein in one of several possible ways. The hormone–receptor complex could bind to a primary response gene that encodes a transcription factor (the intermediary protein) that is necessary to regulate the secondary response gene. Alternatively, the intermediary protein encoded by the primary response gene could be an enzyme, perhaps a kinase, that activates or inactivates a pre-existing protein that is directly or indirectly critical for transcription of the secondary response gene. The activated protein could be a transcription factor. It could also be an mRNA-stabilizing protein, stabilizing an mRNA whose protein product is essential for transcription of the secondary response gene. Because synthesis of an intermediary protein is required, the responses are inhibited by cycloheximide. Secondary response genes do not show a significant change in mRNA steady-state levels until 1 or more hours after steroid administration; for this reason, they are often referred to as 'late genes'.

Delayed primary response genes directly bind the hormone–receptor complex and yet exhibit a delayed induction that requires attendant protein synthesis. This type of gene is exemplified by the vitamin D-responsive *osteocalcin* gene and the retinoic acid-responsive β-*laminin* gene. The mechanisms involved in the induction of these genes are unclear.

6.8.5 Receptor domains

Based on amino acid sequence similarity, the protein structures of the receptors can be divided into six domains, designated A to F (Fig. 6.17). The A/B domain is at the amino (N) terminus of the molecule and the F domain is at the carboxy (C) terminus. Significant sequence homology is found among the members of the nuclear receptor superfamily; those domains exhibiting strong homology have been conserved during evolution.

The most highly conserved domain is the C domain, which contains the DNA binding site and regions that contribute to receptor dimerization and nuclear localization. Part of the peptide chain in the C domain is folded into two loops separated by a linker region of 15 to 17 amino acids. Each loop is anchored by a single zinc atom tetrahedrally coordinated by the sulphydryl groups of four cysteine residues. The two loops are commonly referred to as 'zinc fingers' – a misnomer, as they are actually folded together to form a compact, interdependent structure (Glass, 1994). Each zinc coordination complex initiates an α-helix and these helices cross at right angles to form the core of the DNA binding site. The first helix acts as the DNA recognition helix; it contains a sequence of amino acid residues (the P box) that make base-specific contacts with the major groove of DNA. Other regions located at the carboxy-terminal side of the second zinc finger make multiple phosphate backbone contacts and

	N-terminus			C-terminus	
A/B	C	D	E	F

	A/B	C	D	E	F
DNA binding		+			
Ligand binding				+	
Nuclear localization		+		+	
Dimerization		+		+	
Activation	+ (AF-1)			+ (AF-2)	
Repression[a]				+	
Heat-shock protein association[b]				+	

Fig. 6.17 General functional organization of steroid receptors into six domains, A–F. [a]not steroid hormone receptors; [b]not RAR, VDR and TR.

may establish the orientation and position of the first helix with respect to the hormone response element half-site. The second helix stabilizes the recognition helix. A sequence of amino acid residues (the D box) located within the second zinc finger forms a portion of a dimerization interface (Glass, 1994).

The functionally complex E domain encompasses about 250 amino acids and contains subdomains responsible for ligand binding, dimerization, nuclear localization and transcriptional activation. In addition, TR and RAR contain a CoR box, and steroid hormone receptors contain a region responsible for heat-shock protein association. The peptide chain in the ligand binding region contains many hydrophobic amino acids and is folded to form a hydrophobic ligand-binding pocket. The major dimerization region is localized in the C-terminal half of the E domain. This region contains nine heptad sequences of hydrophobic amino acids putatively organized into five discontinuous α-helices (Forman & Samuels, 1990). These helices form multiple independent dimerization interfaces at which two receptor molecules become joined through coil–coil interactions. A region essential for transcriptional activation, AF-2, is one of two activation functions. The core motif for AF-2 is highly conserved and is present in all nuclear receptors for which a specific ligand has been identified. The motif forms an amphipathic α-helix consisting of a glutamic acid residue flanked by hydrophobic amino acid residues.

The A/B domain is highly variable in size, ranging from 25 (VDR) to 603 amino acids (MR), and exhibits negligible sequence conservation. It contains the second activation function, AF-1, whose length and sequence are highly variable and unique to each specific receptor isoform. AF-1 functions independently of ligand, as opposed to AF-2, which is ligand-inducible. Although only weakly active by itself, AF-1 synergizes with and modulates the activity of AF-2.

The D domain is a flexible 'hinge' region, allowing a degree of rotation within the protein molecule. The F domain is a variable region for which no specific function has been identified and is completely lacking in the PR.

6.8.6   Structural basis for ligand binding to receptor

The three-dimensional structures of the ligand-binding domains (LBDs) of unliganded (apo)-RXR

(Bourguet et al. 1995), liganded (holo)-RARγ (Renaud et al., 1995) and holo-TRα (Wagner et al., 1995) have been reported. The overall structure of each receptor's LBD is similar, consisting almost entirely of twelve α-helices arranged in three layers to form an antiparallel α-helical sandwich. However, there is one striking difference between the structures of apo and holo LBDs with regard to the position of helix 12, which contains the conserved AF-2 core. Whereas helix 12 protrudes beyond the main body of the protein in apo-RXR, this helix is folded back in holo-RAR and holo-TR and makes direct contact with the bound ligands buried deep within a hydrophobic binding pocket. Comparison of the apo and holo LBD structures has led to the proposal of a 'mouse trap' mechanism by which the ligand-induced conformational change renders the receptor transcriptionally active (Wurtz et al., 1996). According to this proposal, the mouse (ligand), tempted into the trap (ligand-binding pocket) by the bait (electrostatic forces), pushes a lever (helix 11) thus springing the trap mechanism (release of helix 12 from the Ω-loop) and causing the lid (helix 12) to seal the trap and imprison the mouse. Despite the apparently higher structural stability of the liganded receptor, an equilibrium must exist that allows the ligand to dissociate from the protein. The conformational change upon ligand binding creates new interfaces, allowing for interaction with coactivators; it also disrupts pre-existing interfaces, causing the release of co-repressors. The relief of nucleosomal repression and recruitment of coactivators results in activation of gene transcription. It is likely that at least some of the ligands that function as antagonists of transcription prevent the correct realignment of helix 12 and fail to create the proper interacting surfaces.

6.8.7   Repressive effect of COUP-TF

The chicken ovalbumin upstream promoter transcription factor (COUP-TF) is an orphan member of the nuclear receptor superfamily. This receptor was originally characterized in chick oviduct extracts, where it bound as a homodimer to a DR-1 response element in the ovalbumin gene promoter and activated transcription. COUP-TF I and COUP-TF II are close homologues, which are also known as ear-3 and ARP-1, respectively (Qui et al., 1994). COUP-TF is expressed ubiquitously in vertebrates, especially in the liver. The structural flexibility of the COUP-TF molecule allows it to bind to different arrangements of the AGGTCA consensus core half-site. It can bind to both direct repeats and palindromes with different nucleotide spacings between the half-sites (Cooney *et al.*, 1992), the highest preference being toward DR1 elements (Kliewer *et al.*, 1992). By virtue of their promiscuous DNA binding, COUP-TFs repress ligand-induced transcriptional activity of RAR, RXR, TR, VDR and PPAR.

Four mechanisms have been proposed to address COUP-TF's repressive ability.

1   Direct competition between COUP-TF and other nuclear receptors for binding to common response elements (Tran *et al.*, 1992). Support for this proposal is the observed release of repression when the expression of RAR is increased.

2   Competition for RXR between COUP-TF and other receptors (Cooney *et al.*, 1993). The reduction in available RXR caused by its sequestration in functionally inactive heterodimers with COUP-TF indirectly decreases the DNA-binding affinity of RAR, VDR and TR and thereby interferes with the potential of these receptors to activate their target genes. Over-expression of RXR relieves the COUP-TF inhibition.

3   Transrepression, in which COUP-TF is tethered to a promoter via dimerization with RAR, RXR and TR so that it represses their ligand-dependent transcriptional activity (Leng *et al.*, 1996).

4   Active repression mediated by co-repressors, such as N-CoR and SMRT, which interact with a silencing function (CoR box) localized in the extreme carboxy terminus of the E domain of COUP-TF (Shibata *et al.*, 1997).

Further reading

Aranda, A. & Pascual, A. (2001) Nuclear hormone receptors and gene expression. *Physiological Reviews*, **81**, 1269–304.

Chen, J. D. & Li, H. (1998) Coactivation and corepression in transcriptional regulation by steroid/nuclear hormone receptors. *Critical Reviews in Eukaryotic Gene Expression*, **8**, 169–90.

Glass, C. K., Rose, D. W. & Rosenfeld, M. G. (1997) Nuclear receptor coactivators. *Current Opinion in Cell Biology*, **9**, 222–32.

Hassig, C. A. & Schreiber, S. L. (1997) Nuclear histone acetylases and deacetylases and transcriptional regulation: HATs off to HDACs. *Current Opinion in Chemical Biology*, **1**, 300–8.

Kadonaga, J. T. (1998) Eukaryotic transcription: an interlaced network of transcription factors and chromatin-modifying machines. *Cell*, **92**, 307–13.

Moras, D. & Gronemeyer, H. (1998) The nuclear receptor ligand-binding domain: structure and function. *Current Opinion in Cell Biology*, **10**, 384–91.

Parker, M. G. (1993) Steroid and related receptors. *Current Opinion in Cell Biology*, **5**, 499–504.

Tsai, M.-J. & O'Malley, B. W. (1994) Molecular mechanisms of action of steroid/thyroid receptor superfamily members. *Annual Review of Biochemistry*, **63**, 451–86.

Workman, J. L. & Kingston, R. E. (1998) Alteration of nucleosome structure as a mechanism of transcriptional regulation. *Annual Review of Biochemistry*, **67**, 545–79.

Yu, V. C., Näär, A. M. & Rosenfeld, M. G. (1992) Transcriptional regulation by the nuclear receptor superfamily. *Current Opinion in Biotechnology*, **3**, 597–602.

Zawel, L. & Reinberg, D. (1995) Common themes in assembly and function of eukaryotic transcription complexes. *Annual Review of Biochemistry*, **64**, 533–61.

References

Angel, P. & Karin, M. (1991) The role of Jun, Fos and the AP-1 complex in cell-proliferation and transformation. *Biochimica et Biophysica Acta*, **1072**, 129–57.

Angel, P., Baumann, I., Stein, B., Delius, H., Rahmsdorf, H. J. & Herrlich, P. (1987) 12-*O*-Tetradecanoyl-phorbol-13-acetate induction of the human collagenase gene is mediated by an inducible enhancer located in the 5′ flanking region. *Molecular and Cell Biology*, **7**, 2256–66.

Arias, J., Alberts, A. S., Brindle, P., Claret, F. X., Smeal, T., Karin, M., Feramisco, J. & Montminy, M. (1994) Activation of cAMP and mitogen responsive genes relies on a common nuclear factor. *Nature*, **370**, 226–9.

Bourguet, W., Ruff, M., Chambon, P., Gronemeyer, H. & Moras, D. (1995) Crystal structure of the ligand-binding domain of the human nuclear receptor RXR-α. *Nature*, **375**, 377–82.

Boyle, W. J., Smeal, T., Defize, L. H. K., Angel, P., Woodgett, J. R., Karin, M. & Hunter, T. (1991) Activation of protein kinase C decreases phosphorylation of c-Jun at sites that negatively regulate its DNA-binding activity. *Cell*, **64**, 573–84.

Brown, T. A. (1999) *Genomes*. Bios Scientific, Oxford.

Brownell, J. E., Zhou, J., Ranalli, T., Kobayashi, R., Edmondson, D. G., Roth, S. Y. & Allis, C. D. (1996) Tetrahymena histone acetyltransferase A: a homolog to yeast Gcn5p linking histone acetylation to gene activation. *Cell*, **84**, 843–51.

Cooney, A. J., Tsai, S. Y., O'Malley, B. W. & Tsai, M.-J. (1992) Chicken ovalbumin upstream promoter transcription factor (COUP-TF) dimers bind to different GGTCA response elements, allowing COUP-TF to repress hormonal induction of the vitamin D, thyroid hormone, and retinoic acid receptors. *Molecular and Cellular Biology*, **12**, 4153–63.

Cooney, A. J., Leng, X., Tsai, S. Y., O'Malley, B. W. & Tsai, M.-J. (1993) Multiple mechanisms of chicken ovalbumin upstream promoter transcription factor-dependent repression of transactivation by the vitamin D, thyroid hormone, and retinoic acid receptors. *Journal of Biological Chemistry*, **268**(6), 4152–60.

Cosma, M. P., Tanaka, T. & Nasmyth, K. (1999) Ordered recruitment of transcription and chromatin remodeling factors to a cell cycle- and developmentally regulated promoter. *Cell*, **97**, 299–311.

Csordas, A. (1990) On the biological role of histone acetylation. *Biochemical Journal*, **265**, 23–38.

Dean, D. M. & Sanders, M. M. (1996) Ten years after; reclassification of steroid-responsive genes. *Molecular Endocrinology*, **10**,

1489–95.

Forman, B. M. & Samuels, H. H. (1990) Interactions among a subfamily of nuclear hormone receptors: the regulatory zipper model. *Molecular Endocrinology*, **4**, 1293–301.

Glass, C. L. (1994) Differential recognition of target genes by nuclear receptor monomers, dimers, and heterodimers. *Endocrine Reviews*, **15**, 391–407.

Green, N. P. O., Stout, G. W. & Taylor, D. J. (1990) *Biological Science*, 2nd edn. Cambridge University Press.

Hibi, M., Lin, A., Smeal, T., Minden, A. & Karin, M. (1993) Identification of an oncoprotein- and UV-responsive protein kinase that binds and potentiates the c-Jun activation domain. *Genes & Development*, **7**, 2135–48.

Karin, M. (1994) Signal transduction from the cell surface to the nucleus through the phosphorylation of transcription factors. *Current Opinion in Cell Biology*, **6**, 415–24.

Kerppola, T. K. & Curran, T. (1991) Fos–Jun heterodimers and Jun homodimers bend DNA in opposite orientations: implications for transcription factor cooperativity. *Cell*, **66**, 317–26.

Kliewer, S. A., Umesono, K., Heyman, R. A., Mangelsdorf, D. J., Dyck, J. A. & Evans, R. M. (1992) Retinoid X receptor–COUP-TF interactions modulate retinoic acid signaling. *Proceedings of the National Academy of Sciences of the U.S.A.*, **89**, 1448–52.

Koleske, A. J. & Young, R. A. (1995) The RNA polymerase II holoenzyme and its implications for gene regulation. *Trends in Biochemical Sciences*, **20**, 113–16.

Kollmar, R. & Farnham, P. J. (1993) Site-specific initiation of transcription by RNA polymerase II. *Proceedings of the Society for Experimental Biology and Medicine*, **203**, 127–39.

Kuo, M.-H., Zhou, J., Jambeck, P., Churchill, M. E. A. & Allis, C. D. (1998) Histone acetyltransferase activity of yeast Gcn5p is required for the activation of target genes in vivo. *Genes & Development*, **12**, 627–39.

Laird, P. W. & Jaenisch, R. (1994) DNA methylation and cancer. *Human Molecular Genetics*, **3**, 1487–95.

Leng, X., Cooney, A. J., Tsai, S. Y. & Tsai, M.-J. (1996) Molecular mechanisms of COUP-TF-mediated transcriptional repression: evidence for transrepression and active repression. *Molecular and Cellular Biology*, **16**, 2332–40.

Ng, H.-H. & Bird, A. (1999) DNA methylation and chromatin modification. *Current Opinion in Genetics & Development*, **9**, 158–63.

Pazin, M. J. & Kadonaga, J. T. (1997) SWI2/SNF2 and related proteins: ATP-driven motors that disrupt protein–DNA interactions? *Cell*, **88**, 737–40.

Qiu, Y., Tsai, S. Y. & Tsai, M.-J. (1994) COUP-TF. An orphan member of the steroid/thyroid hormone receptor superfamily. *Trends in Endocrinology and Metabolism*, **5**, 234–9.

Renaud, J.-P., Rochel, N., Ruff, M., Vivat, V, Chambon, P., Gronemeyer, H. & Moras, D. (1995) Crystal structure of the RAR-ligand-binding domain bound to all-*trans* retinoic acid. *Nature*, **378**, 681–9.

Roberts, S. G. E. & Green, M. R. (1994) Activator-induced conformational change in general transcription factor TFIIB. *Nature*, **371**, 717–20.

Roberts, S. M. & Winston, F. (1997) Essential functional interactions of SAGA, a *Saccharomyces cerevisiae* complex of SPt, Ada, and Gcn5 proteins, with the Snf/Swi and Srb/mediator complexes. *Genetics*, **147**, 451–65.

Roeder, R. G. (1996) The role of general initiation factors in transcription by RNA polymerase II. *Trends in Biochemical Sciences*, **21**, 327–35.

Sheldon, M. & Reinberg, D. (1995) Tuning-up transcription. *Current Biology*, **5**, 43–6.

Shemshedini, L., Knauthe, R., Sassone-Corsi, P., Pornon, A. & Gronemeyer, H. (1991) Cell-specific inhibitory and stimulatory effects of Fos and Jun on transcription activation by nuclear receptors. *EMBO Journal*, **10**, 3839–49.

Shibata, H., Nawaz, Z., Tsai, S. Y., O'Malley, B. W. & Tsai, M.-J. (1997) Gene silencing by chicken ovalbumin upstream promoter-transcription factor 1 (COUP-TF1) is mediated by transcriptional corepressors, nuclear receptor-corepressor (N-CoR) and silencing mediator for retinoic acid receptor and thyroid hormone receptor (SMRT). *Molecular Endocrinology*, **11**, 714–24.

Tran, P., Zhang, X. K., Salbert, G., Hermann, T., Lehmann, J. M. & Pfahl, M. (1992) COUP orphan receptors are negative regulators of retinoic acid response pathways. *Molecular and Cellular Biology*, **12**, 4666–76.

Varga-Weisz, P. D. & Becker, P. B. (1998) Chromatin-remodeling factors: machines that regulate? *Current Opinion in Cell Biology*, **10**, 346–53.

Wagner, R. L., Apriletti, J. W., McGrath, M. E., West, B. L., Baxter, J. D. & Fletterick, R. J. (1995) A structural role for hormone in the thyroid hormone receptor. *Nature*, **378**, 690–7.

Wang, L., Liu, L. & Berger, S. L. (1998) Critical residues for histone acetylation by Gcn5, functioning in Ada and SAGA complexes, are also required for transcriptional function in vivo. *Genes & Development*, **12**, 640–53.

Wurtz, J.-M., Bourguet, W., Renaud, J.-P., Vivat, V., Chambon, P., Moras, D. & Gronemeyer, H. (1996) A canonical structure for the ligand-binding domain of nuclear receptors. *Nature Structural Biology*, **3**, 87–94.

7
Vitamin A: Retinoids and Carotenoids

Key discussion topics

- Ingested provitamin A carotenoids, after absorption, are converted first to retinaldehyde and then to retinol in the enterocytes.
- Retinoic acid, the metabolite responsible for most of the nonvisual functions of vitamin A, is produced intracellularly by oxidation of diet-derived retinol via retinaldehyde and also from β-carotene.
- Various types of retinoid-binding proteins transport the hydrophobic retinoids within aqueous extracellular, cytosolic and nuclear compartments.
- Vitamin A is stored in the liver as retinyl esters and mobilized for use in a highly regulated process.
- Circulating retinol concentrations are homeostatically regulated to remain constant.
- The function of vitamin A in vision is based upon the binding of 11-*cis* retinaldehyde with the protein opsin to form the visual pigment, rhodopsin.
- All-*trans* retinoic acid and 9-*cis* retinoic acid are hormonal metabolites of vitamin A that mediate tissue-specific expression of target genes through their binding to two types of nuclear retinoid receptors.
- When bound to DNA, retinoic acid receptor (RAR) functions as a transcriptional activator in the presence of its hormonal ligand, and as a repressor in the absence of ligand.
- Heterodimer formation between the retinoid X receptor (RXR) and the nuclear receptors for retinoic acid, thyroid hormone and vitamin D_3 allow RXR to function as a master controller for signals from various converging hormonal pathways.
- The COUP-TF orphan receptors act as negative regulators of retinoid hormone response pathways.
- Retinoid receptors antagonize the AP-1 activator thereby preventing excessive cell proliferation.
- Retinoic acid induces the transcription of many genes encoding proteins that are involved in cell differentiation and a variety of biochemical processes.
- Disrupted expression patterns of retinoid-responsive cytokine genes account for impaired antibody-mediated immunity in vitamin A deficiency.
- Retinoic acid exerts profound effects on pattern formation during embryogenesis.
- Carotenoids act as biological antioxidants by trapping peroxyl free radicals and deactivating singlet oxygen.
- The cancer-preventing action of retinoids correlates with enhanced gap junctional communication of growth controlling signals.

7.1   Historical overview

In 1912, McCollum and, independently, Osborne and Mendel, separated in almost pure form the proteins, fats, carbohydrates, mineral matter and water from a variety of foods. Mixtures of the isolated nutrients were then fed to animals which soon sickened and died. It was concluded that the food from which the nutrients were derived contained some additional factor that is necessary to sustain life. In 1915 McCollum and Davis isolated from animal fats and fish oils a 'fat-soluble A' that was essential to rats for growth and also cured eye disorders. In 1921 Bloch reported that a diet containing full milk and cod-liver oil cured xerophthalmia in infants and concluded that the eye affliction was due to the absence of the fat-soluble A in the diet. In the meantime it was discovered that green vegetables also possess fat-soluble A activity and in 1930 Moore provided evidence that carotene was converted to vitamin A in the body. The provitamin role of β-carotene became obvious after Karrer elucidated the structures of β-carotene and retinol.

The biochemical function of vitamin A in vision was established by Wald in 1935.

In 1987, two independent research groups led by Pierre Chambon in Paris and Ronald Evans in California made the important discovery that retinoic acid acts in the manner of a steroid hormone through binding to a specific nuclear receptor.

7.2   Chemistry and biological functions

Vitamin A-active compounds, defined as compounds having qualitatively the biological activity of retinol, are represented by retinoids and provitamin A carotenoids. The retinoids comprise retinol, retinaldehyde and retinoic acid, together with their naturally occurring and synthetic analogues. The naturally occurring retinoids are sometimes referred to as preformed vitamin A because they do not require metabolic conversion, as do carotenoids, in order to become biologically active. Carotenoids are represented by β-carotene and chemically related pigments that are responsible for the colour of many vegetables and fruits. From a nutritional viewpoint, these pigments are classified as provitamin A carotenoids and inactive carotenoids. In nature, carotenoids are synthesized exclusively by higher plants and photosynthetic microorganisms, in which they function as accessory light-harvesting pigments to chlorophyll. Although animals are unable to synthesize carotenoids, they can assimilate them through their diet.

Vitamin A is required for several essential life processes, including metabolism, haematopoiesis, bone development, pattern formation during embryogenesis, the maintenance of differentiated epithelia, and immunocompetence. These processes can be supported by all forms of vitamin A, including the provitamin A carotenoids. The other vitamin A-dependent processes, namely vision and reproduction, specifically require either retinol or retinaldehyde. Retinoic acid cannot support these functions because it cannot be reduced back metabolically to retinaldehyde. Hence animals maintained on retinoic acid as the only source of vitamin A become both blind and sterile, but are otherwise in good general health.

Retinoids promote the differentiation of a variety of cell lines in culture, including epithelial cells and chondrocytes. That this function occurs *in vivo* is demonstrated by the replacement of secretory cells in epithelia by keratin-producing cells when an animal is deprived of vitamin A. The effects of vitamin A on cellular differentiation are due to the control of gene expression by retinoic acid in selected tissues, the protein products being responsible for the effects. Not all vitamin A-responsive genes are up-regulated by retinoic acid; some are down-regulated.

In this text the precise terms 'retinoids' and 'carotenoids' are used where the specificity is known. The non-specific term 'vitamin A' is used in the sense of vitamin A activity and therefore accounts for provitamin A carotenoids as well as retinoids.

7.2.1   Preformed vitamin A

The structures of three physiologically important retinoids are shown in Fig. 7.1. The parent vitamin A compound, retinol, comprises a cyclohexenyl (β-ionone) ring attached at the carbon-6 position to a polyene side chain. The four double bonds in the side chain give rise to *cis/trans* isomerization. The predominant isomer, all-*trans* retinol, possesses maximal (100%) vitamin A activity and is frequently accompanied in foodstuffs by smaller amounts of 13-*cis* retinol, which has 75% relative activity. An aldehyde form, 11-*cis* retinaldehyde, is the chromophore in the retina of the eye, while all-*trans* and 9-*cis* retinoic acid are active metabolites of retinol found in most if not all tissues. Changes in the molecular state of oxidation and *cis/trans* isomerization are of physiological importance in modifying the biological activity of retinoids.

7.2.2   Provitamin A carotenoids

Carotenoids are classified chemically as carotenes, which are hydrocarbons, and xanthophylls, which have one or more oxygen-containing groups (e.g. hydroxyl) either on the ring or in the chain. Most naturally occurring carotenoids contain 40 carbon atoms. In some instances, C_{40}-carotenoids undergo partial oxidative cleavage in the plant tissues to give shortened molecules known as apocarotenoids. The majority of xanthophylls in plant tissues occur as mono or bis esters of saturated long-chain fatty acids (e.g. palmitic acid).

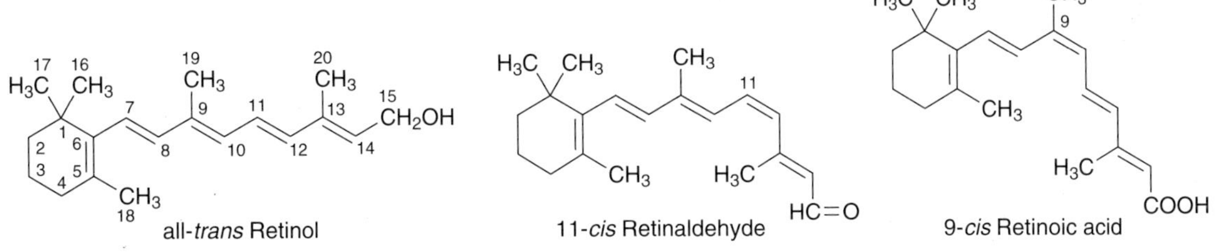

Fig. 7.1 Structures of some physiologically important retinoids.

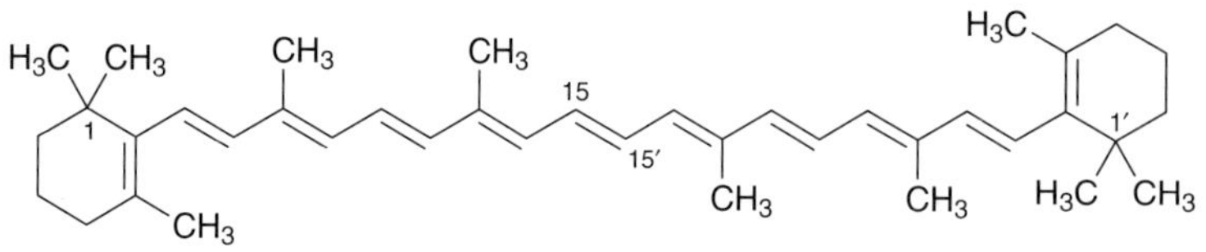

Fig. 7.2 Structure of β-carotene.

For a carotenoid to have vitamin A activity, its structure must incorporate a molecule of retinol, i.e. an unsubstituted β-ionone ring with an 11-carbon polyene chain. The most ubiquitous and nutritionally most important carotenoid, β-carotene (Fig. 7.2), is composed of two molecules of retinol joined tail to tail, thus β-carotene possesses maximal provitamin A activity. The structures of all other provitamin carotenoids incorporate only one molecule of retinol, hence theoretically contribute 50% of the biological value of β-carotene. Over 500 naturally occurring carotenoids have been isolated and characterized; of these, about 50 possess provitamin A activity in varying degrees.

In plant and animal tissues the carotenoids are usually found associated with lipid fractions in noncovalent association with membranes and lipoproteins, and they accumulate in the chloroplasts of green leaves. In nature, carotenoids exist mainly as their all-*trans* forms. Food processing and preservation methods, especially canning, induce *cis*–*trans* isomerization, leading to a reduced vitamin A potency.

7.3   Dietary sources

All natural sources of vitamin A in the diet are derived ultimately from provitamin A carotenoids. For much of the world's human population, and particularly in parts of the developing world, vegetables and fruits provide the main dietary sources of vitamin A in the form of β-carotene and other provitamin carotenoids. In other parts of the world, milk, butter, cheese and eggs are important dietary sources of vitamin A. The liver of meat animals is a particularly rich source as this organ stores the vitamin for the body's use. Preformed vitamin A is present in animal tissues and in milk as a consequence of the enzymatic conversion of ingested provitamin carotenoids in the intestinal wall of the animal. Dietary preformed vitamin A consists mainly of retinol esterified with long chain fatty acids, particularly palmitic acid. Retinyl esters are also found in processed foods supplemented with vitamin A.

7.4   Absorption, transport and metabolism

7.4.1   Overview

Retinol in the free state can enter the lipid bilayer of biological membranes and disrupt membrane structure and function. In order to permit transport within an aqueous environment and to limit its level in membranes, retinol (and other retinoids) are bound to proteins, both extracellularly and intracellularly. The intracellular retinol–protein complex is the metabolically active form of retinol. Alternatively, retinol is esterified with long-chain fatty acids for transport in lipoproteins or storage in cytoplasmic lipid droplets. Protein binding and esterification prevent the disruptive action of free retinol on membrane structure and function, whilst also protecting retinoids from unwanted metabolic processing and decomposition.

In the human, the main events that take place from absorption of dietary vitamin A to cellular metabolism in the target tissues are as follows. Ingested retinyl esters and carotenoids are incorporated into mixed micelles in the intestinal lumen and the retinyl esters are hydrolysed. The micelles dissociate and the retinol and carotenoids are absorbed. Within the enterocytes, varying proportions of the provitamin carotenoids are converted first to retinaldehyde and then to retinol, which is subsequently esterified. Some of the retinaldehyde is oxidized irreversibly to retinoic acid. Retinoic acid can also be produced from β-carotene via apo-carotenals of varying chain length without involving retinaldehyde as an intermediate. The absorbed retinol is also esterified and the combined retinyl esters, accompanied by varying small amounts of unchanged carotenoids, are released into the bloodstream via the lymphatic system as components of chylomicrons. The absorption of β-carotene and retinyl ester and principal metabolic events within the enterocyte are shown diagrammatically in Fig. 7.3.

The circulating chylomicrons undergo lipolysis and the resultant chylomicron remnants are taken up by the liver and to a lesser extent by extrahepatic

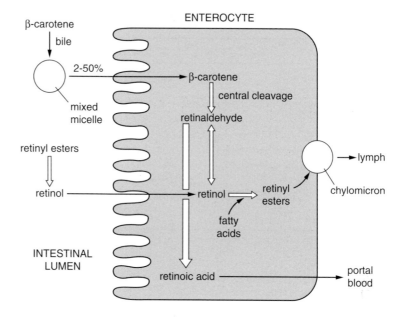

Fig. 7.3 Intestinal absorption and metabolism of β-carotene and retinyl esters. See text for additional metabolic reactions. Reproduced, with permission, from Erdman *et al.* (1993), *Annals of the New York Academy of Sciences*, Vol. 691, pp 76–85, © 1993, New York Academy of Sciences.

tissues. Within the liver the chylomicron remnant retinyl esters are hydrolysed and most of the retinol is transferred from hepatocytes to stellate cells where it is esterified and stored. Remnant carotenoids do not accumulate in liver cells: they are released into the circulation as components of very low density lipoproteins (VLDLs) and ultimately stored intact in adipose tissues and in various organs of the body. Upon demand, the retinyl esters in the liver are hydrolysed and the retinol is released into the bloodstream bound to retinol-binding protein (RBP), which is synthesized in the liver. In the plasma the retinol–RBP complex forms a larger complex with a protein called transthyretin (formerly known as prealbumin), which also transports thyroid hormone. The retinol–RBP–transthyretin complex delivers retinol to a cell-surface receptor expressed in vitamin A-requiring cells. RBP is recognized by the receptor and, after negotiating the lipid bilayer of the plasma membrane, the retinol interacts with a specific cellular binding protein. Cytoplasmic retinol is subject to a variety of metabolic fates, including oxidation to retinoic acid. Cellular binding proteins play major roles in controlling retinol metabolism and may regulate the movement of retinoic acid to the nucleus where it acts as a hormone to affect gene expression.

7.4.2 Retinoid-binding proteins

A number of retinoid-binding proteins (Table 7.1) play an essential role in transporting the hydrophobic retinoids within aqueous extracellular, cytosolic and nuclear compartments. The binding proteins in their free uncomplexed state are referred to as apo-proteins (e.g. apoRBP); when complexed with their ligand they are referred to as holo-proteins (e.g. holoRBP).

Retinol-binding protein (RBP) is a single polypeptide of molecular weight 21 kDa, which specifically binds retinol for transport in the plasma. The protein is synthesized in the liver as a larger molecular weight preRBP, which is rapidly processed to the 21-kDa molecule by the removal of a 3.5-kDa peptide. RBP is also synthesized in a large number of extrahepatic tissues. The protein molecule has a barrel core that completely encapsulates a single retinol molecule, with the β-ionone ring lying deep in the hydrophobic pocket and the polyene tail extending almost to the surface. This arrangement protects the retinol from oxidation and exposure to enzymes during transport. The ligand is tightly bound and can only be removed *in vitro* by extraction with organic solvents or by denaturing the protein.

RBP possesses two additional binding sites: one for attachment to transthyretin and the second for linking to receptors on the surface of target cells. Transthyretin, which is also synthesized in the liver, is

Table 7.1   Principal retinoid-binding proteins involved in vitamin A metabolism.

Binding protein	Major ligand	Location
Intercellular transport		
Retinol-binding protein, RBP	all-*trans* retinol	Synthesized in hepatocytes, circulates in plasma
Interphotoreceptor or interstitial retinol-binding protein, IRBP	all-*trans* and 11-*cis* retinol	Matrix between pigment epithelium and photoreceptor cells of the retina
Intracellular transport		
Cellular retinol-binding protein type I, CRBP-I	all-*trans* retinol	Proximal epididymis, liver, kidney (1), bone (2)
Cellular retinol-binding protein type II, CRBP-II	all-*trans* retinol and retinaldehyde	Intestine (enterocytes), liver and intestine of developing embryo
Cellular retinoic acid-binding protein type I, CRABP-I	all-*trans* retinoic acid	Developing embryo seminal vesicle, vas deferens, skin (1)
Cellular retinoic acid-binding protein type II, CRABP-II	all-*trans* retinoic acid	Developing embryo, adult skin cells
Cellular retinaldehyde-binding protein, CRALBP	11-*cis* retinaldehyde	Retina

(1) Kato *et al.* (1985). CRBP-I and CRABP-I were found in every rat tissue tested (21 tissues in males, 18 in females). Those listed are the top three locations.
(2) Harada *et al.* (1995).

a tetrameric protein composed of apparently identical subunits, each with a molecular weight of 14 kDa, and possesses a single thyroid hormone-binding site. Although transthyretin would seem to be capable of binding four molecules of RBP, it only binds one. Apparently, the binding of one molecule of RBP to one transthyretin subunit causes the remaining subunits to lose their affinity for RBP. Hence, under normal physiological conditions, with transthyretin in molar excess, holoRBP–transthyretin exists as a 1:1 molar complex. In blood, approximately 95% of the retinol–RBP is complexed with transthyretin – the rest is free. As will become evident, retinol nutritional status strikingly influences the metabolism and tissue levels of RBP.

The cellular retinoid-binding proteins (CRBPs) facilitate normal vitamin A metabolism by delivering retinoids to the appropriate enzyme reaction sites within the cell. These cytoplasmic proteins are distinct from plasma RBP. The four cellular proteins for binding retinol and retinoic acid share a high degree of homology and have molecular weights in the range 15.0–15.7 kDa. CRBP-I and CRABP-I have been found in all rat tissues and organs tested, suggesting that they are involved in essential cellular processes throughout the body. The levels vary widely among different tissues, the highest concentrations being found in tissues of the reproductive tract. They have an additional role in delivering their respective ligands to specific binding sites within the nucleus. CRABP-I also sequesters

retinoic acid, in excess of cellular needs, and facilitates its catabolism into a variety of polar metabolites. Tissue distribution of CRBP-II and CRABP-II is much more restricted. The former is found mainly in the enterocytes of the small intestine, where it is involved in the metabolism of newly absorbed or newly formed retinol. The unique proteins, CRALBP and IRBP, are found only in visual tissue; their respective molecular weights are 36.0 kDa and 135.0 kDa.

There is a problem in studies of retinoid metabolism of promiscuity of retinoids *in vitro*. For example, a plethora of non-specific enzymes, including alcohol dehydrogenases, convert 'free' retinol into retinoic acid *in vitro*, but have no access to the protein-bound retinol *in vivo*. To ensure that only the physiologically relevant enzymes catalyse retinoid metabolism in the body, the substrate is not the retinoid *per se*, but the holo-cellular retinoid-binding protein, and the enzyme recognizes the substrate through protein–protein interaction. The enzyme forms a transient complex with the holo-binding protein and the retinoid is transferred directly from the binding protein to the active site of the enzyme without diffusing into the aqueous medium (Napoli, 1993).

With regard to CRBP-I and CRABP-I, the amount and availability of their respective ligands, retinol and retinoic acid, does not influence the tissue levels of these cellular binding proteins. Thus a low dietary supply of vitamin A is accompanied by a concomitant increase in the level of apoCRBP-I relative to holoCRBP-I – this is an important concept in retinol metabolism. It has been demonstrated that tissue levels of both CRBP-I and CRABP-I are maintained constant in the face of considerable differences in retinoid nutritional status (Kato *et al.*, 1985; Blaner *et al.*, 1986). However, tissue levels of CRBP-I (but not CRABP-I) are decreased if the diet is totally devoid of retinoid.

7.4.3 Intestinal absorption

Ingested retinyl esters and provitamin A carotenoids are liberated from their association with membranes and lipoproteins by the action of pepsin in the stomach and of proteolytic enzymes in the small intestine. In the stomach the free carotenoids and retinyl esters congregate in fatty globules, which then pass into the duodenum. In the presence of bile salts, the globules are broken up into smaller globules, which renders them more easily digestible by a variety of pancreatic lipases and results in the formation of mixed micelles. Extensive hydrolysis of retinyl esters takes place within the duodenum, catalysed mainly by a non-specific pancreatic hydrolase that can act on a wide variety of esters as substrates. Retinyl ester hydrolysis is completed by brush-border hydrolases. With the exception of esterified xanthophylls, which are hydrolysed by esterases, carotenoids are absorbed without prior metabolic conversion.

The retinol and carotenoids contained within the mixed micelles cross the unstirred layer of the intestinal lumen and are released as a result of micelle dissociation in the brush-border region. Physiological concentrations of retinol derived from natural food sources are absorbed by facilitated diffusion; at higher concentrations a process of simple diffusion takes over. The carrier-mediated absorption of retinol shows specificity toward all-*trans* retinol and 3-dehydroretinol; uptake of 9-*cis* and 13-*cis* retinol and retinaldehyde takes place by simple diffusion (Dew & Ong, 1994). Carotenoid absorption is also by simple diffusion.

Preformed vitamin A and provitamin A carotenoids (provitamins) of dietary origin differ in their efficiency of absorption. When foods containing normal physiological amounts of these compounds are ingested, retinol is absorbed with an efficiency of 70–90% compared with 20–50% for the provitamins. The

absorption efficiency of retinol remains high as the amount ingested increases beyond physiological levels, whereas that of the provitamins falls markedly with increased ingestion to less than 10%. Whereas crystalline β-carotene in antioxidant-stabilized commercial form is absorbed with an efficiency of about 50%, the absorption of carotenoids from raw carrot can be as low as 1%. The cooking of vegetables increases absorption, probably as a result of dissociation of carotenoids from plant cell membranes and lipoproteins.

In a human study of β-carotene absorption, Blomstrand & Werner (1967) fed single small doses of radioactive β-carotene dissolved in vegetable oil to hospitalized patients in whom cannulae had been inserted into the thoracic duct. The percentages of administered radioactivity recovered in the lymph of three patients were 14.6, 8.7 and 16.8. In these patients most of the radioactivity was found in the retinyl ester fraction which contained 68 to 88% of the total radioactivity in the lymph lipids. Smaller amounts of radioactivity (1.7, 11.3 and 27.9%) were recovered in the β-carotene fractions. These results demonstrate that only a part of β-carotene consumed is absorbed in the intestine. Most of that absorbed is converted in the enterocytes to retinaldehyde and further to retinol and retinyl esters; some remains as intact β-carotene.

There is a large variability, three- to four-fold among healthy male humans, in efficiency of carotenoid absorption (Brown *et al.*, 1989). In some people there is no plasma response to a single oral dose of β-carotene. Johnson & Russell (1992) measured β-carotene concentrations in plasma and various lipoproteins in healthy males for 10 days after a single oral dose (120 mg) of β-carotene in capsule form. Seven of the eleven subjects were nonresponders, showing little or no increase in plasma β-carotene and only a small response in chylomicrons. This lack of response may be caused by inefficient uptake of luminal β-carotene by enterocytes, inefficient incorporation of β-carotene into chylomicrons, or extensive conversion of β-carotene to retinyl esters. Of interest with the four responders was that surges of chylomicron β-carotene occurred every few days following the single dose, suggesting delayed release of β-carotene from enterocytes. It is possible that these surges were the result of re-uptake of β-carotene from the intestinal lumen following sloughing off of the epithelial cells.

7.4.4   Metabolic events in the intestine

Esterification of retinol

Within enterocytes retinol becomes bound in a 1:1 molar ratio to CRBP-II, which is present exclusively and abundantly in these cells. CRBP-II binds all-*trans* and 13-*cis* retinol with high affinity; it also binds retinaldehyde, but not retinoic acid. The protein-bound retinol is esterified with saturated long-chain fatty acids, preferentially palmitic acid. The esterification uses a different pool of fatty acids and hence different enzymes than are used for the synthesis of triglycerides. Two microsomal enzymes are involved in the esterification of retinol, namely acyl coenzyme A:retinol acyltransferase (ARAT) and lecithin:retinol acyltransferase (LRAT). The substrates for the ARAT-catalysed reaction are free retinol and acyl-CoAs; retinol bound to CRBP-II is not a substrate for ARAT. LRAT is an unusual enzyme in that it utilizes a membrane phospholipid, phosphatidylcholine (lecithin), as an endogenous donor of fatty acids for esterification. The enzyme activity shows positional selectivity as only the fatty acid from position 1 of the phospholipid is transferred to retinol. Position 1 is usually occupied by a saturated fatty acid (palmitic or stearic acid), which explains the predominance of saturated fatty acids in the retinyl esters. Unlike ARAT, LRAT can utilize CRBP-II-bound retinol as well as free retinol. However, because of the abundance of CRBP-II in enterocytes, the majority of retinol will be bound and thus restricted to esterification by LRAT.

Whether ARAT or LRAT is involved in retinol esterification depends on the amount of available retinol. LRAT is responsible for the esterification of retinol–CRBP-II when normal loads of vitamin A are ingested. In contrast, ARAT activity is important if the amount of retinol absorbed exceeds the saturation level of CRBP-II. It seems that CRBP-II functions both to direct retinol to the microsomes for esterification by LRAT and to prevent retinol from participating in the ARAT reaction.

Conversion of provitamin carotenoids to retinoids

Both central and excentric (asymmetric) oxidative cleavage of provitamin carotenoids have been proposed for the biosynthesis of retinaldehyde in enterocytes (Fig. 7.4). In the central cleavage reaction, molecular oxygen reacts with carbon atoms 15 and 15′ of the polyene chain, after which the central double bond is cleaved. This reaction would be expected to generate two molecules of retinaldehyde from one molecule of β-carotene (or one molecule of retinal-

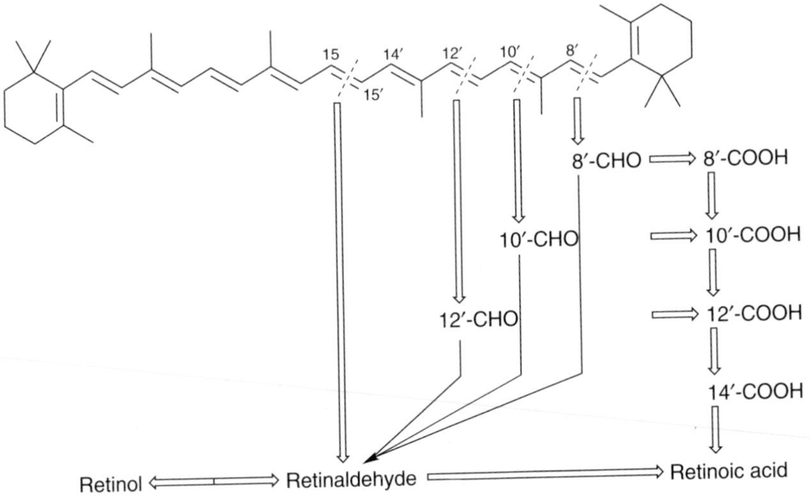

Fig. 7.4 Intestinal metabolism of β-carotene. The enzyme β-carotenoid-15,15′-dioxygenase forms retinaldehyde directly. Cleavage at other double bonds forms β-apocarotenals (e.g. 8′-CHO), which can be shortened to retinaldehyde. β-Apocarotenals may be oxidized to β-apocarotenoic acids (e.g. 8′-COOH), which can form retinoic acid. Retinol is esterified, incorporated in chylomicrons together with some intact β-carotene, and secreted into lymph. Retinoic acid enters portal blood accompanied by other polar metabolites. Reprinted from *Biochimica et Biophysica Acta*, Vol. 486, Sharma *et al.*, Studies on the metabolism of β-carotene and apo-β-carotenoids in rats and chickens, pp. 183–94, © 1977, with permission from Elsevier.

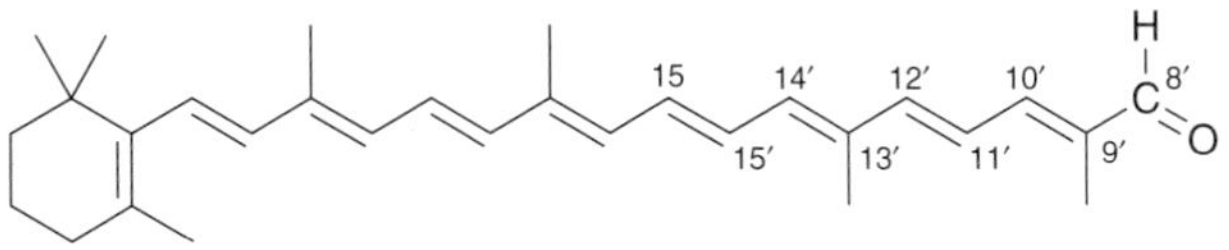

Fig. 7.5 Structure of β-apo-8′-carotenal.

dehyde in the case of other provitamin carotenoids). However, the reaction fails to produce the theoretical amount of retinoids *in vivo* because of incomplete absorption of β-carotene from the intestinal lumen and (in humans) inefficient conversion in the mucosa. Metabolism of carotenoids to retinoic acid as a result of excentric cleavage may account for some of the discrepancy in humans.

In the excentric cleavage of β-carotene described by Glover (1960) one molecule of β-carotene ultimately yields one molecule of retinaldehyde. The initial reaction is cleavage of the terminal 7′–8′ double bond to produce β-apo-8′-carotenal (Fig. 7.5). The stepwise degradation of this compound is postulated to take place by a β-oxidative-type enzyme system. All of the β-apocarotenals formed from β-carotene can be shortened to retinaldehyde.

There is good evidence for the existence of both central and excentric cleavage of carotenoids (Wolf, 1995). The enzyme responsible for central cleavage, β-carotenoid-15,15′-dioxygenase, is found in both intestine and liver. However, because of lability during attempts to purify it, the pure enzyme has not yet been isolated. Bile salts have been found to be essential for β-carotene cleavage. Enzyme(s) seem to be involved in excentric cleavage: amounts of β-apocarotenals and retinoids were markedly reduced when NAD^+ was replaced by NADH and their formation was completely inhibited by an inhibitor of sulphydryl-containing enzymes (Wang *et al.*, 1991). However, no enzyme(s) specifically responsible for excentric cleavage has yet been found. It is not known whether different specific dioxygenases cleave the different double bonds of the polyene chain or whether the β-carotenoid-15,15′-dioxygenase is rather non-specific and can attack other double bonds also.

Most of the retinaldehyde formed from carotenoids becomes bound to CRBP-II and reversibly reduced to retinol by retinaldehyde reductase – a relatively non-specific aldehyde reductase which does not appear to be zinc-dependent (Fidge & Goodman, 1968). The resulting retinol–CRBP-II complex is then used as a substrate for esterification by LRAT.

The bioconversion of provitamins to retinoids may be regulated both up and down at the level of the intestinal cleavage enzyme. Using a dioxygenase assay, van Vliet *et al.* (1992) found a 130% higher cleavage activity in hamsters fed a low vitamin A diet compared with normally fed controls. This up-regulation was confirmed in rats by van Vliet *et al.* (1996) who also found that a high intake of either retinyl ester or β-carotene down-regulated (decreased) cleavage activity.

7.4.5 Tissue uptake of chylomicron remnant retinyl esters

The chylomicrons, containing retinyl esters and small amounts of intact carotenoids, are released from enterocytes by exocytosis into the lymph. They enter the bloodstream where lipase activity and apolipoprotein exchange result in their conversion to chylomicron remnants, which are taken up primarily by the parenchymal cells (hepatocytes) of the liver. Uptake appears to involve binding of the chylomicron remnants to lipoprotein receptors in the space of Disse, followed by lipolytic processing and receptor-mediated endocytosis. After uptake of chylomicron remnants, the constituent retinyl esters are hydrolysed, probably by a hydrolase located in the plasma membrane of hepatocytes and/or in early endosomes. In contrast to many other ligands that are transferred to lysosomes after endosomal processing, retinol is transferred from endosomes to the endoplasmic reticulum, where apoRBP is found in high concentration. Whether this transfer occurs via vesicular transport or via CRBP-I in the cytosol is not known.

Although chylomicron remnants are mainly cleared by the liver, uptake of remnants also takes place in the bone marrow and spleen, and to a lesser extent in adipose tissue, skeletal muscle, testes, lungs and kidneys. Considering the role of retinoids in cell differentiation, chylomicron remnants may be important for delivering retinyl esters to tissues with intensive cell proliferation and differentiation such as bone marrow and spleen.

7.4.6   Metabolic events in the liver

Esterification of retinol

Within hepatic stellate cells, retinol binds to CRBP-I which directs retinol to LRAT for esterification when the vitamin is present in normal amounts. When retinol is present at high levels and the pool of CRBP-I becomes saturated, ARAT may esterify the excess. Thus, as in the intestine, both enzymes may be involved in hepatic retinol esterification, depending on the amount of retinol present and on whether it is bound to CRBP-I.

Storage of retinyl esters

Vitamin A is unique among vitamins because it is massively stored by the liver. The level of stored retinyl ester fluctuates in accordance with dietary intake. Normally, most of the newly absorbed retinol is transferred within 2–4 hours from hepatocytes to stellate cells for storage. However, during periods of vitamin A insufficiency, newly absorbed retinol is secreted from hepatocytes, as holoRBP, directly into the blood to satisfy the immediate needs of the tissues.

The transfer of newly absorbed retinol from hepatocytes to stellate cells within the liver is mediated by RBP, thus other components of chylomicron remnants, such as cholesterol and vitamin D, are not transferred. Binding of retinol to RBP in hepatocytes initiates a translocation of holoRBP from the endoplasmic reticulum to the Golgi apparatus, followed by secretion of the retinol complex from the cell. Within stellate cells, retinol is esterified and the esters are stored in cytoplasmic lipid droplets. The storage capacity of hepatic stellate cells is high and accounts for about 50 to 80% of the total body pool of vitamin A. The normal reserve of vitamin A in stellate cells is adequate to last for several months in humans. Stellate cells are also found in the intestine, kidney, heart, large blood vessels, ovaries and testes; these cells store retinyl esters when large amounts of vitamin A are consumed. When the stellate cells contain so much retinol that they can accept no more, hypervitaminosis A occurs.

The amount of vitamin A stored in the liver influences retinol utilization by extrahepatic tissues, and therefore hepatic liver reserves are a true indication of vitamin A status. Green et al. (1987) determined the retinol utilization rate in rats provided with different intakes of vitamin A, such that the rats had low,

marginal or high liver vitamin A reserves. Vitamin A-depleted rats exhibited a lower utilization rate, which was positively correlated with the size of the plasma retinol pool; i.e. the lower the plasma retinol concentration, the lower the vitamin A utilization rate. The increased rate of utilization observed in rats of higher vitamin A status was reflected in an increased rate of retinol catabolism. It appeared that some minimal utilization rate is maintained as long as dietary supply and/or liver stores of vitamin A can maintain normal plasma retinol concentrations. The decreased utilization rate in depleted states could be a way of conserving vitamin A for its most critical functions, whereas in vitamin A sufficiency increased catabolism prevents excessive accumulation of retinol. Accelerated catabolism as a function of increase in liver vitamin A stores was also reported in rats fed excessive amounts of vitamin A (Leo et al., 1989).

Mobilization of retinol

The vitamin A stored in stellate cells can be readily mobilized for use in a highly regulated process. Thus an individual's plasma vitamin A levels remain quite constant over a wide range of dietary intakes and liver stores. Only when liver reserves of vitamin A are nearly depleted do plasma concentrations of retinol decrease significantly. A kinetic model of retinol dynamics in rats (Green et al., 1993) predicted that the stellate cell retinol pool responsible for the secretion is small and rapidly turning over. This is compatible with the relatively small amounts of apoRBP observed in stellate cells (more than 90% of the apoRBP in liver is found in hepatocytes). Upon demand, the retinyl esters are hydrolysed to retinol, which then combines with RBP to form holoRBP. This complex is secreted into the bloodstream where it becomes reversibly complexed in a 1:1 molar ratio with transthyretin. The formation of the larger retinol–RBP–transthyretin complex minimizes the loss of holoRBP in the urine during its passage through the kidney.

One factor that specifically regulates the release of holoRBP from the liver is the dietary intake of vitamin A. Studies in the rat (Muto et al., 1972; Smith et al., 1973) showed that in the retinol-depleted state, the secretion of holoRBP from the liver was blocked, resulting in the accumulation of an enlarged pool of apoRBP in the liver and a concomitant decline in plasma RBP levels (as holoRBP–transthyretin). Oral administration of retinyl acetate to the depleted rats stimulated the rapid secretion of holoRBP from the expanded liver pool into the plasma and within 5 hours after administration the plasma RBP levels had returned to normal. This effect of retinol upon RBP secretion took place without affecting RBP synthesis (Soprano et al., 1982); this is unusual as the synthesis of other binding proteins (e.g. transferrin, ferritin and zinc metallothionein) is controlled by their specific ligands. These experiments demonstrated that the livers of vitamin A-deficient animals contain a pool of previously formed apoRBP, which can be released rapidly into the plasma, as holoRBP, as soon as vitamin A becomes available. The delayed (5 h) response to oral administration of vitamin A is due to the processes of intestinal absorption, hepatic uptake of chylomicron remnant retinyl ester, and hydrolysis of ester to provide retinol.

The rapid release of holoRBP from the liver in response to vitamin A dosing during vitamin A deficiency provides the basis of the relative dose response (RDR) test, which measures the amount by which plasma retinol levels are below normal due to inadequate liver stores (Loerch et al., 1979). The liver stores reflect tissue needs and therefore the test is a true indicator of vitamin A nutritional status. In subjects with low hepatic vitamin A reserves, a test dose of vitamin A will provoke a prominent increase in plasma retinol because of accumulated apoRBP in the liver. The test entails taking an initial blood sample from the fasted subject and administering a large oral dose of retinyl acetate or palmitate in oil immediately afterwards. A second blood sample is collected 5 hours after dosing and the RDR is calculated as follows:

$$RDR = \frac{(A_5 - A_0)}{A_5} \times 100\%$$

where A_0 and A_5 = concentrations of retinol in the initial and 5-h blood samples, respectively.

RDR values higher than 50% are characteristic of acute vitamin A deficiency; values between 20 and 50% indicate marginal nutritional status; and values lower than 20% indicate adequate status.

7.4.7   Regulation of retinol metabolism in the liver and intestine

The activity of hepatic LRAT is regulated by vitamin A nutritional status. LRAT activity decreased to un-

detectable levels in the livers of vitamin A-depleted rats and returned to normal levels on repletion with an oral dose of retinyl ester (Randolph & Ross, 1991). This decrease would inhibit liver storage of vitamin A in the chronically deficient state. Retinoic acid was shown to be more potent than an equimolar dose of retinol in restoring hepatic LRAT activity (Matsuura & Ross, 1993). The dose of retinoic acid required to restore the activity (2–20 μg) is consistent with physiological concentrations of this retinoid in tissues. The increase in LRAT activity in response to retinoic acid dosing was blocked completely by both actinomycin D and cycloheximide, which are inhibitors of RNA and protein synthesis, respectively. It can be inferred from these results that the vitamin A metabolite, retinoic acid, regulates the esterification of newly available retinol in the liver through an induction of LRAT, which requires synthesis of both new RNA and new protein. In contrast, neither the activity of intestinal LRAT nor that of ARAT in either liver or intestine was affected by vitamin A deficiency (Randolph & Ross, 1991).

In vitro experiments using liver microsomes have shown that when the ratio of apoCRBP-I to retinol exceeds 1, apoCRBP-I inhibits the esterification of retinol by LRAT (Herr & Ong, 1992). Working in concert with the inhibition of hepatic LRAT is the ability of apoCRBP-I to stimulate retinyl ester hydrolysis in liver microsomes (Boerman & Napoli, 1991). The changing ratio of apo- to holoCRBP-I during variable vitamin A status could regulate vitamin A storage and mobilization in the liver, as shown in Fig. 7.6. During times of low vitamin A intake or deficiency, when apoCRBP-I will predominate over holoCRBP-I, hydrolysis of stored retinyl esters will be stimulated and esterification of retinol will be inhibited, leading to mobilization of vitamin A. Any retinol arriving at the liver during such times would be immediately released, bound to RBP, for distribution to other organs, rather than stored in the liver as retinyl esters. When the supply of exogenous retinol becomes plentiful, holoCRBP-I will predominate over apoCRBP-I, hydrolysis of esters will not be stimulated and synthesis of esters will not be inhibited, leading to net storage. The inhibitory and stimulatory effects of apoCRBP-I on retinol esterification and ester hydrolysis respectively provide a mechanism for the animal to respond more rapidly to changes in intracellular retinol levels.

In the intestine, esterification of retinol is essential for completion of the absorptive process because the

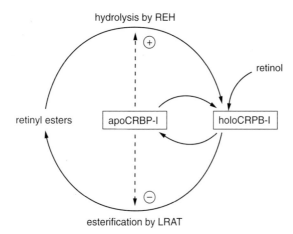

Fig. 7.6 Effect of the apo-/holoCRBP-I ratio on retinol esterification and hydrolysis in the liver. HoloCRBP-I, which is formed as a result of an influx of exogenous retinol, serves as substrate for LRAT to facilitate liver storage of retinyl esters. ApoCRBP-I, resulting from depletion of holoCRBP-I, stimulates retinyl ester hydrolase (REH) and inhibits LRAT, leading to mobilization of vitamin A.

esters are then incorporated into chylomicrons for release and distribution to the rest of the body. Not surprisingly, therefore, apoCRBP-II has relatively little effect on the rate of esterification. The difference between hepatic and intestinal LRAT in their response to vitamin A deficiency is attributable to the different ways in which the holo forms of CRBP-I and CRBP-II interact with LRAT. This difference fulfils the physiological needs of the animal during vitamin A deficiency by allowing efficient intestinal processing of the low vitamin A intake, while minimizing the storage of retinyl esters in the liver.

7.4.8 Turnover and recycling of plasma retinol

For many years it was assumed that, once retinol left the plasma, it was taken up by tissues and irreversibly utilized. It has now been established that retinol recycles extensively among liver, plasma, interstitial fluid and extrahepatic tissues. Recycling is a means of conserving vitamin A by the body and, indeed, excretory loss of the vitamin in vitamin A-depleted animals is much reduced relative to the loss in vitamin A-sufficient animals. The rate of plasma retinol turnover is 9–10 times the rate of irreversible utilization of retinol, and this ratio is not affected by vitamin A status. This means that a relatively small and constant fraction

(approximately 10%) of retinol molecules that leaves the plasma is irreversibly utilized, and approximately 90% is recycled to plasma for distribution to liver and to other target organs or tissues. More than half of the retinol secreted by the liver as holoRBP is provided by recycled plasma retinol.

Retinol recycling involves cellular uptake of circulating retinol, interaction with CRBP, possible esterification and hydrolysis, and then a transfer to apoRBP and secretion of holoRBP. Changes in the dynamics of retinol recycling allow for rapid adjustment in vitamin A distribution in response to changes in nutritional, metabolic or physiological conditions. The vehicle for retinol recycling is RBP, which is synthesized in adequate amounts in a wide variety of extrahepatic tissues, including the kidneys and adipose tissue, as well as in the liver. Little of the RBP associated with retinol recycling to the liver is degraded in the liver; rather it too is recycled to the plasma. Thus there are adequate amounts of apoRBP in plasma to complex with retinol that has been reabsorbed by the kidney.

In the rat, retinol taken up by tissues is recycled to the blood an average of 7–13 times before irreversible utilization. The recycling number is not significantly influenced by vitamin A status. The kidneys contribute 40–50% of plasma retinol; this is after glomerular filtration of holoRBP that is not bound to transthyretin and subsequent tubular reabsorption of retinol. Only 20% of the input of retinol into plasma is predicted to be from the liver, leaving a 30% contribution from extrahepatic/extrarenal tissues. In rats with normal versus marginal versus nearly depleted liver vitamin A stores, the recycling time for retinol averages 8.4, 1.7–2.0 and 0.6–0.7 days, respectively (R. Blomhoff *et al.*, 1992). That is, once retinol leaves the plasma, it may take more than a week to recycle to the plasma in a normal rat. Most of this time would presumably be spent in retinyl ester pools.

Green & Green (1994) developed a simple three-compartmental model (Fig. 7.7) to provide information on vitamin A utilization and other aspects of retinol dynamics in rats with low or marginal vitamin A status. The equivalent of 10–14 pools of plasma retinol were predicted to be transferred to the fast turning-over extravascular compartment each day. All fractional transfer coefficients were significantly affected by diet (i.e. vitamin A status). The model predicted that rats that had almost depleted liver stores of vitamin A and lowered plasma retinol concentrations

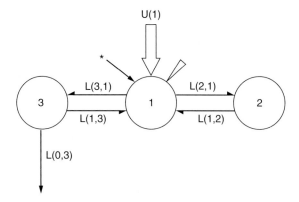

Fig. 7.7 Model proposed by Green & Green (1994) for vitamin A turnover in rats. Compartments: 1 represents the pool of plasma retinol bound to RBP and is the compartment into which the tracer ([³H]retinol-labelled plasma) is introduced (see asterisk); 2 represents a smaller, fast turning-over extravascular pool of retinol that consists mainly of retinol in interstitial fluid and retinol present in the lumen of the Bowman's capsule as a result of renal filtration; 3 represents a larger, slow turning-over extravascular pool of retinol that consists mainly of retinyl ester stores and from which vitamin A is irreversibly utilized. U(1) denotes input of retinol into plasma from the diet via chylomicron remnants. L(3,1), L(2,1) etc. are fractional transfer coefficients; for example, L(3,1) is the fraction of compartment 1's tracer transferred to compartment 3 per day. The triangle shows the site of sampling. Reproduced, with permission, from Green, M. H. & Green, J. B., *Journal of Nutrition*, Vol. 124, pp. 2477–85, © 1994, American Society for Nutritional Sciences.

were able to draw upon extrahepatic reserves of vitamin A. Data suggested that vitamin A absorption efficiency is similar in rats with low or marginal vitamin A status, whereas vitamin A utilization seems to be up- and down-regulated.

7.4.9   Homeostasis of circulating retinol

Circulating retinol concentrations are homeostatically regulated to remain constant, despite great variations in the dietary supply and liver stores of vitamin A. The controlled release of vitamin A from liver stores is necessary to provide tissues with optimal amounts of retinol, without releasing excessive amounts which would lead to toxicity. Although various schemes for the homeostasis of circulating retinol have been proposed, an unequivocal mechanism has not yet been established.

The concentration of retinol bound to plasma RBP is maintained within a normal range of concentrations, referred to as its homeostatic set point, as long as there is some minimal concentration of vitamin A

in the liver and in extrahepatic tissues. Thus rats fed a vitamin A-deficient diet maintained a relatively stable plasma retinol level, which did not drop below 30 µg per 100 mL until liver reserves fell below 10 µg g⁻¹ tissue (Underwood *et al.*, 1979). Control of plasma retinol concentration is mediated by factors that affect the balance between retinol input to plasma and retinol output from plasma. Controlling factors include the enzymes that esterify retinol and hydrolyse retinyl esters in the tissues. The activity of hydrolytic enzymes is enhanced during vitamin A deprivation, releasing holoRBP into the bloodstream. The activity of esterifying enzymes, on the other hand, is enhanced when vitamin A intake is plentiful, allowing surplus vitamin A to be stored. Ultimately, the set point for plasma retinol depends on the rate of release of holoRBP from the liver. Underwood proposed that hepatic secretion of retinol is controlled by a signal generated in proportion to the uptake or utilization of retinol in extrahepatic target tissues.

The plasma retinol homeostatic set point is influenced by several dietary and hormonal factors; these include protein, calorie and zinc nutriture, and fluctuating steroid hormone levels that occur during the oestrous cycle or as a result of stress. It is likely that steroid hormones act by influencing the synthesis of RBP (Borek *et al.*, 1981). Ahluwalia *et al.* (1980) used hypophysectomized rats to demonstrate that without growth there was no vitamin A utilization. They showed that, in addition to dietary protein, growth hormone was required for mobilization of liver vitamin A stores. The data suggested that growth hormone may play an important role in vitamin A homeostasis by regulating retinol entry at the tissue level.

It is well documented that humans with chronic renal failure have elevated plasma levels of retinol. Gerlach & Zile (1990), using rats with surgically induced acute renal failure, established that the rise in plasma retinol was almost entirely due to an increase in retinol associated with RBP. The source of the elevated plasma holoRBP was shown to be an increased hepatic release of the complex and not peripheral uptake (Gerlach & Zile, 1991a). These findings suggest that the kidney has a physiological role in regulating the homeostatic set point for circulating retinol concentrations, possibly by modulating the release of holoRBP from the liver.

Gerlach & Zile (1991b) postulated the following regulatory mechanisms. (1) The intact kidney provides a specific regulatory substance (negative feedback signal) which prevents the release of hepatic holoRBP. In the absence of kidney function the decreased signal will allow the release of holoRBP. (2) A regulatory substance originating in the peripheral tissues (positive feedback signal) is normally removed by the kidney and therefore hepatic holoRBP will not be released. In renal failure the substance will accumulate and elicit the release of holoRBP.

Gerlach & Zile (1991b) investigated the possibility that retinoic acid might be a negative feedback signal released by the kidney or a positive feedback signal from peripheral tissues. The negative feedback hypothesis was tested by administering an exogenous supply of near physiological amounts of retinoic acid to rats with renal failure to compensate for the absence of retinoic acid in circulation owing to lack of kidney function. If this hypothesis was valid, adding retinoic acid to the circulation would restore the negative feedback and plasma retinol levels would be lowered to the normal levels of intact animals. However, the administration of retinoic acid did not alter the elevated plasma retinol levels that occurred in renal failure. The positive feedback hypothesis was tested by increasing the serum levels of retinoic acid at concentrations approximating the upper physiological limit. If this hypothesis was valid, rats with renal failure would respond with a substantial increase in serum retinol concentrations, whereas animals with renal failure that were not treated with retinoic acid would respond in a less pronounced manner. It was found that administration of retinoic acid had no significant effect on the existing serum retinol concentration and it was therefore concluded that retinoic acid does not serve as a negative or positive feedback signal for the release of hepatic retinol.

Another possibility considered by Gerlach & Zile (1991b) was that a positive peripheral feedback signal molecule other than retinoic acid regulates the release of hepatic retinol into circulation. This hypothesis was tested by greatly increasing the serum retinoic acid concentration so that it would be expected to provide peripheral tissues with a sustained high concentration of retinoic acid. Under these conditions, retinoic acid can partially substitute for retinol requirement in peripheral tissues, i.e. exert a sparing effect on retinol utilization. Consequently, peripheral target tissues would have a reduced requirement for retinol and the signal for hepatic retinol release

would be decreased. In rats with renal failure a higher amount of this positive feedback signal would remain in circulation compared to the amounts in rats with intact kidneys because the signal is not removed by the kidney. Therefore, if this hypothesis is valid, under conditions of retinoic acid sparing effect on retinol utilization, intact rats as well as rats with renal failure should have lower serum retinol concentrations than their respective controls not given retinoic acid. This depression (sparing effect) should be significantly smaller in rats with renal failure compared with that obtained in intact rats. These effects were indeed observed with decreases in serum retinol concentration of 29% and 19% relative to controls in rats with intact kidney function and with renal failure, respectively. The data supported the hypothesis that a positive peripheral feedback signal other than retinoic acid regulates the release of hepatic retinol.

Gerlach & Zile (1991b) postulated that the positive feedback signal molecule from the periphery is apoRBP, which returns to circulation after retinol–RBP–transthyretin is delivered to target tissues and would be a sensitive indicator of the physiological needs of retinol by tissues. The lack of removal of apoRBP by the kidney in renal failure would cause it to accumulate in the circulation, triggering an enhanced release of hepatic retinol. The hypothesis was tested by adding apoRBP to the circulation of rats with renal failure. An observed increase in plasma retinol concentration above that already caused by renal failure was evidence that apoRBP is a positive physiological feedback signal from the periphery for the regulation of release of hepatic retinol into circulation.

7.4.10   Cellular uptake of circulating retinol

Because of the disruptive effects of free (uncomplexed) retinol on membrane structure and function (Roels et al., 1969), it is desirable to discourage non-specific uptake of retinol by cells that have no particular requirement for it. This might be achieved by means of specific RBP receptors on the plasma membrane of vitamin A-requiring cells, which recognize holoRBP, bind it, and facilitate the transfer of holoRBP or free retinol across the membrane and into the cytoplasm.

RBP binding to cell membranes has been reported in the following specific locations: the choroidal surface of retinal pigment epithelial cells, but not in rod outer segments (Heller, 1975); interstitial cells of testes, but not on epithelial cells of seminiferous tubules (McGuire *et al.*, 1981); human placental cells (Sivaprasadarao & Findlay, 1988a) and epithelial cells of the choroid plexus, signifying movement of retinol across the blood–brain barrier (MacDonald *et al.*, 1990). Evidence of RBP receptor-mediated uptake of retinol has also been reported in enterocytes of the small intestine (Rask & Peterson, 1976) and testicular Sertoli cells (Shingleton *et al.*, 1989). Among these locations, cellular uptake of retinol without a concomitant uptake of the RBP has been reported to take place in retinal pigment epithelium (Chen & Heller, 1977), enterocytes (Rask & Peterson, 1976) and Sertoli cells (Shingleton *et al.*, 1989). The latter authors found that the amount of retinol accumulated by cultured Sertoli cells from holoRBP was approximately equal to the cellular content of CRBP-I. This implied that the ligand saturation of CRBP-I may be the factor regulating the cellular uptake of retinol.

There appears to be two entirely different mechanisms for receptor-mediated uptake of circulating retinol by the cells of target tissues. The first mechanism applies to the tissues mentioned above, at least some of which have been shown to take up retinol unaccompanied by RBP. Upon recognition and binding by a cell-surface receptor, holoRBP releases its retinol molecule and, as a result, undergoes a conformational change which reduces its affinity for both the receptor and transthyretin. The transthyretin portion of the holoRBP–transthyretin complex is not involved in the recognition process. Indeed, transthyretin has been found to inhibit the binding of RBP to plasma membranes *in vitro* (Sivaprasadarao & Findlay, 1988a). Retinol is internalized into the cytoplasm where it interacts with its specific cytoplasmic binding protein, CRBP-I. The low-affinity form of apoRBP is circulated to the kidneys where it is filtered at the glomerulus, endocytosed in the cells of the proximal convoluted tubules, and degraded in lysosomes within the tubular cells.

Sivaprasadarao & Findlay (1988b) suggested that the ratio of apo- to holoRBP levels in the plasma can regulate retinol distribution among various tissues. Vitamin A deficiency can effect a change in this ratio: holoRBP levels decrease to almost zero while apoRBP levels remain unchanged. Since apoRBP has poor affinity for transthyretin, most of it will exist in the free state. As both holo- and apoRBP bind to the cell-surface receptor, the high ratio of apo- to holoRBP in the plasma would not only result in the decreased uptake of retinol by most tissues, but actually stimulate the secretion of retinol by extrahepatic tissues. The retinol so liberated might then be used for critically dependent tissues such as the eye and gonads.

The second mechanism of retinol uptake, exemplified in the liver and kidney, also involves the interaction of holoRBP with a specific cell-surface receptor, but the entire retinol–RBP complex is internalized by receptor-mediated endocytosis. Evidence for this uptake mechanism was provided by Senoo *et al.* (1990), who studied the *in vivo* uptake of RBP in rat liver cells by immunocytochemistry at the electron microscopic level using ultra-thin cryosections. Rats were injected intravenously with human RBP and simultaneously, for comparison, with asialo-orosomucoid, a protein known to be taken up by hepatocytes by receptor-mediated endocytosis. The native, unmodified RBP was subsequently identified in the liver sections by a sheep anti-human RBP antibody, which does not recognize endogenous rat RBP. Ten minutes after injection, RBP was found in close contact with the plasma membrane of parenchymal and stellate cells. Ten minutes later, RBP was also found attached to the membranes of small vesicles near the cell surface. At 2 hours after injection, RBP was detected in larger vesicles deeper in the cytoplasm, remote from the vesicle membranes as though dissociated from its putative receptor. Asialo-orosomucoid was also localized in these larger vesicles.

Blomhoff's research group (Gjøen *et al.*, 1987) studied the uptake of RBP in various organs at different times. RBP was labelled with ^{125}I-tyramine cellobiose (^{125}I-TC-RBP) and injected intravenously into rats. (The advantage of using ^{125}I-TC-RBP is that the radioactive degradation products do not escape from the cells in which the protein is degraded, as is the case for proteins radioiodinated directly.) Of all the organs tested (liver, kidneys, intestine, spleen, heart, lungs, etc.) the liver contained the most radioactivity, followed by the kidneys. After 1 hour, approximately 20% and 10% of the injected dose was recovered in the liver and kidneys, respectively; other organs contained less than 3%. Of the liver cell types, parenchymal and stellate cells took up about equal amounts of ^{125}I-TC-RBP when calculated per gram of liver; Kupffer cells and endothelial cells accumulated insignificant amounts. The liver was shown to be the main organ for tissue catabolism of plasma RBP. The same laboratory (Senoo *et al.*, 1990) labelled RBP and several other proteins with ^{125}I-TC and compared their *in vivo* uptake in different rat liver cell types. RBP was the only protein that was taken up selectively by parenchymal and stellate cells. The data from these two studies suggest that hepatic parenchymal and stellate cells and cells in kidneys contain receptors for RBP, and that RBP is internalized in these cells, probably by receptor-mediated endocytosis.

Proof of an RBP receptor-mediated uptake of circulating retinol requires isolation and characterization of an RBP receptor. An abundant 63-kDa terminally glycosylated membrane protein which specifically binds RBP has been identified as the RBP receptor in microsomal membranes of retinal pigment epithelial cells (Båvik *et al.*, 1991) and further characterized (Båvik *et al.*, 1992, 1993). The receptor cannot discriminate between the apo- and the holo-form of RBP. Particularly large numbers of receptor-binding sites were also found in microsome fractions of liver and kidney, whereas lung and muscle contained few, if any. The abundance of RBP receptors in retinal pigment epithelium and in liver and kidney cells is in accordance with the responsibility of these cells for the uptake and transport of large amounts of retinol for functional purposes. In contrast, it is expected that only relatively small amounts of retinol are needed in cells where accumulated retinol is used mainly for the synthesis of retinoic acid.

7.4.11 Biosynthesis of retinoic acid

The *in situ* synthesis of retinoic acid has been demonstrated in a wide array of tissues and in a variety of species. Despite its physiological importance, retinoic acid is a quantitatively minor metabolite of retinol. One pathway, outlined in Fig. 7.8, begins with the hydrolysis of retinyl esters to release retinol. The irreversible nature of the terminal oxidation step (Step 3) explains the observation that retinoic acid is unable to support those processes, namely vision and reproduction, that specifically require either retinol or retinaldehyde.

In view of the known existence of over 150 dehydrogenases in mammalian cells, the possibility of *in vivo* conversion of retinol to retinoic acid by non-specific dehydrogenases has been considered. The failure of an inhibitor of alcohol dehydrogenase (4-methylpyrazole) to prevent retinoic acid synthesis suggests that alcohol dehydrogenase has no significant role. Moreover, cytosol from a mutant strain of deermouse devoid of alcohol dehydrogenase was able to convert retinol into retinoic acid (Napoli *et al.*, 1991). The current view is that the pathway for retinoic acid synthesis from retinol involves specific retinoid dehydrogenases that recognize holoCRBP-I as substrate. As most of the tissue retinoids are bound to cellular binding proteins, non-specific enzymes, such as alcohol dehydrogenase, would not have access to retinoids *in vivo*.

The retinyl ester hydrolysis in Step 1 is catalysed by a microsomal retinyl ester hydrolase. The actual hydrolase responsible has no requirement for cholate and is distinct from the frequently studied cholate-dependent hydrolase which has greater activity with nonretinoid esters, such as cholesteryl esters. In Step 2, the rate-limiting step, two alternative pathways appear to oxidize retinol to retinaldehyde. One pathway involves a NADP-dependent microsomal retinol dehydrogenase that is not inhibited by apoCRBP-I

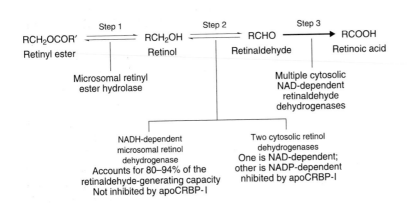

Fig. 7.8 Biosynthesis of retinoic acid from retinyl ester.

and the other involves a cytosolic retinol dehydrogenase that is inhibited by apoCRBP-I (Boerman & Napoli, 1996). There are actually two cytosolic retinol dehydrogenases, one being NAD-dependent and the other NADP-dependent. Under physiological conditions, in the presence of both holo- and apoCRBP-I, microsomal retinol dehydrogenase accounted for 80–94% of the retinaldehyde-generating capacity in the four rat tissues tested (liver, kidney, testis and lung). Because cytosolic retinol dehydrogenase would normally be inhibited by the apoCRBP-I present, the question arises as to what its role in the body might be. Boerman & Napoli (1996) speculated that the enzyme might be a reductase capable of reducing retinaldehyde generated by provitamin carotenoids into retinol. Inhibiting such an enzyme during vitamin deficiency, when apoCRBP-I would be prevalent, would provide increased retinaldehyde from carotenoids for conversion into retinoic acid. In Step 3, the retinaldehyde is converted into retinoic acid by multiple cytosolic NAD-dependent retinaldehyde dehydrogenases that recognize retinaldehyde–CRBP-I as substrate and are inhibited partially by apoCRBP-I (Boerman & Napoli, 1996). In this reaction retinaldehyde is a ligand for CRBP-I, although its binding affinity is less than that of retinol (Posch et al., 1992).

In vitro studies using ferret liver led Wang et al. (1993a) to suggest that retinoic acid regulates its own synthesis via feedback inhibition of retinol oxidation to retinaldehyde and stimulation of retinol esterification. This suggestion is supported by the observation that addition of retinoic acid to a vitamin A-deficient rat diet resulted in an increase in hepatic retinyl ester concentration and a concomitant decrease in plasma retinol concentration (Bhat & Lacroix, 1991).

A second pathway of retinoic acid synthesis arises from the excentric cleavage of β-carotene that is independent of the well-controlled mobilization of retinol from liver stores. The β-apocarotenals thus produced are oxidized to their corresponding β-apocarotenoic acids and these in turn undergo a stepwise oxidation to retinoic acid (see Fig. 7.4). Evidence for this pathway is provided by the following in vitro and in vivo studies. Retinoic acid was a quantitatively significant metabolite of β-carotene in cytosol fractions or homogenates prepared from small intestine, liver, kidney, testes and adipose tissue from humans, rats, ferrets and monkeys (Napoli & Race, 1988; Wang et al., 1991). Folman et al. (1989) reported elevated concentrations of retinoic

acid after feeding β-carotene to rabbits. Citral (3,7-dimethyl-2,6-octadienal), which inhibits the oxidation of retinaldehyde to retinoic acid, did not inhibit the formation of retinoic acid from β-apo-8′-carotenal and β-apo-12′-carotenal in human intestinal homogenate (Wang et al., 1992). Perfusion of β-carotene through jejunal segments of ferret in vivo raised the retinoic acid level in portal blood (Wang et al., 1993b).

7.4.12   Transport of retinoic acid to the nucleus

Retinoic acid synthesised in the cytoplasm moves to the nucleus where it binds to a nuclear retinoid receptor. The binding protein CRABP-I may be important in establishing equilibrium between the cytoplasmic and nuclear concentrations of retinoic acid.

7.4.13   Fate of unmetabolized carotenoids

Intact carotenoids taken up by the liver as components of chylomicron remnants are secreted from hepatocytes into the bloodstream as components of VLDLs. Triglyceride stripping of VLDLs results in a transfer of carotenoids to low density lipoproteins (LDLs), which are the major vehicles for transport of hydrocarbon carotenoids (carotenes) in plasma. The intact carotenoids are ultimately stored in adipose tissues, liver and other organs without a toxic effect. Cellular uptake of plasma carotenes might be mediated by LDL receptors. Recycling of carotenoids from tissues back to plasma takes place among VLDL, LDL and high-density lipoproteins (HDL). Carotenoid accumulation in tissues does not seem to be homeostatically regulated, but is related to plasma levels.

Rats absorb β-carotene in a different manner to humans. When rats are fed radioactive β-carotene, the β-carotene is converted almost entirely to retinyl esters, and there is no labelled β-carotene in the lymph (Huang & Goodman, 1965). This means that accumulation of β-carotene in rat tissues does not occur and neither does it occur in the tissues of mice, hamsters, guinea pigs, rabbits, chickens, pigs or sheep. The low tissue concentrations of β-carotene in rats, mice and hamsters confounds experimental studies on the putative anti-cancer activity of β-carotene. In the search for a more suitable animal model, the ferret has been found to resemble the human in its ability to absorb and accumulate intact carotenoids (Ribaya-Mercado et al., 1989).

7.4.14   Catabolism and excretion

In the liver and extrahepatic tissues, most of the catabolism of retinol involves the production of retinoic acid as an intermediate. Retinoic acid is inactivated biologically, for example, by hydroxylation of the cyclohexenyl ring at the C-4 position or by epoxidation at the C-5,6 positions, and conjugated with taurine or β-glucuronic acid to form water-soluble products which can be excreted.

Approximately 5–20% of ingested vitamin A and a larger percentage of carotenoids are not absorbed from the intestinal tract and are eliminated from the body in the faeces. Some 10–40% of the absorbed vitamin A is oxidized and/or conjugated in the liver and then is secreted into the bile. Although some of these biliary metabolites, such as retinoyl β-glucuronide, are reabsorbed to some extent and returned to the liver in an enterohepatic cycle, most of the biliary metabolites are eliminated in the faeces.

7.5   Nutritional factors that influence vitamin A status

Among various nutrients which influence vitamin A nutritional status, fat and protein are the most important.

7.5.1   Fat deficiency

The presence of adequate amounts of dietary fat is essential in forming micelles and providing a lipid vehicle for vitamin A absorption and transport. The absorption of retinol and carotenoids is markedly lower than normal when diets contain very little fat (less than 5 g per day). A study conducted in a Rwandan village area in Africa showed that supplementation of the carotenoid-sufficient but low-fat diet with 18 g per day of olive oil increased the absorption of vegetable carotenoids from 5% to 25% in boys showing clear signs of vitamin A deficiency (Roels *et al.*, 1958).

7.5.2   Protein deficiency

In cases of severe protein–energy malnutrition, the lack of dietary protein leads to an impairment of all stages of vitamin A metabolism due to a depressed synthesis of enzymes, retinoid-binding proteins and receptors. Even where dietary carotenoids are abundant, a reduced enzymatic cleavage of carotenoids will result in vitamin A deficiency. Furthermore, liver stores of vitamin (even if plentiful) will not be released into the bloodstream due to the depressed synthesis of RBP.

7.5.3   Zinc deficiency

Zinc is an essential cofactor for many enzymes, some of which are directly critical to vitamin A metabolism; for example, zinc deficiency significantly reduces the enzymatic oxidation of retinol to retinaldehyde in the retina (Huber & Gershoff, 1975). Other zinc-dependent enzymes are involved in the synthesis of proteins, including perhaps retinoid-binding proteins and receptors. The synthesis of one particular protein, opsin in the rod cells of the eye, is depressed in zinc-deficient rats (Dorea & Olson, 1986). The consequent depression in rhodopsin levels, rather than a depressed enzymatic oxidation of retinol, probably explains the impaired dark adaptation found in zinc-deficient humans.

Zinc-deficient animals exhibit low plasma vitamin A levels even if large supplements of vitamin A are given. Zinc deficiency also reduces food intake, with a consequent impairment of growth, and these parameters confound experiments on zinc–vitamin A interactions. Smith *et al.* (1976) showed that a severely food-restricted group of rats fed a zinc-adequate diet had plasma vitamin A levels similar to zinc-deficient rats. They concluded that either zinc deficiency or growth depression decreases plasma vitamin A levels, and postulated that zinc deficiency *per se* may impair hepatic RBP synthesis. It was not possible from their data to establish if the reduction in plasma vitamin A in the zinc-deficient animals was a result of zinc deficiency *per se* or a secondary effect of reduced food intake accompanying zinc deficiency.

7.5.4   Vitamin E

It is generally recognized that vitamin E is necessary for optimal utilization of vitamin A. More vitamin A is stored in the liver when the diet contains vitamin E than when the diet is deficient in vitamin E (Ames, 1969).

7.6   The role of vitamin A in vision

7.6.1   Overview

The function of vitamin A in vision is based upon the binding of 11-*cis* retinaldehyde with the protein opsin to form rhodopsin (visual purple) in the rod cells of the retina. Light energy induces the decomposition (bleaching) of rhodopsin through several unstable intermediates. Rhodopsin must regenerate in the dark to prepare for another response to light. This is accomplished via isomerization reactions of retinoids in the visual cycle.

7.6.2   Structure and function of the retina

The retina is composed of nervous tissue forming a photosensitive inner lining within the posterior half of the eyeball. The actual light receptor cells – the rods and cones – are modified neurons. The layers of the retina are shown in Fig. 7.9. The retinal pigment epithelium is a monolayer of cells interposed between the rich choroidal blood supply and the neural retina. This epithelial monolayer creates the blood–retina barrier, which prevents blood proteins and many other substances of lower molecular weight from entering the retinal interstitial space.

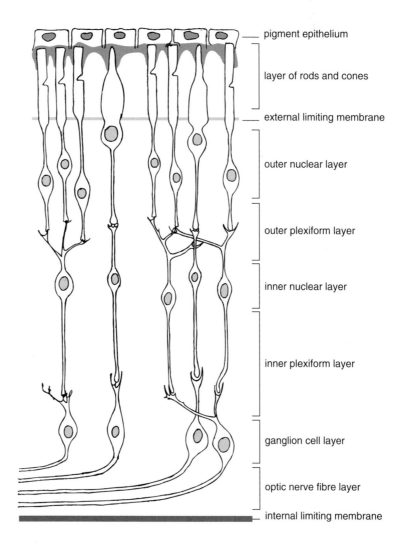

Fig. 7.9 Diagram showing the layers of the retina. Only visual receptors and direct conducting neurons are illustrated. Reprinted from *Histology*, 2nd edn., Leeson & Leeson, Figure 20.13, © 1970, with permission from Elsevier.

The human retina contains about 3 million cones and 100 million rods. Rod cells make it possible to form black-and-white images in dim light, while cones are responsible for colour vision in bright light. Both rods and cones are divided into inner and outer segments situated outside the external limiting membrane, and a conducting nucleated portion lying within the outer nuclear layer. The rods and cones make synaptic connections with dendrites of bipolar neurons of the inner nuclear layer and with axons of horizontal neurons. The inner plexiform layer marks the junction between the bipolar neurons and the ganglion cells. These cells give rise to the optic nerve fibres which run as the innermost layer of the retina towards the optic nerve head.

The rod cell is a long, thin structure divided into two parts – the outer segment and the inner segment (Fig. 7.10). The outer segment consists of a narrow tube filled with a stack of some 2000 tiny discs that contain the light-absorbing pigment rhodopsin. The discs originate near the bottom of the tube as invaginations of the plasma membrane. They gradually migrate toward the top, replacing those that are shed and phagocytosed. The inner segment contains organelles that generate energy and renew the molecules required for light absorption.

7.6.3   Rhodopsin

Rhodopsin is a stereospecific combination of a chromophore (11-*cis* retinaldehyde) and a protein (opsin), joined covalently in a Schiff base linkage by the condensation of the aldehyde group of retinaldehyde with the ε-amino group of a lysine residue (Fig. 7.11). The bent shape of the 11-*cis* isomer of retinaldehyde allows it to fit snugly into the opsin molecule and also holds the protein in the conformation specific to rhodopsin. No other stereoisomer of retinaldehyde

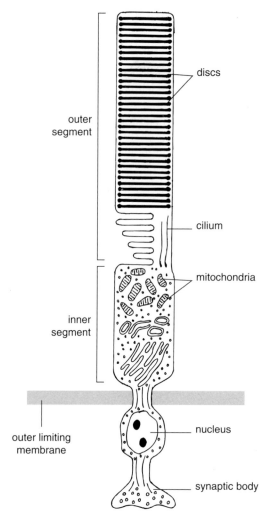

Fig. 7.10 Diagram of a rod cell. The visual pigment rhodopsin is contained in the discs that are stacked in the outer segment.

11-*cis* Retinaldehyde   Lysine residue   Schiff base

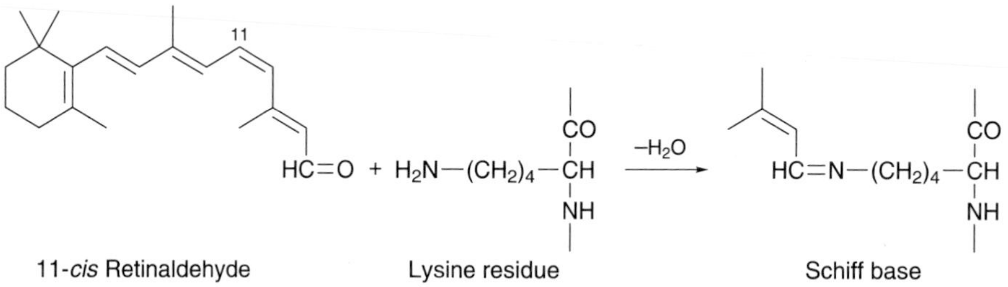

Fig. 7.11 Schiff base formation between 11-*cis* retinaldehyde and a lysine residue in opsin.

can combine with opsin in this manner. Whereas free 11-*cis* retinaldehyde in solution absorbs radiation in the ultraviolet (UV) region of the spectrum (maximal absorbance at a wavelength of 380 nm), the chromophore in rhodopsin absorbs the much more plentiful radiation in the visible (green) region (maximal absorbance, 498 nm).

7.6.4 The excitatory cascade

Rod vision is described here, as it has been studied more extensively than cone vision. The series of events

in cone cells is presumed to be analogous to that occurring in rod cells.

A rod cell can be excited by a single photon. Excitation initiates an amplification cascade of molecular events which lead ultimately to the conductance of a nerve impulse from the eye to the brain (Fig. 7.12). A photoactivated form of the visual pigment rhodopsin (metarhodopsin II) interacts with transducin – a specific disc protein with three subunits, α (alpha), β (beta) and γ (gamma). In response, the α-subunit of transducin binds guanosine triphosphate (GTP) in place of endogenously associated guanosine

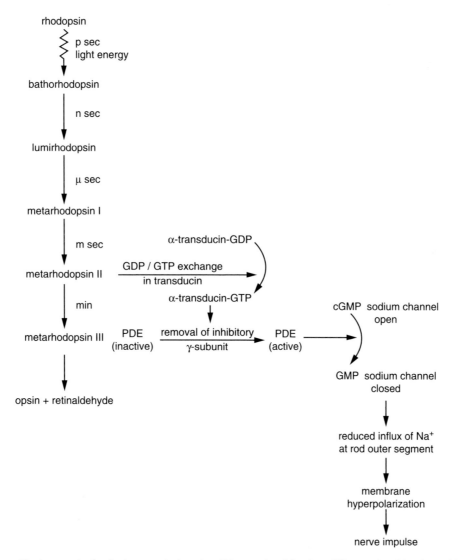

Fig. 7.12 The amplification cascade of molecular events in the retina. GDP, guanosine diphosphate; GTP, guanosine triphosphate; cGMP, 3′,5′-cyclic guanosine monophosphate (cyclic GMP); PDE, phosphodiesterase.

diphosphate (GDP). The production of hundreds of α-transducin–GTP complexes by a single molecule of activated rhodopsin is the first stage of amplification in vision. α-Transducin with its GTP then triggers the activity of a phosphodiesterase enzyme which hydrolyses 3′,5′-cyclic guanosine monophosphate (cyclic GMP) to the noncyclic form (GMP). Activation of the phosphodiesterase takes place because it is subject to an inhibitory constraint. When the α-subunit of transducin with its attached GTP binds to the phosphodiesterase, it carries away an inhibitory γ-subunit of the enzyme. The departure of this subunit unleashes the catalytic activity of the phosphodiesterase. That activity is powerful: each activated enzyme molecule can hydrolyse 4200 molecules of cyclic GMP per second. Because cyclic GMP specifically maintains the sodium channels in the plasma membrane of the rod cell in an open state, a decrease in its concentration closes the channels, leading to a marked reduction in the influx of sodium ions into the rod outer segment. The membrane consequently becomes hyperpolarized and the change in membrane potential is passed along the plasma membrane to the synaptic terminal at the other end of the rod, where the nerve impulse arises.

The biochemical system must be turned off and reset after nerve propagation. A GTPase intrinsic to the α-subunit of transducin terminates the activated state by converting the bound GTP to GDP. During this hydrolysis step the α-subunit of transducin releases the inhibitory γ-unit of phosphodiesterase. The γ-unit returns to the phosphodiesterase, binds to it and restores the enzyme to the quiescent state. Transducin is then restored to its pre-activation form by the recombination of the α-subunit and the joined β-γ unit. At the same time the light-stimulated rhodopsin is desensitized by the binding of arrestin following phosphorylation catalysed by rhodopsin kinase.

7.6.5   The visual cycle

The essential isomerization reactions of the visual cycle are shown in Fig. 7.13. When a photon strikes the dark-adapted retina, the rhodopsin is converted to the first of several unstable intermediates, bathorhodopsin, in which the 11-*cis* retinaldehyde is converted to a distorted all-*trans* configuration. This initial photochemical reaction occurs within picoseconds (10^{-12} s) of illumination and is the only light-dependent step in the visual cycle; all subsequent steps are

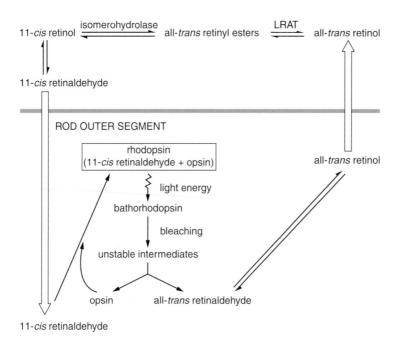

Fig. 7.13 The visual cycle. Two-way arrows indicate reversible enzymatic reactions; solid arrows represent transport mediated by interphotoreceptor retinoid-binding protein (IRBP); LRAT, lecithin:retinol acyltransferase.

thermal reactions proceeding in the dark. Hydrolysis of the Schiff base linkage and release of all-*trans* retinaldehyde takes several minutes. The breakdown of rhodopsin is called bleaching because of the loss of colour as the retinaldehyde pulls away from the opsin.

After its dissociation from opsin, all-*trans* retinaldehyde is reduced to all-*trans* retinol by a membrane-bound, NADP-dependent retinol dehydrogenase in the rod outer segment. The all-*trans* retinol is then transported by interphotoreceptor retinol-binding protein (IRBP) to the pigment epithelium; the opsin remains in the rod outer segment. The isomerization of all-*trans* retinol to 11-*cis* retinol in the pigment epithelium is a thermodynamically unfavourable process because intramolecular steric repulsion between the C-10 hydrogen atom and the methyl group at C-13 imposes a strain in the 11-*cis* isomer (Fig. 7.14). The energy requirement is provided for by coupling the negative free energy of ester hydrolysis to the isomerization reaction. In a minimal two-step reaction, all-*trans* retinol is first esterified by lecithin: retinol acyltransferase (LRAT) and the all-*trans* retinyl ester (mainly retinyl palmitate) is converted to 11-*cis* retinol by an isomerohydrolase (Rando, 1991). Since retinyl esters are themselves generated by the transfer of acyl groups from a membrane phospholipid (lecithin), the energy for the isomerization reaction originates in the membrane itself. The 11-*cis* retinol thus formed is oxidized to 11-*cis* retinaldehyde while the substrate is bound to CRALBP. The 11-*cis* retinaldehyde is transported by IRBP to the rod outer segment where it spontaneously combines with opsin to form rhodopsin. Additional small amounts of 11-*cis* retinaldehyde are available from the degradation of phagocytosed discs shed from the distal end of the rod outer segment.

The bleaching–regeneration cycle regulates the amount of rhodopsin present in the rods, allowing the visual system to alter its sensitivity according to the amount of available light. The increase in sensitivity which occurs while the eyes are in darkness or near darkness is called dark adaptation, and the decrease in sensitivity caused by exposure to bright light is called light adaptation. In cases of chronic vitamin A deficiency, dark adaptation is slow and the ability to see in poor light is impaired.

All-*trans* retinol in the form of holoRBP is taken up from the blood by receptor-mediated endocytosis at the pigment epithelium. It is then esterified in the pigment epithelium and stored in lipid globules pending conversion to 11-*cis* retinaldehyde when required. The vitamin A stored in the eye can exchange fairly rapidly with the general metabolic pool of vitamin A as long as the pool is adequate. If a rat is maintained on a low vitamin A diet, its eyes take up retinol much more avidly than other tissues which also have a need for it. Moreover, the eyes can hold tenaciously to their stores of esterified vitamin long after other tissues are depleted.

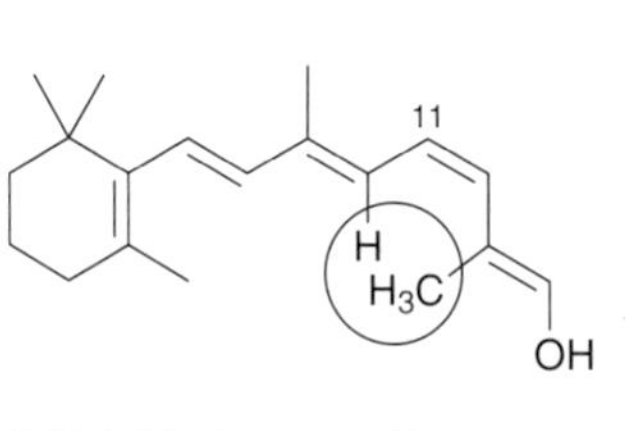

7.7 Retinoids as regulators of gene expression

Background information can be found in Chapter 6.

7.7.1 Nuclear retinoid receptors

Nuclear retinoid receptors are implicated in various aspects of cell growth, development and homeostasis by controlling expression of specific genes through their hormonal ligands, which act as signals. The two classes of receptor – retinoic acid receptors (RARs) and retinoid X receptors (RXRs) – differ in their primary structure, their binding affinity to retinoids, and their ability to regulate expression of different target genes. The retinoid receptors belong to a subfamily of the superfamily of receptors that function as ligand-dependent transcription factors; the subfamily includes receptors for steroid hormones, thyroid hormone and vitamin D.

In contrast to steroid hormone receptors, which are encoded by single-copy genes located on separate chromosomes, the RARs and RXRs are each encoded by three distinct genes, giving rise to receptor subtypes α, β and γ. The receptors show characteristic patterns of distribution in adult and embryonic tissues (Table 7.2). The three RAR subtypes within a given animal

Fig. 7.14 Methyl–hydrogen repulsion as a source of strain in 11-*cis* retinol.

Table 7.2   Distribution of RAR and RXR in mammalian adult and embryonic tissues.

Receptor	Adult	Developing embryo
RARα	Ubiquitous	Ubiquitous
RARβ	Kidney, adrenal glands, pituitary gland, prostate gland, spinal cord, brain, muscle, bone	Neural crest cells Developing peripheral nervous system Epithelia of lungs, intestine and genital tract
RARγ	Skin, bone	Neural crest craniofacial domains Differentiating squamous and mucous epithelia
RXRα	Skin, liver, kidney, lung, spleen, muscle, bone	Epithelia of digestive tract, liver, skin
RXRβ	Ubiquitous	Ubiquitous
RXRγ	Liver, kidney, adrenal glands, lung, brain, muscle	Discrete areas of developing central nervous system, pituitary gland

species have very similar amino acid sequences in their DNA-binding C domains and ligand-binding E domains. The same is true for the three RXR subtypes. The lack of similarity among domains A/B, D and F suggests that functional differences between subtypes may be conferred by these regions. Between species (mouse and human) the sequence of a particular subtype is nearly 100% conserved through domains A–F. The sequence homology between RARs and RXRs is not strong, the most conserved region lying in the C domain. Somewhat surprisingly, there is greater homology between RARs and thyroid hormone receptors than between RARs and RXRs.

The diversity of the retinoid signalling pathways is further increased by the presence of two promoters for each of the six genes that encode the α, β and γ subtypes of RAR and RXR, giving rise to two alternative primary mRNA transcripts for each gene. These transcripts generate receptor isoforms, which are identified by numbers behind the Greek letter. Isoforms for a given receptor subtype differ only in the amino acid sequences of their amino-terminal A regions. Further isoforms are generated post-translationally by the alternative splicing of the primary transcripts. At least seven isoforms of RARγ, for example, have been identified in the mouse, but RARγ3 to γ7 are

minor and lack the A region altogether (Zelent *et al.*, 1991). The major isoforms of the RARs and RXRs are listed in Table 7.3. Some target genes are activated preferentially by one RAR isoform over another and antagonism between various isoforms has been demonstrated (Husmann *et al.*, 1991).

The RARs bind both all-*trans* retinoic acid and 9-*cis* retinoic acid with approximately the same high affinity and activate transcription as a consequence of this binding. The two ligands compete with each other for binding to distinct but overlapping binding sites within AF-2 of RARα (Tate *et al.*, 1994). The RXRs are incapable of high-affinity binding to all-*trans* retinoic acid, but they bind and are activated by 9-*cis* retinoic acid. In addition, the 9-*cis* isomer of 3,4-didehydro-retinoic acid, but not the all-*trans* isomer, is an activating ligand for RXRs (Allenby *et al.*, 1993). The ability of 9-*cis* retinoic acid to serve as a bifunctional ligand for RARs and RXRs may have physiological significance. Interconversion of the all-*trans* and 9-*cis* retinoic acid isomers by an as yet undiscovered specific isomerase at localized sites could provide a means for cell-specific regulation of retinoid signalling.

RARs are unable to form functional homodimers, and require heterodimerization with RXRs for efficient DNA binding and transcriptional activity. In contrast, the RXRs can function both as heterodimers and homodimers. The ability of the RXRs to homodimerize is attributable to a unique third helix in the C/D domain (Lee *et al.*, 1993) and is dependent upon the binding of its ligand, 9-*cis* retinoic acid.

Table 7.3   Major isoforms of RAR and RXR α, β, and γ subtypes (according to Chambon, 1996).

RAR		
Type 1	Type 2	RXR
α1	α2	α1, α2
β1, β3	β2, β4	β1, β2
γ1	γ2	γ1, γ2

Type 1 and type 2 RAR isoforms are transcribed from an upstream promoter (P1) and a downstream promoter (P2), respectively. The two pairs of RARβ isoforms (β1/β3 and β2/β4) are generated by alternative splicing. The isoforms of RXRα, RXRβ and RXRγ are also transcribed from different promoters.

7.7.2 Role of retinoid receptors in transcriptional regulation

RAR, in dimeric combination with RXR, binds in a ligand-independent manner to a retinoic acid response element (RARE) on the DNA. The RARE is an enhancer type of regulatory element and the RAR is an activator protein. In the absence of its ligand (retinoic acid), the RAR partner of the DNA-bound heterodimer interacts via its repressor function (the CoR box) with either or both of the co-repressors N-CoR and SMRT, which in turn interact with a Sin3–histone deacetylase (HDAC) complex to repress transcription. The binding of ligand to RAR causes a conformational change in the helix 12 of the receptor's ligand-binding domain. This triggers release of the co-repressor–Sin 3–HDAC complex and exposes the activation surface of the receptor's AF-2 motif. The conformational change also prompts the simultaneous recruitment of a coactivator complex containing combinations of CBP/p300, PCAF, SRC-1 and ACTR, all of which exhibit histone acetyltransferase (HAT) activity. The relief of repression resulting from dismissal of HDAC, together with HAT-induced changes in nucleosomal structure and the chromatin remodelling activity of Swi/Snf, allows recruitment of the transcription machinery to the promoter. Thus RAR functions as a transcriptional activator in the presence of its ligand and as a repressor in the absence of ligand (Fig. 7.15). RXR does not respond to its ligand in the manner of RAR and acts as a silent partner. The receptor dimers and promoter-bound complex are brought together by DNA looping or bending. The stable pre-initiation complex is now poised for rapid and repeated initiation of transcription by RNA polymerase II.

7.7.3 Specifying the retinoic acid response

The retinoic acid responses can be limited to certain cell types because the retinoid receptors can influence the magnitude of response. For instance, the RARγ1 isoform can inhibit the activation of the βRARE by other RARs (Husmann et al., 1991). βRARE is a response element found in the promoter of the *RARβ* gene. It is located adjacent to the TATA box in CV-1 cells and is therefore part of a natural minimal retinoic acid-responsive promoter that may not require other transcription factors beyond those associated with the TATA box (Hoffmann et al., 1990). The RARγ1-mediated inhibition is isoform-specific, as RARγ2 activates the βRARE. The inhibition is also dose-dependent and may involve competition among receptors for the response element. Thus in cells that

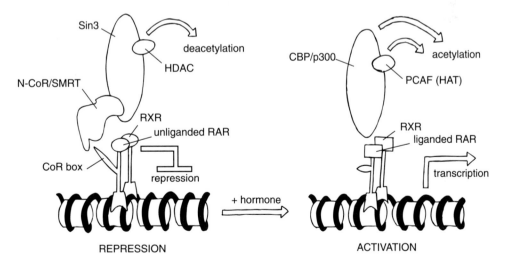

Fig. 7.15 Function of an RAR as a transcriptional activator in the presence of ligand or as a repressor in the absence of ligand. The N-CoR/SMRT-Sin3 combination is the co-repressor complex to which is linked a histone deacetylase (HDAC). The CBP/p300–PCAF coactivator complex contains inherent histone acetyltransferase (HAT) activity. Binding of ligand (retinoic acid) to the RAR partner of the DNA-bound heterodimer results in the release of the co-repressor complex and the recruitment of the coactivator complex. The HAT activity of the coactivators loosens the nucleosomal structure, thereby permitting access of the transcription machinery to the promoter. Reprinted from Hassig & Schreiber (1997), *Current Opinion in Chemical Biology*, Vol. 1, pp. 30–308, copyright 1997, with permission from Elsevier Science.

produce RARγ1, retinoic acid-responsive genes that contain βRARE-like response elements may show a reduced or complete lack of response to retinoic acid.

A given RAR–RXR heterodimer can have different ligand affinities, and thus different levels of activation, depending on the relative polarity of the two receptors and the exact structure of the DNA binding site. It is therefore the receptor–response element complex and not the receptor alone that determines the hormonal response. The diversity of RAREs, together with tissue- and cell type-specific expression patterns of the various RAR and RXR subtypes and isoforms, allows for a pleiotropic and fine-tuned hormonal response.

La Vista-Picard et al. (1996) further showed that synthetic retinoids with restricted molecular conformations can be highly selective for binding to certain receptor–RARE combinations, and could serve as gene-selective activators. Because of their limited biological activity, such compounds could have therapeutic value since they would have fewer side effects than the flexible natural compounds with their broad-spectrum activities.

7.7.4   Interaction between the thyroid hormone receptor and the retinoic acid receptor

The thyroid hormone receptors (TR) are encoded by two different genes, giving rise to subtypes α and β. Thyroid hormone response elements (TRE) are typically composed of two or more sequences of a consensus AGGTCA half-site arranged as an inverted repeat (palindrome), everted repeat or direct repeat (Ribeiro et al., 1995), thereby allowing a great flexibility in half-site arrangement and orientation. Palindromic TREs are responsive to both thyroid hormone (triiodothyronine) and retinoic acid. The two hormones interact co-operatively to stimulate transcription of the growth hormone gene in the rat pituitary gland (Bedo et al, 1989; Morita et al., 1989, 1990). The presence or absence of thyroid hormone dictates how these dual-responsive elements are regulated. In the presence of thyroid hormone, TRs activate the TRE and also allow some degree of positive co-operativity with RARs. In the absence of thyroid hormone, the unliganded TR functions as a repressor, preventing either TR and RAR from activating the TRE. The unliganded RAR does not show a negative effect upon TR (Brent et al., 1989; Graupner et al., 1989). The repres-

sive effect of unliganded TR on retinoic acid-induced gene expression through a common response element could account for well-characterized developmental abnormalities associated with hypothyroidism.

7.7.5   Experimental use of embryonal carcinoma cells

The establishment of retinoic acid-responsive genes has been facilitated by the use of cultured mouse teratocarcinoma stem cells, also known as embryonal carcinoma (EC) cells. These cells exhibit many features of normal cell differentiation pathways and cell–cell interactions. EC cell lines can be isolated from tumours (teratocarcinomas) that arise when normal pre-implantation (1- to 7.5-day-old) inbred mouse embryos (blastocysts) are transplanted to an extra-uterine site such as the kidney or testis of an adult mouse (Martin, 1981) or by injecting cultured embryonic stem cells taken from late blastocysts into mice (Evans & Kaufman, 1981). A typical mouse teratocarcinoma contains undifferentiated stem cells (the EC cells) interspersed in a disorganized mixture of differentiated cell types. The continued proliferation of the EC cell population is responsible for the malignant properties of teratocarcinomas. EC cells share morphological, biochemical and genetic properties with pluripotent stem cells from the inner cell mass of mouse blastocysts. (Pluripotent stem cells are capable of forming derivatives of all three primary germ layers, namely, endoderm, mesoderm and ectoderm.) Many murine EC cell lines are capable of undergoing a controlled differentiation in culture in a manner that closely parallels the normal behaviour of embryonic cells. The EC cells therefore provide an in vitro model for biochemical studies of cellular differentiation and early embryonic development.

Cultures of mouse EC cells can either proliferate exponentially in an undifferentiated state or, if stimulated, differentiate into cells similar to definitive embryonic cells. Retinoic acid is a potent inducer of differentiation in a number of EC cell lines, including F9 and P19. Differentiation of these stem cells is accompanied by a decrease in the rate of proliferation and also by the induction of expression of several genes.

The particular type of differentiated cell depends on the EC cell line, the manner in which the cells are cultured, and the concentration of retinoic acid added. Treatment of low-density monolayer cultures of F9 stem cells with retinoic acid converts the cells to primitive endoderm cells, and subsequent treatment with dibutyryl cyclic AMP induces further differentiation to parietal endoderm (Strickland, 1981). If F9 cells are grown as suspension aggregates or as high-density monolayer cultures, treatment with retinoic acid converts the outer surface cells to visceral rather than parietal endoderm (Hogan *et al.*, 1981). Retinoic acid treatment of P19 stem cells in monolayer cultures results in fibroblasts or, in the case of aggregate cultures, in neurons and glial cells (Jones-Villeneuve *et al.*, 1982). The effect of retinoic acid concentration was demonstrated by Edwards & McBurney (1983) using a subclone of the P19 cell line in aggregate culture. A concentration of 10^{-9} M retinoic acid induced an abundance of cardiac muscle; at a higher concentration (10^{-8} M) skeletal muscle became abundant, and at 10^{-7} to 10^{-5} M neurons and glial cells appeared.

7.7.6   Retinoic acid-responsive genes

Retinoic acid-responsive genes in which a RARE has been identified fall into the category of primary response genes or, in some cases, delayed primary response genes. These genes, by definition, bind the hormone–receptor complex – in this case, the RAR–RXR heterodimer – and produce the hormone responsive protein with no requirement for ongoing protein synthesis. Primary response genes produce mRNA within minutes to a few hours after addition of retinoic acid to cell cultures, whereas delayed primary response genes produce mRNA only after several hours. Vitamin A-responsive genes, which apparently have no RARE and which produce mRNA only after several hours, are categorized as secondary response genes. These genes, by definition do not bind the hormone–receptor complex. They may be regulated by a transcription factor produced by a primary response gene or they may be regulated at the post-transcriptional level. In the latter case, for example, retinol acts by stabilizing newly synthesized alkaline phosphatase transcripts (Zhou *et al.*, 1994), regulating the processing of interleukin-1 precursor transcripts into mature mRNA (Jarrous & Kaempfer, 1994) and increasing the half-life of connexin43 by inducing adhesion molecules (Bex *et al.*, 1995).

The many retinoic acid-responsive genes encode proteins having very diverse functions. The proteins include nuclear retinoid receptors, cellular retinoid-binding proteins, transcription factors, enzymes, extracellular matrix proteins and growth factors (Table 7.4). The RAREs that are present in primary response genes frequently consist of direct repeats of two core recognition motifs with consensus sequence AGGTCA separated by 5, 2 or 1 base pairs and designated DR5, DR2 and DR1 elements, respectively. Sequence differences from the consensus do occur and generally result in a reduced transcriptional response to retinoic acid owing to a lower receptor binding affinity. RAREs are not exclusively of the direct repeat type: everted repeat elements were identified in the genes encoding γF-crystallin (Tini *et al.*, 1993) and medium-chain acyl-coenzyme A dehydrogenase (Raisher *et al.*, 1992). In the latter gene, the response element was activated by RXRα in preference to RARα or RARβ and thus could be described as an RXRE.

The promoters of some genes contain composite response elements which can selectively bind and initiate transcription from multiple nuclear hormone receptors, thereby allowing cross-talk between different hormonal pathways. For example, the rat oxytocin promoter contains a RARE that is predominantly responsive to retinoic acid, but also permits binding of TR and ER (oestrogen receptor) to mediate transcription in the presence of thyroid hormone and oestradiol (Adan *et al.*, 1993). Kato *et al.* (1995) described a novel class of response elements which are widely spaced (10 to 200 base pairs) direct repeats of the consensus AGGTCA motif (DR10 to DR200) and which act as promiscuous transactivation sites for ER, RAR–RXR and VDR–RXR, but not TR–RXR.

In the following discussion, special attention is given to the genes encoding the retinoid receptors and the cellular retinoid-binding proteins, as these proteins are physiologically important in vitamin A function. Also discussed are the homeobox and *oct* genes, which are involved in embryonic development.

Genes encoding the retinoid receptors

All three genes coding for the RAR proteins (subtypes α, β and γ) contain a RARE in one of their two promoters and have been shown to be transcriptionally up-regulated in response to all-*trans* and 9-*cis* retinoic acid. This form of autoregulation may amplify a retinoic acid signal by increasing the number of available receptors in target tissues. Target gene responsiveness is cell type specific (Davis & Lazar,

Table 7.4 A selection of retinoic acid-responsive genes.

Gene or gene product	Stimulated (↑) or repressed (↓) by retinoic acid	Type of gene (if known)	Type of RARE* (if identified) or AP-1 binding site	References
Nuclear receptors				
RARα2 (M)	↑	Primary response	DR5*	Leroy *et al.* (1991a,b)
RARβ2 (H)	↑	Primary response	DR5*	de Thé *et al.* (1989, 1990)
RARγ2 (H)	↑	Primary response	DR5*	Lehmann *et al.* (1992)
Cellular retinoid-binding proteins				
CRBP-I (R)	↑	Primary response	DR2*	Husmann *et al.* (1992)
CRBP-II (M)	↑	Primary response	DR1* and DR2*	Nakshatri & Chambon (1994)
CRABP-I (M)	↑	Secondary response		Wei *et al.* (1989, 1995)
CRABP-II (H)	↑	Primary response	DR5*	Åström *et al.* (1994)
Homeobox genes				
Hoxa-1 (M)	↑	Primary response	DR5*	Langston & Gudas (1992)
HOXB1 (H)	↑	Primary response	Two DR2* elements	Ogura & Evans (1995b)
Hoxd-4 (M)	↑	Primary response	DR5*	Pöpperl & Featherstone (1993)
Enzymes				
PEPCK (R)	↑	Primary response	DR1* and DR5*	Scott *et al.* (1996)
MCAD (H)	↑	Primary response	Complex*	Raisher *et al.* (1992)
Alcohol dehydrogenase (H)	↑	Primary response	DR5*	Duester *et al.* (1991)
Alkaline phosphatase (M)	↑	Secondary response		Gianni *et al.* (1991)
Collagenase (H)	↓	Primary response	AP-1	Lafyatis *et al.* (1990)
Stromelysin (R)	↓	Primary response	AP-1	Nicholson *et al.* (1990)
Transglutaminase (M)	↑	Primary response	Not identified	Chiocca *et al.* (1988)
Extracellular matrix proteins				
Laminin B1 (M)	↑	Delayed primary response	Complex*	Vasios *et al.* (1989, 1991)
Collagen type IV (M)	↑	Secondary response		Gudas *et al.* (1990)
Matrix Gla protein (H)	↓	Primary response	Novel*[a]	Kirfel *et al.* (1997)
Growth factors and their receptors				
IGF-I (R)	↓	Secondary response		Lowe *et al.* (1992)
Interleukin-2 (H)	↓	Secondary response		Felli *et al.* (1991)
PDGF-Rα (M)	↑	Primary response	Not identified	Wang *et al.* (1990)
Gap-junctional protein				
Connexin 43 (M)	↑	Secondary response		Guo *et al.* (1992)
Other proteins				
Complement factor H (M)	↑	Primary response	DR5*	Muñoz-Cánoves *et al.* (1990)
Apolipoprotein A1 (H)	↑	Primary response	DR2*	Rottmann *et al.* (1991)
Lactoferrin (H)	↑	Primary response	DR1*	Lee *et al.* (1995)
γF-crystallin (M)	↑	Primary response	ER8*	Tini *et al.* (1993)

(M), mouse; (R), rat; (H), human.

DR, direct repeat motif with 1, 2 or 5 base pair spacers between half-sites; ER, everted repeat motif.

PEPCK, phosphoenolpyruvate carboxykinase; MCAD, medium-chain acyl-coenzyme A dehydrogenase; IGF-I, insulin-like growth factor-I; PDGF-Rα, platelet-derived growth factor receptor-α.

[a]Novel negative response element (NRE).

1993). Autoregulation of RARs has not only been demonstrated in tissue culture cell lines (Zelent *et al.*, 1991), but also in the adult rat (Haq *et al.*, 1991). Each RAR subtype is known to contain at least one isoform that can control its own synthesis. The RARE in the *RARβ2* gene promoter confers the greatest sensitivity to transcriptional activation. This element is located only about one helical turn from the TATA box in comparison with RAREs from other genes which are located further upstream. The induction of *RARβ* transcription is a direct response to retinoic acid treatment in that it does not require new protein synthesis. In this respect the *RARβ* gene is a primary response gene whose induction occurs within 3 hours of retinoic acid addition. The βRARE is a target for all three RAR subtypes, but not for TR or VDR (Sucov *et al.*, 1990). However, RARγ1 can repress the activation of the βRARE by other RARs, thereby limiting the autoregulated stimulation of *RARβ* expression (Husmann *et al.*, 1991). The induction of RARs by their retinoid ligands provides another possible mechanism by which retinoic acid can control the availability of RXR for other nuclear receptors. The induced increase in RAR molecules is likely to encourage RAR–RXR heterodimerization and, under conditions where RXR molecules are limited, this could impair signal responses mediated by other nuclear receptors that require RXR for DNA binding.

Genes encoding the cellular retinoid-binding proteins

CRBP-I

Several whole animal studies have examined the effects of oral administration of retinyl acetate or retinoic acid on CRBP-I mRNA levels in various tissues. Rajan *et al.* (1990) reported that the levels of CRBP-I mRNA in certain tissues (lung, testis, spleen and small intestine) of vitamin A-deficient rats were lower than those in normally-fed rats. Oral repletion with retinyl acetate restored the levels to normal. Retinoid deficiency did not affect the levels of CRBP-I mRNA in the three tissues with the highest content of CRBP-I protein and CRBP-I mRNA (proximal epididymis, liver and kidney). Haq & Chytil (1988) showed that administration of retinoic acid to vitamin A-deficient rats elicited a more rapid response than observed with retinyl acetate, with a two- to three-fold increase in CRBP-I mRNA in lung tissue within 1 hour. Increased expression of CRBP-I was also demonstrated in the lung tissue of normally-fed, vitamin A-replete rats after oral administration of retinoic acid (Rush *et al.*, 1991). Consistent with these studies was the demonstration that topical application of retinol or retinoic acid to adult human skin led to increased levels of CRBP-I mRNA and protein (Fisher *et al.*, 1995). These

experiments indicate that, in certain tissues at least, dietary retinol (or more directly retinoic acid) directly induces the expression of the *CRBP-I* gene. Thus organs in which CRBP-I expression is depressed during vitamin A deficiency are able to respond rapidly to retinoids as soon as they become available.

The expression of CRBP-I can be modulated in the vitamin A-replete animal by glucocorticoid hormones. The administration of dexamethasone to vitamin A-replete rats decreased the levels of CRBP-I mRNA levels in lung and liver tissues. In addition, the increase in CRBP-I mRNA induced by oral administration of retinoic acid was blocked when dexamethasone was administered at the same time (Rush *et al.*, 1991). This effect may be maintained by putative glucocorticoid-response elements identified in the promoter of the *CRBP-I* gene.

The hormonal changes that occur during pregnancy and lactation also affect the expression of CRBP-I. Towards the end of pregnancy in the rat, the level of CRBP-I mRNA in the maternal liver rises markedly then drops abruptly at term (Levin *et al.*, 1987). This event coincides with a significant mobilization of hepatic vitamin A stores so that the milk of the lactating rat can meet the vitamin A needs of the suckling pups.

Wei *et al.* (1989) demonstrated that treatment of tissue cultures with retinoic acid induced an increase in CRBP-I mRNA followed by the protein itself. The 3-hour lag period and the nondependence on concomitant protein synthesis identified the *CRBP-I* gene as a primary response gene. CRBP-I induction occurred both at 10^{-7} and 10^{-9} M retinoic acid in EC cells that differentiate into neurons and extra-embryonic endoderm and also in a non-EC cell that differentiates into glial cells.

The rapid synthesis of the CRBP-I protein in response to retinoic acid, observed for the whole animal as well as in cultured cells, suggested that the *CRBP-I* gene would contain a RARE. Such a response element has been demonstrated in the mouse (Smith *et al.*, 1991) and the rat (Husmann *et al.*, 1992). In both species, the RARE is located 1 kilobase upstream of the transcription start site. The RARE in the rat *CRBP-I* gene is a DR2 type element and is activated *in vitro* by the RAR–RXR heterodimer. The presence of a RARE in the *CRBP-I* gene indicates that CRBP-I protein levels are regulated primarily at the level of transcription.

CRBP-II

In the adult, expression of the *CRBP-II* gene is essentially confined to the small intestinal enterocytes. In contrast to CRBP-I, whose expression is decreased in various organs during vitamin A deficiency, expression of intestinal CRBP-II is actually increased. Rajan *et al.* (1990) reported an increase in the CRBP-II mRNA level of 42% in the small intestine of the vitamin A-deficient rat. The contrasting expression profiles of these two similar proteins reflect the physiological needs of the animal. During vitamin A deficiency, the animal conserves its precious supply of retinoids to maintain only essential functions, allowing the animal to hunt for food. In addition, the intestine is kept at the ready to receive dietary vitamin A as soon as the animal finds it.

During the last 5 days of pregnancy in the rat, mRNA for CRBP-II in the small intestine shows a four-fold increase, accompanying the increase observed for CRBP-I in the maternal liver. Intestinal CRBP-II levels remain elevated during the suckling period and return to normal by 1 week post-weaning (Quick & Ong, 1989). This increase in production of intestinal CRBP-II, like that of hepatic CRBP-I, is an adaptive response, ensuring that sufficient vitamin A reaches the mammary gland during lactation.

Nakshrati & Chambon (1994) showed that the mouse *CRBP-II* gene contains three response elements, which they designated RE1, RE2 and RE3. The elements RE2 and RE3, which have DR2 and DR1 sequence motifs, respectively, are putative RAREs and are conserved in the rat and mouse *CRBP-II* gene 5′-flanking regions. The more distal RE1 element, which also has a DR1 motif, is a truncated form of an element previously found in the rat and designated an RXRE by Mangelsdorf *et al.* (1991). Nakshatri & Chambon (1994) showed that RE2 and RE3 were required for maximal RAR–RXR-mediated retinoic acid inducibility to the mouse CRBP-II promoter in transfection experiments. RE2 had no effect on its own, but co-operated with RE3. RE1 was not involved in the induction; if anything, it exerted a slight inhibitory effect. Thus RE3 appeared to be the only element within the mouse CRBP-II promoter which responded on its own to RAR and RXR. The RE3 and RE1 response elements have a much higher affinity for HNF-4 and ARP-1 than for RAR–RXR heterodimers and RXR homodimers. HNF-4 and ARP-1 are members of the nuclear receptor superfamily and

are expressed in liver and intestinal cells. Nakshatri & Chambon (1994) showed that HNF-4 constitutively activates the mouse CRBP-II promoter, whereas ARP-1 competitively represses its activation by RAR, RXR and HNF-4. Although the data reported by Nakshatri & Chambon (1994) and also by Mangelsdorf *et al.* (1991) show that the mouse and rat CRBP-II promoters can respond to over-expressed RXR and RAR in co-transfection experiments, for these results to be physiologically relevant, it must be demonstrated that expression of the *CRBP-II* gene can be stimulated by retinoic acid treatment *in vivo*. There are no available data concerning a possible retinoic acid induction of CRBP-II mRNA or protein in adult intestine and in prenatal liver or intestine, which are also known to express the *CRBP-II* gene (Nakshatri & Chambon, 1994). It appears that HNF-4 is the major transcriptional activator of the *CRBP-II* gene *in vivo*. Inducement of the *CRBP-II* gene by retinoic acid may only take place in tissues where HNF-4 and ARP-1 are lacking or present in low amounts.

CRABP-I

CRABP-I is ubiquitously expressed in adult animal tissues at a low basal level, except in several retinoic acid-sensitive tissues such as the eye and the testis where the expression is highly elevated. In adult rats, neither CRABP-I protein nor mRNA levels were affected by dietary vitamin A deficiency (Rajan *et al.*, 1991), suggesting that the binding protein is not regulated by overall vitamin A status. CRABP-I is also constitutively expressed at a required level in certain regions of the developing embryo and at certain times of development. In the developing mouse, CRABP-I mRNA has been detected in the neural crest, the eye region and the craniofacial region (Perez-Castro *et al.*, 1989) and in rudimentary limbs (Dollé *et al.*, 1989).

Wei *et al.* (1989), using tissue cultures, showed that expression of the *CRABP-I* gene was induced by 10^{-7} M (but not 10^{-9} M) retinoic acid in a manner that required the synthesis of new protein. A detectable increase in CRABP-I mRNA was not observed until 12 hours after retinoic acid treatment. These observations, and the absence of a RARE with any known consensus sequence, place the *CRABP-I* gene in the category of secondary response genes. Induction occurred in cells, which differentiate into neurons, but not in cells which differentiate into extra-embryonic endoderm or glial cells.

CRABP-II

Transcription of the human *CRABP-II* gene was markedly induced by retinoic acid in skin *in vivo* and in skin fibroblasts *in vitro*. Retinoic acid had no such effect on cultured lung fibroblasts, demonstrating cell-specific regulation of the *CRABP-II* gene (Åström *et al.*, 1991). In the cultured skin fibroblasts, the increase in CRABP-II mRNA was detected 1 hour after addition of retinoic acid. The level peaked at 2 hours and returned to basal levels within 6 hours. Ongoing protein synthesis was required for this transient increase of transcription (Åström *et al.*, 1992). The human CRABP-II contains one far upstream RARE of the DR5 type that binds the RAR–RXR heterodimer (Åström *et al.*, 1994). The binding of receptor to the response element and the early response are consistent with *CRABP-II* being a primary response gene, but the ongoing protein synthesis is inconsistent with this definition. Interestingly, the mouse *CRABP-II* gene contains two co-operating response elements, a DR2 RARE and a DR1 RXRE, mediating differential induction of transcription in response to both all-*trans* and 9-*cis* retinoic acid (Durand *et al.*, 1992).

Homeobox genes

In embryonic development, the process of segmentation and the specification of segment identity along the body axis are controlled by an organized system of regulatory genes, which encode DNA-binding transcription factors. One important family of such genes is the homeobox (*Hox*) gene family whose members encode proteins containing a helix–turn–helix DNA-binding domain known as the homeodomain. Each of four specific chromosomes contains a linear array of *Hox* genes clustered within a restricted region called the *Hox* locus. The four gene clusters (*Hoxa*, *Hoxb*, *Hoxc* and *Hoxd*) contain at least nine genes arranged in the same order along the chromosome (3′ to 5′ direction) as they are expressed along the anterior–posterior body axis of the developing embryo. The expression of at least some of the *Hox* genes is induced by exposure to retinoic acid in cultured EC cells. The non-requirement for concomitant protein synthesis and the binding of RAR to RARE places the *Hox* genes in the category of primary response genes. The products of these genes alter cellular behaviour, either directly or by inducing the expression of secondary response genes such as those encoding laminin and collagen IV.

Treatment of cultured EC cells with physiological concentrations of retinoic acid induces the transcription of the murine *Hoxa-1* gene in a dose-dependent manner. This gene, originally designated *Era-1* and later *Hox-1.6*, is located at the 3′ end of the A cluster on mouse chromosome 6. Two distinct proteins arise as a result of alternative splicing of the primary transcript, one containing the homeodomain and the other lacking this motif (LaRosa & Gudas, 1988). Possibly, the protein lacking the homeodomain could act as a competitive inhibitor of the complete Hox protein by competing for interaction with regulatory factors, while being unable itself to bind to DNA. Langston & Gudas (1992) demonstrated the presence of a DR5-type RARE within a retinoic acid-responsive enhancer located approximately 5 kilobases downstream (3′) of the *Hoxa-1* promoter. This RAR-binding element was necessary and sufficient for retinoic acid to activate the *Hoxa-1* gene in EC cells.

Ogura & Evans (1995a, 1995b) produced *in vitro* evidence for two distinct retinoic acid response pathways for regulation of the human *HOXB1* gene (Fig. 7.16). The first pathway depends upon a retinoic acid-responsive site located toward the 5′ end of the gene. This site has two functional components: a DR2 RARE, which is the direct target of a RAR–RXR heterodimer, and an upstream response element (URE), which serves as a binding site for a coactivator termed retinoid-inducible protein (RIP). The second pathway depends upon a 3′ site comprising a second DR2 RARE and a downstream response element (DRE) capable of binding another coactivator called retinoid-activating protein (RAP). Retinoic acid activates the *HOXB1* gene through the 5′ or 3′ RARE and the coactivators modulate the activation. The two coactivators are cell-specific: RIP is induced by retinoic acid in P19 cells but not in NT2/D1 cells, whilst RAP is constitutively expressed in NT2/D1 and P19 cells but not in CV-1 cells. This cell specificity enables selective tissues to respond to retinoic acid in the different time courses of development. In a third autoregulatory pathway, the *HOXB1* gene is activated by its encoded protein. The experimental data suggest that retinoic acid is required to initiate activation, after which gene expression is maintained by the autoregulatory loop.

Retinoic acid has been shown to induce at least one *Hox* gene *in vivo*. Insertion of a retinoic acid bead in the anterior of a limb bud induces expression of *Hoxc-6* in the area around the bead (Oliver *et al.*, 1990).

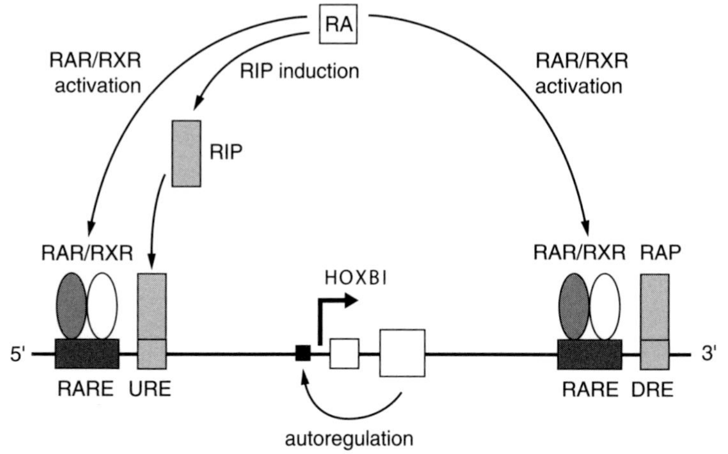

Fig. 7.16 Activation of the human *HOXB1* gene by retinoic acid. Retinoic acid (RA) activates *HOXB1* through the 5′ or 3′ RARE in two distinct pathways modulated by the coactivators RIP and RAP, respectively. RIP itself is induced by retinoic acid. *HOXB1* is activated by its encoded protein, creating an autoregulatory loop. RIP, retinoid-inducible protein; RAP, retinoid-activating protein; URE, upstream response element; DRE downstream response element. Reproduced, with permission, from Ogura, T. & Evans, R. M. Evidence for two distinct retinoic acid response pathways for *HOXB1* gene regulation. *Proceedings of the National Academy of Sciences of the U.S.A.*, **92**, 392–6. Copyright 1995 National Academy of Sciences, U.S.A.

The oct-3/4 gene

The *oct* genes form another important family of regulatory genes involved in embryonic development. Members of this family encode transcription factors (Oct proteins), which bind to the octamer DNA sequence ATTTGCAT in a variety of genes. The *oct3* and *oct4* genes are expressed in embryonic stem cells some time before 3.5 days after coitus and then repressed within a few days afterwards, the exact day of repression depending on the cell lineage. The presence or absence of Oct-3/4 protein in developing embryonic cells probably influences the fate of the cells.

The expression of the *oct-3/4* gene is rapidly down-regulated *in vitro* when both embryonic stem (ES) cells and EC cells are induced to differentiate by treatment with retinoic acid. The down-regulation is the result of a specific inhibition of expression by retinoic acid. Okazawa *et al.* (1991) reported that two sequences (designated RARE1A and RARE1B) in the *oct-3* enhancer region were targets for retinoic acid-mediated repression. These sequences did not contain a typical RAR recognition site and the loss of enhancer activity did not involve binding of RARs.

In addition to the RARE1A/B situated in the enhancer, a novel element has been identified in the *oct-3/4* gene promoter which contains a putative Sp1 binding site juxtaposed to a DR1-type RARE (designated RAREoct) (Pikarsky *et al.*, 1994; Schloorlemmer *et al.*, 1994). Mutations in the Sp1 site drastically diminish expression of *oct-3/4* in P19 cells, showing that the binding of an Sp1 protein or related protein is essential for maximal activation. In the absence of retinoic acid, RAREoct mediates transcriptional activation, but, when cells are

treated with retinoic acid, RAREoct functions as a binding site for a negative regulator. RAREoct, being responsive to both positive and negative regulatory proteins, is therefore a point of integration of several signalling pathways influencing *oct-3/4* gene expression.

COUP-TFs have been identified as candidate endogenous repressors of the *oct4* gene promoter (Schloorlemmer *et al.*, 1994). However, repression is exerted by a different mechanism from the interference by COUP-TFs of retinoic acid-induced transcriptional activation via DR1 elements, since the RAREoct is transactivated neither by all-*trans* nor by 9-*cis* retinoic acid.

Thus, the down-regulation of *oct-3/4* expression by retinoic acid in embryonic stem cells involves two independent mechanisms: deactivation of a stem cell-specific enhancer by a mechanism not clearly defined and promoter silencing by COUP orphan receptors. The enhancer and promoter elements involved are shown in Fig. 7.17.

Genes encoding extracellular matrix proteins

Laminin and collagen type IV are extracellular matrix proteins and are major constituents of basal lamenae. Laminin comprises three polypeptide subunits (A, B1 and B2) and collagen IV comprises two subunits (proα1 and proα2). The subunits of both proteins are the products of separate genes. Synthesis of the laminin B proteins and collagen type IVα2 is stimulated in F9 teratocarcinoma stem cells after treatment of the cells with retinoic acid (Wang & Gudas, 1983). In the case of the *laminin* gene, the requirement for protein synthesis during the late transcriptional response and the presence of an RARE define this gene as a delayed

Fig. 7.17 Map of the 5′ region of the *oct-3/4* gene showing the RARE1A and RARE1B sequences in the enhancer region (E) and a novel element containing an Sp1 binding site and RAREoct in the promoter region (P). The arrowheads indicate the initiation sites of transcription. Reproduced, with permission, from Pikarsky, *et al.*, *Molecular and Cellular Biology*, Vol. 14, pp. 1026–38, © 1994, American Society for Microbiology.

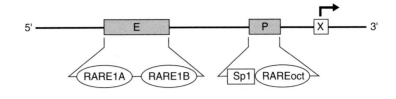

primary response gene. The RARE consists of three directly repeated TGACC-related motifs (Vasios *et al.*, 1989, 1991) but the distinguishing features responsible for the late response have not been determined. The gene encoding collagen type IV is a straightforward secondary response gene.

Gene encoding a gluconeogenesis enzyme

Phosphoenolpyruvate carboxykinase (PEPCK) catalyses a rate-controlling step (oxaloacetate to phosphoenolpyruvate) in gluconeogenesis. The *PEPCK* gene contains two RAREs; RARE1 is a DR1 and RARE2 is a DR5 type of element (Scott *et al.*, 1996). RARE1 is a binding site for TRs as well as for RARs. This allows thyroid hormone to regulate *PEPCK* gene transcrip-

tion through RARE1 in the following manner (Fig. 7.18). During hyperthyroidism, intracellular levels of retinoic acid may be elevated owing to a stimulatory effect of thyroid hormone on activities of liver enzymes responsible for retinoic acid synthesis (Kishore *et al.*, 1971). The elevated retinoic acid levels lead to direct enhancement of *PEPCK* gene transcription. Expression of TRs is reduced during hyperthyroidism owing to negative feedback regulation of TR synthesis by thyroid hormone, thus there is little antagonism of the RAR-mediated effect. In contrast, during hypothyroidism, TR levels are increased, leading to the binding of nonfunctional TR–RAR heterodimers to the RARE1. This form of repression is not acutely relieved by re-administration of thyroid hormone to

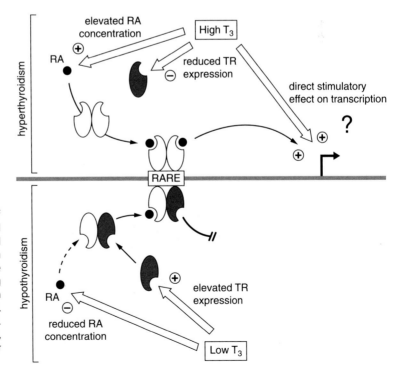

Fig. 7.18 Model for *in vivo* regulation of hepatic PEPCK gene transcription by thyroid hormone. The PEPCK gene promoter is depicted with the known RARE1. Hormonal regulation during hyperthyroidism is depicted above the promoter diagram, and events occurring during hypothyroidism are shown below. RARs, open ovals; TRs, darkened ovals. For details, see text. Reproduced, with permission, from Lucas *et al.* (1991), *Molecular and Cellular Biology*, Vol. 11, pp. 5164–70, © 1991, American Society for Microbiology.

a hypothyroid animal because the ligand-bound TR is still capable of repressing RAR activation of *PEPCK* gene transcription through RARE1.

The dependence of PEPCK on adequate vitamin A status explains the well-documented connection between vitamin A deficiency and hepatic glycogen depletion caused by reduced glucogenesis.

7.7.7   RXR – the master controller of transcription

General features of dimerization
RXR can mediate two distinct retinoid signalling pathways activated by all-*trans* or 9-*cis* retinoic acid through RAR–RXR heterodimer or RXR–RXR homodimer formation. In addition to partnering RARs, the RXRs are obligate heterodimeric partners to several other members of the type II nuclear receptor family, including TR, VDR and PPAR. Heterodimerization of RXR with TR or RAR leads to enhanced DNA binding *in vitro*, altered DNA recognition patterns, and increased transcriptional activity *in vivo* (Marks *et al.*, 1992). Het-

erodimerization provides one way of diversifying the transcriptional response to hormonal signalling in the face of constantly changing physiological events.

RXR-dependent heterodimers can be divided into two categories, permissive and non-permissive, depending on whether or not RXR is able to bind its ligand and activate transcription. In the case of non-permissive heterodimers, such as RAR–RXR and TR–RXR, the ability of RXR to bind ligand is prevented because of an allosteric alteration of the ligand-binding pocket by interaction with the partner. In such instances, RAR or TR is said to be the active partner and RXR the silent partner; that is, the heterodimer can activate gene expression in response to RAR- or TR-specific ligands, but not in response to RXR-specific ligands. Permissive heterodimers are those in which the partner to RXR has no known hormonal ligand, allowing RXR to be activated by 9-*cis* retinoic acid.

The 5′ → 3′ polarity of binding of an RXR-dependent heterodimer to DNA is a critical determinant for ligand-induced activation. Figure 7.19 shows how N-CoR functions as a polarity-specific co-repressor. In

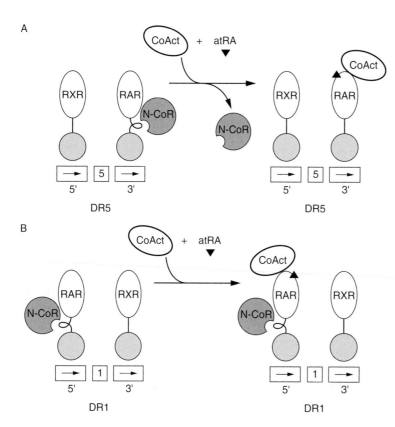

Fig 7.19 Effects of reversing the polarity of RAR-RXR heterodimer binding to DNA. (A) On a DR5 response element, RAR binds to the 3′ half-site. Ligand binding to RAR induces both the dissociation of co-repressor (N-CoR) and recruitment of coactivators (CoAct), resulting in transcriptional activation. (B) On a DR1 response element, RAR binds to the 5′ half-site and remains associated with N-CoR in the presence or absence of ligand. Even in the presence of coactivators, transcription is suppressed on DR1 elements, implying that co-repressors are dominant over coactivators. Reprinted with permission from Perlmann & Vennström (1995), The sound of silence. *Nature*, Vol. 377, pp. 387–8, copyright 1995, Macmillan Magazines Limited.

the case of RAR–RXR heterodimers on DR5 RAREs, the silent partner (RXR) occupies the 5′-upstream half-site and the active partner (RAR) occupies the 3′-downstream half-site. In this case, the heterodimer can be activated by the binding of either all-*trans* or 9-*cis* retinoic acid to RAR. Unlike the heterogeneity of the RAREs, the RXREs are almost exclusively of the DR1 type. The RAR–RXR heterodimer can also bind to the DR1 element, but the polarity is reversed as compared with that on a DR5 element. On DR1 elements, N-CoR remains associated with RAR–RXR heterodimers, even in the presence of RAR ligands, resulting in constitutive repression. These observations show that hormone response elements can allosterically regulate RAR–co-repressor interactions to determine positive or negative regulation of gene transcription (Kurokawa *et al.*, 1995).

The dimerization properties of RXR and RAR on DR1 response elements are complicated by the fact that the controlling ligands are metabolically related. Thus, while 9-*cis* retinoic acid induces the formation of and activates the RXR homodimer, it is formed by the isomerization of all-*trans* retinoic acid, which only activates the RAR subunit of the RAR–RXR heterodimer. The level of complexity is increased by the ability of the RAR–RXR heterodimer to repress RXR homodimer formation (Fig. 7.20). It would appear therefore that the ratio of RXR to RAR in a cell must be very high if the RXR–RXR signalling pathway is to take preference over the RAR–RXR pathway. Hormonal signalling through RXR has been demonstrated *in vitro* under conditions in which RXR is artificially over-expressed. *In vivo* evidence of RXR-mediated signalling under natural conditions was provided by Davis *et al.* (1994). Using a synthetic retinoid known to be selective for RXR homodimers, these authors showed that endogenous RXRs can function independently as a ligand-activated receptor in GH3 pituitary gland cells, activating transcription of the rat growth hormone gene.

The fact that RXR is a common dimeric partner for many receptors suggests that various receptors compete with each other for heterodimerization with limited amounts of RXR. *In vitro* studies (Barettino *et al.*, 1993) showed that unliganded TR efficiently competes with RAR for RXR and is able to dissociate a high-affinity RAR–RXR–RARE complex. In addition, RXR homodimers, formed in the presence of 9-*cis* retinoic acid, compete with heterodimers for RXR

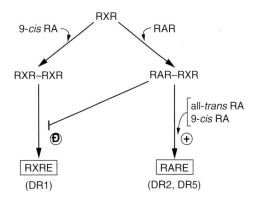

Fig. 7.20 Regulation of two retinoid signalling pathways by RXR. At high intracellular concentrations, 9-*cis* retinoic acid stabilizes the RXR homodimer on DR1 RXREs, thus favouring the transcriptional activation of RXRE target genes. Under conditions of low 9-*cis* retinoic acid and/or high RAR concentrations, the RAR–RXR heterodimer is stabilized. As a heterodimer, RXR functions as a silent partner to RAR in mediating all-*trans*- and 9-*cis* retinoic acid responses through DR5 and DR2 RAREs. Since the RAR–RXR heterodimer has a higher affinity for DNA than does the RXR homodimer, the heterodimer out-competes the homodimer for binding to RXREs, and forms a transcriptionally inactive complex on the DR1 element.

molecules. Lehmann *et al.* (1993) observed that the thyroid hormone response of several TRE-containing genes was strongly repressed by 9-*cis* retinoic acid. Evidently, 9-*cis* retinoic acid shunted the RXR molecules from TR–RXR heterodimers into RXR homodimers, thereby depleting TR–RXR required to mediate the thyroid hormone response. Conversely, RXR homodimerization could be inhibited by an excess of TR, leading to a reduced RXR–RXR-mediated gene activation. Thus the relative concentrations of RXR and TR and the dimerization status of RXR determine the magnitude of the hormone response. The vitamin D$_3$ response of the *osteocalcin* gene was also repressed by 9-*cis* retinoic acid in a similar manner (MacDonald *et al.*, 1993). Therefore there may exist a form of transcriptional repression, known as ligand-induced squelching, which controls the availability of RXR molecules for dimerization with other receptors. It should be noted that these observations are the results of gene transfer experiments and it is not known whether such interactions take place *in vivo*.

Heterodimerization between TR and RXR allows differential thyroid hormone sensitivity of thyroid hormone-responsive genes within a cell. Genes with a complex TRE composed of both direct and inverted repeat half-sites (e.g. the rat growth hormone gene) are activated synergistically by thyroid hormone and 9-*cis* retinoic acid. In contrast, when the TRE consists only of direct repeat half-sites, unliganded RXR enhances thyroid hormone responsiveness but 9-*cis* retinoic acid induces no additional activation (Rosen *et al.*, 1992). Thus, genes with appropriate TREs will show amplification of the thyroid hormone response by 9-*cis* retinoic acid in the presence of RXRs; other thyroid hormone-responsive genes will be influenced by RXRs, but not by 9-*cis* retinoic acid. The ability of 9-*cis* retinoic acid to synergize with thyroid hormone on certain response elements is likely to reflect a heterodimer conformation that is optimized for interaction with other transcription factors.

Lu *et al.* (1993) provided evidence that RAR–RXR and TR–RXR heterodimer and RXR–RXR homodimer complexes induce directed DNA bending when bound to their cognate response elements. The overall bending orientation for RXR-containing complexes is directed toward the major groove of the DNA helix at the centre of hormone response elements.

Heterodimerization between RXR and orphan receptors

A large number of orphan receptors dimerize with RXR and allow ligand binding to RXR, thereby switching RXR from a silent to an active heterodimerization partner. The ability of orphan receptors to allow RXR to bind and be activated by ligand (9-*cis* retinoic acid) increases the diversity of 9-*cis* retinoic acid signalling through RXR. The many different orphan receptors confer DNA-specific binding of the heterodimer to a variety of response elements, including DR1, DR4 and DR5 types.

COUP-TF–RXR

The COUP-TFs inhibit retinoid hormone-mediated transcription on several response elements that are activated by RAR–RXR heterodimers or RXR homodimers (Tran *et al.*, 1992). Possible mechanisms of this repressive effect are discussed in Section 6.8.7. DR1 response elements have been the most extensively studied. COUP-TFs are expressed only in selected tissues or cell types, such as liver and enterocytes. In the developing embryo, they are expressed in a spatially and temporally regulated manner. Furthermore, COUP-TFs antagonize only certain subsets of retinoid receptors; for instance, they do not repress RARβ2-mediated transcription (Tran *et al.*, 1992).

Overall, the ability of COUP-TFs to block transcription from certain RAREs and RXREs provides an important mechanism of restricting the broad spectrum of responses to retinoid hormones.

A member of the apolipoprotein (apo) gene family, *apoAI*, is an example of a gene containing a DR1 RXRE. The encoded protein, apoAI, is the major protein constituent of plasma HDL (high-density lipoprotein), which is involved in the transport of cholesterol and other lipids in the plasma. Widom *et al.* (1992) studied the effects of ARP-1 (apoAI regulatory protein, a homologue of COUP-TFII) on the responsiveness of the *apoAI* gene in human liver cells to RXRα and its ligand 9-*cis* retinoic acid. ARP-1 and RXRα were found to bind individually to the RXRE with similar affinity. These receptors also bound to the same site as heterodimers with an affinity approximately 10 times greater than that of either ARP-1 or RXRα alone. Repression of gene transcription by ARP-1 was overcome by over-expression of RXRα in the presence of 9-*cis* retinoic acid. These observations indicate that regulation of *apoAI* gene expression is controlled by the balance of the intracellular levels of ARP-1 and liganded RXRα. High plasma HDL concentrations are believed to protect against premature atherosclerosis. This demonstration that retinoic acid transactivates *apoAI* gene expression raises the possibility that vitamin A plays an important role in atherosclerosis prevention.

Retinoic acid (either all-*trans* or 9-*cis*) induces high levels of inhibitory COUP-TFI and II during differentiation of P19 EC cells (Jonk *et al.*, 1994), thus creating a negative feedback system involved in the down-regulation of retinoic acid-activated genes.

LXR–RXR

The orphan receptor LXR in heterodimeric complex with RXR binds to a specific DR-4-type response element, the LXRE. The complex is activated by the RXR ligand 9-*cis* retinoic acid, there being no observable repression in the absence of ligand. Ligand binding induces a conformational change in the entire heterodimer complex, exposing the AF-2 of LXR, and allowing transcription through interaction with coactivator proteins (Willy & Mangelsdorf, 1997).

OR1–RXR

The orphan receptor OR1 is also known as ubiquitous receptor (UR), RIP15 and NER. Heterodimeric interaction between OR1 and RXRα on a DR4 response element activates transcription in both the absence and presence of 9-*cis* retinoic acid. The activation potential is mainly dependent on the AF-2 of OR1, which is unmasked by a dimerization-induced conformational change (Wiebel & Gustafsson, 1997). The DR4-type response element is shared by the TR–RXR heterodimer and therefore OR1 has the potential to modulate the thyroid hormone signal pathway.

RLD-1–RXR

The particular response element recognized by the RLD-1–RXR heterodimer is a unique DR4, which is also capable of binding RAR–RXR and TR–RXR heterodimers. Retinoids and thyroid hormone can induce transcription through the RLD-1 response element in the presence of RAR–RXR or TR–RXR heterodimers, but only in the absence of TRs or RARs can the RLD-1–RXR heterodimer constitutively mediate transcription. In contrast to OR1, the presence of 9-*cis* retinoic acid inhibits the activity of RLD-1–RXR (Apfel *et al.*, 1994). These observations suggest a highly specific role for RLD-1 within the network of gene regulation by the TR/RAR subfamily.

NGFI-B–RXR

The orphan receptors NGFI-B (also called nur77) and the closely related nurr-1 can initiate transcription on binding both as monomers and heterodimers to DNA. NGFI-B is found in a variety of tissues, including the muscle, brain, heart, ovary and testis, while nurr-1 expression is restricted to the brain. NGFI-B binds as a monomer to a specific response element that contains a single extended half-site, 5′-AAAG-GTCA-3′. The receptor's zinc fingers interact with the consensus half-site (AGGTCA), while an unusual amino acid motif (the A box) interacts with the two A/T base pairs immediately 5′ of the consensus half-site (Wilson *et al.*, 1993). NGFI-B and nurr-1, as monomers, are constitutively active, but in heterodimeric complex with RXR they require 9-*cis* retinoic acid in order to activate transcription (Perlmann & Jansson, 1995). The heterodimers bind selectively to DR-5 response elements, with RXR occupying the 5′ half-site. NGFI-B and nurr-1 are encoded by primary response genes, which are ultimately induced by various growth factors. From a physiological point of view, the heterodimeric interaction of these receptors with RXR

indicates a novel mechanism for convergence between retinoid and growth factor signalling pathways.

MB67–RXR

Another orphan receptor, MB67, which occurs predominantly in liver, can heterodimerize with RXR and activate transcription from DR-5 response elements in the absence of a ligand. Baes *et al.* (1994) demonstrated this constitutive activity in RAREs that control expression of the RARβ2 and alcohol dehydrogenase 3 genes. Activation of the βRARE by the MB67–RXR heterodimer is weaker than that conferred by RAR–RXR heterodimers, possibly because MB67 essentially lacks the A/B domain, which contains amino acid sequences necessary for full transcriptional activation. The lack of dependence upon a retinoid ligand suggests that MB67 acts to stimulate expression of retinoid-responsive genes (i.e. those containing a DR-5 element) when retinoic acid levels are low. In this respect, MB67 activation of the βRARE could contribute to the basal level of expression of RARβ2 mRNA observed in the livers of retinol-deficient rats (Haq *et al.*, 1991).

FXR–RXR

Some nuclear receptors, in heterodimeric association with RXR, are activated by non-hormonal intracellular metabolites, thereby transducing metabolic cues into genomic responses. Although referred to as orphan receptors, the metabolites may possibly act as their ligands. One such receptor, FXR, is activated by farnesol and related metabolites, the transcriptional response being determined by the FXR component of the FXR–RXR complex (Forman *et al.*, 1995). Farnesyl pyrophosphate is a key intermediate in the mevalonate pathway leading to the biosynthesis of cholesterol.

Transcriptional synergy between RXR and PPAR

The peroxisome proliferator-activated receptor (PPAR), of which there are three known subtypes (α, β and γ), regulates expression of genes involved in modulation of lipid homeostasis, including the metabolism of long-chain fatty acids and conversion of cholesterol to bile salts. PPAR functions as a heterodimer with RXR on peroxisome proliferator response elements (PPREs), which are exclusively of the DR1 type. RXR occupies the 3′ half-site of the DR1 element, which is consistent with the idea that replacement of RAR by PPAR over the 5′ half-site switches RXR from a silent heterodimeric partner to a ligand-dependent activator. The PPAR–RXR heterodimer permits dual activation by the RXR ligand (9-*cis* retinoic acid) and PPAR-specific ligands (peroxisome proliferators) in a unique synergistic fashion (Schulman *et al.*, 1998). Peroxisome proliferators increase both the size and number of peroxisomes. The enzyme acyl coenzyme A oxidase is widely used as a marker of peroxisome proliferator action and is the rate-limiting step in peroxisomal fatty acid β-oxidation. Certain polyunsaturated fatty acids are potent activators of PPAR and thereby exert positive feedback regulation of fatty acid β-oxidation. Thus, the PPAR–RXR heterodimer represents a single bifunctional transcription factor that integrates peroxisome proliferator and retinoid signalling pathways. A physiological role for 9-*cis* retinoic acid as a hypolipidaemic agent is therefore evident.

7.7.8 Transcriptional cross-modulation with the AP-1 pathway

Cross-modulation can take place between the retinoid receptors and the AP-1 signalling pathways, allowing one type of transcription factor to regulate the function of the other and increasing the level of complexity. Since, in the main, retinoids induce cell differentiation and AP-1 induces cell proliferation, cross-modulation provides a molecular switch, allowing a finely tuned balance between these cellular activities.

Retinoic acid stimulates the production of several protein components of the extracellular matrix, including collagen, fibronectin and laminin. The extracellular matrix forms a substrate for cell attachment and migration, directs cell form and function, and forms a barrier which must be removed in order for tumour invasion to occur. A controlled rate of turnover of the extracellular matrix (remodelling) must accompany the changes which occur during development and other events such as wound healing. Remodelling requires the action of extracellular proteolytic enzymes such as the family of metalloproteases. This family includes collagenase, which degrades interstitial collagens (types I, II and III) and stromelysin, which, less specifically, degrades fibronectin, collagen types III, IV and V, laminin and proteoglycans. The ability to modulate the activity of

collagenase and stromelysin, in addition to regulating the level of their gene transcription, underlines the importance of these enzymes in controlling the rate of extracellular matrix turnover. Uncontrolled degradation of the extracellular matrix can have severe pathological consequences. In rheumatoid arthritis, for example, the cells (synoviocytes) in the synovial fluid lubricating the joints produce an excess of collagenase and stromelysin which degrade the connective tissue and cause impairment of the joints.

Transcription of the collagenase gene is stimulated independently by interleukin-1 (a cytokine) and the tumour-promoting TPA and inhibited by liganded RAR (Lafyatis *et al.*, 1990). Both positive and negative regulatory effects are mediated by the AP-1 binding site. The inhibitory effect of RAR on AP-1 activity is thought to be responsible for the clinical effects of retinoids as anti-neoplastic, anti-arthritic and immunosuppressive agents. In the case of the stromelysin gene, inhibition can occur in the absence of protein synthesis, indicating a primary transcriptional response (Nicholson *et al.*, 1990). All three subtypes of RAR (α, β and γ) can repress transcriptional induction of the human collagenase gene (Schüle *et al.*, 1991). RXR in the presence of its ligand, 9-*cis* retinoic acid, has also been shown to inhibit AP-1 activation (Salbert *et al.*, 1993). Multiple regions of RAR, including the DNA-binding domain, are required for inhibitory activity and both c-Jun homodimers and c-Jun/c-Fos heterodimers can be repressed. The inhibitory effect of retinoic acid can be removed by treatment of cells with TPA and also by treatment with both c-Jun and c-Fos (Yang-Yen *et al.*, 1991). At least *in vitro*, inhibition of AP-1 activity requires an excess of ligand-activated RAR, whereas removal of inhibition requires an excess of AP-1 protein. This reciprocal effect is due to an interaction between RAR and AP-1 proteins that results in mutual loss of DNA-binding activity. The interaction appears to be weak in that a stable complex between c-Jun and RARβ could not be detected in the absence of a chemical cross-linking agent (Yang-Yen *et al.*, 1991). In spite of the apparently weak interaction, however, endogenous RAR levels appear sufficient to allow inhibition of AP-1 activity. The RARβ2 isoform is particularly strongly up-regulated in many epithelial tissues by retinoic acid and could thus be an important modulator of AP-1 activity in these tissues.

The mechanism of nuclear receptor/AP-1 interaction has not been established, but it does not involve direct DNA contact. Most likely it involves indirect interaction through cell-type specific transcription factors that could stabilize the receptor/AP-1 complex. Based on the demonstration by Kamei *et al.* (1996) that CBP can act as a transcriptional coactivator for nuclear receptors and AP-1, these authors suggested that competition for limiting amounts of CBP could account for the inhibitory action of liganded RAR on AP-1 activation. Another hypothesis proposed by Caelles *et al.* (1997) is that nuclear receptors inhibit the activity of Jun amino-terminal kinase (JNK), thereby interfering with the c-Jun activation step that is required for recruitment of CBP. Zhou *et al.* (1999) proposed a novel mechanism in which liganded retinoid receptors are able to interfere with the homo- and heterodimerization properties of c-Jun and c-Fos and in this way prevent the formation of AP-1 complexes capable of DNA binding. These authors showed that human RARα disrupted *in vivo* c-Jun–c-Fos dimerization in a ligand-dependent manner. Inhibition of dimerization was cell specific, occurring only in those cells that exhibit retinoic acid-induced repression of AP-1 activity. Furthermore, the glucocorticoid receptor did not affect dimerization, suggesting that this mechanism is specific for the retinoid receptors.

As already discussed, the retinoid receptors mediate two distinct types of action: (1) cell differentiation by transcriptional activation through specific response elements on the DNA and (2) anti-proliferative activity by inhibition of AP-1. Because the two types of action are mechanistically distinct, various laboratories have investigated whether novel retinoids can be synthesized that inhibit AP-1 but do not activate transcription. The potential advantage of such 'dissociated' retinoids as receptor ligands is that they could be therapeutically useful in the treatment of hyperproliferative and inflammatory diseases without the side effects resulting from the activation of retinoid-responsive genes. Synthetic retinoids having this dissociation ability have been described (Fanjul *et al.*, 1994; Chen *et al.*, 1995; Nagpal *et al.*, 1995), but they display distinct receptor selectivities and their differential action is limited to only some of the RAR subtypes or isoforms. The aim is to discover retinoids that are completely specific for AP-1 antagonism through all the retinoid receptors.

7.8 Effects of vitamin A on the immune system

7.8.1 Introduction

Vitamin A deficiency is strongly associated with depressed immunity (Smith *et al.*, 1987) and therefore a combination of deficiency and infectious disease is potentially fatal, especially among infants and children. Randomized trials in Sumatran (Tarwotjo *et al.*, 1987) and Indian (Rahmathullah *et al.*, 1990) preschool-age children showed that vitamin A supplementation decreased mortality due to infection by 96% and 54%, respectively.

7.8.2 Lymphocytes

Retinoic acid was shown to stimulate, and retinaldehyde to inhibit, the activity of protein kinase C derived from T cells (Isakov, 1988). This enzyme has a major role in transmembrane signal transduction and therefore its regulation by retinoids could account for the modulatory effects of vitamin A on T-cell function. Retinoic acid induces the expression of the RARα gene in unstimulated cloned mouse T cells and increases proliferation of these cells in the presence of antigen (Friedman *et al.*, 1993). Cytotoxic T cells recognize antigens in association with MHC class I molecules. Retinoic acid mediates the regulation of MHC class I gene expression via a nuclear hormone receptor (Nagata *et al.*, 1992). Expression of the intercellular adhesion molecule-1 (ICAM-1) gene is up-regulated by retinoic acid in a RARβ/RXRα-dependent fashion (Aoudjit *et al.*, 1994, 1995). Retinoic acid can enhance the functional responses of human T lymphocytes via transcriptional up-regulation of IL-2 receptors (Sidell *et al.*, 1993).

Retinol is essential for proliferation of activated human B cells (Buck *et al.*, 1990) and, moreover, is a normal modulator of B-cell function (H. Blomhoff *et al.*, 1992). In a study of the effects of retinoids on B-cell immune function in newborn infants (Ballow *et al.*, 1996), retinoic acid enhanced the synthesis of IgM in antigen-stimulated umbilical cord blood mononuclear cells, whereas in adult peripheral blood mononuclear cells it enhanced the synthesis of IgG. IgM is the first antibody produced during a primary immune response and is 15 times more effective than

IgG in activating the complement cascade. Highly purified T cells pre-incubated with retinoic acid released a factor (probably a cytokine) which acted on cord blood B cells to augment IgM synthesis.

Antibody production in the vitamin A deficiency state

Infantile tetanus arising from infection with *Clostridium tetanii* remains a significant cause of morbidity and mortality in parts of the developing world (Henderson *et al.*, 1988), even though it is preventable by vaccination with tetanus toxoid (TT). Kinoshita *et al.* (1991) reported that vitamin A deficiency in the rat led to a decreased production of TT-specific IgM and IgG antibodies in both the primary and secondary responses. However, levels of total plasma IgG (as opposed to anti-TT IgG) were abnormally elevated. When the rats were repleted with retinol 1 day after primary immunization with tetanus toxoid, anti-TT IgM and IgG concentrations in both the primary and secondary responses reached vitamin A-sufficient control levels. When the deficient rats were repleted 2 days before the booster immunization, the secondary response was normal in terms of antibody concentrations and class switching from anti-TT IgM to IgG. These experiments showed that immunological memory to TT could be established and maintained in the vitamin A-deficient rat. In the early retinol-repleted rats, the increase in anti-TT IgG production during the secondary response persisted for 26 days without any additional retinol in the interim. This strong secondary response was specific for the IgG2a and IgG2b subclasses of IgG and reflected the previous development of subclass-specific memory B cells (Kinoshita & Ross, 1993). These authors showed that vitamin A deficiency most likely impaired the process of B cell differentiation, either from the naive B cell to the antibody-secreting plasma cell during the primary response and/or from the quiescent memory B cell to the plasma cell during the secondary response. The observation that the total plasma IgG of vitamin A-deficient rats is elevated above normal shows that the B cells are at least capable of producing antibodies, albeit not the *specific* antibodies required to deal with a particular antigen. This would explain reports of decreased host defence against certain types of infection in human vitamin A deficiency.

Pasatiempo *et al.* (1990) studied the effects of vitamin A deficiency on the antibody response to T-independent type 1 and type 2 bacterial antigens and to protein T-dependent antigens (see Table 7.9 for summary). The type 2 antigens were capsular polysaccharides from *Streptococcus pneumoniae*, type III and *Neisseria meningitidis*, serotype C. The former causes meningitis and otitis media as well as pneumonia in humans, while the latter causes meningitis. The type 1 antigens were lipopolysaccharides from *Pseudomonas aeruginosa*, an opportunistic pathogen associated with respiratory and ocular infections, and from *Serratia marcescens*. The T-dependent protein antigens were tetanus toxoid and sheep red blood cells. Young growing male rats raised on vitamin A-deficient or sufficient diets were immunized either near 40 days of age, before signs of vitamin A deficiency were apparent, or near 47 days when symptoms of deficiency were beginning to manifest. The results showed that asymptomatic vitamin A-deprived rats, immunized when they were still growing, had a markedly reduced specific antibody response to the bacterial polysaccharides (type 2 antigens) and to T-dependent protein antigens. Symptomatic vitamin A-deprived rats, immunized later, were essentially unable to produce specific antibodies to these antigens. Repletion of vitamin A-deficient rats with retinol near the time of immunization restored antibody production to control quantities. In striking contrast, vitamin A-deprived rats immunized with bacterial lipopolysaccharides (type 1 antigens) produced an antibody response indistinguishable from vitamin A-sufficient animals. In summary, specific antibody production in response to T-independent, type 2 antigens and T-dependent antigens depends on adequate vitamin A status. Antibody responses to type 1 antigens (at least those tested) are not affected by vitamin A status.

Lipopolysaccharide (LPS), a component of the outer surface of Gram-negative bacteria, is a mitogen, which can stimulate B-cell proliferation. Many of the immunogenic actions of LPS are mediated by macrophages through the release of cytokines, principally TNF-α and IL-1β, that in turn stimulate release of additional soluble factors. Arora & Ross (1994) showed that co-immunization with tetanus toxoid and LPS significantly elevated the IgG concentration in the plasma of vitamin A-sufficient and deficient rats as compared with identical rats immunized with tetanus toxoid alone. In a similar set of experiments, Pasatiempo *et al.* (1994) showed that even symptomatic vitamin A-deficient rats were able to mount a strong

Table 7.5 Antibody production in vitamin A-depleted rats after immunization with bacterial or protein antigens.

Bacterium	Antigen		Antibody production in vitamin A-depleted rats
	Composition	Type	
Streptococcus pneumoniae, type III	Polysaccharide (SSS-III)	TI, type 2	Impaired
Neisseria meningitidis, serotype C	Polysaccharide	TI, type 2	Impaired
Pseudomonas aeruginosa, FD-type 1	Lipopolysaccharide	TI, type 1	Normal
Serratia marcescens	Lipopolysaccharide	TI, type 1	Normal
–	Tetanus toxoid (protein)	TD	Impaired
–	Sheep red blood cells (protein)	TD	Impaired

TI, T-independent; TD, T-dependent.

antibody response to SSS-III after co-immunization with SSS-III and LPS. These observations were not unexpected in view of the normal antibody response to LPS (Table 7.5) and its known adjuvant properties (McGhee *et al.*, 1979). Arora & Ross (1994) further showed that the adjuvant effect of LPS is mediated through the release of TNF-α. TNF-α is known to augment the capacity of macrophages to release IL-1 and prostaglandin E_2, among many other effects. These results demonstrate that vitamin A-deficient rats fail to produce specific antibodies to protein antigens and type 2 antigens because TNF-α and probably other soluble factors are missing or non-functional. Stimulation of cytokines by co-immunization with LPS induces specific antibody responses in vitamin A-deficient rats.

Wiedermann *et al.* (1993) studied the *in vivo* and *in vitro* immune responses in vitamin A-deficient rats to parenterally administered antigens. The serum IgG and IgM antibody responses to a T-cell-dependent antigen (β-lactoglobulin) were significantly lower in the deficient rats than in the pair-fed controls, but there were no such differences in the IgG and IgM responses to a type 2, T-cell-independent antigen (Ficoll conjugated to picrylsulphonic acid). This observation indicates that B-cell function is not directly affected by vitamin A deficiency and the decreased antibody response to the T-cell-dependent antigen might be due to cytokine production by T helper cells. However, the biliary IgA and the serum IgE antibodies against both antigens were decreased in the deficient animals. In the *in vitro* experiments, IL-2 and IFN-γ levels in supernatants from mitogen-stimulated lymphocytes from vitamin A-deficient rats were higher than control levels, whereas IL-6 levels were lower. Il-2 and IFN-γ are produced by Th1 cells, while IL-6

is produced by Th2 cells. IgE production is dependent on the presence of IL-4, which is also produced by Th2 cells. These results indicate an up-regulation of Th1 cell function and a down-regulation of Th2 cell function. Despite an increase in T cell proliferation *in vitro*, vitamin A-deficient rats had a lower delayed-type hypersensitivity than the control rats as well as suppressed antibody production.

Smith & Hayes (1987) reported that in vitamin A-deficient mice, the IgG1 and IgG3 responses to a protein antigen (haemocyanin) were impaired earlier and to a greater extent than were IgM responses. The impaired responses were attributable to fewer antibody-secreting cells (plasma cells) rather than to a decreased secretion rate per cell. The reduction in plasma cell number resulted from a defect in the ability of T helper cells to provide stimulatory signals to B cells (Carman *et al.*, 1989). The IgG responses were restored by adding retinyl acetate to the murine diet (Chun *et al.*, 1992). Carman & Hayes (1991) reported that the T cells of vitamin A-deficient mice produced excess interferon-γ (IFN-γ).

Carman *et al.* (1992) investigated the immunological effects of vitamin A deficiency in mice infected with the parasitic helminth *Trichinella spiralis*. They showed that vitamin A deficiency shifts the immune response toward an early Th1-type response and delays the development of a Th2-type response. The normal Th2 response to *T. spiralis* infection is characterized by high levels of parasite-specific IgG antibodies and increased bone marrow synthesis of eosinophils, the cells that specialize in killing extracellular parasites. The inappropriate Th1 response elicits high levels of IFN-γ, low Th2 and IgG-secreting cell frequencies and impaired eosinophil production. Th2 cells secrete IL-5, which induces growth and differentiation of eosinophils;

therefore, by suppressing Th2 cell growth through excess production of IFN-γ, one would expect decreased eosinophil production in vitamin A deficiency. Further investigations (Cantorna et al., 1994, 1995) confirmed that the imbalance between Th1 and Th2 responses in vitamin A deficiency was caused by a distorted pattern of cytokine gene expression, in particular an excessive production of IFN-γ and IL-12. IFN-γ, by antagonizing IL-4, can inhibit proliferation of Th2 cells; it can also inhibit B-cell proliferation, activation and immunoglobulin class switching. IL-12 stimulates the differentiation of Th1 cells. Excessive production of IFN-γ was due to dysregulation of IFN-γ gene expression and excess antigen-presenting capacity for IFN-γ stimulation. Vitamin A repletion decreased the synthesis of IFN-γ and IL-12, limited the antigen presentation capacity to stimulate IFN-γ and increased the Th2 cell frequency, thereby restoring the Th1/Th2 balance to normal. Retinoic acid was 100-fold more active than retinol for restoring IgG responses in vitamin A-deficient cell cultures (Chun et al., 1992). Retinoic acid was shown to inhibit IFN-γ gene transcription through its role as a ligand for nuclear retinoic acid receptor (RAR) (Cantorna et al., 1996).

7.8.3 Natural killer cells

Vitamin A deficiency in rats reduced the absolute number of natural killer (NK) cells in blood and to a lesser extent in spleen. The activity per NK cell was normal in blood and only slightly, but significantly, reduced in the spleen (Zhao et al., 1994). NK cytotoxicity was increased in vitamin A-deficient rats when their production of cytokines was stimulated by polyinosinic acid:cytidylic acid (Ross, 1996). When vitamin A-deficient rats were fed a retinoic acid supplement, the number of NK cells equalled those of control rats and NK cytotoxicity was significantly elevated (Zhao & Ross, 1995). Thus, as for antibody production, adequate vitamin A status is required to ensure the correct pattern of cytokine gene expression.

7.8.4 Neutrophils

The neutrophils of vitamin A-deficient rats showed impaired chemotaxis, lower rate of adhesion to pathogenic organisms, and impaired respiratory burst activity. Neutrophil function was restored to normal 8 days after vitamin A administration (Twining et al., 1997).

7.8.5 Monocytes/macrophages

Retinoic acid increased the proliferation of granulocyte/macrophage precursor cells even in the presence of maximally stimulating concentrations of colony-stimulating factor (Tobler et al., 1986). Retinoids can modulate macrophage function by enhancing phagocytosis and IL-1 production (Dillehay et al., 1988). An increase in transglutaminase activity during macrophage activation is thought to contribute to the enhanced functional capacity of activated macrophages. Moore et al. (1984) reported that physiological concentrations of retinoic acid specifically induced the synthesis of transglutaminase by cultured mouse macrophages. Retinoic acid stimulated the capacity of macrophages to phagocytose and kill the unicellular parasite *Trypanosoma cruzi* (Wirth & Kierszenbaum, 1986). Transglutaminase activity appeared to be involved in the retinoid effect, because inhibition of the enzyme activity cancelled the effect. Retinoic acid at physiological concentrations does not act alone in inducing IL-1β production in human monocytes; rather it strongly enhances phorbol ester-induced IL-1β production at the level of transcription (Matikainen et al., 1991). This effect of phorbol ester is mediated through the activation of its cellular receptor, protein kinase C. Macrophages from normal healthy donors are usually not cytotoxic to tumour cells *in vitro*, but they can be rendered tumoricidal by interaction *in vitro* with bacterial products, lymphokines or vitamin A (retinyl palmitate) (Tachibana et al., 1984). Macrophages from rats or mice receiving very high intakes of retinyl palmitate also exhibit an increased ability to kill tumour cells (Tachibana et al., 1984; Moriguchi et al., 1985).

7.9   Role of vitamin A in bone metabolism and embryonic development

7.9.1   Effects of vitamin A on bone metabolism

The gene expression of the nuclear retinoid receptors (RARα, RARβ, RARγ, RXRα, RXRβ but not RXRγ) and one of the cellular retinoid-binding proteins (CRBP-I) has been demonstrated in adult rat tibia (Harada et al., 1995). Retinoic acid (either all-*trans* or 9-*cis*) increased the mRNA levels of the *RARβ* and *CRBP-I* genes. These observations indicate that, in bone, the actions of vitamin A are exerted through these nuclear receptors by regulating target gene expression, and through CRBP-1 by modulating the intracellular transport of vitamin A.

The regulatory effects of vitamin A on bone metabolism appear somewhat contradictory. Oreffo *et al.* (1988) reported that retinol and all-*trans* retinoic acids stimulate bone resorption through direct effects on osteoclasts. On the other hand, retinoic acid acts as an inducer of osteocalcin (Oliva *et al.*, 1993), matrix Gla protein (Cancela & Price, 1992) and bone morphogenetic proteins (Rogers *et al.*, 1992).

7.9.2   Consequences of retinoid imbalance during embryogenesis

All-*trans* retinoic acid, and also 9-*cis* retinoic acid, 4-*oxo*-all-*trans* retinoic acid and 3,4-didehydro-all-*trans* retinoic acid, are implicated in pattern formation, i.e. the development of the embryo in a spatially organized fashion. In particular, endogenous retinoids play a role in the anterior–posterior development of the central body axis and in limb development. The concentrations of retinoic acid and nuclear retinoid receptors in the developing embryo are highly regulated, both spatially and temporally. Treatment of embryos with exogenous retinoids produces teratogenic effects, while maternal insufficiency of vitamin A during pregnancy results in either fetal death or severe congenital malformations.

After the formation of the primary tissue layers in vertebrate embryogenesis (gastrulation), the anterior–posterior axis is established with the formation of the neural tube. Cranial neural crest cells arising from the developing hindbrain migrate and differentiate to form parts of the face, both jaws, periocular tissues, bones of the ear, the thymus, and the septa of the heart and its major arteries. Many of the malformations resulting from retinoic acid excess occur in tissues whose origins can be traced back to the early development of the neural tube. Malformations may arise through the premature induction of gene transcription by retinoic acid or through death of many neural crest cells by apoptosis. Abnormalities are frequently found in craniofacial structures, the central nervous system, the heart and the thymus.

The developing eye is the most sensitive organ to vitamin A deprivation. The eye may be completely absent; otherwise, the lens is reduced in diameter and the lens cells fail to elongate and form the necessary crystallin fibres. Cardiovascular defects include failure of closure of the interventricular septum in the heart. In the developing central nervous system, vitamin A deficiency leads to incomplete formation of the myelencephalon (part of the posterior hindbrain) and a failure of the neural tube to extend neurites into the periphery. Development of the lungs, diaphragm and urinogenital tract is also impaired. The above effects have been reported in animals. Vitamin A deficiency sufficient to cause morphological abnormalities in human embryonic development is rare, although functional defects, especially of the lungs, are quite common.

Boylan & Gudas (1992) showed that the level of CRABP-I expression influences the metabolism of retinoic acid in the cytoplasm of differentiating embryonic stem cells: the higher the CRABP-I level, the faster the metabolism of retinoic acid to inactive metabolites. Retinoic acid not immediately metabolized presumably moves to the nuclear receptors and initiates the activation of responsive genes, leading to differentiation. The level of CRABP-I expression also influences the sensitivity of the stem cells to the addition of retinoic acid: the higher level of CRABP-I, the greater the concentration of retinoic acid required to initiate differentiation (Boylan & Gudas, 1991). It appears, therefore, that the function of CRABP-I in embryonic stem cells is to regulate the concentration of intracellular retinoic acid. This function is very important in the developing embryo where excessive retinoic acid could lead to teratogenesis.

The distributions of the nuclear retinoid receptors (RARs and RXRs) in the mammalian embryo are shown in Table 7.2. The characteristic spatial and temporal expression of the different receptor subtypes correlates with pattern formation, suggesting that they play a role in morphogenesis and other developmental events (Underhill *et al.*, 1995).

7.9.3   Anterior–posterior development of the central body axis

Pattern formation along the central anterior–posterior axis is determined by the expression patterns of *Hox* genes in the developing embryo. Within the Hox locus of the chromosome, *Hox* genes are arranged in decreasing order of sensitivity to retinoic acid in the 3′ to 5′ direction. Similarly, *Hox* genes at the 3′ ends of the cluster are expressed earlier in embryonic development and in more anterior regions, while *Hox* genes closer to the 5´ ends of the cluster are expressed at later times in development and in posterior regions of the embryo. The order of induction will correspond to the gene expression patterns (anterior to posterior) and will be influenced by the concentration of retinoic acid (Gudas, 1994).

7.9.4 Limb development

Three regions of the developing limb bud have been identified that profoundly influence limb development, namely the zone of polarizing activity (ZPA), the apical ectodermal ridge (AER) and the progress zone. The ZPA regulates the anterior–posterior axis, whereas the AER is required for proper formation of structures along the anterior–posterior axis. The progress zone receives signals from both the ZPA and the AER and translates this information into distinct cell identities (Johnson *et al.*, 1994). Several members of the fibroblast growth factor (FGF) family are expressed in the AER and these may initiate the proliferation of the mesenchyme in normal limb development.

Transplantation of mesenchyme from the ZPA results in mirror-image duplication of the limb along the anterior–posterior axis, a property called polarizing activity. A secreted protein called Sonic hedgehog has been identified as the likely mediator of polarizing activity within the limb bud. The expression of Sonic hedgehog is regulated by *Hoxb-8*, a primary response gene whose expression is induced by retinoic acid (Tabin, 1995). When a bead containing retinoic acid is placed on the anterior of a limb bud, it causes polarizing activity by inducing an ectopic ZPA adjacent to the bead. This effect is due to the retinoic acid-induced expression of *Sonic hedgehog*, which is localized and does not extend around the bead.

7.10 Vitamin A and cancer

7.10.1 Retinoids and apoptosis

Apoptosis is a tightly regulated natural process of cell death, which involves changes in the expression of distinct genes. The physiological role of apoptosis in cancer prevention is to eliminate DNA-damaged cells

that would otherwise replicate and lead to mutations and possibly cancer. Retinoic acid induces apoptosis in many tumour cell types and therefore retinoids have potential use for cancer chemotherapy and prevention. According to Warrell *et al.* (1993), all-*trans* retinoic acid appears to be the most effective single agent for the treatment of any type of acute leukaemia. The relationship between terminal differentiation and apoptosis may conform to one of the following: (1) retinoids first induce differentiation, and then the differentiated cells undergo apoptosis; (2) retinoids induce differentiation and apoptosis concurrently; (3) retinoids induce apoptosis in a process that is independent of differentiation (Lotan, 1995).

7.10.2 Anti-cancer effects

A majority of primary human cancers arise in epithelial tissues that depend upon retinoids for normal cellular differentiation. The inhibition of carcinogenesis by retinoids in various epithelial tissues is well documented. Retinoids suppress malignant transformation of cells in culture irrespective of whether the transformation is induced by ionizing radiation or by chemical carcinogens. Moreover, retinoids are potent inhibitors of phorbol ester-induced tumour promotion. Other studies have demonstrated a relationship between retinoid deficiency and cancer. Unfortunately, chronic pharmacological administration of retinoids is limited by their potential toxicity.

In humans, a significant body of epidemiological evidence correlates the intake of carotenoid-rich fruits and vegetables with protection from some forms of cancer. The potential use of carotenoids for the chemoprevention of cancer in humans would appear to be of great significance as β-carotene is essentially non-toxic. However, data obtained from experimental studies using rats or mice (the well-defined cancer models) cannot be extrapolated to humans on account of the rodent's limited ability to absorb carotenoids as intact molecules and by the rapid metabolism of any absorbed carotenoid.

Studies of carotenoids in cell culture have been hindered in the past by difficulties in supplying the highly lipophilic carotenoids in a bioavailable form. Bertram *et al.* (1991) overcame this problem by the use of tetrahydrofuran as solvent, allowing the delivery of diverse carotenoids to cultured cells at high concentration in a bioavailable, micelle-like form. Using this delivery system and the 10T½ line of transformable mouse fibroblasts, Bertram's group demonstrated that many dietary carotenoids can inhibit neoplastic transformation in the post-initiation phase of carcinogenesis.

7.10.3 Carotenoids as biological antioxidants

The anticarcinogenic effect of carotenoids may be due, at least partly, to their antioxidant activity. This is attributable to two main properties of carotenoids: (1) the ability to trap peroxyl free radicals implicated in lipid peroxidation (Burton & Ingold, 1984) and (2) the ability to deactivate singlet oxygen by physical quenching (Foote & Denny, 1968). The extensive conjugated double bond system of carotenoids is important for both of these properties, but provitamin A activity is irrelevant.

Trapping of peroxyl radicals

β-Carotene acts as a chain-breaking antioxidant in lipid peroxidation by trapping the chain-propagating lipid peroxyl radical, LOO•, in an addition reaction (reaction 7.1). The chain-breaking activity of β-carotene is weak compared with that of α-tocopherol, the major lipid-soluble antioxidant.

$$LOO^{\bullet} + \beta\text{-carotene} \rightarrow LOO\text{-}\beta\text{-carotene}^{\bullet} \qquad (7.1)$$

The carbon-centred β-carotenyl radical thus formed is resonance-stabilized because of the delocalization of the unpaired electron in the conjugated polyene system. The β-carotenyl radical can react with another peroxyl radical, leading to a termination reaction (reaction 7.2).

$$\begin{aligned} LOO\text{-}\beta\text{-carotene}^{\bullet} + LOO^{\bullet} \rightarrow LOO\text{-}\beta\text{-carotene-OOR} \\ (\text{non-radical}) \qquad (7.2) \end{aligned}$$

Alternatively, the β-carotenyl radical can react with molecular oxygen to form a β-carotene–peroxyl radical (reaction 7.3).

$$LOO\text{-}\beta\text{-carotene}^{\bullet} + O_2 \rightleftharpoons LOO\text{-}\beta\text{-carotene-OO}^{\bullet} \qquad (7.3)$$

Reaction 7.3 is reversible and dependent on the partial pressure of oxygen (pO_2) in the system. If pO_2 is sufficiently low, the equilibrium shifts to the left, reducing the amount of β-carotene–peroxyl radical. On the other hand, if pO_2 is high, the equilibrium shifts to the right, increasing the amount of β-carotene–peroxyl radical, which is capable of propagating the lipid peroxidation chain reaction. The physiological pO_2 in most tissues is below 20 torr, but in lung it is much higher – around 160 torr. Kennedy & Liebler (1992) investigated the effect of pO_2 on the ability of β-carotene to inhibit peroxidation in phospholipid liposomes (a model membrane bilayer). They found β-carotene to be an effective antioxidant up to 160 torr oxygen, with no difference in effectiveness between 160 and 15 torr; at 760 torr inhibition of peroxidation markedly declined. These data imply that β-carotene could be as effective an antioxidant in lung as in other tissues. Canthaxanthin and astaxanthin, which possess oxo groups at the 4 and 4′-positions in the β-ionone ring, are purported to be more effective than β-carotene in trapping peroxyl radicals (Terao, 1989). It may be no coincidence that the length of the β-carotene molecule approximates to the width of a typical cell membrane. With an orientation perpendicular to the plane of the membrane, the conjugated double bond system of the carotene molecule could trap radicals at any depth in the membrane.

Quenching of singlet oxygen

Carotenoids deactivate singlet oxygen ($^1O_2$) by physical quenching, which involves the transfer of excitation energy from $^1O_2$ to the carotenoid, forming ground state triplet oxygen ($^3O_2$) and triplet excited carotenoid (reaction 7.4).

$$^1O_2 + \text{carotenoid} \rightarrow {}^3O_2 + {}^3\text{carotenoid} \qquad (7.4)$$

The energy is harmlessly dissipated through rotational and vibrational interactions between the triplet carotenoid and the surrounding medium to regenerate ground state carotenoid (reaction 7.5).

$$^3\text{carotenoid} \rightarrow \text{carotenoid} + \text{thermal energy (heat)} \qquad (7.5)$$

The rate of quenching is a function of the length of the conjugated polyene chain and parallels the protective action of carotenoids (Foote et al., 1970). Lycopene, an open chain carotenoid, is approximately twice as effective as β-carotene in quenching $^1O_2$ (Di Mascio et al., 1989).

Prooxidant actions of carotenoids

The antioxidant activity of carotenoids may shift into pro-oxidant activity, depending on the redox potential of the carotenoid molecules as well as on the biological environment in which they act. If an inappropriate prooxidant activity were to develop in normal cells, the reactive oxygen metabolites generated would lead to damage of cellular lipids, proteins and DNA, and possibly induce neoplastic transformation. In contrast, if carotenoids were to act as prooxidants in already transformed cells, the production of cytotoxic products would be beneficial (Palozza, 1998).

7.10.4 Induction of gap junctional communication

There is increasing evidence that one biochemical mechanism underlying the chemopreventive action of retinoids is enhanced gap junctional communication of growth controlling signals. Hossain *et al.* (1989) showed good correlation between retinoid inhibition of neoplastic transformation and enhanced gap junctional communication in carcinogen-initiated 10T½ cells. Retinoid-enhanced junctional communication is achieved in mouse 10T½ fibroblasts (Rogers *et al.*, 1990) and in human skin (Guo *et al.*, 1992) through the synthesis of the gap junction protein, connexin43, and its mRNA.

Zhang *et al.* (1991) demonstrated excellent correlation between the inhibition of neoplastic transformation of 10T½ cells by carotenoids and their ability to enhance gap junctional communication. The magnitude of induced junctional communication was similar to that induced by retinoids, but required higher concentrations of carotenoids (up to 1000-fold) and longer treatment times (3–4 days vs. 1 day for retinoids). The order of potency was β-

carotene/canthaxanthin (approximately equipotent), lutein, lycopene and α-carotene. The antioxidant activity of the carotenoids was found not to correlate with their ability to inhibit neoplastic transformation or their ability to enhance junctional communication. Furthermore, the antioxidant α-tocopherol exhibited only limited activity in the transformation assay and methyl-bixin was inactive (Table 7.6). These data suggest that the antioxidant properties of carotenoids are not significant in their action as inhibitors of neoplastic transformation of 10T½ cells. Three of the carotenoids tested (canthaxanthin, lutein and lycopene) are reported to be without provitamin A activity in mammals, thus their activity in the 10T½ cells is presumably not attributable to conversion to retinoids. The carotenoids enhanced gap junctional communication by up-regulating *connexin43* gene expression (Zhang *et al.*, 1992). This effect appeared unrelated to their provitamin A or antioxidant properties. Whereas a synthetic retinoid up-regulated expression of the *RARβ* gene at the message level (as expected), canthaxanthin did not produce this effect. These results imply that carotenoids and retinoids function through separate but overlapping pathways.

7.11   Vitamin A deficiency and toxicity

7.11.1   Deficiency

Animals

The first sign of vitamin A deficiency is loss of appetite. In young animals, the decreased food intake

Table 7.6   Relations among various biological properties of carotenoids and α-tocopherol (from Zhang *et al.*, 1991).

Compound	Provitamin A status[a]	Chemopreventive activity in 10T½ cells	Induction of gap junctional communication	Relative inhibition of lipid peroxidation
β-Carotene	++++	++++	++++	++
Canthaxanthin	–	++++	++++	+++
Lutein	–	+	+++	+++
α-Carotene[b]	++	++	+	+
Lycopene	–	+	++	++
Methyl-bixin	–	–	–	+++
α-Tocopherol	NA	+	±[c]	++++

[a]Assessed by a classical method involving growth rate determination of rodents deficient in vitamin A.
[b]α-Carotene is much less stable in cell culture than β-carotene.
[c]Tendency to enhance junctional communication, but does not reach statistical significance.
NA, not applicable.

results in lack of growth. Controlled experiments using laboratory animals have shown that loss of appetite is not due to poor palatability of the vitamin A-deficient diet, nor is it due to impaired taste function (Anzano *et al.*, 1979). Metabolic disturbances caused by vitamin A deficiency may be sufficiently detrimental to the animal that it reduces its food intake in order to minimize these disturbances; however, the neurophysiological control systems are unknown.

When rats are deprived of vitamin A, mucus-secreting epithelia such as found in the trachea, certain parts of the urinogenital tract and the conjunctiva are replaced by a keratin-producing squamous epithelium that is not secretory. This results in a drying-up (xerosis) of the mucous membranes with loss of function and a greater susceptibility to infection. Goblet cells in the intestinal crypts are also reduced in number. Reproductive changes in the male rat include shrinkage of the testes and atrophy of the accessory sex organs. The effects on the seminiferous tubules include degeneration of the germinal epithelium, decrease in tubule size and a halting of spermatogenesis. These histological and reproductive changes can be prevented or corrected by restoring vitamin A to the animal's diet. Female rats deprived of vitamin A fail to maintain pregnancy and may resorb their fetuses. This is more likely to be a direct effect on the fetus than a reduction in placental transport of nutrients (Anon, 1977).

In adult cattle, a mild deficiency of vitamin A is associated with roughened hair and scaly skin. Prolonged deficiency affects the cornea, which becomes dry, soft and cloudy. Bulls continue to produce viable spermatozoa even when blindness through xerophthalmia has developed. Continued vitamin A deprivation leads to degeneration of the seminiferous tubules, with a consequent reduction in semen volume and sperm count, and an increased production of abnormal spermatozoa. The lack of protective mucus in the alimentary and respiratory tracts of cattle leads to scours and pneumonia, resulting often in death. In pigs, compression of the brain, due to improper modelling of bone, gives rise to nervous disorders such as uncoordinated movements and convulsions. Vitamin A-deficient poultry suffer a high mortality rate. Early signs of deficiency include retarded growth, weakness, ruffled plumage and a staggering gait (ataxia). The keratinization of intestinal epithelia leads to parasitic infestations and the impaired production of antibodies reduces the bird's resistance to infections such as coccidiosis. In mature birds suffering from severe vitamin A deficiency, egg production and hatchability are reduced.

Humans

The clinical effects of vitamin A deficiency in adults are usually seen only in people whose diet has been deficient for a long time in both dairy produce and vegetables. An early sign of vitamin A deficiency is night blindness, which is caused by an insufficient amount of visual purple in the retina. In more advanced deficiency, the epithelial cells of the skin and mucous membranes lining the respiratory, gastrointestinal and urinogenital tracts cease to differentiate, and lose their secretory function. The undifferentiated cells are flattened and multiply at an increased rate, so that the cells pile up on one another and the surface becomes keratinized. This condition promotes dry skin and loss of hair sheen. The lack of protective mucus in the affected mucosae leads to an increased susceptibility to infections. Xerophthalmia, a disease which mainly affects very young children, refers to keratinization of the conjunctiva, which later spreads to the cornea causing ulceration. The ultimate condition is keratomalacia which, if not treated, leads to permanent blindness.

7.11.2   Toxicity

An excessive intake of preformed vitamin A produces symptoms of toxicity, either acute or chronic. In either case, toxicity results from the indiscriminate use of pharmaceutical supplements, and not from the consumption of usual diets. The only naturally occurring products that contain sufficient vitamin A to induce toxicity in humans are the livers of animals at the top of long food chains, such as large marine fish and carnivores (e.g. bear and dog).

Acute toxicity results from the ingestion of a single or several closely spaced very large doses of vitamin A, usually more than 100 times the recommended intake. Such doses produce a variety of toxic signs that include vomiting, severe headache, dizziness, blurred vision, muscular incoordination and malaise. These signs are usually transient and disappear within a few days. In acute hypervitaminosis A, the excess retinol circulating in the bloodstream is not subject to the normal regulation of RBP binding, and the unbound retinol disrupts the integrity of the cell membranes.

Chronic toxicity results from the recurrent ingestion over a period of weeks to years of excessive doses of vitamin A that are usually more than 10 times the recommended intake. Toxic signs commonly include headache, bone and joint pain, hair loss, nose bleed, bleeding lips, and cracking and peeling skin. After terminating dosing, most patients recover fully from toxicity. Prolonged dosing may eventually result in cirrhosis of the liver.

The most serious consequences of an excessive intake of vitamin A are its teratogenicity. Fetal resorption, abortion, and malformed fetuses or infants are the most serious teratogenic effects. The acidic retinoids, both synthetic and natural, are more powerful teratogens than are retinol and its esters.

Carotenoids in foods are not known to be toxic, even when ingested in large amounts. Hypercarotenosis, a benign condition characterized by a jaundice-like yellowing of the skin, can result when large amounts of carotene-rich foods (e.g. carrot juice) are ingested regularly.

Further reading

Ross, A. C. (1992) Vitamin A status; relationship to immunity and the antibody response. *Proceedings of the Society for Experimental and Biological Medicine*, **200**, 303–20.
Zhang, X.-K. & Pfahl, M. (1993) Regulation of retinoid and thyroid hormone action through homodimeric and heterodimeric receptors. *Trends in Endocrinology and Metabolism*, **4**, 156–62.

References

Adan, R. A. H., Cox, J. J., Beischlag, T. V. & Burbach, J. P. H. (1993) A composite hormone response element mediates the transactivation of the rat oxytocin gene by different classes of nuclear hormone receptors. *Molecular Endocrinology*, **7**, 47–57.
Ahluwalia, G. S., Kaul, L. & Ahluwalia, B. S. (1980) Evidence of facilitory effect of growth hormone on tissue vitamin A uptake in rats. *Journal of Nutrition*, **110**, 1185–93.
Allenby, G., Bocquel, M.-T., Saunders, M., Kazmer, S., Speck, J., Rosenberger, M., Lovey, A., Kastner, P., Grippo, J. F., Chambon, P. & Levin, A. A. (1993) Retinoic acid receptors and retinoid X receptors: interactions with endogenous retinoic acids. *Proceedings of the National Academy of Sciences of the U.S.A.*, **90**, 30–4.
Ames, S. R. (1969) Factors affecting absorption, transport, and storage of vitamin A. *American Journal of Clinical Nutrition*, **22**, 934–5.
Anon (1977) Vitamin A and retinol-binding protein in fetal growth and development of the rat. *Nutrition Reviews*, **35**, 305–9.
Anzano, M. A., Lamb, A. J. & Olson, J. A. (1979) Growth, appetite, sequence of pathological signs and survival following the induction of rapid, synchronous vitamin A deficiency in the rat. *Journal of Nutrition*, **109**, 1419–31.

Aoudjit, F., Bossé, M., Stratowa, C., Voraberger, G. & Audette, M. (1994) Regulation of intercellular adhesion molecule-1 expression by retinoic acid: analysis of the 5′ regulatory region of the gene. *International Journal of Cancer*, **58**, 543–9.
Aoudjit, F., Brochu, N., Morin, N., Poulin, G., Stratowa, C. & Audette, M. (1995) Heterodimeric retinoic acid receptor-β and retinoid X receptor-α complexes stimulate expression of the intercellular adhesion molecule-1 gene. *Cell Growth and Differentiation*, **6**, 515–21.
Apfel, R., Benbrook, D., Lernhardt, E., Ortiz, M. A., Salbert, G. & Pfahl, M. (1994) A novel orphan receptor specific for a subset of thyroid hormone-responsive elements and its interaction with the retinoid/thyroid hormone receptor subfamily. *Molecular and Cellular Biology*, **14**, 7025–35.
Arora, D. & Ross, A. C. (1994) Antibody response against tetanus toxoid is enhanced by lipopolysaccharide or tumor necrosis factor-alpha in vitamin A-sufficient and deficient rats. *American Journal of Clinical Nutrition*, **59**, 922–8.
Åström, A., Tavakkol, A., Pettersson, U., Cromie, M., Elder, J. T. & Voorhees, J. J. (1991) Molecular cloning of two human cellular retinoic acid-binding proteins (CRABP). Retinoic acid-induced expression of CRABP-II but not CRABP-I in adult human skin *in vivo* and in skin fibroblasts *in vitro*. *Journal of Biological Chemistry*, **266**(26), 17662–6.
Åström, A., Pettersson, U. & Voorhees, J. J. (1992) Structure of the human cellular retinoic acid-binding protein II gene. Early transcriptional regulation by retinoic acid. *Journal of Biological Chemistry*, **267**(35), 25 251–5.
Åström, A., Pettersson, U., Chambon, P. & Voorhees, J. J. (1994) Retinoic acid induction of human cellular retinoic acid-binding protein-II gene transcription is mediated by retinoic acid receptor-retinoid X receptor heterodimers bound to one far upstream retinoic acid-responsive element with 5-base pair spacing. *Journal of Biological Chemistry*, **269**(35), 22 334–9.
Baes, M., Gulick, T., Choi, H.-S., Martinoli, M. G., Simha, D. & Moore, D. D. (1994) A new orphan member of the nuclear hormone receptor superfamily that interacts with a subset of retinoic acid response elements. *Molecular and Cellular Biology*, **14**, 1544–52.
Ballow, M., Wang, W. & Xiang, S. (1996) Modulation of B-cell immunoglobulin synthesis by retinoic acid. *Clinical Immunology and Immunopathology*, **80**, S73–S81.
Barettino, D., Bugge, T. H., Bartunek, P., Vivanco Ruiz, M. d. M., Sonntag-Buck, V., Beug, H., Zenke, M. & Stunnenberg, H. G. (1993) Unliganded T_3R, but not its oncogenic variant, v-erbA, suppresses RAR-dependent transactivation by titrating out RXR. *EMBO Journal*, **12**, 1343–54.
Båvik, C.-O., Eriksson, U., Allen, R. A. & Peterson, P. A. (1991) Identification and partial characterization of a retinal pigment epithelial membrane receptor for plasma retinol-binding protein. *Journal of Biological Chemistry*, **266**(23), 14 978–85.
Båvik, C.-O., Busch, C. & Eriksson, U. (1992) Characterization of a plasma retinol-binding protein membrane receptor expressed in the retinal pigment epithelium. *Journal of Biological Chemistry*, **267**(32), 23 035–42.
Båvik, C.-O., Lévy, F., Hellman, U., Wernstedt, C. & Eriksson, U. (1993) The retinal pigment epithelial membrane receptor for plasma retinol-binding protein. Isolation and cDNA cloning of the 63-kDa protein. *Journal of Biological Chemistry*, **268**(27), 20 540–6.
Bedo, G., Santisteban, P. & Aranda, A. (1989) Retinoic acid regulates growth hormone gene expression. *Nature*, **339**, 231–4.
Bertram, J. S., Pung, A., Churley, M., Kappock, T. J., IV, Wilkins, L. R. & Cooney, R. V. (1991) Diverse carotenoids protect against chemically induced neoplastic transformation. *Carcinogenesis*, **12**, 671–8.

Bex, V., Mercier, T., Chaumontet, C., Gaillard-Sanchez, I., Flechon, B., Mazet, F., Traub, O. & Martel, P. (1995) Retinoic acid enhances connexin43 expression at the post-transcriptional level in rat liver epithelial cells. *Cell Biochemistry and Function*, **13**, 69–77.

Bhat, P. V. & Lacroix, A. (1991) Effects of retinoic acid on the concentrations of radioactive metabolites of retinol in tissues of rats maintained on a retinol-deficient diet. *Canadian Journal of Physiology and Pharmacology*, **69**, 826–30.

Blaner, W. S., Das, K., Mertz, J. R., Das, S. R. & Goodman, D. S. (1986) Effects of dietary retinoic acid on cellular retinol- and retinoic acid-binding protein levels in various rat tissues. *Journal of Lipid Research*, **27**, 1084–8.

Blomhoff, H. K., Smeland, E. B., Erikstein, B., Rasmussen, A. M., Skrede, B., Skjønsberg, C. & Blomhoff, R. (1992) Vitamin A is a key regulator for cell growth, cytokine production, and differentiation in normal B cells. *Journal of Biological Chemistry*, **267**(33), 23 988–92.

Blomhoff, R., Green, M. H. & Norum, K. R. (1992) Vitamin A: physiological and biochemical processing. *Annual Review of Nutrition*, **12**, 37–57.

Blomstrand, R. & Werner, B. (1967) Studies on the intestinal absorption of radioactive β-carotene and vitamin A in man. *Scandinavian Journal of Clinical and Laboratory Investigation*, **19**, 339–45.

Boerman, M. H. E. M. & Napoli, J. L. (1991) Cholate-independent retinyl ester hydrolysis. Stimulation by apo-cellular retinol-binding protein. *Journal of Biological Chemistry*, **266**(33), 22 273–8.

Boerman, M. H. E. M. & Napoli, J. L. (1996) Cellular retinol-binding protein-supported retinoic acid synthesis. Relative roles of microsomes and cytosol. *Journal of Biological Chemistry*, **271**(10), 5610–16.

Borek, C., Smith, J. E., Soprano, D. R. & Goodman, D. S. (1981) Regulation of retinol-binding protein metabolism by glucocorticoid hormones in cultured H_4IIEC$_3$ liver cells. *Endocrinology*, **109**, 386–91.

Boylan, J. F. & Gudas, L. J. (1991) Overexpression of the cellular retinoic acid binding protein-I (CRABP-I) results in a reduction in differentiation-specific gene expression in F9 teratocarcinoma cells. *Journal of Cell Biology*, **112**, 965–79.

Boylan, J. F. & Gudas, L. J. (1992) The level of CRABP-I expression influences the amounts and types of all-*trans* retinoic acid metabolites in F9 teratocarcinoma stem cells. *Journal of Biological Chemistry*, **267**(30), 21 486–91.

Brent, G. A., Dunn, M. K., Harney, J. W., Gulik, T., Larsen, P. R. & Moore, D. D. (1989) Thyroid hormone aporeceptor represses T3-inducible promoters and blocks activity of the retinoic acid receptor. *New Biologist*, **1**, 329–36.

Brown, E. D., Micozzi, M. S., Craft, N. E., Bieri, J. G., Beecher, G., Edwards, B. K., Rose, A., Taylor, P. R. & Smith, J. C. Jr. (1989) Plasma carotenoids in normal men after a single ingestion of vegetables or purified β-carotene. *American Journal of Clinical Nutrition*, **49**, 1258–65.

Buck, J., Ritter, G., Dannecker, L., Katta, V., Cohen, S. L., Chait, B. T. & Hämmerling, U. (1990) Retinol is essential for growth of activated human B cells. *Journal of Experimental Medicine*, **171**, 1613–24.

Burton, G. W. & Ingold, K. U. (1984) β-Carotene: an unusual type of lipid antioxidant. *Science*, **224**, 569–73.

Caelles, C., González-Sancho, J. M. & Munoz, A. (1997) Nuclear hormone receptor antagonism with AP-1 by inhibition of the JNK pathway. *Genes & Development*, **11**, 3351–64.

Cancela, M. L. & Price, P. A. (1992) Retinoic acid induces matrix Gla protein gene expression in human cells. *Endocrinology*, **130**, 102–8.

Cantorna, M. T., Nashold, F. E. & Hayes, C. E. (1994) In vitamin A deficiency multiple mechanisms establish a regulatory T helper cell imbalance with excess Th1 and insufficient Th2 function. *Journal of Immunology*, **152**, 1515–22.

Cantorna, M. T., Nashold, F. E. & Hayes, C. E. (1995) Vitamin A deficiency results in a priming environment conducive for Th1 cell development. *European Journal of Immunology*, **25**, 1673–9.

Cantorna, M. T., Nashold, F. E., Chun, T. Y. & Hayes, C. E. (1996) Vitamin A down-regulation of IFN-γ synthesis in cloned mouse Th1 lymphocytes depends on the CD28 costimulatory pathway. *Journal of Immunology*, **156**, 2674–9.

Carman, J. A. & Hayes, C. E. (1991) Abnormal regulation of IFN-γ secretion in vitamin A deficiency. *Journal of Immunology*, **147**, 1247–52.

Carman, J. A., Smith, S. M. & Hayes, C. E. (1989) Characterization of a helper T lymphocyte defect in vitamin A-deficient mice. *Journal of Immunology*, **142**, 388–93.

Carman, J. A., Pond, L., Nashold, F., Wassom, D. L. & Hayes, C. E. (1992) Immunity to *Trichinella spiralis* infection in vitamin A-deficient mice. *Journal of Experimental Medicine*, **175**, 111–20.

Chambon, P. (1996) A decade of molecular biology of retinoic acid receptors. *FASEB Journal*, **10**, 940–54.

Chen, C.-C. & Heller, J. (1977) Uptake of retinol and retinoic acid from serum retinol-binding protein by retinal pigment epithelial cells. *Journal of Biological Chemistry*, **252**(15), 5216–21.

Chen, J.-Y., Penco, S., Ostrowski, J., Balaguer, P., Pons, M., Starrett, J. E., Reczek, P., Chambon, P. & Gronemeyer, H. (1995) RAR-specific agonist/antagonists which dissociate transactivation and AP1 transrepression inhibit anchorage-independent cell proliferation. *EMBO Journal*, **14**, 1187–97.

Chiocca, E. A., Davies, P. J. A. & Stein, J. P. (1988) The molecular basis of retinoic acid action. Transcriptional regulation of tissue transglutaminase gene expression in macrophages. *Journal of Biological Chemistry*, **263**(23), 11 584–9.

Chun, T. Y., Carman, J. A. & Hayes, C. E. (1992) Retinoid repletion of vitamin A-deficient mice restores IgG responses. *Journal of Nutrition*, **122**, 1062–9.

Davis, K. D. & Lazar, M. A. (1993) Induction of retinoic acid receptor-β by retinoic acid is cell specific. *Endocrinology*, **132**, 1469–74.

Davis, K. D., Berrodin, T. J., Stelmach, J. E., Winkler, J. D. & Lazar, M. A. (1994) Endogenous retinoid X receptors can function as hormone receptors in pituitary cells. *Molecular and Cellular Biology*, **14**, 7105–10.

de Thé, H., Marchio, A., Tiollais, P. & Dejean, A. (1989) Differential expression and ligand regulation of the retinoic acid receptor α and β genes. *EMBO Journal*, **8**, 429–33.

de Thé, H., Vivanco-Ruiz, M. d. M., Tiollais, P., Stunnenberg, H. & Dejean, A. (1990) Identification of a retinoic acid responsive element in the retinoic acid receptor β gene. *Nature*, **343**, 177–80.

Dew, S. E. & Ong, D. E. (1994) Specificity of the retinol transporter of the rat small intestine brush border. *Biochemistry*, **33**, 12 340–5.

Dillehay, D. L., Walia, A. S. & Lamon, E. W. (1988) Effects of retinoids on macrophage function and IL-1 activity. *Journal of Leukocyte Biology*, **44**, 353–60.

Di Mascio, P., Kaiser, S,. & Sies, H. (1989) Lycopene as the most efficient biological carotenoid singlet oxygen quencher. *Archives of Biochemistry and Biophysics*, **274**, 532–8.

Dollé, P., Ruberte, E., Kastner, P., Petkovich, M., Stoner, C. M., Gudas, L. J. & Chambon, P. (1989) Differential expression of genes encoding α, β, and γ retinoic acid receptors and CRABP in the developing limbs of the mouse. *Nature*, **342**, 702–5.

Dorea, J. G. & Olson, J. A. (1986) The rate of rhodopsin regeneration in the bleached eyes of zinc-deficient rats in the dark. *Journal of Nutrition*, **116**, 121–7.

Duester, G., Shean, M. L., McBride, M. S. & Stewart, M. J. (1991) Retinoic acid response element in the human alcohol dehydrogenase gene *ADH3*: implications for regulation of retinoic acid synthesis. *Molecular and Cellular Biology*, **11**, 1638–46.

Durand, B., Saunders, M., Leroy, P., Leid, M. & Chambon, P. (1992) All-trans and 9-*cis* retinoic acid induction of CRABPII transcription is mediated by RAR–RXR heterodimers bound to DR1 and DR2 repeated motifs. *Cell*, **71**, 73–85.

Edwards, M. K. S. & McBurney, M. W. (1983) The concentration of retinoic acid determines the differentiated cell types formed by a teratocarcinoma cell line. *Developmental Biology*, **98**, 187–91.

Erdman, J. W. Jr., Bierer, T. L. & Gugger, E. T. (1993) Absorption and transport of carotenoids. *Annals of the New York Academy of Sciences*, **691**, 76–85.

Evans, M. J. & Kaufman, M. H. (1981) Establishment in culture of pluripotent cells from mouse embryos. *Nature*, **292**, 154–6.

Fanjul, A., Dawson, M. I., Hobbs, P. D., Jong, L., Cameron, J. F., Harlev, E., Graupner, G., Lu, X.-P. & Pfahl, M. (1994) A new class of retinoids with selective inhibition of AP-1 inhibits proliferation. *Nature*, **372**, 107–11.

Felli, M. P., Vacca, A., Meco, D., Screpanti, I., Farina, A. R., Maroder, M., Martinotti, S., Petrangeli, E., Frati, L. & Gulino, A. (1991) Retinoic acid-induced down-regulation of the interleukin-2 promoter via *cis*-regulatory sequences containing an octamer motif. *Molecular and Cellular Biology*, **11**, 4771–8.

Fidge, N. H. & Goodman, D. S. (1968) The enzymatic reduction of retinal to retinol in rat intestine. *Journal of Biological Chemistry*, **243**(16), 4372–9.

Fisher, G. J., Reddy, A. P., Datta, S. C., Kang, S., Yi, J. Y. & Chambon, P. (1995) All-*trans* retinoic acid induces cellular retinol-binding protein in human skin *in vivo*. *Journal of Investigative Dermatology*, **105**, 80–6.

Folman, Y., Russell, R. M., Tang, G. W. & Wolf, G. (1989) Rabbits fed on β-carotene have higher serum levels of all-*trans* retinoic acid than those receiving no β-carotene. *British Journal of Nutrition*, **62**, 195–201.

Foote, C. S. & Denny, R. W. (1968) Chemistry of singlet oxygen. VII. Quenching by β-carotene. *Journal of the American Chemical Society*, **90**, 6233–5.

Foote, C. S., Chang, Y. C. & Denny, R. W. (1970) Chemistry of singlet oxygen. X. Carotenoid quenching parallels biological protection. *Journal of the American Chemical Society*, **92**, 5216–18.

Forman, B. M., Goode, E., Chen, J., Oro, A. E., Bradley, D. J., Perlmann, T., Noonan, D. J., Burka, L. T., McMorris, T., Lamph, W. W., Evans, R. M. & Weinberger, C. (1995) Identification of a nuclear receptor that is activated by farnesol metabolites. *Cell*, **81**, 687–93.

Friedman, A., Halevy, O., Schrift, M., Arazi, Y. & Sklan, D. (1993) Retinoic acid promotes proliferation and induces expression of retinoic acid receptor-α gene in murine T lymphocytes. *Cellular Immunology*, **152**, 240–8.

Gerlach, T. H. & Zile, M. H. (1990) Upregulation of serum retinol in experimental acute renal failure. *FASEB Journal*, **4**, 2511–17.

Gerlach, T. H. & Zile, M. H. (1991a) Metabolism and secretion of retinol transport complex in acute renal failure. *Journal of Lipid Research*, **32**, 515–20.

Gerlach, T. H. & Zile, M. H. (1991b) Effect of retinoic acid and apo-RBP on serum retinol concentration in acute renal failure. *FASEB Journal*, **5**, 86–92.

Gianni, M., Studer, M., Carpani, G., Terao, M. & Garattini, E. (1991) Retinoic acid induces liver/bone/kidney-type alkaline phosphatase gene expression in F9 teratocarcinoma cells. *Biochemical Journal*, **274**, 673–8.

Gjøen, T., Bjerkelund, T., Blomhoff, H. K., Norum, K. R., Berg, T. & Blomhoff, R. (1987) Liver takes up retinol-binding protein from plasma. *Journal of Biological Chemistry*, **262**(23), 10 926–30.

Glover, J. (1960) The conversion of β-carotene into vitamin A. *Vitamins and Hormones*, **18**, 371–86.

Graupner, G., Wills, K. N., Tzukerman, M., Zhang, X.-K. & Pfahl, M. (1989) Dual regulatory role for thyroid-hormone receptors allows control of retinoic-acid receptor activity. *Nature*, **340**, 653–6.

Green, M. H. & Green, J. B. (1994) Vitamin A intake and status influence retinol balance, utilization and dynamics in rats. *Journal of Nutrition*, **124**, 2477–85.

Green, M. H., Green, J. B. & Lewis, K. C. (1987) Variation in retinol utilization rate with vitamin A status in the rat. *Journal of Nutrition*, **117**, 694–703.

Green, M. H., Green, J. B., Berg, T., Norum, K. R. & Blomhoff, R. (1993) Vitamin A metabolism in rat liver: a kinetic model. *American Journal of Physiology*, **264**, G509–21.

Gudas, L. J. (1994) Retinoids and vertebrate development. *Journal of Biological Chemistry*, **269**(22), 15 399–402.

Gudas, L. J., Grippo, J. F., Kim, K.-W., LaRosa, G. J. & Stoner, C. M. (1990) The regulation of the expression of genes encoding basement membrane proteins during the retinoic acid-associated differentiation of murine teratocarcinoma cells. *Annals of the New York Academy of Sciences*, **580**, 245–51.

Guo, H., Acevedo, P., Parsa, F. D. & Bertram, J. S. (1992) Gap-junctional protein connexin 43 is expressed in dermis and epidermis of human skin: differential modulation by retinoids. *Journal of Investigative Dermatology*, **99**, 460–7.

Haq, R. & Chytil, F. (1988) Retinoic acid rapidly induces lung cellular retinol-binding protein mRNA levels in retinol deficient rats. *Biochemical and Biophysical Research Communications*, **156**, 712–16.

Haq, R., Pfahl, M. & Chytil, F. (1991) Retinoic acid affects the expression of nuclear retinoic acid receptors in tissues of retinol-deficient rats. *Proceedings of the National Academy of Sciences of the U.S.A.*, **88**, 8272–6.

Harada, H., Miki, R., Masushige, S. & Kato, S. (1995) Gene expression of retinoic acid receptors, retinoid-X receptors, and cellular retinol-binding protein I in bone and its regulation by vitamin A. *Endocrinology*, **136**, 5329–35.

Hassig, C. A. & Schreiber, S. L. (1997) Nuclear histone acetylases and deacetylases and transcriptional regulation: HATs off to HDACs. *Current Opinion in Chemical Biology*, **1**, 300–8.

Heller, J. (1975) Interactions of plasma retinol-binding protein with its receptor. Specific binding of bovine and human retinol-binding protein to pigment epithelium cells from bovine eyes. *Journal of Biological Chemistry*, **250**(10), 3613–19.

Henderson, R. H., Keja, J., Hayden, G., Galazka, A., Clements, J. & Chan, C. (1988) Immunizing the children of the world: progress and prospects. *Bulletin of the World Health Organization*, **66**, 535–43.

Herr, F. M. & Ong, D. E. (1992) Differential interaction of lecithin-retinol acyltransferase with cellular retinol binding proteins. *Biochemistry*, **31**, 6748–55.

Hoffmann, B., Lehmann, J. M., Zhang, X.-K., Hermann, T., Husmann, M., Graupner, G. & Pfahl, M. (1990) A retinoic acid receptor-specific element controls the retinoic acid receptor-β promoter. *Molecular Endocrinology*, **4**, 1727–36.

Hogan, B. L. M., Taylor, A. & Adamson, E. (1981) Cell interactions modulate embryonal carcinoma cell differentiation into parietal or visceral endoderm. *Nature*, **291**, 235–7.

Hossain, M. Z., Wilkens, L. R., Mehta, P. P., Loewenstein, W. & Bertram, J. S. (1989) Enhancement of gap junctional communication by retinoids correlates with their ability to inhibit neoplastic transformation. *Carcinogenesis*, **10**, 1743–8.

Huang, H. S. & Goodman, D. S. (1965) Vitamin A and carotenoids. 1. Intestinal absorption and metabolism of ¹⁴C-labeled vitamin A alcohol and β-carotene in the rat. *Journal of Biological Chemistry*, **240**(7), 2839–44.

Huber, A. M. & Gershoff, S. N. (1975) Effects of zinc deficiency on the oxidation of retinol and ethanol in rats. *Journal of Nutrition*, **105**, 1486–90.

Husmann, M., Lehmann, J., Hoffmann, B., Hermann, T., Tzukerman, M. & Pfahl, M. (1991) Antagonism between retinoic acid receptors. *Molecular and Cellular Biology*, **11**, 4097–103.

Husmann, M., Hoffmann, B., Stump, D. G., Chytil, F. & Pfahl, M. (1992) A retinoic acid response element from the rat CRBPI promoter is activated by an RAR/RXR heterodimer. *Biochemical and Biophysical Research Communications*, **187**, 1558–64.

Isakov, N. (1988) Regulation of T-cell-derived protein kinase C activity by vitamin A derivatives. *Cellular Immunology*, **115**, 288–98.

Jarrous, N. & Kaempfer, R. (1994) Induction of human interleukin-1 gene expression by retinoic acid and its regulation at processing of precursor transcripts. *Journal of Biological Chemistry*, **269**(37), 23 141–9.

Johnson, E. J. & Russell, R. M. (1992) Distribution of orally administered β-carotene among lipoproteins in healthy men. *American Journal of Clinical Nutrition*, **56**, 128–35.

Johnson, R. L., Riddle, R. D. & Tabin, C. J. (1994) Mechanisms of limb patterning. *Current Opinion in Genetics and Development*, **4**, 535–42.

Jones-Villeneuve, E. M. V., McBurney, M. W., Rogers, K. A. & Kalnins, V. I. (1982) Retinoic acid induces embryonal carcinoma cells to differentiate into neurons and glial cells. *Journal of Cell Biology*, **94**, 253–62.

Jonk, L. J. C., de Jonge, M. E. J., Vervaart, J. M. A., Wissink, S. & Kruijer, W. (1994) Isolation and developmental expression of retinoic-acid-induced genes. *Developmental Biology*, **161**, 604–14.

Kamei, Y., Xu, L., Heinzel, T., Torchia, J., Kurokawa, R., Gloss, B., Lin., S.-C., Heyman, R. A., Rose, D. W., Glass, C. K. & Rosenfeld, M. G. (1996) A CBP integrator complex mediates transcriptional activation and AP-1 inhibition by nuclear receptors. *Cell*, **85**, 403–14.

Kato, M., Blaner, W. S., Mertz, J. R., Das, K., Kato, K. & Goodman, D. S. (1985) Influence of retinoid nutritional status on cellular retinol- and cellular retinoic acid-binding protein concentrations in various rat tissues. *Journal of Biological Chemistry*, **260**(8), 4832–6.

Kato, S., Sasaki, H., Suzawa, M., Masushige, S., Tora, L., Chambon, P. & Gronemeyer, H. (1995) Widely spaced, directly repeated PuGGTCA elements act as promiscuous enhancers for different classes of nuclear receptors. *Molecular and Cellular Biology*, **15**, 5858–67.

Kennedy, T. A. & Liebler, D. C. (1992) Peroxyl radical scavenging by β-carotene in lipid bilayers. Effect of oxygen partial pressure. *Journal of Biological Chemistry*, **267**(7), 4658–63.

Kinoshita, M. & Ross, A. C. (1993) Vitamin A status and immunoglobulin G subclasses in rats immunized with tetanus toxoid. *FASEB Journal*, **7**, 1277–82.

Kinoshita, M., Pasatiempo, A. M. G., Taylor, C. E. & Ross, A. C. (1991) Immunological memory to tetanus toxoid is established and maintained in the vitamin A-depleted rat. *FASEB Journal*, **5**, 2473–81.

Kirfel, J., Kelter, M., Cancela, L. M., Price, P. A. & Schüle, R. (1997) Identification of a novel negative retinoic acid responsive element in the promoter of the human matrix Gla protein gene. *Proceedings of the National Academy of Sciences of the U.S.A.*, **94**, 2227–32.

Kishore, G. S., Perumal, A. S. & Cama, H. R. (1971) The effect of thyroid activity on the enzymes of vitamin A metabolism and on the stability of lysosomes. *International Journal for Vitamin and Nutrition Research*, **41**, 171–9.

Kurokawa, R., Söderström, M., Hörlein, A., Halachmi, S., Brown, M., Rosenfeld, M. G. & Glass, C. K. (1995) Polarity-specific activities of retinoic acid receptors determined by a co-repressor. *Nature*, **377**, 451–4.

Lafyatis, R., Kim, S.-J., Angel, P., Roberts, A. B., Sporn, M. B., Karin, M. & Wilder, R. L. (1990) Interleukin-1 stimulates and all-*trans*-retinoic acid inhibits collagenase gene expression through its 5′ activator protein-1-binding site. *Molecular Endocrinology*, **4**, 973–80.

Langston, A. W. & Gudas, L. J. (1992) Identification of a retinoic acid responsive enhancer 3′ of the murine homeobox gene Hox-1.6. *Mechanisms of Development*, **38**, 217–27.

LaRosa, G. J. & Gudas, L. J. (1988) Early retinoic acid-induced F9 teratocarcinoma stem cell gene *ERA-1*: alternate splicing creates transcripts for a homeobox-containing protein and one lacking the homeobox. *Molecular and Cellular Biology*, **8**, 3906–17.

La Vista-Picard, N., Hobbs, P. D., Pfahl, M., Dawson, M. I. & Pfahl, M. (1996) The receptor-DNA complex determines the retinoid response: a mechanism for the diversification of the ligand signal. *Molecular and Cellular Biology*, **16**, 4137–46.

Lee, M.-O., Liu, Y. & Zhang, X.-K. (1995) A retinoic acid response element that overlaps an estrogen response element mediates multihormonal sensitivity in transcriptional activation of the lactoferrin gene. *Molecular and Cellular Biology*, **15**, 4194–207.

Lee, M. S., Kliewer, S. A., Provencal, J., Wright, P. E. & Evans, R. M. (1993) Structure of the retinoid X receptor α DNA binding domain: a helix required for homodimeric DNA binding. *Science*, **260**, 1117–21.

Lehmann, J. M., Zhang, X.-K., & Pfahl, M. (1992) RARγ2 expression is regulated through a retinoic acid response element embedded in Sp1 sites. *Molecular and Cellular Biology*, **12**, 2976–85.

Lehmann, J. M., Zhang, X.-K., Graupner, G., Lee, M.-O., Hermann, T., Hoffmann, B. & Pfahl, M. (1993) Formation of retinoid X receptor homodimers leads to repression of T_3 response: hormonal cross talk by ligand-induced squelching. *Molecular and Cellular Biology*, **13**, 7698–707.

Leo, M. A., Kim, C.-I. & Lieber, C. S. (1989) Role of vitamin A degradation in the control of hepatic levels in the rat. *Journal of Nutrition*, **119**, 993–1000.

Leroy, P., Krust, A., Zelent, A., Mendelsohn, C., Garnier, J.-M., Kastner, P., Dierich, A. & Chambon, P. (1991a) Multiple isoforms of the mouse retinoic acid receptor α are generated by alternative splicing and differential induction by retinoic acid. *EMBO Journal*, **10**, 59–69.

Leroy, P., Nakshatri, H. & Chambon, P. (1991b) Mouse retinoic acid receptor α2 isoform is transcribed from a promoter that contains a retinoic acid response element. *Proceedings of the National Academy of Sciences of the U.S.A.*, **88**, 10 138–42.

Levin, M. S., Li, E., Ong, D. E. & Gordon, J. I. (1987) Comparison of the tissue-specific expression and developmental regulation of two closely linked rodent genes encoding cytosolic retinol-binding proteins. *Journal of Biological Chemistry*, **262**(15), 711–24.

Loerch, J. D., Underwood, B. A. & Lewis, K. C. (1979) Response of plasma levels of vitamin A to a dose of vitamin A as an indicator of hepatic vitamin A reserves in rats. *Journal of Nutrition*, **109**, 778–86.

Lotan, R. (1995) Retinoids and apoptosis: implications for cancer chemoprevention and therapy. *Journal of the National Cancer Institute*, **87**, 1655–7.

Lowe, W. L. Jr, Meyer, T., Karpen, C. W. & Lorentzen, L. R. (1992) Regulation of insulin-like growth factor I production in rat C6 glioma cells: possible role as an autocrine/paracrine growth factor. *Endocrinology*, **130**, 2683–91.

Lu, X. P., Eberhardt, N. L. & Pfahl, M. (1993) DNA bending by retinoid X receptor-containing retinoid and thyroid hormone receptor complexes. *Molecular and Cellular Biology*, **13**, 6509–19.

Lucas, P. C., Forman, B. M., Samuels, H. H. & Granner, D. K. (1991) Specificity of a retinoic acid response element in the phosphoenolpyruvate carboxykinase gene promoter: consequences of both retinoic acid and thyroid hormone receptor binding. *Molecular and Cellular Biology*, 11, 5164–70.

MacDonald, P. N., Bok, D. & Ong, D. E. (1990) Localization of cellular retinol-binding protein and retinol-binding protein in cells comprising the blood-brain barrier of rat and human. *Proceedings of the National Academy of Sciences of the U.S.A.*, 87, 4265–9.

MacDonald, P. N., Dowd, D. R., Nakajima, S., Galligan, M. A., Reeder, M. C., Haussler, C. A., Ozato, K. & Haussler, M. R. (1993) Retinoid X receptors stimulate and 9-*cis* retinoic acid inhibits 1,25-dihydroxyvitamin D_3-activated expression of the rat osteocalcin gene. *Molecular and Cellular Biology*, 13, 5907–17.

McGhee, J. R., Farrar, J. J., Michalek, S. M., Mergenhagen, S. E. & Rosenstreich, D. L. (1979) Cellular requirements for lipopolysaccharide adjuvanticity. A role for both T lymphocytes and macrophages for in vitro responses to particulate antigens. *Journal of Experimental Medicine*, 149, 793–807.

McGuire, B. W., Orgebin-Christ, M.-C. & Chytil, F. (1981) Autoradiographic localization of serum retinol-binding protein in rat testis. *Endocrinology*, 108, 658–67.

Mangelsdorf, D. J., Umesono, K., Kliewer, S. A., Borgmeyer, U., Ong, E. S. & Evans, R. M. (1991) A direct repeat in the cellular retinol-binding protein type II gene confers differential regulation by RXR and RAR. *Cell*, 66, 555–61.

Marks, M. S., Hallenbeck, P. L., Nagata, T., Segars, J. H., Appella, E., Nikodem, V. M. & Ozato, K. (1992) H-2RIIBP (RXRβ) heterodimerization provides a mechanism for combinatorial diversity in the regulation of retinoic acid and thyroid hormone responsive genes. *EMBO Journal*, 11, 1419–35.

Martin, G. R. (1981) Isolation of a pluripotent cell line from early mouse embryos cultured in medium conditioned by teratocarcinoma stem cells. *Proceedings of the National Academy of Sciences of the U.S.A.*, 78, 7634–8.

Matikainen, S., Serkkola, E. & Hurme, M. (1991) Retinoic acid enhances IL-1β expression in myeloid leukemia cells and in human monocytes. *Journal of Immunology*, 147, 162–7.

Matsuura, T. & Ross, A. C. (1993) Regulation of hepatic lecithin:retinol acyltransferase activity by retinoic acid. *Archives of Biochemistry and Biophysics*, 301, 221–7.

Moore, W. T., Murtaugh, M. P. & Davies, P. J. A. (1984) Retinoic acid-induced expression of tissue transglutaminase in mouse peritoneal macrophages. *Journal of Biological Chemistry*, 259(20), 12 794–802.

Moriguchi, S., Werner, L. & Watson, R. R. (1985) High dietary vitamin A (retinyl palmitate) and cellular immune functions in mice. *Immunology*, 56, 169–77.

Morita, S., Fernandez-Mejia, C. & Melmed, S. (1989) Retinoic acid selectively stimulates growth hormone secretion and messenger ribonucleic acid levels in rat pituitary cells. *Endocrinology*, 124, 2052–6.

Morita, S., Matsuo, K., Tsuruta, M., Leng, S., Yamashita, S., Izumi, M. & Nagataki, S. (1990) Stimulatory effect of retinoic acid on GH gene expression: the interaction of retinoic acid and triiodothyronine in rat pituitary cells. *Journal of Endocrinology*, 125, 251–6.

Muñoz-Cánoves, P., Vik, D. P. & Tack, B. F. (1990) Mapping of a retinoic acid-responsive element in the promoter region of the complement factor H gene. *Journal of Biological Chemistry*, 265(33), 20 065–8.

Muto, Y., Smith, J. E., Milch, P. O. & Goodman, D. S. (1972) Regulation of retinol-binding protein metabolism by vitamin A status in the rat. *Journal of Biological Chemistry*, 247(8), 2542–50.

Nagata, T., Segars, J. H., Levi, B.-Z. & Ozato, K. (1992) Retinoic acid-dependent transactivation of major histocompatibility complex class I promoters by the nuclear hormone receptor H-2RIIBP in undifferentiated embryonal carcinoma cells. *Proceedings of the National Academy of Sciences of the U.S.A.*, 89, 937–41.

Nagpal, S., Athanikar, J. & Chandraratna, R. A. S. (1995) Separation of transactivation and AP1 antagonism functions of retinoic acid receptor α. *Journal of Biological Chemistry*, 270(2), 923–7.

Nakshatri, H. & Chambon, P. (1994) The directly repeated RG(G/T)TCA motifs of the rat and mouse cellular retinol-binding protein II genes are promiscuous binding sites for RAR, RXR, HNF-4, and ARP-1 homo- and heterodimers. *Journal of Biological Chemistry*, 269(2), 890–902.

Napoli, J. L. (1993) Biosynthesis and metabolism of retinoic acid: roles of CRBP and CRABP in retinoic acid homeostasis. *Journal of Nutrition*, 123, 362–6.

Napoli, J. L. & Race, K. R. (1988) Biogenesis of retinoic acid from β-carotene. Differences between the metabolism of β-carotene and retinal. *Journal of Biological Chemistry*, 263(33), 17 372–7.

Napoli, J. L., Posch, K. P., Fiorella, P. D. & Boerman, M. H. E. M. (1991) Physiological occurrence, biosynthesis and metabolism of retinoic acid: evidence for roles of cellular retinol-binding protein (CRBP) and cellular retinoic acid-binding protein (CRABP) in the pathway of retinoic acid homeostasis. *Biomedicine and Pharmacotherapy*, 45, 131–43.

Nicholson, R. C., Mader, S., Nagpal, S., Leid, M., Rochette-Egly, C. & Chambon, P. (1990) Negative regulation of the rat stromelysin gene promoter by retinoic acid is mediated by an AP1 binding site. *EMBO Journal*, 9, 4443–54.

Ogura, T. & Evans, R. M. (1995a) A retinoic acid-triggered cascade of *HOXB1* gene activation. *Proceedings of the National Academy of Sciences of the U.S.A.*, 92, 387–91.

Ogura, T. & Evans, R. M. (1995b) Evidence for two distinct retinoic acid response pathways for *HOXB1* gene regulation. *Proceedings of the National Academy of Sciences of the U.S.A.*, 92, 392–6.

Okazawa, H., Okamoto, K., Ishino, F., Ishino-Kaneko, T., Takeda, S., Toyoda, Y., Muramatsu, M. & Hamada, H. (1991) The *oct3* gene, a gene for an embryonic transcription factor, is controlled by a retinoic acid repressible enhancer. *EMBO Journal*, 10, 2997–3005.

Oliva, A., Ragione, F. D., Fratta, M., Marrone, G., Palumbo, R. & Zappia, V. (1993) Effect of retinoic acid on osteocalcin gene expression in human osteoblasts. *Biochemical and Biophysical Research Communications*, 191, 908–14.

Oliver, G., De Robertis, E. M., Wolpert, L. & Tickle, C. (1990) Expression of a homeobox gene in the chick wing bud following application of retinoic acid and grafts of polarizing region tissue. *EMBO Journal*, 9, 3093–9.

Oreffo, R. O. C., Teti, A., Triffitt, J. T., Francis, M. J. O., Carano, A. & Zallone, A. Z. (1998) Effect of vitamin A on bone resorption: evidence for direct stimulation of isolated chicken osteoclasts by retinol and retinoic acid. *Journal of Bone and Mineral Research*, 3, 203–10.

Palozza, P. (1998) Prooxidant actions of carotenoids in biologic systems. *Nutrition Reviews*, 56, 257–65.

Pasatiempo, A. M. G., Kinoshita, M., Taylor, C. E. & Ross, A. C. (1990) Antibody production in vitamin A-depleted rats is impaired after immunization with bacterial polysaccharide or protein antigens. *FASEB Journal*, 4, 2518–27.

Pasatiempo, A. M. G., Kinoshita, M., Foulke, D. T. & Ross, A. C. (1994) The antibody response of vitamin A-deficient rats to pneumococcal polysaccharide is enhanced through coimmunization with lipopolysaccharide. *Journal of Infectious Diseases*, 169, 441–4.

Perez-Castro, A. V., Toth-Rogler, L. E., Wei, L.-N. & Nguyen-Huu,

M. C. (1989) Spatial and temporal pattern of expression of the cellular retinoic acid-binding protein and the cellular retinol-binding protein during mouse embryogenesis. *Proceedings of the National Academy of Sciences of the U.S.A.*, **86**, 8813–7.

Perlmann, T. & Jansson, L. (1995) A novel pathway for vitamin A signaling mediated by RXR heterodimerization with NGFI-B and NURR1. *Genes & Development*, **9**, 769–82.

Perlmann, T. & Vennström, B. (1995) The sound of silence. *Nature*, **377**, 387–8.

Pikarsky, E., Sharir, H., Ben-Shushan, E. & Bergman, Y. (1994) Retinoic acid represses Oct-3/4 gene expression through several retinoic acid-responsive elements located in the promoter-enhancer region. *Molecular and Cellular Biology*, **14**, 1026–38.

Pöpperl, H. & Featherstone, M. S. (1993) Identification of a retinoic acid response element upstream of the murine *Hox-4.2* gene. *Molecular and Cellular Biology*, **13**, 257–65.

Posch, K. C., Burns, R. D. & Napoli, J. L. (1992) Biosynthesis of all-*trans*-retinoic acid from retinal. Recognition of retinal bound to cellular retinol binding protein (type I) as substrate by a purified cytosolic dehydrogenase. *Journal of Biological Chemistry*, **267**(27), 19 676–82.

Quick, T. C. & Ong, D. E. (1989) Levels of cellular retinol-binding proteins in the small intestine of rats during pregnancy and lactation. *Journal of Lipid Research*, **30**, 1049–54.

Rahmathullah, L., Underwood, B. A., Thulasiraj, R. D., Milton, R. C., Ramaswamy, K., Rahmathullah, R. & Babu, G. (1990) Reduced mortality among children in southern India receiving a small weekly dose of vitamin A. *New England Journal of Medicine*, **323**, 929–35.

Raisher, B. D., Gulick, T., Zhang, Z., Strauss, A. W., Moore, D. D. & Kelly, D. P. (1992) Identification of a novel retinoid-responsive element in the promoter region of the medium chain acyl-coenzyme A dehydrogenase gene. *Journal of Biological Chemistry*, **267**(28), 20 264–9.

Rajan, N., Blaner, W. S., Soprano, D. R., Suhara, A. & Goodman, D. S. (1990) Cellular retinol-binding protein messenger RNA levels in normal and retinoid-deficient rats. *Journal of Lipid Research*, **31**, 821–9.

Rajan, N., Kidd, G. L., Talmage, D. A., Blaner, W. S., Suhara, A. & Goodman, D. S. (1991) Cellular retinoic acid-binding protein messenger RNA: levels in rat tissues and localization in rat testis. *Journal of Lipid Research*, **32**, 1195–204.

Rando, R. R. (1991) Membrane phospholipids as an energy source in the operation of the visual cycle. *Biochemistry*, **30**, 595–602.

Randolph, R. K. & Ross, A. C. (1991) Vitamin A status regulates hepatic lecithin:retinol acyltransferase activity in rats. *Journal of Biological Chemistry*, **266**(25), 16 453–7.

Rask, L. & Peterson, P. A. (1976) *In vitro* uptake of vitamin A from the retinol-binding plasma protein to mucosal epithelial cells from the monkey's small intestine. *Journal of Biological Chemistry*, **251**(20), 6360–6.

Ribaya-Mercado, J. D., Holmgren, S. C., Fox, J. G. & Russell, R. M. (1989) Dietary β-carotene absorption and metabolism in ferrets and rats. *Journal of Nutrition*, **119**, 665–8.

Ribeiro, R. C. J., Apriletti, J. W., West, B. L., Wagner, R. L., Fletterick, R. J., Schaufele, F. & Baxter, J. D. (1995) The molecular biology of thyroid hormone action. *Annals of the New York Academy of Sciences*, **758**, 366–89.

Roels, O. A., Trout, M. & Dujacquier, R. (1958) Carotene balances on boys in Rwanda where vitamin A deficiency is prevalent. *Journal of Nutrition*, **65**, 115–27.

Roels, O. A., Anderson, O. R., Lui, N. S. T., Shah, D. O. & Trout, M. E. (1969) Vitamin A and membranes. *American Journal of Clinical Nutrition*, **22**, 1020–32.

Rogers, M., Berestecky, J. M., Hossain, M. Z., Guo, H., Kadle, R., Nicholson, B. J. & Bertram, J. S. (1990) Retinoid-enhanced gap junctional communication is achieved by increased levels of connexin 43 mRNA and protein. *Molecular Carcinogenesis*, **3**, 335–43.

Rogers, M. B., Rosen, V., Wozney, J. M. & Gudas, L. J. (1992) Bone morphogenetic proteins-2 and -4 are involved in the retinoic acid-induced differentiation of embryonal carcinoma cells. *Molecular Biology of the Cell*, **3**, 189–96.

Rosen, E. D., O'Donnell, A. L. O. & Koenig, R. J. (1992) Ligand-dependent synergy of thyroid hormone and retinoid X receptors. *Journal of Biological Chemistry*, **267**(31), 22 010–13.

Ross, A. C. (1996) Vitamin A deficiency and retinoid repletion regulate the antibody response to bacterial antigens and the maintenance of natural killer cells. *Clinical Immunology and Immunopathology*, **80**, S63–S72.

Rottman, J. N., Widom, R. L., Nadal-Ginard, B., Mahdavi, V. & Karathanasis, S. K. (1991) A retinoic acid-responsive element in the apolipoprotein AI gene distinguishes between two different retinoic acid response pathways. *Molecular and Cellular Biology*, **11**, 3814–20.

Rush, M. G., Haq, R. & Chytil, F. (1991) Opposing effects of retinoic acid and dexamethasone on cellular retinol-binding protein ribonucleic acid levels in the rat. *Endocrinology*, **129**, 705–9.

Salbert, G., Fanjul, A., Piedrafita, F. J., Lu, X. P., Kim, S.-J., Tran, P. & Pfahl, M. (1993) Retinoic acid receptors and retinoid X receptor-α down-regulate the transforming growth factor-β$_1$ promoter by antagonizing AP-1 activity. *Molecular Endocrinology*, **7**, 1347–56.

Schoorlemmer, J., van Puijenbroek, A., van den Eijnden, J. L., Pals, C. & Kruijer, W. (1994) Characterization of a negative retinoic acid response element in the murine Oct promoter. *Molecular and Cellular Biology*, **14**, 1122–36.

Schüle, R., Rangarajan, P., Yang, N., Kliewer, S., Ransone, L. J., Bolado, J., Verma, I. M. & Evans, R. M. (1991) Retinoic acid is a negative regulator of AP-1-responsive genes. *Proceedings of the National Academy of Sciences of the U.S.A.*, **88**, 6092–6.

Schulman, I. G., Shao, G. & Heyman, R. A. (1998) Transactivation by retinoid X receptor–peroxisome proliferator-activated receptor γ (PPARγ) heterodimers: intermolecular synergy requires only the PPARγ hormone-dependent activation function. *Molecular and Cellular Biology*, **18**, 3483–94.

Scott, D. K., Mitchell, J. A. & Granner, D. K. (1996) Identification and characterization of a second retinoic acid response element in the phosphoenolpyruvate carboxykinase gene promoter. *Journal of Biological Chemistry*, **271**(11), 6260–4.

Senoo, H., Stang, E., Nilsson, A., Kindberg, G. M., Berg, T., Roos, N., Norum, K. R. & Blomhoff, R. (1990) Internalization of retinol-binding protein in parenchymal and stellate cells of rat liver. *Journal of Lipid Research*, **31**, 1229–39.

Sharma, R. V., Mathur, S. N., Dmitrovskii, A. A., Das, R. C. & Ganguly, J. (1977) Studies on the metabolism of β-carotene and apo-β-carotenoids in rats and chickens. *Biochimica et Biophysica Acta*, **486**, 183–94.

Shingleton, J. L., Skinner, M. K. & Ong, D. E. (1989) Characteristics of retinol accumulation from serum retinol-binding protein by cultured Sertoli cells. *Biochemistry*, **28**, 9641–7.

Sidell, N., Chang, B. & Bhatti, L. (1993) Upregulation by retinoic acid of interleukin-2-receptor mRNA in human T lymphocytes. *Cellular Immunology*, **146**, 28–37.

Sivaprasadarao, A. & Findlay, J. B. C. (1988a) The interaction of retinol-binding protein with its plasma-membrane receptor. *Biochemical Journal*, **255**, 561–9.

Sivaprasadarao, A. & Findlay, J. B. C. (1988b) The mechanism of uptake of retinol by plasma-membrane vesicles. *Biochemical Journal*, **255**, 571–9.

Smith, J. C. Jr., Brown, E. D., McDaniel, E. G. & Chan, W. (1976) Alterations in vitamin A metabolism during zinc deficiency and food and growth restriction. *Journal of Nutrition*, **106**, 569–74.

Smith, J. E., Muto, Y., Milch, P. O. & Goodman, D. S. (1973) The effects of chylomicron vitamin A on the metabolism of retinol-binding protein in the rat. *Journal of Biological Chemistry*, **248**(5), 1544–9.

Smith, S. M. & Hayes, C. E. (1987) Contrasting impairments in IgM and IgG responses of vitamin A-deficient mice. *Proceedings of the National Academy of Sciences of the U.S.A.*, **84**, 5878–82.

Smith, S. M., Levy, N. S. & Hayes, C. E. (1987) Impaired immunity in vitamin A-deficient mice. *Journal of Nutrition*, **117**, 857–65.

Smith, W. C., Nakshatri, H., Leroy, P., Rees, J. & Chambon, P. (1991) A retinoic acid response element is present in the mouse cellular retinol binding protein I (mCRBPI) promoter. *EMBO Journal*, **10**, 2223–30.

Soprano, D. R., Smith, J. E. & Goodman, D. S. (1982) Effect of retinol status on retinol-binding protein biosynthesis rate and translatable messenger RNA level in rat liver. *Journal of Biological Chemistry*, **257**(13), 7693–7.

Strickland, S. (1981) Mouse teratocarcinoma cells: prospects for the study of embryogenesis and neoplasia. *Cell*, **24**, 277–8.

Sucov, H. M., Murakami, K. K. & Evans, R. M. (1990) Characterization of an autoregulated response element in the mouse retinoic acid receptor type β gene. *Proceedings of the National Academy of Sciences of the U.S.A.*, **87**, 5392–6.

Tabin, C. (1995) The initiation of the limb bud: growth factors, *Hox* genes, and retinoids. *Cell*, **80**, 671–4.

Tachibana, K., Stone, S., Tsubura, E. & Kishino, Y. (1984) Stimulatory effect of vitamin A on tumoricidal activity of rat alveolar macrophages. *British Journal of Cancer*, **49**, 343–8.

Tarwotjo, I., Sommer, A., West, K. P. Jr., Djunaedi, E., Mele, L., Hawkins, B. & the Aceh Study Group (1987) Influence of participation on mortality in a randomized trial of vitamin A prophylaxis. *American Journal of Clinical Nutrition*, **45**, 1466–71.

Tate, B. F., Allenby, G., Janocha, R., Kazmer, S., Speck, J., Sturzenbecker, L. J., Abarzúa, P., Levin, A. A. & Grippo, J. F. (1994) Distinct binding determinants for 9-*cis* retinoic acid are located within AF-2 of retinoic acid receptor α. *Molecular and Cellular Biology*, **14**, 2323–30.

Terao, J. (1989) Antioxidant activity of β-carotene-related carotenoids in solution. *Lipids*, **24**, 659–61.

Tini, M., Otulakowski, G., Breitman, M. L., Tsui, L.-C. & Giguère, V. (1993) An everted repeat mediates retinoic acid induction of the γF-crystallin gene: evidence of a direct role for retinoids in lens development. *Genes & Development*, **7**, 295–307.

Tobler, A., Dawson, M. I. & Koeffler, H. P. (1986) Retinoids. Structure–function relationship in normal and leukemic hematopoiesis in vitro. *Journal of Clinical Investigation*, **78**, 303–9.

Tran, P., Zhang, X.-K., Salbert, G., Hermann, T., Lehmann, J. M. & Pfahl, M. (1992) COUP orphan receptors are negative regulators of retinoic acid response pathways. *Molecular and Cellular Biology*, **12**, 4666–76.

Twining, S. S., Schulte, D. P., Wilson, P. M., Fish, B. L. & Moulder, J. E. (1997) Vitamin A deficiency alters rat neutrophil function. *Journal of Nutrition*, **127**, 558–65.

Underhill, T. M., Kotch, L. E. & Linney, E. (1995) Retinoids and mouse embryonic development. *Vitamins and Hormones*, **51**, 403–57.

Underwood, B. A., Loerch, J. D. & Lewis, K. C. (1979) Effects of dietary vitamin A deficiency, retinoic acid and protein quantity and quality on serially obtained plasma and liver levels of vitamin A in rats. *Journal of Nutrition*, **109**, 796–806.

van Vliet, T., van Schaik, F. & van den Berg, H. (1992) Beta-carotene metabolism: the enzymatic cleavage to retinal. *Voeding*, **53**, 186–90.

van Vliet, T., van Vlissingen, M. F., van Schaik, F. & van den Berg, H. (1996) β-Carotene absorption and cleavage in rats is affected by the vitamin A concentration of the diet. *Journal of Nutrition*, **126**, 499–508.

Vasios, G. W., Gold, J. D., Petkovich, M., Chambon, P. & Gudas, L. J. (1989) A retinoic acid-responsive element is present in the 5′-flanking region of the laminin B1 gene. *Proceedings of the National Academy of Sciences of the U.S.A.*, **86**, 9099–103.

Vasios, G., Mader, S., Gold, J. D., Leid, M., Lutz, Y., Gaub, M.-P., Chambon, P. & Gudas, L. (1991) The late retinoic acid induction of laminin B1 gene transcription involves RAR binding to the responsive element. *EMBO Journal*, **10**, 1149–58.

Wang, C., Kelly, J., Bowen-Pope, D. F. & Stiles, C. D. (1990) Retinoic acid promotes transcription of the platelet-derived growth factor α-receptor gene. *Molecular and Cellular Biology*, **10**, 6781–4.

Wang, S.-Y. & Gudas, L. J. (1983) Isolation of cDNA clones specific for collagen IV and laminin from mouse teratocarcinoma cells. *Proceedings of the National Academy of Sciences of the U.S.A.*, **80**, 5880–4.

Wang, X.-D., Tang, G.-W., Fox, J. G., Krinsky, N. I. & Russell, R. M. (1991) Enzymatic conversion of β-carotene into β-apo-carotenals and retinoids by human, monkey, ferret, and rat tissues. *Archives of Biochemistry and Biophysics*, **285**, 8–16.

Wang, X.-D., Krinsky, N. I., Tang, G. & Russell, R. M. (1992) Retinoic acid can be produced from excentric cleavage of β-carotene in human intestinal mucosa. *Archives of Biochemistry and Biophysics*, **293**, 298–304.

Wang, X.-D., Krinsky, N. I. & Russell, R. M. (1993a) Retinoic acid regulates retinol metabolism via feedback inhibition of retinol oxidation and stimulation of retinol esterification in ferret liver. *Journal of Nutrition*, **123**, 1277–85.

Wang, X.-D., Russell, R. M., Marini, R. P., Tang, G., Dolnikowski, G. D., Fox, J. G. & Krinsky, N. I. (1993b) Intestinal perfusion of β-carotene in the ferret raises retinoic acid level in portal blood. *Biochimica et Biophysica Acta*, **1167**, 159–64.

Warrell, R. P. Jr., de Thé, H., Wang, Z.-Y. & Degos, L. (1993) Acute promyelocytic leukemia. *New England Journal of Medicine*, **329**, 177–89.

Wei, L.-N., Blaner, W. S., Goodman, D. S. & Nguyen-Huu, M. C. (1989) Regulation of the cellular retinoid-binding proteins and their messenger ribonucleic acids during P19 embryonal carcinoma cell differentiation induced by retinoic acid. *Molecular Endocrinology*, **3**, 454–63.

Wei, L.-N., Lee, C.-H. & Chang, L. (1995) Retinoic acid induction of mouse cellular retinoic acid-binding protein-I gene expression is enhanced by sphinganine. *Molecular and Cellular Endocrinology*, **111**, 207–11.

Widom, R. L., Rhee, M. & Karathanasis, S. K. (1992) Repression by ARP-1 sensitizes apolipoprotein AI gene responsiveness to RXRα and retinoic acid. *Molecular and Cellular Biology*, **12**, 3380–9.

Wiebel, F. F. & Gustafsson, J.-Å. (1997) Heterodimeric interaction between retinoid X receptor α and orphan nuclear receptor OR1 reveals dimerization-induced activation as a novel mechanism of nuclear receptor activation. *Molecular and Cellular Biology*, **17**, 3977–86.

Wiedermann, U., Hanson, L. Å., Kahu, H. & Dahlgren, U. I. (1993) Aberrant T-cell function *in vitro* and impaired T-cell dependent antibody response *in vivo* in vitamin A-deficient rats. *Immunology*, **80**, 581–6.

Willy, P. J. & Mangelsdorf, D. J. (1997) Unique requirements for retinoid-dependent transcriptional activation by the orphan receptor LXR. *Genes & Development*, **11**, 289–98.

Wilson, T. E., Fahrner, T. J. & Milbrandt, J. (1993) The orphan receptors NGFI-B and steroidogenic factor 1 establish monomer binding as a third paradigm of nuclear receptor-DNA interaction. *Molecular and Cellular Biology*, **13**, 5794–804.

Wirth, J. J. & Kierszenbaum, F. (1986) Stimulatory effects of retinoic acid on macrophage interaction with blood forms of *Trypanosoma cruzi*: involvement of transglutaminase activity. *Journal of Immunology*, **137**, 3326–31.

Wolf, G. (1995) The enzymatic cleavage of β-carotene: still controversial. *Nutrition Reviews*, **53**, 134–7.

Yang-Yen, H.-F., Zhang, X.-K., Graupner, G., Tzukerman, M., Sakamoto, B., Karin, M. & Pfahl, M. (1991) Antagonism between retinoic acid receptors and AP-1: implications for tumor promotion and inflammation. *New Biologist*, **3**, 1206–19.

Zelent, A., Mendelsohn, C., Kastner, P., Krust, A., Garnier, J.-M., Ruffenach, F., Leroy, P. & Chambon, P. (1991) Differentially expressed isoforms of the mouse retinoic acid receptor β are generated by usage of two promoters and alternative splicing. *EMBO Journal*, **10**, 71–81.

Zhang, L.-X., Cooney, R. V. & Bertram, J. S. (1991) Carotenoids enhance gap junctional communication and inhibit lipid peroxidation in C3H/10T1/2 cells: relationship to their cancer chemopreventive action. *Carcinogenesis*, **12**, 2109–14.

Zhang, L.-X., Cooney, R. V. & Bertram, J. S. (1992) Carotenoids up-regulate *connexin43* gene expression independent of their provitamin A or antioxidant properties. *Cancer Research*, **52**, 5707–12.

Zhao, Z. & Ross, A. C. (1995) Retinoic acid repletion restores the number of leukocytes and their subsets and stimulates natural cytotoxicity in vitamin A-deficient rats. *Journal of Nutrition*, **125**, 2064–73.

Zhao, Z., Murasko, D. M. & Ross, A. C. (1994) The role of vitamin A in natural killer cell cytotoxicity, number and activation in the rat. *Natural Immunity*, **13**, 29–41.

Zhou, H., Manji, S. S., Findlay, D. M., Martin, T. J., Heath, J. K. & Ng, K. W. (1994) Novel action of retinoic acid. Stabilization of newly synthesized alkaline phosphatase transcripts. *Journal of Biological Chemistry*, **269**(35), 22 433–9.

Zhou, X.-F., Shen, X.-Q. & Shemshedini, L. (1999) Ligand-activated retinoic acid receptor inhibits AP-1 transactivation by disrupting c-Jun/c-Fos dimerization. *Molecular Endocrinology*, **13**, 276–85.

8
Vitamin D

Key discussion topics

- Humans obtain their vitamin D mainly by photosynthesis in the skin.
- Within target cells, 1α,25-dihydroxyvitamin D_3 binds to the nuclear vitamin D receptor, which acts as a transcription factor in the regulation of gene expression.
- 1α,25-Dihydroxyvitamin D_3 exerts rapid, nongenomic effects in target cells by second messenger

pathways mediated by a specific membrane receptor.
- 24R,25-Dihydroxyvitamin D_3 plays a crucial role in bone formation and repair of bone fractures.
- The main physiological role of 1α,25-dihydroxyvitamin D_3 is maintaining calcium homeostasis.
- Vitamin D metabolites have immunoregulatory properties.

8.1 Historical overview

The discovery of vitamin D arose from research into rickets – a bone disease of infancy and early childhood that reached epidemic proportions in the industrial cities of Europe and the United States of America during the industrial revolution. The beneficial effect of sunlight in curing rickets had been recognized in the early nineteenth century. It was the work of Sir Edward Mellanby published in 1919 that finally led to the acceptance of rickets as a nutritional disease. In the same year, Huldschinsky cured four children with severe rickets by exposing them to the rays of a mercury quartz lamp, thus demonstrating that UV radiation from an artificial source was equally effective as solar radiation. Huldschinsky further showed that the effect was not localized, since exposing one of each child's arms to the radiation resulted in the healing of both arms. Two years later, Powers showed that cod-liver oil and UV radiation had similar curative effects on rachitic rats, thus establishing the dual source for antirachitic activity – diet and UV radiation.

In 1922 McCollum and associates published the results of experiments designed to determine whether the antirachitic factor in cod-liver oil was identical to or distinct from the previously discovered 'fat-soluble vitamin A'. They found that cod-liver oil retained its antirachitic properties after destruction of the vitamin A by heating and aeration. Thus, in addition to vitamin A, cod-liver oil contained a new fat-soluble vitamin, which McCollum later (1925) called 'fat-soluble vitamin D'. Zucker and co-workers in 1922 found that vitamin D was present in the unsaponifiable fraction of cod-liver oil, and suggested that it was closely related to cholesterol.

In 1923, Goldblatt and Soames irradiated rachitic rats and fed their livers to other rachitic rats which were not irradiated. The latter rats were cured of their rickets, thereby demonstrating that exposure to UV radiation induces the production of an antirachitic substance in the liver. Later, in a similar experiment, Hess and Weinstock fed small portions of irradiated skin to rachitic rats and noted a curative effect. In 1924, Steenbock and Black discovered that rat rations exposed to UV radiation had the same beneficial effects as when rachitic rats were irradiated. A year later, Hess and Weinstock induced antirachitic activity by irradiating such foods as milk, butter, bread and meats. It was further demonstrated that it is the sterols in foods that are activated and converted to vitamin D. It was finally realized that skin and certain foods contain a precursor of vitamin D that can be converted to the active vitamin by exposure to UV irradiation.

Irradiation of ergosterol, a sterol obtained from yeast, led to the isolation of a photo-product that was originally designated as vitamin D_1. It was later realized that vitamin D_1 was a mixture of substances, which explains its non-existence as a D vitamer in present nomenclature. Further purification of the irradiation mixture by Askew in 1931 yielded a single compound which was called ergocalciferol or vitamin D_2. It was assumed at the time that the vitamin D produced in human skin during exposure to UV radiation was vitamin D_2. However, in the following year, Steenbock noted that rachitic chickens did not respond to irradiated ergosterol, but did so to irradiated cholesterol preparations and cod-liver oil. This observation led to the discovery of 7-dehydrocholesterol as the vitamin D precursor in the cholesterol preparations and the isolation of cholecalciferol (vitamin D_3) by Windaus in 1936. Vitamin D_3, unlike vitamin D_2, had antirachitic activity in both chicks and rats. It was concluded that 7-dehydrocholesterol, rather than ergosterol, was the precursor for vitamin D_3 in the skin.

A major breakthrough in our understanding of vitamin D function arose from the discovery of the biologically active metabolite, $1\alpha,25$-dihydroxyvitamin D_3. This event was initiated by Carlsson who, in 1952, noted a lag between the time of vitamin D administration and the appearance of its physiological response, namely intestinal calcium transport. The discovery of a metabolite of vitamin D_3 in intestinal mucosa chromatin was published by Norman's group in 1968, and its biological significance was reported in 1970 by the same group. In 1970, Fraser and Kodicek showed that the kidney was the source of synthesis of the newly discovered metabolite. The chemical characterization of $1\alpha,25$-dihydroxyvitamin D_3 was reported in 1971 simultaneously by three independent laboratories, those of Norman, Kodicek, and Deluca, all within a six-week period in February/March of that year. The major circulating metabolite of vitamin D_3, 25-hydroxyvitamin D_3, was identified by DeLuca's group in 1968 and subsequently was shown to be produced primarily in the liver.

In 1969, Norman's group reported the existence of the vitamin D receptor in the chromatin fraction of the intestinal mucosa. The interaction of the receptor with the transcriptional machinery inside vitamin D target cells demonstrated that $1\alpha,25$-dihydroxyvitamin D_3 has a similar mechanism of action to that of steroid hormones.

8.2   Chemistry and biological functions

Vitamin D is represented by cholecalciferol (vitamin D_3) and ergocalciferol (vitamin D_2), which are structurally similar secosteroids derived from the UV irradiation of provitamin D sterols. (Secosteroids are steroids in which one of the rings has broken.) In vertebrates, vitamin D_3 is produced *in vivo* by the action of sunlight on 7-dehydrocholesterol in the skin. Vitamin D_2 is produced in plants, fungi and yeasts by the solar irradiation of ergosterol.

Vitamin D_3 and vitamin D_2 differ structurally only in the C-17 side chain, which in vitamin D_2 has a double bond and an additional methyl group (Fig. 8.1). Irradiation of the parent steroid results in breakage of the B ring at the 9,10-carbon bond, resulting in the conjugated triene system of double bonds. The vitamin D structures retain their numbering from the parent compound, cholesterol. Asymmetric carbon atoms are designated by using the *R,S* notation.

The vitamin D_2 and D_3 molecules are biologically inactive and their conversion to active, hormonal forms (Fig. 8.2) involves successive hydroxylations at the same carbon atoms. Vitamin D (D_2 or D_3) of endogenous or dietary origin arrives at the liver where it is hydroxylated at carbon 25 to yield 25-hydroxyvitamin D [25(OH)D]. This compound circulates in the blood and, in passing through the kidney, is hydroxylated at the α-position of carbon 1 to generate $1\alpha,25$-dihydroxyvitamin D [$1\alpha,25(OH)_2D$]. The dihydroxylated vitamin D_2 and D_3 metabolites are the active hormones; they show the same physiological activities as one another in mammals, including the maintenance of calcium and phosphate homeostasis, regulation of bone remodelling, and modulation of cell proliferation and differentiation. The vitamin D_2/D_3 hormones also function in the immune system. Another metabolite, 24R,25-dihydroxyvitamin D_3 [$24R,25OH)_2D_3$] is the initial product in the catabolism of $1\alpha,25(OH)_2D_3$ and in bone tissue may function as a hormone in an autocrine or paracrine fashion.

The potency of vitamin D_2 is (for humans) considered to be equivalent to that of D_3 and vitamin D_2 has been commonly used as a dietary substitute for D_3 (Parrish, 1979). Birds and New World monkeys respond efficiently only to vitamin D_3; thus they are apparently able to discriminate against the vitamin D_2 series of compounds. Horst *et al.* (1982) demonstrated for the first time that the pig and rat also discriminate in their metabolism of the two forms of vitamin D. Discrimination by the pig, a species which evolved with adequate exposure to sunlight, is predictably in

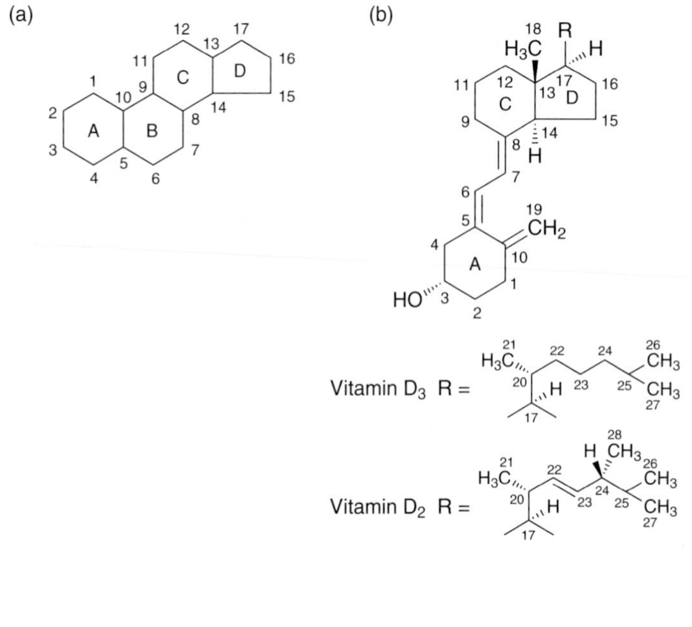

Fig. 8.1 Structural relationship of (a) the parent steroid nucleus to (b) vitamin D.

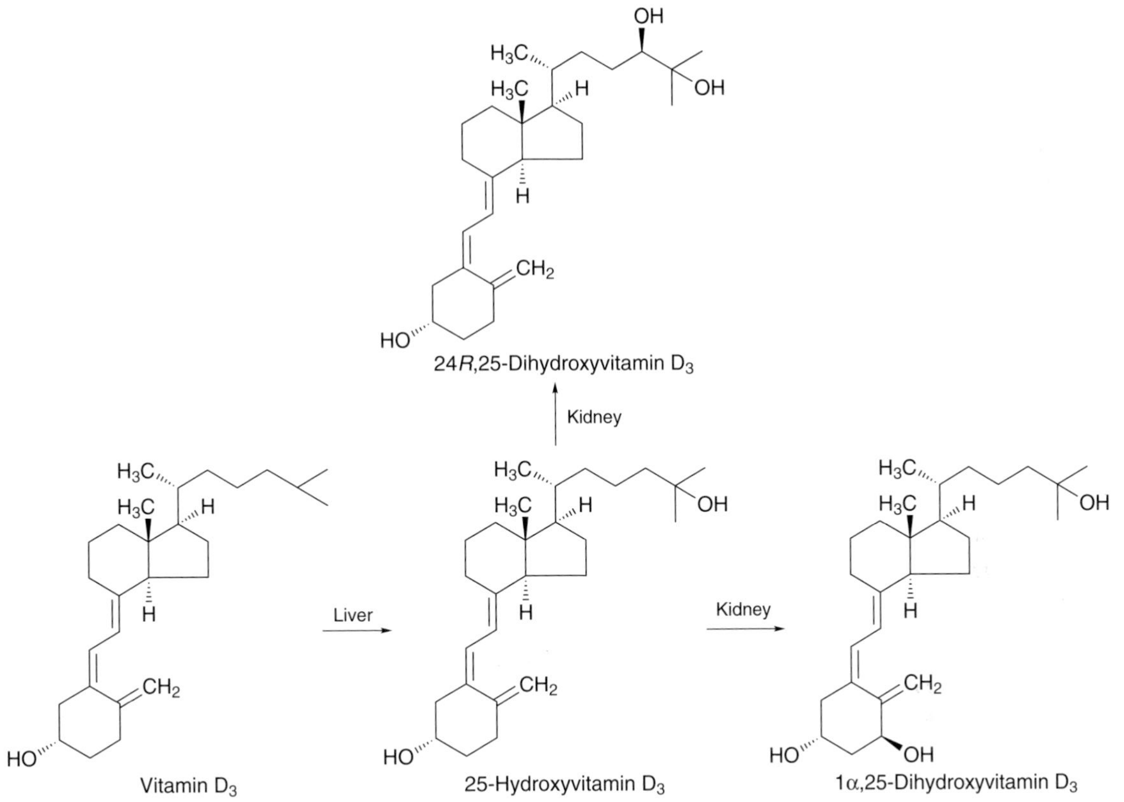

Fig. 8.2 Conversion of vitamin D_3 to hormonal metabolites.

favour of a vitamin D_3 metabolite. The rat, on the other hand, discriminates in favour of a vitamin D_2 metabolite, perhaps because it evolved as a nocturnal animal consuming grains (which contain predominantly vitamin D_2) as a significant part of its diet.

Although, in humans, vitamins D_2 and D_3 are comparable in their metabolism and the potency of their metabolites, the D_3 designation is used throughout much of this chapter because the experimental work has been done on the D_3 form. The distinguishing subscript is not used where the situation applies to either vitamin D_2 or D_3.

8.3   Dietary sources

The vitamin D activity in the human diet is contributed mainly by vitamin D itself and its immediate metabolite, 25(OH)D. The proportion of vitamin D obtained from the diet is normally very small compared with that synthesized in skin in response to

sunlight. The richest natural sources of vitamin D_3 are fish-liver oils, especially halibut-liver oil. Fatty fish, such as herring, sardines, pilchards and tuna, are rich natural food sources; smaller amounts of the vitamin are found in mammalian liver, eggs and dairy products. Cereals, vegetables and fruit contain no vitamin D, whilst meat, poultry and white fish contribute insignificant amounts.

Foodstuffs commonly enriched with vitamin D include margarine, skimmed milk powder, evaporated milk, milk-based beverages, breakfast cereals, dietetic products of all kinds, baby foods and soup powders.

8.4   Cutaneous synthesis, intestinal absorption, transport and metabolism

8.4.1   Overview

Solar radiation converts 7-dehydrocholesterol in the skin to previtamin D_3, which in turn is converted by body heat to vitamin D_3. Vitamins D_2 and D_3 can be obtained orally from natural and fortified foods, commercial fish-liver oil preparations and vitamin tablets. Unlike excessive ingestion of vitamin D supplements, the cutaneous source of vitamin D_3 does not result in toxicity when the skin is overexposed to sunlight. Vitamin D of both cutaneous and dietary origin is converted in the liver to 25(OH)D, the major circulating form of the vitamin. The 25(OH)D is converted in the kidney to $1\alpha,25(OH)_2D$, which circulates at low concentrations and acts in the manner of a steroid hormone.

8.4.2   The vitamin D-binding protein

In the plasma, 25(OH)D, and indeed all vitamin D metabolites, are mainly bound to a specific glycoprotein, known as the vitamin D-binding protein (DBP). Much smaller amounts of circulating vitamin D metabolites are bound with low affinity to albumin. DBP is synthesized principally in the liver and belongs to the same gene family as albumin. It has a molecular weight of 58 kDa and contains a single binding site for vitamin D metabolites. At normal circulating concentrations of vitamin D metabolites, less than 5% of the available binding sites on DBP are occupied. The features of the secosteroid molecule necessary for binding activity are the three conjugated double bonds and a hydroxyl group at C-25. The binding affinities of the DBP for vitamin D and its metabolites are $25(OH)D_3$ = $24R,25(OH)_2D_3$ = $25,26(OH)_2D_3$ > $1\alpha,25(OH)_2D_3$ > vitamin D_3. The difference in the dissociation constants for $25(OH)D_3$ and $1\alpha,25(OH)_2D_3$ is about 10-fold. In mammals, the metabolites of vitamins D_2 and D_3 exhibit the same relative affinities for DBP (Brown et al. 2000).

8.4.3   Cutaneous synthesis of vitamin D_3

Structural organization of the epidermis
The skin is composed of two layers: the epidermis and the underlying dermis. The bulk of the epidermal cells (keratinocytes) undergo a process of keratinization, resulting in the formation of the dead superficial layers of skin. Other cells, melanocytes, which produce the melanin pigment, do not undergo keratinization. The superficial keratinized cells are continuously sloughed from the surface and must be replaced by cells that proliferate in the basal layers of the epider-

mis. The newly formed cells are displaced to higher levels and as they move upward their cytoplasm is replaced by keratin. Thus the structural organization of the epidermis into layers reflects stages in the dynamic processes of cell proliferation and differentiation.

The epidermis consists of five layers, as shown in Fig. 8.3. Melanin is present mainly in the stratum basale and in the deeper layer of the stratum spinosum. Exposure of the skin to UV radiation increases the enzymatic activity of melanocytes, leading to tanning. The Malpighian layer is responsible for cell proliferation and for initiation of the keratinization process.

Photosynthesis
Vitamin D_3 is synthesized in the skin from 7-dehydrocholesterol (provitamin D_3) during exposure to sunlight by strictly chemical (i.e. nonenzymatic) reactions (Fig. 8.4). Exposure to increasing doses of solar radiation results in a corresponding increase in serum vitamin D_3 concentration within 24–48 h and a return to baseline concentration by 7 days (Adams et al., 1982). In young white adults, at least 30 µg of vitamin D_3 is made in the skin and released into the circulation from each square metre of body surface after exposure to 1 minimal erythema dose (MED), i.e. a dose causing minimal sunburn (Holick, 1987).

7-Dehydrocholesterol is converted photochemically to previtamin D_3, which is then converted to vitamin D_3 by a temperature-dependent process. The provitamin is equally distributed between the epidermis and the dermis, but because the penetrating radiation reaches the epidermis first, approximately 90% of the total cutaneous previtamin D_3 is made in the epidermis, mostly in the Malpighian layer. The waveband of solar radiation responsible for the conversion of the provitamin to the previtamin is that between 290 and 315 nm, known as the UV-B band. The optimum radiation was experimentally determined to be between 295 and 300 nm, with an apparent maximum near 297 nm (MacLaughlin et al., 1982). Solar radiation below 290 nm is prevented from reaching the Earth's surface by the ozone layer in the stratosphere. Complete cloud cover reduces UV energy by only 50% (Lawson, 1985).

The high-energy photons of the UV-B radiation are absorbed by the conjugated 6,7-diene in the B-ring of 7-dehydrocholesterol, resulting in ring opening at C9–C10 to produce previtamin D_3. Previtamin D_3, which is biologically inactive and thermodynami-

SKIN SURFACE

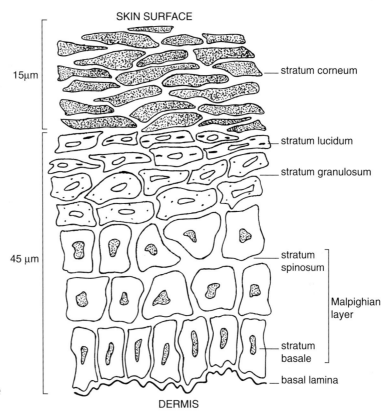

15μm

stratum corneum

stratum lucidum

stratum granulosum

45 μm

stratum spinosum

Malpighian layer

stratum basale

basal lamina

DERMIS

Fig. 8.3 Diagrammatic representation of the epidermis.

cally unstable, undergoes temperature-dependent isomerization to vitamin D_3. In human skin *in vitro* at 37°C, it took only 24 h for the conversion of previtamin D_3 to vitamin D_3 to reach equilibrium, compared to 7 to 10 days in hexane. The $t_{1/2}$ for the conversion in skin was 2.5 h compared to 30 h in hexane (Tian *et al.*, 1993). The selective removal of vitamin D_3 from its site of synthesis to the blood capillaries in the dermis might be at least partly attributable to its preferential binding to DBP on reaching the blood.

During a single prolonged exposure to the sun, the synthesis of previtamin D_3 reaches a plateau at about 10 to 15% of the original cutaneous 7-dehydrocholesterol concentration. At this point, the previtamin, instead of converting to vitamin D_3, undergoes photoisomerization to two biologically inactive products, lumisterol and tachysterol. Tachysterol formation also plateaus (at about 5% of the original 7-dehydrocholesterol concentration), whereas lumisterol formation continues to increase. These events take place regardless of the amount of skin pigmentation. Lumisterol and tachysterol have little or no affinity for DBP and

so fail to enter the circulation; they are eventually discarded during the sloughing off of old epidermal cells. As soon as previtamin D_3 stores are depleted, exposure of cutaneous lumisterol and tachysterol to solar UV radiation may promote their isomerization back to previtamin D_3 (Holick *et al.*, 1981). The photochemical conversion of previtamin D_3 to lumisterol and tachysterol is the first line of defence against the production of toxic levels of vitamin D after excessive exposure to sunlight. A second line of defence is the conversion of vitamin D_3 itself to 5,6-*trans*-vitamin D_3 and biologically inactive suprasterols (Webb *et al.*, 1989). These photochemical mechanisms for regulating the total cutaneous production of vitamin D_3 presumably account for the absence of reported cases of solar-induced vitamin D toxicity.

It is evident that only short exposures to bright sunlight produce sufficient vitamin D_3 in white people. After the initial beneficial exposure, use of a sunscreen is recommended to prevent the harmful effects of the sun. Individuals who have limited or no access to direct sunlight throughout the year are at risk from

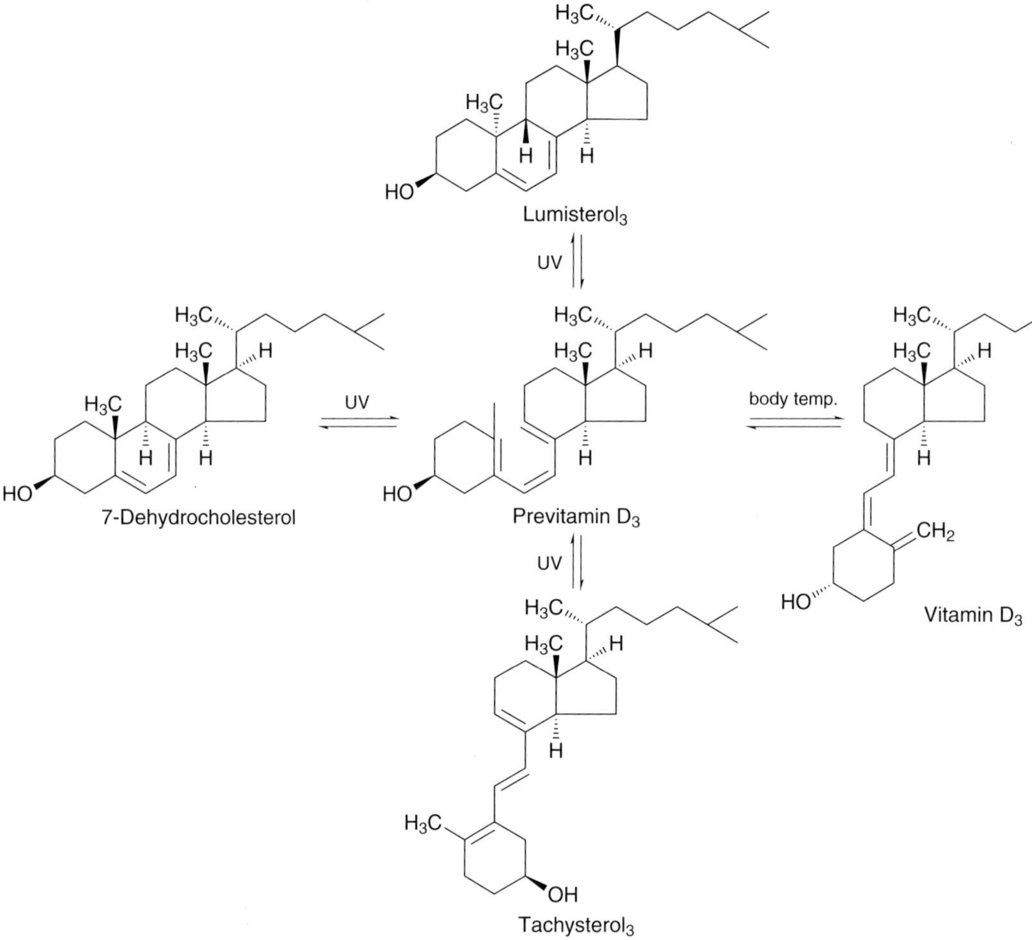

Fig. 8.4 The cutaneous synthesis of vitamin D₃.

vitamin D deficiency unless they have an adequate dietary supply of the vitamin. Window glass does not transmit radiation of wavelengths below 334 nm, therefore natural sunlight that is transmitted indoors is of no benefit for cutaneous vitamin D₃ production. Fluorescent tubes emit short wavelength radiation (λ < 280 nm) but this is filtered out by the glass or plastic fixtures in which they are mounted.

Factors affecting vitamin D₃ production

Various biological and environmental factors affect the cutaneous photosynthesis of vitamin D₃, including ageing, degree of skin pigmentation, occlusive clothing, duration of exposure to sunlight, the use of topical sunscreens, cloud cover, air pollution, season of year and latitude.

Ageing

After about 20 years of age, age-related changes in skin take place (Montagna & Carlisle, 1979) and the skin becomes progressively thinner. The concentration of epidermal 7-dehydrocholesterol also decreases with age and young adults can produce two to three times more previtamin D₃ in their skin than can elderly individuals (MacLaughlin & Holick, 1985). When healthy young and elderly volunteers were exposed to the same amount of simulated sunlight, serum vitamin D concentrations in the young subjects increased to a maximum of 30 ng mL^{-1} within 24 h after exposure, whereas the elderly subjects achieved a maximum of only 8 ng mL^{-1} (Holick et al., 1989). The results of a study of 433 postmenopausal women (Need et al., 1993) showed that the tendency for serum 25(OH)D to fall with age is due in part to the age-related decline in skin thickness.

Degree of skin pigmentation

At relatively low levels of solar radiation, skin pigmentation is a limiting factor for previtamin D_3 synthesis because melanin competes with 7-dehydrocholesterol in absorbing UV-B radiation (Holick et al., 1981). When surgical specimens of white skin and a range of black skins were exposed to the same dose of simulated sunlight (1.5 MED), the exposure times necessary to maximize previtamin D_3 formation increased with increasing skin pigmentation (Holick et al., 1981). The 1.5 MED induced a >30-fold increase in serum vitamin D in white-skinned subjects, but did not alter serum vitamin D in heavily pigmented black subjects. Re-exposure of one black subject to 9 MED increased serum vitamin D to a concentration similar to those recorded in the white subjects after exposure to 1.5 MED (Clemens et al., 1982). Hence black individuals have the same capacity as whites to produce vitamin D_3, but require a longer exposure to, or higher intensity of, solar radiation to do so.

Use of sunscreens

Sunscreen lotions play an important role in protecting against sunburn, photo-ageing and skin cancer. The problem with sunscreens is that they filter out the same radiation that is responsible for vitamin D synthesis in the skin. When young white adults were entirely covered with a protection factor 8 sunscreen, they were unable to elevate their serum vitamin D_3 levels after a whole-body exposure to a dose of simulated sunlight that caused marked elevations of serum vitamin D_3 in unprotected subjects (Matsuoka et al., 1987).

Season and latitude

Webb et al. (1988) investigated the effect of season and latitude on the cutaneous production of vitamin D_3 in Boston, USA (42°N) and Edmonton, Canada (52°N). In Boston, the conversion of 7-dehydrocholesterol to previtamin D_3 is greatest in June and July and gradually declines after August. Between November and February, exposure to sunlight on cloudless days for about 5 hours does not result in any significant conversion. Previtamin D_3 synthesis resumes in the middle of March. In Edmonton (10° north of Boston), the photosynthesis of previtamin D_3 ceases in October and is not resumed until April. These observations are explained by an increase in the zenith angle of the sun during the winter months and with latitude. Filtration of sunlight through the ozone layer takes place through an increased path length, decreasing the UV-B radiation that reaches the Earth's surface.

8.4.4   Intestinal absorption and transport

The vitamin D activity in the human diet is contributed mainly by free vitamin D, with 25(OH)D making a quantitatively small but nutritionally significant contribution. Animal tissues contain a small proportion of vitamin D esterified with both saturated and unsaturated fatty acids. Ingested vitamin D is solubilized within mixed micelles in the duodenum and esters of vitamin D, if present, are hydrolysed during solubilization (van den Berg, 1997). Solubilization is highly bile salt-dependent and patients with intraluminal bile salt deficiency have inefficient absorption of vitamin D. The micelles dissociate in the acidic microclimate of the unstirred layer and the liberated vitamin D is absorbed in the jejunum by simple diffusion, along with other lipids (Hollander et al., 1978). Vitamin D is incorporated into chylomicrons within the enterocytes and, when released, the chylomicrons convey the vitamin in the mesenteric lymph to the systemic circulation. During the journey in the lymph, an appreciable amount of the vitamin D in the chylomicrons is transferred to the DBP (Dueland et al., 1982). After lipolysis of the chylomicrons, the vitamin D remaining on the chylomicron remnants, and also the vitamin D bound to protein, is initially taken up by the liver (Dueland et al., 1983a). Approximately 80% of ingested vitamin D enters the body via the lymphatic system.

Absorption of 25(OH)D is faster than that of vitamin D in normal humans and in patients with fat malabsorption syndromes (Davies et al., 1980). Dueland et al. (1983b) compared the distribution of [^{14}C]vitamin D_3 and 25-[^{3}H]hydroxyvitamin D_3 in mesenteric lymph after simultaneous instillation of these compounds in the duodenum of rats. They showed that vitamin D_3 is carried mainly with chylomicrons, whereas 25(OH)D_3 is carried mainly by protein (Table 8.1). The protein responsible for carrying the bulk of 25(OH)D and part of vitamin D is very likely DPB, which has a greater affinity for 25(OH)D than for vitamin D. The results suggested

Protein fraction	[^{14}C]vitamin D$_3$	25-[^{3}H]hydroxyvitamin D$_3$
Chylomicrons, $d < 1.006$ g mL^{-1}	79.6 ± 7.5	5.4 ± 1.2
LDL/HDL, $1.006 < d < 1.21$ g mL^{-1}	1.9 ± 0.9	0.8 ± 0.5
Protein fraction, $d > 1.21$ g mL^{-1}	18.6 ± 7.7	93.8 ± 1.3

Table 8.1   Distribution of [^{14}C]vitamin D$_3$ and 25-[^{3}H]hydroxyvitamin D$_3$ in mesenteric lymph.

Values are means $\pm$ SD of duplicate samples from 3 different animals and are given as percentage of distribution of the activity recovered in the mesenteric lymph. [^{14}C]vitamin D$_3$ and 25-[^{3}H]hydroxyvitamin D$_3$ were given simultaneously through a duodenal tube. Lymph continuously collected between 2 and 24 hours was centrifuged at different densities (d). From Dueland *et al.* (1983b).

that the portal circulation plays only a minor role in the total absorption of vitamin D and 25(OH)D. The association of 25(OH)D with DBP rather than with chylomicrons implies that absorption of 25(OH)D is far less dependent on bile salts. Thus 25(OH)D is an important pharmacological agent in cases of bile salt deficiency.

8.4.5   Functional metabolism

Three key enzymes are involved in the conversion of vitamin D to active hormonal forms: vitamin D-25-hydroxylase in the liver converts vitamin D to 25(OH)D; a multicatalytic 1α-hydroxylase in the kidney converts 25(OH)D to 1α,25(OH)$_2$D; and 24*R*-hydroxylase, another renal multicatalytic enzyme, converts 25(OH)D to 24*R*,25(OH)$_2$D. These enzymes are mitochondrial mixed-function oxidases that require molecular oxygen and a source of electrons. The electron transport chain of the mitochondria reduces NAD to NADH and a transferase uses the NADH to reduce NADP to NADPH. The NADPH provides the electrons required for the reduction of molecular oxygen. The mechanism of enzyme action is shown in Fig. 8.5. The enzymes have three components which facilitate the transfer of electrons: ferredoxin reductase (a flavoprotein), ferredoxin (an iron sulphur protein) and a terminal cytochrome P450, which is embedded

in the inner mitochondrial membrane. The cytochrome P450 transfers electrons to molecular oxygen, one atom of which is reduced to form water and the other reduced to the hydroxyl group to be incorporated into the secosteroid substrate. All of the three enzymes use the same system of electron transfer, the specificity being conferred by differences in the cytochrome P450.

The mammalian liver does not store vitamin D to any significant extent and any vitamin D which is not metabolized in the liver is stored in the adipose tissue and skeletal muscle (Mawer *et al.*, 1972). The liver metabolite, 25(OH)D$_3$, is the major circulating form of vitamin D$_3$ and is a good indicator of the combined effects of exposure to sunlight and dietary intake of vitamin D.

Chylomicron remnants transfer vitamin D to liver cells more rapidly than does DBP. Therefore, lymph-borne dietary vitamin D bound to chylomicron remnants is taken up more rapidly by the liver than is blood-borne DBP-bound vitamin D of cutaneous origin. In the liver, the vitamin D of both cutaneous and dietary origin is hydroxylated to 25(OH)D or is catabolized to inactive compounds for excretion in the bile. In contrast to the rapid hepatic uptake of dietary vitamin D and inactivation of surplus amounts, the supply of cutaneous vitamin D to the liver is gradual, allowing continuous, prolonged production of 25(OH)D. Thus, the plasma concentration of this metabolite is maintained even when exposure of the skin to sunlight occurs only intermittently. The hydroxylating enzyme, vitamin D-25-hydroxylase, is only loosely regulated and circulating concentrations of 25(OH)D continue to rise in response to ingestion of pharmacological doses of vitamin D. Levels can rise to more than 400 ng mL^{-1}, leading to vitamin D toxicity. In contrast, extensive UV irradiation of the skin does not cause hypervitaminosis D and raises

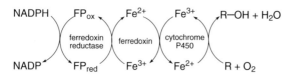

Fig. 8.5 Mechanism of mitochondrial steroid hydroxylation used by vitamin D-25-hydroxylase, 1α-hydroxylase and 24*R*-hydroxylase. R, secosteroid substrate.

25(OH)D levels in plasma to no more than 80 ng mL^{-1} (Fraser, 1983). Increasing the oral intake of vitamin D results in progressively smaller changes in 25(OH)D levels, showing that partial saturation of 25(OH)D production can be achieved *in vivo*.

Almost all of the 25(OH)D produced in the liver is released without delay into the bloodstream, where it becomes tightly bound to DBP. The normal concentration range of plasma 25(OH)D is 10–40 ng mL^{-1}. The blood constitutes the largest single body pool of 25(OH)D, since extrahepatic tissues take up only small amounts. During vitamin D deprivation the 25(OH)D blood pool is maintained through the prolonged release of vitamin D from its skin reservoir and from storage sites in muscle and adipose tissue.

On arrival at the kidney, the 25(OH)D/DBP complex is filtered through the glomerulus and reabsorbed by the epithelial cells of the proximal tubule by receptor-mediated endocytosis. The DBP is degraded in lysosomes while 25(OH)D is hydroxylated in the mitochondria and the products secreted into the circulation. The receptor responsible for the endocytosis is megalin. Mice bred with an absence of megalin are unable to retrieve the 25(OH)D/DBP complex from the glomerular filtrate and develop vitamin D deficiency and bone disease (Nykjaer *et al.*, 1999).

The metabolic fate of 25(OH)D in the kidney is dependent on the calcium and phosphorus requirements of the animal. An urgent need for either element results in the formation of $1\alpha,25(OH)_2D$, whereas during states of adequate calcium or phosphate balance, 25(OH)D is converted predominantly to $24R,25(OH)_2D$ (see Fig. 8.2). The latter metabolite circulates in the bloodstream bound to DBP at concentrations ranging from 1 to 4 ng mL^{-1}. Parathyroid hormone is involved in these enzymatic responses to changing plasma calcium and phosphate levels, as discussed in Sections 8.6.9 and 8.6.10.

The placenta has the capacity to provide additional $1\alpha,25(OH)_2D$ to fulfil the need during pregnancy. Hollis *et al.* (1989) could find no evidence for the existence of 1α- and $24R$-hydroxylases in the trophoblastic portion of the human placenta and postulated that $1\alpha,25(OH)_2D$ production in this tissue depends on free radical chemistry.

Plasma concentrations of the highly potent $1\alpha,25(OH)_2D_3$ are kept within the range 25–70 pg mL^{-1} by reciprocal changes in the rates of synthesis and degradation at the cellular level. $1\alpha,25$-Dihydroxyvitamin D_3 acts on the 1α-hydroxylase in a classical feedback mechanism to inhibit its own production (Henry *et al.*, 1974). $1\alpha,25$-Dihydroxyvitamin D_3 can also elicit its own degradation by inducing $24R$-hydroxylase, as reported in cultures of intestinal epithelial cells (Armbrecht *et al.*, 1993; Koyama *et al.*, 1994), renal tubular cells (Chen *et al.*, 1993; Armbrecht *et al.*, 1997), osteoblastic cells (Armbrecht & Hodam, 1994) and keratinocytes (Chen *et al.*, 1994). The protein kinase C signalling system is indispensable to the $1\alpha,25(OH)_2D_3$-dependent transcription of the $24R$-hydroxylase gene (Koyama *et al.*, 1994). The hydroxylated product, $1\alpha,24R,25(OH)_3D_3$, is ten times less biologically active than $1\alpha,25(OH)_2D_3$. The induced increase in $24R$-hydroxylase mRNA in renal and bone cells requires new protein synthesis, whereas induction in intestinal cells does not (Armbrecht *et al.*, 1997). The continuous production of a labile protein may be necessary for the transcription and/or stabilization of the mRNA in kidney and bone.

The formation of $1\alpha,24R,25(OH)_3D_3$ is the first step in the C-24 oxidation pathway (Fig. 8.6), which represents a self-induced mechanism for limiting the action of $1\alpha,25(OH)_2D$ once the initial wave of gene expression has been initiated. Each oxidation step leads to a progressive loss of biological activity, culminating in the inactive water-soluble product, calcitroic acid, which is excreted in the urine.

8.4.6 Excretion

The liver has a large capacity for catabolizing vitamin D into highly polar inactivation products and excreting these catabolites in bile. Many of these excretion products are conjugated with glucuronic acid. Only a negligible proportion of injected radioactively labelled vitamin D appears in the bile as unchanged vitamin D or 25(OH)D (Clements *et al.*, 1984). An enterohepatic circulation of vitamin D catabolites exists (Arnaud *et al.*, 1975) but, as the catabolites have only trivial biological activity, it does not constitute a functional mechanism for conserving vitamin D (Fraser, 1983). In conclusion, the majority of vitamin D degradation products is excreted in the faeces via the bile, with only a few percent appearing in the urine.

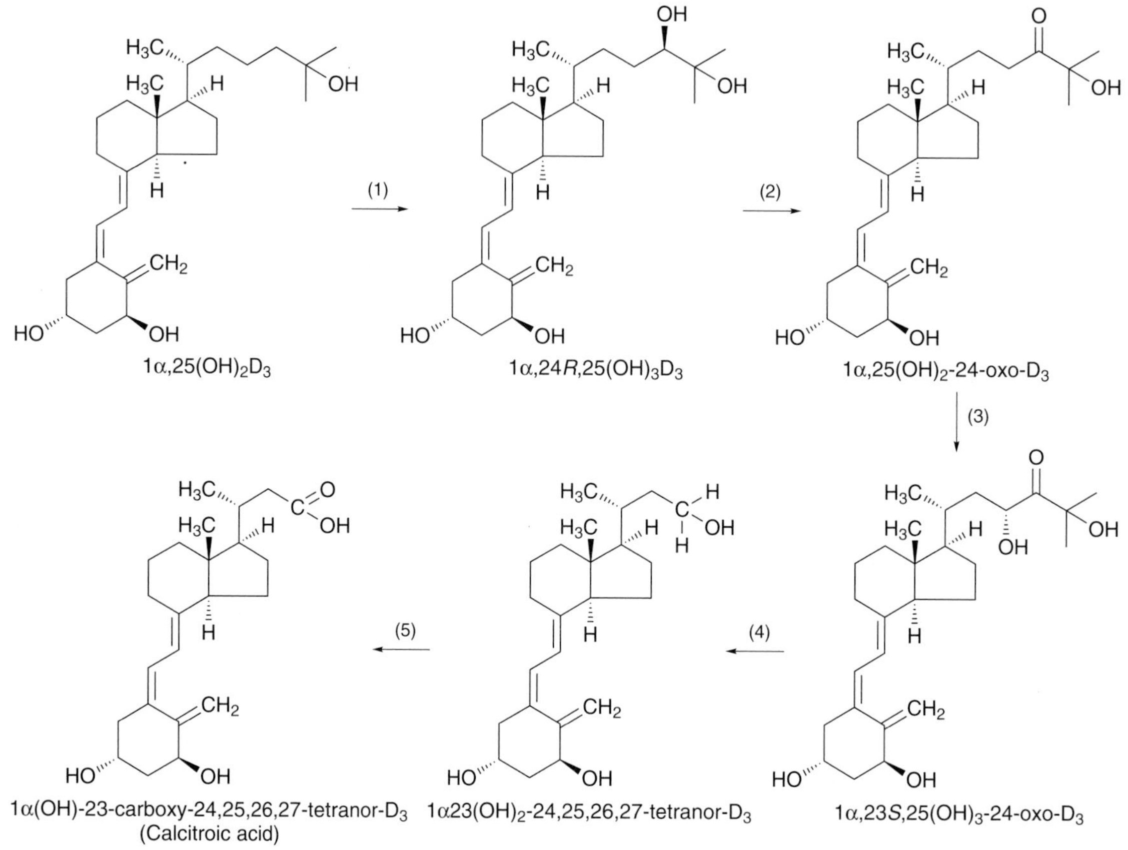

Fig 8.6 The carbon-24 (C-24) oxidation pathway of $1\alpha,25$-dihydroxyvitamin D_3 degradation. Steps: (1) Hydroxylation at C-24, (2) oxidation of the C-24 hydroxyl group to a ketone, (3) hydroxylation at C-23, (4) cleavage of the C-23–C-24 bond and (5) oxidation of the C-23 hydroxyl group to a carboxyl group. Steps 1 to 5 are catalysed by $24R$-hydroxylase.

8.5 Molecular action of the vitamin D hormones

8.5.1 Introduction

$1\alpha,25$-Dihydroxyvitamin D_3, also known as calcitriol, exerts its effects in cells by both genomic and nongenomic mechanisms. These involve long-term modulation of gene expression and short-term activation of intracellular signalling pathways, respectively. The genomic actions are mediated by the vitamin D receptor (VDR) which, on binding the hormone, interacts with the DNA to induce or inhibit new protein synthesis. Nongenomic actions are mediated by a membrane receptor that is distinct from the VDR. The binding of $1\alpha,25(OH)_2D_3$ to the membrane receptor triggers signal transduction pathways which involve second messengers and which modulate the genomic actions of the hormone.

Historically, $24R,25(OH)_2D_3$ has been considered by many to possess little or no intrinsic activity, its formation serving only to divert the metabolism of $25(OH)D_3$ away from $1\alpha,25(OH)_2D_3$. However, several reports indicate that $24R,25(OH)_2D_3$ is a functionally independent hormone and plays a crucial role in intramembranous and endochondral bone formation and in the repair of bone fractures.

8.5.2 Genomic actions of $1\alpha,25$-dihydroxyvitamin D_3

Background information can be found in Chapter 6.

The genomic action of $1\alpha,25(OH)_2D_3$ is mediated by the VDR, which functions as a ligand-activated transcription factor in the cells of target tissues. The sequence of events involved in the control of gene transcription by the VDR is (1) binding of $1\alpha,25(OH)_2D_3$ to the VDR in the cytosol, (2) translocation of the hormone–receptor complex to the nucleus, (3) binding of VDR–RXR heterodimers (RXR, retinoid X receptor) or, less commonly, VDR homodimers to the vitamin D response element (VDRE) in the promoter of primary vitamin D-responding genes and (4) recruitment of other nuclear proteins into the transcriptional pre-initiation complex. The VDRE functions as a transcriptional enhancer.

One must always bear in mind that an increase in the level of mRNA is not necessarily due to increased transcription: an increased mRNA stability will also lead to its accumulation.

Expression and regulation of the VDR

The VDR is a protein of 53 kDa which selectively binds $1\alpha,25(OH)_2D_3$ with high affinity. The protein is a type II member of the nuclear hormone receptor superfamily and possesses the characteristic two zinc finger motifs in the DNA binding site (see Section 6.8.5). The VDR is present in most tissues that have been examined, including activated immune cells such as T lymphocytes, where it plays a role in modulating the levels of cytokines such as interleukin-2. Bone, kidney and especially small intestine have high levels of receptor compared to other tissues. There are no isoforms of the VDR. The level of VDR expression in a cell determines the magnitude of the response evoked by $1\alpha,25(OH)_2D_3$. Within each target tissue, the level of VDR is not fixed but rather it is dynamically regulated by multiple factors. These include $1\alpha,25(OH)_2D_3$, which up-regulates the amount of receptor (homologous regulation), and other hormones and growth factors which may cause up- or down-regulation of receptor abundance (heterologous regulation). The mechanisms underlying the regulation of VDR abundance include alterations in the rate of transcription of the VDR gene, the stability of the VDR mRNA and post-translational events. The protein kinase A (PKA) and protein kinase C (PKC) signal transduction pathways interact at the level of VDR regulation. Activation of the PKA pathway by forskolin up-regulates VDR gene expression whereas activation of the PKC pathway by phorbol ester down-

regulates VDR gene expression (Krishnan & Feldman, 1991, 1992). There are profound tissue- and cell-specific variations in VDR regulation.

Post-translational modification of the VDR by phosphorylation

The binding of $1\alpha,25(OH)_2D_3$ to the VDR results in a substantial increase in phosphorylation of the receptor (Brown & DeLuca, 1990). Two sites of serine (Ser) phosphorylation on the human VDR have been identified, each with a different function. Ser-51 in the zinc finger region is phosphorylated by PKC (Hsieh et al., 1991), a post-translational modification that inhibits the receptor's ability to interact with the VDRE (Hsieh et al., 1993). Phosphorylation of Ser-208 in the ligand-binding domain by casein kinase II enhances the transcriptional activating capacity of the receptor, with no effect on receptor–ligand binding, receptor partitioning into the nucleus or association of receptor with a VDRE (Jurutka et al., 1996). Replacement of Ser-51 or Ser-208 with amino acids that are incapable of being phosphorylated does not affect DNA binding or attenuate $1\alpha,25(OH)_2D_3$-mediated transcriptional activation. This demonstrates that phosphorylation of the two serine residues is not an obligatory switch for VDR function; rather, these modifications represent both positive (casein kinase II) and negative (PKC) modulatory mechanisms that apparently govern receptor activity under appropriate cellular conditions. Jurutka et al. (1996) envisaged two populations of liganded VDR: one that is hypophosphorylated at Ser-208, yet still active in transcriptional enhancement, and a superactive, hyperphosphorylated form that is even more effective at co-operatively recruiting coactivators and/or basal transcription factors.

Desai et al. (1995) used staurosporine, an inhibitor of PKC and related protein kinases, and okadaic acid, an inhibitor of protein phosphatases, to investigate the contribution of VDR phosphorylation/dephosphorylation to vitamin D-stimulated transcription of the rat osteocalcin gene. The results suggested the presence of at least two functionally distinct phosphorylation sites on the VDR. At one site, staurosporine inhibits a phosphorylation event that is specifically required for the intrinsic transactivation function of VDR–RXR heterodimers. At the other site, okadaic acid inhibits a post-translational dephosphorylation event that is required for VDRE binding of VDR-containing transcription factor complexes.

Nuclear localization of the liganded VDR

The unoccupied VDR exists in equilibrium between the cytosolic and nuclear compartments of the target cell. Receptor–hormone binding shifts this equilibrium to favour nuclear localization (Walters *et al.*, 1986). The hormone–receptor complex rapidly translocates to the nucleus along microtubules facilitated by specialized motor proteins. Disruption of microtubular integrity impairs the genomic response to 1α,25-dihydroxyvitamin D_3 in human monocytes, which clearly underlines the physiological importance of the intracellular tubulin transport system (Kamimura *et al.*, 1995).

Role of ligands in VDR–RXR heterodimer binding to DNA

Thompson *et al.* (1998) investigated the molecular function of 1α,25(OH)$_2$D$_3$ and 9-*cis* retinoic acid ligands in the binding of the VDR and RXR to mouse osteopontin and rat osteocalcin VDREs. Efficient binding to either VDRE occurred as a VDR–RXR heterodimer, not as a VDR homodimer. 1α,25-Dihydroxyvitamin D_3 dramatically enhanced heterodimer–VDRE interaction, whereas somewhat higher concentrations of 9-*cis* retinoic acid inhibited this association. A possible explanation for this inhibition is that the binding of 9-*cis* retinoic acid to the RXR partner destabilizes the heterodimer and induces RXR homodimer formation. MacDonald *et al.* (1993) offered this explanation when they demonstrated that 9-*cis* retinoic acid repressed vitamin D_3-induced transactivation of the osteocalcin gene. Thus liganded RXR is diverted from vitamin D-activated transcription toward expression of vitamin A-dependent genes.

Thompson *et al.* (1998) showed that the transcriptional response to hormone depends on the sequential order in which the components assemble. They proposed the existence of two alternative allosteric pathways for VDR–RXR association and response to ligand. (1) An unliganded VDR associates with RXR to form an apo-heterodimer in solution. Subsequent binding of 1α,25(OH)$_2$D$_3$ induces a conformational change in the heterodimer, which results in enhanced binding to the VDRE. The RXR partner can readily be dissociated from the DNA-bound heterodimer by the addition of 9-*cis* retinoic acid, leading to the formation of RXR homodimers that mediate retinoid-responsive pathways. This 9-*cis* retinoic acid-receptive conformation is proposed to exist also in monomeric RXR and in the apo-VDR–RXR. (2) When VDR binds 1α,25(OH)$_2$D$_3$ before heterodimer formation, it is postulated to acquire a conformation distinct from that in the first pathway. After heterodimerization, the liganded VDR allosterically alters the ligand-binding domain of its RXR partner, rendering the RXR unable to bind its own ligand and thus making the heterodimer resistant to 9-*cis* retinoic acid-elicited dissociation.

Interaction of the VDR with basal transcription factor TFIIB

In the formation of the pre-initiation complex on a gene promoter, the binding of the basal transcription factor TFIIB to the TATA-binding protein is a requisite for the recruitment of RNA polymerase II (Section 6.5.3). VDR interacts with TFIIB through a highly specific, ligand-independent, direct protein–protein contact and enhances transcription in the manner of an activator (Blanco *et al.*, 1995; MacDonald *et al.*, 1995).

Vitamin D-responsive genes containing VDREs

Although over 50 genes have been reported to be regulated by 1α,25(OH)$_2$D$_3$, only a few have been shown to contain VDREs. More than half of the known natural VDREs have a direct repeat structure of two six-nucleotide half-sites with a specific three-nucleotide spacer (DR3). Other natural VDREs have DR4, DR6 or IR9 (inverted palindrome) structures. In most vitamin D-responsive genes, RXR binds to the 5′-half-site and its heterodimeric partner, VDR, binds to the 3′-half-site. A selection of primary vitamin D-responding gene products is listed in Table 8.2.

Genes having a simple DR3-type VDRE include those encoding p21 protein, atrial natriuretic factor, integrin β$_3$ subunit and osteopontin. p21 protein is a potent inhibitor of cyclin-dependent kinases, which are regulators of the cell cycle (Xiong *et al.*, 1993). Atrial natriuretic factor is a peptide hormone released by the atrial walls of the heart when they become stretched and which acts directly on the kidney to greatly increase salt and water excretion. Integrin α$_v$β$_3$ is a receptor that is expressed on the osteoclast plasma membrane and recognizes the bone-residing proteins osteopontin and bone sialoprotein (Medhora *et al.*, 1993). The binding of osteopontin to cell-surface integrin α$_v$β$_3$ initiates signals that elicit osteoclastic actions (Noda & Denhardt, 2002). The carbonic an-

Table 8.2   A selection of protein products encoded by vitamin D-responsive genes.

Gene product	Species	Up- or down-regulated by hormone–VDR	Type of VDRE	Reference
24R-Hydroxylase	Rat	Up	Two DR3s	Zierold et al. (1995)
24R-Hydroxylase	Human	Up	Two DR3s	Chen & DeLuca (1995)
Osteocalcin	Rat	Up	DR3[a]	Demay et al. (1992a)
Osteocalcin	Human	Up	DR3[a]	Ozono et al. (1990)
Osteopontin	Mouse	Up	DR3	Noda et al. (1990)
Osteopontin	Pig	Up	DR3	Zhang et al. (1992)
Fibronectin	Mouse, rat, human	Up	DR6	Polly et al. (1996)
Carbonic anhydrase II	Chicken	Up	DR3	Quélo et al. (1994)
Calbindin-D_{9k}	Rat	Up	DR3	Darwish & DeLuca (1992)
Calbindin-D_{9k}	Human	Up	IP9	Schräder et al. (1995)
Calbindin-D_{28k}	Mouse	Up	DR4	Gill & Christakos (1993)
Na^+/phosphate co-transporter	Human	Up	DR3	Taketani et al. (1997)
Phospholipase C-$\gamma 1$	Human	Up	DR6	Xie & Bikle (1997)
Pit-1	Mouse	Up	DR4	Rhodes et al. (1993)
Integrin β_3 subunit	Chicken	Up	DR3	Cao et al. (1993)
Atrial natriuretic factor	Rat	Up	DR3	Kahlen & Carlberg (1996)
p21	Human	Up	DR3	Liu et al. (1996a)
c-fos	Mouse	Up	IP9	Schräder et al. (1997)
Parathyroid hormone	Chicken	Down	DR3	Liu et al. (1996b)
Parathyroid hormone	Human	Down	DR3	Demay et al. (1992b)
PTH-related peptide	Rat	Down	DR3	Kremer et al. (1996)
Bone sialoprotein	Rat	Down	DR3	Kim et al. (1996)

[a]A DNA sequence which does not bind VDR is essential for the $1\alpha,25(OH)_2D_3$ responsiveness of the rat and human osteocalcin genes (Sneddon et al., 1997).

hydrase isoform II is highly expressed in cells where acid–base regulation is a primary function, i.e. gastric parietal cells, salivary glands, renal tubular cells and osteoclasts. The carbonic anhydrase II DR3-type VDRE is unusual in that the receptor complex binds in 5′-VDR–RXR-3′ polarity, the reverse of that normally found in VDREs (Quélo et al., 1994).

Two functional VDREs have been identified in the promoters of the rat and human 24R-hydroxylase genes – a unique feature among vitamin D-responsive genes. The two response elements function synergistically due to coordinated interaction (Kerry et al., 1996) and the combination represents the most powerful of the VDREs reported to date. Phorbol ester, acting via PKC, can potentiate the effect of $1\alpha,25(OH)_2D_3$ on induction of 24R-hydroxylase in both the kidney and intestine, but not in bone (Armbrecht et al., 1997). There are several possible explanations for this potentiation. The phorbol ester could increase the phosphorylation of VDR by PKC and thus enhance its genomic effect as demonstrated by Hsieh et al. (1991). $1\alpha,25$-Dihydroxyvitamin D_3 may also up-regulate phorbol ester receptors in renal tubular cells as it does in HL-60 leukaemia cells (Martell et al., 1987). This, in turn, could facilitate the effect of phorbol ester on VDR phosphorylation. Phorbol ester can induce transcription of the primary response gene c-fos in renal tubular cells (Chen et al., 1993). The c-fos protein would bind to AP-1 binding sites in the 24-hydroxylase promoter and potentiate the genomic effect of VDR binding to the two VDREs.

Osteocalcin, synthesized exclusively by osteoblasts, is a negative regulator of bone formation (Ducy et al., 1996). The VDRE of the rat osteocalcin gene has been characterized as an imperfect DR3 with the structure GGGTGAATGAGGACA (Demay et al., 1992a). Sneddon et al. (1997) identified a sequence present from –420 to –414 in this gene that markedly enhances VDR-mediated transactivation and is absolutely required for $1\alpha,25(OH)_2D_3$ responsiveness. This sequence is unable to bind the VDR or confer $1\alpha,25(OH)_2D_3$ responsiveness independently of the VDRE. The sequence is also capable of augmenting transcription in concert with either an oestrogen or cyclic AMP response element as shown by an en-hanced transcriptional response to 17β-oestradiol and forskolin. The human osteocalcin gene contains the same augmenting sequence in a similar position relative to the VDRE.

Pit-1, a transcriptional activator of the prolactin and growth hormone genes (Mangalam *et al.*, 1989), has an atypical DR4 VDRE, as does the mouse calbin-din-D_{28} gene. The gene that encodes fibronectin, an important noncollagenous protein in the extracel-lular matrix, has a DR6-type VDRE that specifically binds VDR homodimers (Polly *et al.*, 1996). A DR6-type VDRE has also been identified in the human phospholipase C-γ1 gene.

The product of the c-*fos* gene, c-Fos, pairs with c-Jun to form AP-1, which is the terminal acceptor responsible for converting transient stimuli at the cell surface into long-term transcriptional responses. The mouse c-*fos* gene has an IP9-type VDRE which is bound by VDR–RXR heterodimers and is as function-al as the more common DR3-type elements (Schräder *et al.*, 1997). The human calbindin-D_{9k} gene VDRE is also of the IP9 type.

Repression of the human parathyroid hormone (PTH) gene appears to be attributable to a negative VDRE that preferentially binds a heterodimer con-sisting of VDR and a tissue-specific silencing partner rather than VDR–RXR (Haussler *et al.*, 1998). Simply changing two base pairs in the 3′-half-site of the avian PTH VDRE converted a negative element to a posi-tive one. Binding of the VDR–nonRXR heterodimer to the negative VDRE may change the conformation of the heterodimer, preventing it from recruiting a coactivator, whereas binding to the positive VDRE permits coactivator recruitment. PTH-related pep-tide, which shares a common receptor with PTH, is also down-regulated by $1\alpha,25(OH)_2D_3$. Falzon (1996) identified a region in the gene encoding this protein which resembled the negative VDRE from the PTH gene.

Bone sialoprotein (BSP) initiates hydroxyapatite formation in developing bone. The down-regula-tion of the rat BSP gene appears to be attributable to a VDRE that overlaps a unique inverted TATA box and involves competition between the VDR and the TATA-binding protein. In comparison with activating VDREs, the rat BSP VDRE binds VDR homodimers more avidly than it does VDR–RXR heterodimers (Kim *et al.*, 1996).

Gene regulation

The ligand-activated VDR may function to recruit coactivators that remodel chromatin structure and permit greater accessibility of the transcriptional ma-chinery to DNA. Coactivators shown to interact with liganded VDR include mouse SUG1 (vom Baur *et al.*, 1996), RAC3 (Li *et al.*, 1997), NCoA-62 (Baudino *et al.*, 1998; MacDonald *et al.*, 2001) and a multiprotein complex known as DRIP (Rachez *et al.*, 1998, 1999). There have been no reports as yet of co-repressor pro-teins which bind to the VDR, so it is presently unclear whether the VDR interacts with co-repressors to bring about down-regulation of target genes. At least one co-repressor, N-CoR, fails to interact with the VDR (Hörlein *et al.*, 1995). Determination of whether vi-tamin D hormone action is stimulatory or inhibitory may be tissue-specific or dependent on the state of cellular differentiation. Most vitamin D-responsive genes are up-regulated by $1\alpha,25(OH)_2D_3$, the human PTH gene being one of the few that is down-regulated (see Table 8.2).

Repression of vitamin D-induced transactivation of the osteocalcin gene by YY1

Overlapping the recognition sequences for VDR–RXR within the VDRE of the osteocalcin gene are two bind-ing motifs for the multifunctional transcription factor YY1. This protein can either activate, repress or initiate gene transcription (Shrivastava & Calame, 1994). In the context of the osteocalcin promoter, YY1 represses $1\alpha,25(OH)_2D_3$-induced transcription by competing with VDR–RXR for binding at the VDRE. YYI also in-teracts directly with TFIIB thereby interfering with the transactivation function of the VDR (Guo *et al.*, 1997). This repressive function of YY1 would prevent the pre-cocious induction of osteocalcin gene transcription by VDR-mediated mechanisms under physiological con-ditions in which the gene should not be expressed.

Suppression of osteocalcin gene expression during osteoblast proliferation

The target cell for the hormonal action of vita-min D on bone is the osteoblast. Within this cell, $1\alpha,25(OH)_2D_3$ enhances osteocalcin gene expression at the three principal levels – transcription, mRNA accumulation and protein synthesis. The enhanced transcription is dependent upon basal levels of gene expression (Owen *et al.*, 1991), suggesting that there is a coordinate transactivation involving the contribution of activities at the VDRE and basal elements. Two essential basal elements in the proximal promoter are the TATA box and the osteocalcin box (OC box), a 24-nucleotide sequence that contains a central CCAAT motif (Lian & Stein, 1992). The VDRE is located further upstream between nucleotides −512 and −485 in the human osteocalcin gene promoter (Ozono et al., 1990).

The sequential expression of vitamin D-dependent genes associated with bone tissue development has been studied in cultures of normal diploid rat osteoblasts. The first 10 to 12 days constitute the cell proliferation period, characterized by the expression of genes encoding AP-1 proteins (Jun and Fos) and extracellular matrix proteins. The jun and fos genes are transcribed in response to growth factors and other cell-surface stimuli, and the protein products are responsible for converting the transient stimuli into a long-term transcriptional response. During the following stages, the proliferative activity declines and the genes encoding the AP-1 proteins and extracellular matrix proteins are gradually down-regulated. During the next stage of matrix maturation (days 12 through 18), alkaline phosphatase mRNA and enzyme activity increases more than ten-fold to peak levels, and matrix Gla protein is expressed maximally. Days 16 through 20 are characterized by the progressive mineralization of the extracellular matrix. As the cellular levels of alkaline phosphatase mRNA decline, the accumulation of calcium in the matrix increases coordinately with the up-regulated expression of genes encoding the calcium-binding proteins, osteocalcin and osteopontin (Stein & Lian, 1993).

The modular organization of the human osteocalcin gene promoter explains how gene expression might be suppressed during cell proliferation. Overlapping the VDRE and also within the OC box are AP-1 binding sites which bind Jun–Fos heterodimers and Jun homodimers. During the proliferation of osteoblasts, the Jun and Fos proteins are present at high levels. Occupancy of the AP-1 binding site overlapping the VDRE by Jun and Fos dimers blocks the binding of liganded VDR to its specific site and prevents transcription of the osteocalcin gene. At the end of the proliferation period, the levels of Fos and Jun decline, allowing the VDR to bind to the VDRE and the osteocalcin gene to be expressed. Thus the competition of the VDR and the AP-1 proteins for binding to the composite DNA element determines the activation or suppression of the osteocalcin gene (Lian & Stein, 1992). High levels of Jun and Fos also suppress basal transcription of the osteocalcin gene (Schüle et al., 1990).

Inhibitory effect of the VDR on transactivation of the growth hormone gene by thyroid hormone and retinoic acid

The rat growth hormone gene, located exclusively in the somatotropic pituitary cells, contains a hormone response element that functions both as a retinoic acid response element (RARE) and a thyroid hormone response element (TRE) (García-Villalba et al., 1993). This allows thyroid hormone and retinoic acid to interact co-operatively to stimulate transcription of the growth hormone gene in pituitary cells (Bedo et al., 1989). García-Villalba et al. (1996) reported that incubation of rat pituitary cells with nanomolar concentrations of vitamin D_3 inhibits thyroid hormone and retinoic acid transactivation of the growth hormone gene by interference on the common response element. The results suggested that the liganded VDR can directly affect the pituitary response to other nuclear receptors, thereby contributing to the growth arrest that occurs in hypervitaminosis D. This negative effect on the growth hormone gene is apparently paradoxical, since a deficiency of vitamin D produces a rachitic state associated with a defect in growth.

Repression of VDR-mediated transcription of the osteocalcin and osteopontin genes by the thyroid hormone receptor

Thompson et al. (1999) demonstrated two distinct repressive actions of the TR on VDR-mediated transcription of the rat osteocalcin and mouse osteopontin genes: (1) a thyroid hormone-independent action, perhaps due to TR–RXR out-competing VDR–RXR for binding to the VDREs and (2) a thyroid hormone-dependent repression, likely by diversion of limiting RXR from VDR–RXR toward the formation of TR–RXR heterodimers. The reverse of this phenomenon was indicated by a relatively weak binding of VDR–RXR to the TRE of the myosin heavy chain gene and modest repression by liganded VDR of thyroid hormone-mediated transactivation. This reciprocal inhibition of transactivation by VDR and TR is permitted by the half-site homology between the rat osteocalcin VDRE and the rat myosin heavy chain TRE. The formation of a TR–VDR heterodimer reported by Schräder *et al.* (1994) was not observed by Thompson *et al.* (1999) who concluded that this heterodimer is not biochemically or physiologically relevant. As far as is known, the only relevant heterodimerization among nuclear receptors (excluding RXR) is between the type I mineralocorticoid and glucocorticoid receptors.

8.5.3   Nongenomic actions of 1α,25-dihydroxyvitamin D$_3$ and 24R,25-dihydroxyvitamin D$_3$

Background information can be found in Sections 3.7.6 and 3.7.9.

A large number of responses occur within seconds to minutes following addition of vitamin D metabolites to the *in vitro* system – too rapid to involve changes in gene expression controlled by the VDR. Moreover, such responses are not blocked by inhibitors of transcription (actinomycin D) or protein synthesis (cycloheximide). For these reasons, the rapid responses are described as nongenomic.

1α,25-Dihydroxyvitamin D$_3$

Rapid nongenomic responses to 1α,25(OH)$_2$D$_3$ have been observed in many cell types, including enterocytes, colonocytes, chondrocytes, osteoblasts, hepatocytes, skeletal and cardiac muscle cells, keratinocytes, mammary gland epithelial cells, parathyroid cells and pituitary cells (Norman, 1998). The responses have been most clearly delineated in osteoblast-like osteosarcoma cells. At a molecular level, these include effects on membrane phospholipid metabolism (Grosse *et al.*, 1993), activation of voltage-sensitive calcium channels (Caffrey & Farach-Carson, 1989) and elevation of cytosolic (Baran *et al.*, 1991) and nuclear (Sorensen *et al.*, 1993) Ca^{2+} concentrations.

A number of nongenomic effects of 1α,25(OH)$_2$D$_3$ are concerned with the regulation of intracellular calcium, which is an important second messenger involved in the activation of many target enzymes. Additional effects include stimulation of prostaglandin production (Boyan *et al.*, 1994), increased intracellular pH (Jenis *et al.*, 1993) and increased membrane fluidity (Brasitus *et al.*, 1986).

Regulation of intracellular calcium

Transient increases in intracellular calcium can be initiated in two major ways. (1) Extracellular calcium can enter the cell down its electrochemical gradient by the opening of voltage-gated calcium channels. (2) Calcium can be released from intracellular storage sites associated with mitochondria and the endoplasmic reticulum.

The presence of L-type (dihydropyridine-sensitive) voltage-activated calcium channels has been demonstrated in basolateral membranes of rabbit ileal enterocytes (Homaidan *et al.*, 1989) and in osteosarcoma cells (Guggino *et al.*, 1989). The opening of such channels is the fastest known response of osteoblasts to treatment with nanomolar concentrations of 1α,25(OH)$_2$D$_3$. The hormone enhances the activity of voltage-gated channels in rat pituitary cells (Tornquist & Tashjian, 1989) and rat osteosarcoma cells (Caffrey & Farach-Carson, 1989).

The binding of 1α,25(OH)$_2$D$_3$ to a membrane receptor in a wide range of cell types stimulates the activity of phospholipase C, whose hydrolytic action on membrane phosphoinositides results in the generation of the two second messengers, diacylglycerol and inositol triphosphate (see Fig. 3.31). Cell types examined include osteosarcoma cells (Civitelli *et al.*, 1990), myoblasts (Morelli *et al.*, 1993), enterocytes (Lieberherr *et al.*, 1989), colonocytes (Wali *et al.*, 1990), hepatocytes (Baran *et al.*, 1988), parathyroid cells (Bourdeau *et al.*, 1990) and keratinocytes (MacLaughlin *et al.*, 1990). Diacylglycerol is an activator of PKC, which is involved in a myriad of cellular processes. Inositol triphosphate releases Ca^{2+} from the intracellular storage sites, thereby increasing the concentration of Ca^{2+} in the cytosol.

A rapid increase in calcium translocation, termed transcaltachia, has been described using the perfused chick duodenal loop (Nemere *et al.*, 1984). The involvement of 1α,25(OH)$_2$D$_3$ in the activation of voltage-gated calcium channels appears to be an early effect in transcaltachia. Introduction of a calcium channel antagonist completely abolished the movement of calcium, while a calcium channel agonist mimicked the stimulatory response to 1α,25(OH)$_2$D$_3$ (de Boland *et al.*, 1990). de Boland & Norman (1990) provided evidence for the involvement of PKA and PKC in transcaltachia. Forskolin and phorbol ester, activators of PKA and PKC, respectively, stimulated transcaltachia analogously to 1α,25(OH)$_2$D$_3$. In addition, the transcaltachial response to 1α,25(OH)$_2$D$_3$ was respectively suppressed or abolished by inhibitors of PKA and PKC. Collectively, these observations suggest that $1\alpha,25(OH)_2D_3$ binds to a membrane receptor located in the basolateral membrane of the enterocyte and signal transduction via G proteins, effector proteins and second messengers leads to activation of PKA and PKC. These kinases might stimulate calcium influx via phosphylation-dependent activation of voltage-gated calcium channels at the basolateral membrane.

Evidence for a distinct membrane receptor for $1\alpha,25(OH)_2D_3$

There is strong evidence that the nongenomic responses to $1\alpha,25(OH)_2D_3$ are mediated by a membrane receptor that is biochemically different from the nuclear VDR. Ligand specificity for the rapid actions is different from that for genomic responses (Farach-Carson et al., 1991). Using osteoblasts from mice in which the VDR gene had been genetically ablated, Wali et al. (2003) showed that the $1\alpha,25(OH)_2D_3$-induced rapid increases in intracellular calcium and PKC activity are neither mediated, nor dependent upon, a functional VDR.

A 66-kDa protein that binds vitamin D analogues has been isolated from basolateral membranes of chick intestinal epithelium (Nemere et al., 1994) and from both plasma membranes and matrix vesicles of rat chondrocytes (Nemere et al., 1998). Antibody (Ab99) generated to a $[^3H]1\alpha,25(OH)_2D_3$ binding protein isolated from the basolateral membrane of chick intestinal epithelium blocked the rapid activation of PKC by $1\alpha,25(OH)_2D_3$ in chondrocytes (Nemere et al., 1998) and enterocytes (Nemere et al., 2000). Slater et al. (1995) discovered that physiological concentrations of $1\alpha,25(OH)_2D_3$ can directly activate PKC in artificial membranes. This suggests that the PKC protein itself can act as a membrane-associated receptor for $1\alpha,25(OH)_2D_3$, providing an additional signal transduction pathway to the well-established route in which PKC is activated by diacylglycerol. Baran et al. (2000) reported that annexin II, a 36-kDa protein, can serve as a cell-surface receptor mediating $1\alpha,25(OH)_2D_3$-induced increase in intracellular calcium in osteoblast-like ROS 24/1 cells that lack the functional nuclear VDR. The rapid effects of $1\alpha,25(OH)_2D_3$ to increase intracellular calcium were not observed in cells pre-treated with anti-annexin II antibodies. It is likely that several membrane receptors mediate the rapid actions of $1\alpha,25(OH)_2D_3$ (Brown et al., 1999).

Modulation of the genomic actions of $1\alpha,25(OH)_2D_3$ by nongenomic mechanisms

$1\beta,25$-Dihydroxyvitamin D_3 does not interact with the nuclear VDR and thus has no effect on basal gene transcription. It does, however, inhibit nongenomic effects by competing with $1\alpha,25(OH)_2D_3$ for the membrane receptor. Baran et al. (1992) demonstrated that, in osteosarcoma cells, the 1β epimer inhibits the $1\alpha,25(OH)_2D_3$-induced rapid rise in intracellular calcium and accompanying increase in osteocalcin gene transcription. The inhibition of transcription occurred without interfering with the binding of the $1\alpha,25(OH)_2D_3$–VDR complex to the VDRE. Since $1\beta,25(OH)_2D_3$ has no genomic effects on osteocalcin, yet can block the transcription that accompanies the nongenomic effect of $1\alpha,25(OH)_2D_3$, this study suggests that the nongenomic effects of $1\alpha,25(OH)_2D_3$ can modulate the genomic actions of this hormone in some way.

Khoury et al. (1994) showed that the $1\alpha,25(OH)_2D_3$-induced transcription of osteocalcin and osteopontin genes in osteosarcoma cells is independent of Ca^{2+} influx, suggesting that the nongenomic stimulation of calcium channels by $1\alpha,25(OH)_2D_3$ is not required for target gene activation. Jenis et al. (1993) discovered that the nongenomic $1\alpha,25(OH)_2D_3$-induced increase in intracellular pH is necessary for osteocalcin and osteopontin expression in the osteoblast. The effect upon pH appears to be regulated by the Na^+/H^+ antiporter, since the incubation of cells in a Na^+-free medium eliminated the pH effect and blocked the hormone-induced increase in osteocalcin and osteopontin mRNA steady-state levels.

The genomic response may be modulated by second messengers generated at both the plasma and nuclear membranes in response to the binding of $1\alpha,25(OH)_2D_3$ to membrane receptors (Baran & Sorensen, 1994). $1\alpha,25$-Dihydroxyvitamin D_3 increases PKC activity through stimulation of plasma membrane phosphoinositide and formation of diacylglycerol (Wali et al., 1990). In renal epithelial cells, $1\alpha,25(OH)_2D_3$ specifically induces translocation of PKCβ (but not PKCα) from the plasma membrane to the nuclear membrane, an event which enhances phosphorylation of nuclear proteins (Simboli-Campbell et al., 1994). Phosphorylation of the nuclear VDR by PKC has been shown to down-regulate transcription (Hsieh et al., 1993). Sorensen & Baran (1993) reported that $1\alpha,25(OH)_2D_3$ rapidly enhances phospholipase C activity in the nuclear membrane of osteosarcoma cells, resulting in an increased level of inositol triphosphate, which in turn releases calcium from intranuclear storage sites.

24R,25-Dihydroxyvitamin D$_3$

The importance of 24R,25(OH)$_2$D$_3$ in endochondral bone formation is indicated by its accumulation in growth plate cartilage when normal rats are injected with [^{3}H]25(OH)D$_3$ (Seo et al., 1996).

Effect on calcium current in osteosarcoma cells

Li et al. (1996) demonstrated a dual nongenomic effect of 24R,25(OH)$_2$D$_3$ on the L-type calcium channel current in osteosarcoma cells. At a low physiological concentration (1 × 10^{-8} M), 24R,25(OH)$_2$D$_3$ activated the PKA signal pathway leading to an increase in current amplitude, whereas a higher concentration (1 × 10^{-5} M) reduced the current amplitude via the PKC signal pathway. In comparison, a high concentration of 1α,25(OH)$_2$D$_3$ (1 × 10^{-6} M) increased the current amplitude.

Regulation of chondrocyte maturation and differentiation

Boyan et al. (2001) reviewed the results of their many experiments which examined the biochemical effects of 1α,25(OH)$_2$D$_3$ and 24R,25(OH)$_2$D$_3$ on cultured chondrocytes at two distinct stages of cell development. Cells were selected from the cartilaginous growth plates at the costochondral junction of the ribs of adolescent rats. Resting zone cells are fully committed cartilage cells which undergo proliferation when suitably stimulated. Growth zone cells taken from the prehypertropic/upper hypertropic zones are capable of producing matrix vesicles. Table 8.3 shows differential responses to 1α,25(OH)$_2$D$_3$ and 24R,25(OH)$_2$D$_3$ in the two cell types. In the case of all four biochemical parameters, growth zone chondrocytes respond exclusively to 1α,25(OH)$_2$D$_3$, whereas resting zone chondrocytes respond exclusively to 24R,25(OH)$_2$D$_3$.

The differential effects of the two vitamin D hormones on phospholipase A$_2$ activity are reflected in prostaglandin production, since stimulation of phospholipase A$_2$ releases arachidonic acid from membrane phospholipids and arachidonic is the chief precursor of prostaglandins. Accordingly, 1α,25(OH)$_2$D$_3$ stimulates prostaglandin E$_2$ production in growth zone cells, whereas 24R,25(OH)$_2$D$_3$ inhibits production by resting zone cells. In the case of PKC activation, there is a marked difference in the time course of the two responses. 1α,25-Dihydroxyvitamin D$_3$ exerted its effect within 9 min, whereas the maximal effect of 24R,25(OH)$_2$D$_3$ was noted at 90 min. Use of actinomycin D and cycloheximide demonstrated that the 1α,25(OH)$_2$D effect is nongenomic; in contrast, the 24R,25(OH)$_2$D$_3$ effect is genomic, requiring both new gene transcription and new protein synthesis. The effect of 24R,25(OH)$_2$D$_3$ in stimulating PKC activity is stereospecific since 24S,25(OH)$_2$D$_3$ is unable to elicit the response. The effects of hormone on phospholipid metabolism account for the changes in membrane fluidity, which affect membrane transport processes and the activities of membrane-bound enzymes. In addition, 1α,25(OH)$_2$D$_3$ stimulates Ca^{2+} efflux from growth zone chondrocytes, whereas 24R,25(OH)$_2$D$_3$ inhibits Ca^{2+} efflux from resting zone cells. Overall, 24R,25(OH)$_2$D$_3$ targets less mature cells and 1α,25(OH)$_2$D$_3$ targets more mature cells, thus membrane receptors for these metabolites are differentially expressed as a function of cell maturation.

The rapid, membrane-mediated effects in response to 24R,25(OH)$_2$D$_3$, but not 1α,25(OH)$_2$D$_3$, seen in resting zone chondrocytes suggests that a membrane

Table 8.3 Biochemical responses of chondrocytes to 1α,25(OH)$_2$D$_3$ and 24R,25(OH)$_2$D$_3$.

Parameter	Growth zone cells		Resting zone cells	
	1α,25	24R,25	1α,25	24R,25
Alkaline phosphatase activity	Increase	No response	No response	Increase
PLA$_2$ activity	Increase	No response	No response	Decrease
PKC activity	Increase	No response	No response	Increase
Fluidity of plasma membrane	Increase	No response	No response	Increase

receptor(s) exists which is specific for $24R,25(OH)_2D_3$. Pedrozo et al. (1999) reported that a hybrid analogue of $1\alpha,25(OH)_2D_3$ with <0.1% affinity for the nuclear VDR stimulated PKC activity in plasma membranes from resting zone chondrocytes, and that this effect was not blocked by antibody generated to the $1\alpha,25(OH)_2D_3$ membrane receptor (Ab99). This provided definitive evidence of a membrane receptor for $24R,25(OH)_2D_3$ in the resting zone chondrocytes.

Regulation of matrix vesicles

From their studies of matrix vesicles isolated from cultured chondrocytes, Boyan et al. (1994) proposed that $1\alpha,25(OH)_2D_3$ and $24R,25(OH)_2D_3$ synthesized by chondrocytes diffuse into the extracellular matrix and interact directly with the vesicle membrane receptor. This initiates a cascade of biochemical events which lead to maturation of the matrix vesicle, hydroxyapatite crystal formation, loss of integrity of the vesicle membrane and eventual release of active proteases. The proteases then degrade proteoglycan aggregates in the vicinity of the matrix vesicles, facilitating extracellular matrix calcification. Boyan et al. (1994) discovered that the chondrocyte plasma membrane and matrix vesicle membrane possess different isoforms of PKC: -alpha and -zeta, respectively. This allows chondrocytes to regulate events in matrix vesicles without comparable effect on their plasma membranes.

Bone fracture repair

There is substantial evidence that $24R,25(OH)_2D_3$ at physiological concentration is essential for bone fracture repair. Both the renal 24-hydroxylase activity and the circulating $24R,25(OH)_2D_3$ levels were highly elevated 10–12 days after chick tibial fracture (Seo & Norman, 1997). Oral administration of $24R,25(OH)_2D_3$ in combination with $1\alpha,25(OH)_2D_3$ was effective in healing tibial fracture in chicks, whereas a combination of $24S,25(OH)_2D_3$ and $1\alpha,25(OH)_2D_3$ or $1\alpha,25(OH)_2D_3$ alone resulted in poor healing (Seo et al., 1997). The ability of the bone healing system to distinguish between $24R,25(OH)_2D_3$ and $24S,25(OH)_2D_3$ is further evidence for the presence of a receptor. Accordingly, Kato et al. (1998) separated fracture-healing callus tissue into nuclear, cytosol and membrane fractions and demonstrated the presence of a specific receptor for $24R,25(OH)_2D_3$ in the membrane fraction. Local injection of $24R,25(OH)_2D_3$ into the proximal epiphyseal growth plate of the tibiae of vitamin D-deficient chicks resulted in disappearance of the rachitic lesions in the same leg; there were no signs of healing in response to local injection of $1\alpha,25(OH)_2D_3$ (Lidor et al., 1987). These observations suggest that $24R,25(OH)_2D_3$ may exert effects both locally via autocrine or paracrine mechanisms, or systemically via endocrine mechanisms.

Regulation of intramembranous bone formation

St-Arnaud's group (St-Arnaud, 1999) engineered a strain of mice deficient for the 24-hydroxylase enzyme (24-hydroxylase-ablated or knockout mice) and showed that homozygotes for this mutation cannot effectively clear $1\alpha,25(OH)_2D_3$ from their circulation. This leads to perinatal lethality, most probably secondary to hypercalcaemia caused by sustained elevated levels of $1\alpha,25(OH)_2D_3$. The role of $24R,25(OH)_2D_3$ during development was addressed by breeding mutant animals that had survived to adulthood. When fertile mutant homozygous females are mated to heterozygous males, litters comprise an equal proportion of mutant homozygotes and control heterozygous littermates. Because of the impaired 24-hydroxylase activity of the female, homozygous embryos are completely deprived of vitamin D metabolites hydroxylated at position 24. Heterozygous littermates can synthesize those metabolites because they carry one functional allele of the 24-hydroxylase gene. Histological examination of the bones of homozygous mutants born of homozygous females revealed an accumulation of unmineralized osteoid at sites of intramembranous ossification. Control heterozygous littermates showed normal bone structure. Homozygous mutants born from heterozygous females also showed normal bone histology, presumably because the embryo can receive maternal $24R,25(OH)_2D_3$ via the placenta. These results demonstrate a key role for $24R,25(OH)_2D_3$ in the developmental regulation of intramembranous bone formation. The impairment of matrix calcification in the knockout mice may be due to elevated $1\alpha,25(OH)_2D_3$ levels resulting from altered metabolism rather than a direct action of $24R,25(OH)_2D_3$ (St-Arnaud et al., 2000).

8.6   Calcium and phosphate homeostasis

8.6.1   Introduction

Ionic calcium (Ca^{2+}) is crucial for many cellular functions including neurotransmitter release and nerve impulse propagation; contraction of skeletal, cardiac and smooth muscle; blood clotting; exocrine and endocrine secretory processes; and cell proliferation. Ca^{2+} also acts as a 'second messenger', connecting some stimuli (certain hormones, growth factors and neurotransmitters) with physiological responses. Bones and teeth contain about 99% of the body's calcium; the other 1% is distributed in both intra- and extracellular fluids.

The blood level of Ca^{2+} is very closely regulated: even small changes in Ca^{2+} concentration can be fatal. Acute hypocalcaemia in the human causes essentially no other significant effects besides tetany, because tetany kills the patient before other effects can develop. In tetany, the low concentration of Ca^{2+} in the extracellular fluid causes the nervous system to become progressively more excitable because of increased neuronal membrane permeability. Eventually, peripheral nerve fibres become so excitable that they begin to discharge spontaneously, initiating nerve impulses that pass to the skeletal muscles, where they elicit the muscular spasms of tetany. In hypercalcaemia, the nervous system is depressed, and reflex actions of the central nervous system become sluggish. There is also constipation and lack of appetite, probably because of depressed contractability of the muscular walls of the gastrointestinal tract. Above a certain high level of blood Ca^{2+}, calcium phosphate is likely to precipitate throughout the blood and the soft tissues. Deposition of calcium in the kidney or heart causes death due to renal failure or cardiac arrest.

Phosphorus is a component of hydroxyapatite in the skeleton, of phospholipids in cell membranes, and of the nucleic acids, DNA and RNA. In cells, phosphorus participates in energy metabolism and acid–base regulation. Many signalling molecules depend on the phosphorylation of enzymes to elicit an hormonal response. Approximately 85% of the body's phosphorus is in the skeleton, 14% is associated with soft tissue such as muscle, and 1% is found in the blood and body fluids. Within the physiological range of pH values, inorganic phosphate (Pi) is present in two different ionic species, $H_2PO_4^-$ (monovalent) and HPO_4^{2-} (divalent). The relative concentration of each is dependent on the ambient pH. Thus variation in the pH value may have marked effects on the transport of phosphate by altering the concentration ratio of these phosphate species.

$1\alpha,25$-Dihydroxyvitamin D restores low plasma concentrations of Ca^{2+} and Pi to normal by action at the three major targets, namely intestine, bone and kidney. The hormone (1) stimulates the intestinal absorption of Ca^{2+} and Pi by independent mechanisms, (2) stimulates the transport of Ca^{2+} (accompanied by Pi) from the bone fluid compartment to the extracellular fluid compartment, and (3) facilitates the renal reabsorption of Ca^{2+}. These three mechanisms provide calcium for bone mineralization and prevent hypocalcaemic tetany.

$1\alpha,25$-Dihydroxyvitamin D_3 regulates the synthesis of two classes of calcium-binding proteins (calbindins) found in mammalian intestine and kidney. An intestinal 9-kDa protein (calbindin-D_{9k}) binds two calcium ions per molecule, and a renal 28-kDa protein (calbindin-D_{28k}) binds five to six calcium ions per molecule (Lowe et al., 1992). Gross & Kumar (1990) reviewed extensive evidence that the calbindins are involved in transcellular calcium transport.

8.6.2   Intestinal calcium absorption

Calcium is present in foods and dietary supplements as relatively insoluble salts. Because calcium is absorbed only in its ionized form, it must first be released from the salts. Solubilization of most calcium salts takes place in the acidic medium of the stomach but, on reaching the alkaline environment of the small intestine, some of the Ca^{2+} may complex with minerals or other specific dietary constituents, thereby limiting calcium bioavailability.

The mammalian intestine has developed special vitamin D-dependent mechanisms to ensure the absorption of appropriate amounts of calcium in the face of changing needs and varying dietary calcium intakes. Present knowledge of these mechanisms is rather limited, although it appears that multiple mechanisms are involved. In view of the amount of controversy and continued research into this subject, any model of vitamin D action must be tentative.

Calcium absorption takes place by the translocation of luminal Ca^{2+} through the enterocytes (transcellular route) and between adjacent enterocytes via the tight junctions (paracellular route). Transcellular movement is a saturable, energy-dependent process that is subject to regulation by vitamin D and is confined almost entirely to the duodenum and upper jejunum. In the perfused chick intestine, the stimulation of calcium transport by $1\alpha,25(OH)_2D_3$ is suppressed by $24R,25(OH)_2D_3$ (Nemere, 1999). Paracellular movement is passive, independent of vitamin D status, and exists all along the small intestine (Pansu et al., 1983).

Two models which describe the mechanism of transcellular absorption are the calbindin-based diffusional-active transport model and the vesicular transport model (Wasserman & Fullmer, 1995).

The calbindin-based diffusional-active transport model

This transcellular pathway is a complex process involving three steps: (1) entry by movement of Ca^{2+} from lumen through the brush-border membrane of the enterocyte, (2) intracellular diffusion, and (3) extrusion from the cell across the basolateral membrane. The major action of vitamin D in regulating this process is on the steps involved in Ca^{2+} movement beyond brush-border entry (Roche et al., 1986; Schedl et al., 1994). The concentration of cytosolic Ca^{2+} within the enterocyte is closely controlled at about 10^{-7} M, and this is ultimately a function of the rate of entry and the rate of exit of Ca^{2+} across the cell boundaries. Intracellular organelles, including mitochondria, microsomes and lysosomes, play a major role in controlling cytosolic Ca^{2+} by storing and releasing the cation as appropriate. The overall rate of transcellular movement is determined by the intracellular diffusion, which is the rate-limiting step (Bronner, 1990).

One of the most striking effects of vitamin D is the induction of calbindin-D_{9k}, which is distributed throughout the cytoplasm of the enterocyte. Absence of intestinal calbindin-D_{9k} may be considered a molecular index of vitamin D deficiency (Bronner, 1991).

Entry

This step involves the movement of luminal Ca^{2+} across the brush-border membrane of the enterocyte into the cytosol. The downhill electrochemical gradient permits the entry of luminal Ca^{2+} without the input of metabolic energy.

Fullmer (1992) reviewed data from several laboratories that suggested a 'liponomic regulation' of intestinal calcium transport by $1\alpha,25(OH)_2D_3$. In this model, $1\alpha,25(OH)_2D_3$ alters the phospholipid structure of the brush-border membrane, causing an increase in membrane fluidity, which, in turn, leads to a specific increase in the permeability of the membrane to Ca^{2+}. Among these reports, $1\alpha,25(OH)_2D_3$ enhanced the synthesis of phosphatidylcholine and also increased the incorporation of unsaturated fatty acids into phosphatidylcholine in chick duodenal enterocytes (Matsumoto et al., 1981). Incorporation of methyl cis-vaccinic acid (a fatty acid known to increase membrane fluidity) into brush-border membrane vesicles from vitamin D-deficient chickens caused an increase in rate of vesicular calcium uptake, but there was no such effect in vesicles from $1\alpha,25(OH)_2D_3$-treated chickens. Conversely, methyl trans-vaccinic acid (a fatty acid known to decrease membrane fluidity) caused a decrease in rate of calcium uptake in vesicles from $1\alpha,25(OH)_2D_3$-treated chickens, but no change in vesicles from vitamin D-deficient chickens (Fontaine et al., 1981). Brasitus et al. (1986) demonstrated that the fluidity of the brush-border membrane from vitamin D-deprived rats was lower than that of vitamin D-replete control animals. Treatment with $1\alpha,25(OH)_2D_3$ restored fluidity to control levels within 1–2 hours. The changes in membrane fluidity were associated with appropriate changes in lipid composition, and preceded detectable increases in calcium absorption (demonstrable only during the 5th hour). The lack of temporal correspondence indicates that the early changes in membrane composition attributable to $1\alpha,25(OH)_2D_3$ are probably not a major factor in calcium absorption. The same conclusion was reached by Schedl et al. (1994), who found no significant effect of vitamin D on saturable or nonsaturable uptake of calcium.

The observation that Ca^{2+} uptake at the brush border has a saturable component suggests an interaction with a low-affinity binding site, which might be associated with a calcium channel or a carrier of some sort. The results of in vitro and in vivo studies using calcium channel blocking drugs suggest that voltage-activated calcium channels, such as those found in excitable tissues (nerve, muscle) are unlikely to be present in intestinal brush borders (Favus & Tembe, 1992). This does not exclude the possibility that the brush-border membrane may contain calcium channels with properties distinct from those found in nerve and muscle, although no such channels have as yet been identified in this membrane.

Wilson *et al.* (1989) studied the regulation of saturable Ca^{2+} uptake by rat intestinal brush-border membrane vesicles using the divalent cations strontium (a foreign ion that mimics calcium biologically) and magnesium (a physiologically important ion that resembles calcium physically, although not biologically). Sr^{2+} present outside the vesicle inhibited calcium uptake competitively, while Sr^{2+} inside the vesicle accelerated Ca^{2+} uptake in the manner of countertransport. These events are consistent with the existence in the brush-border membrane of a calcium-transporting protein. Mg^{2+} was a non-competitive inhibitor of saturable Ca^{2+} transport, consistent with a regulatory role in Ca^{2+} uptake by binding to the putative transporter at a locus other than that for Ca^{2+}. The V_{max} of saturable uptake of Ca^{2+} was increased by vitamin D without affecting K_m (Schedl *et al.*, 1994), implying that the response was due to an increase in the number of transporters rather than altered function. Further investigation is needed to confirm the existence and define the nature of the calcium transporter.

Present within the microvillar region of the enterocyte is a relatively high concentration of the ubiquitous calcium-binding protein calmodulin, much of which is associated with the 119-kDa protein in the form of the mechanoenzyme, brush-border myosin I, which is found in the bridges linking the microvillar core bundles of actin filaments with the microvillar plasma membrane. Several studies have demonstrated a role for Ca^{2+} in regulating the mechanochemical activity of brush-border myosin I (Wolenski *et al.*, 1993). Mooseker *et al.* (1991) speculated that brush-border myosin I may somehow affect the permeability of the brush-border membrane through direct tension applied at the cytoplasmic side of the membrane.

In the vitamin D-deficient rat (Sampson *et al.*, 1970) and chick (Chandra *et al.*, 1990) luminal Ca^{2+} readily crosses the brush-border membrane, but remains bound in the microvillus. Vitamin D repletion of the deficient animal results in the mobilization of Ca^{2+} from the microvillar region into the body of the cell. On the basis of these observations and the suggestion of Mooseker *et al.* (1991), Wasserman & Fullmer (1995) proposed the hypothetical mechanism shown in Fig. 8.7 for the control of Ca^{2+} entry. Treatment of Caco-2 cells with the calmodulin antagonist tri-

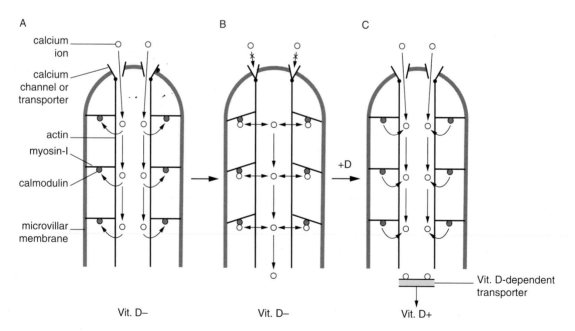

Fig. 8.7 Hypothetical model for the control of calcium entry into the enterocyte. (A) In vitamin D deficiency, part of the calcium that accumulates in the microvillar region reversibly binds to the calmodulin component of brush-border myosin I in the lateral bridges. (B) The activation of myosin I by calcium causes a translocational movement of the actin filaments that results in the closure of putative integral membrane calcium channels to which the filaments are attached. (C) In the vitamin D-replete animal, the calcium is released from calmodulin by preferential binding to the vitamin D-dependent calbindin, causing a deactivation of myosin I and the opening of the calcium channels. Reproduced from Wasserman & Fullmer (1995), *Journal of Nutrition*, Vol. 125, pp. 1971S–9S, with permission from the American Society for Nutritional Sciences.

fluoperazine reduced $1\alpha,25(OH)_2D_3$-stimulated apical-to-basolateral Ca^{2+} transport by 56% (Fleet & Wood, 1999), implicating calmodulin in the transport process.

Intracellular diffusion

This step involves vectorial movement of the transported Ca^{2+} through the cytosol from the apical to the basolateral pole. The rate of unaided Ca^{2+} diffusion through the cytosol of an enterocyte has been calculated to be nearly two orders of magnitude too slow to satisfy the experimentally determined value of V_{max} for transcellular duodenal Ca^{2+} transport (Bronner et al., 1986). This implies that intracellular diffusion will have to be facilitated. A candidate protein for such facilitated diffusion is the vitamin D-inducible protein calbindin-D_{9k}. Active calcium transport rate in everted sacs was proportional to the intestinal concentration of calbindin-D_{9k}; transport was not detectable in vitamin D-deficient rats in which the intestinal calbindin-D_{9k} content is virtually zero (Roche et al. (1986). A model for the intracellular diffusion of Ca^{2+} is shown in Fig. 8.8. The dissociation constants for the brush-border complex, calbindin and the calcium pump favour the apical to basolateral movement of Ca^{2+} (Wasserman & Fullmer, 1995). The sequestration of Ca^{2+} by calmodulin contributes to protection against calcium-mediated cytotoxicity.

Extrusion

The movement of Ca^{2+} out of the cell across the basolateral membrane into the vascular supply of the lamina propria is uphill in terms of both concentration and the prevailing electropotential. An active transport system requiring a source of metabolic energy is therefore needed to pump the Ca^{2+} out of the cell. A basolateral Ca^{2+}-ATPase (calcium pump) identified in enterocytes by Ghijsen et al. (1982) has highest activity in the duodenum with decreasing activity towards the ileum (Ghijsen & van Os, 1982). The calcium pump in the enterocyte basolateral membrane is stimulated by calbindin-D_{9k} (Walters, 1989). It seems reasonable to propose that the binding of Ca^{2+} to calbindin triggers an allosteric activation of the ATPase. A stimulatory effect of $1\alpha,25(OH)_2D_3$ on the ATP-dependent uptake of Ca^{2+} by duodenal basolateral membrane vesicles has been demonstrated in vitamin D-deficient rats (Ghijsen & van Os, 1982;

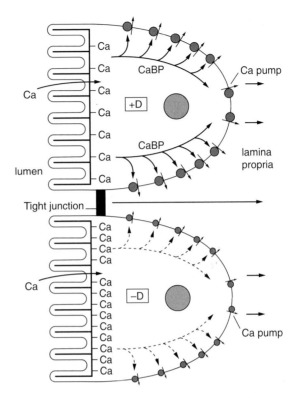

Fig. 8.8 Hypothetical model for the intracellular diffusion of calcium in the enterocyte. (Top) Calcium in the intestinal lumen binds initially to brush-border calmodulin. It is then transferred to cytoplasmic calbindin and thence to the calcium-binding site of the basolateral calcium pump. (Bottom) In vitamin D deficiency, the diffusion rate decreases owing to the reduced cellular content of calbindin. Reproduced from Wasserman & Fullmer (1995), *Journal of Nutrition*, Vol. 125, pp. 1971S–9S, with permission from the American Society for Nutritional Sciences.

Walters & Weiser, 1987; Favus et al., 1989) and chicks (Takito et al., 1990). Immunological studies have shown that feeding vitamin D to chicks previously deprived of the vitamin induces the synthesis of the calcium pump protein (Wasserman et al., 1992). A vitamin D-induced increase in calcium pump mRNA confirmed the effect of vitamin D on gene expression (Zelinski et al., 1991; Armbrecht et al., 1992; Cai et al., 1993). It is noteworthy that $1\alpha,25(OH)_2D_3$ does not stimulate calcium pump activity in vitamin D-replete animals (Favus et al., 1989).

A $3Na^+:1Ca^{2+}$ antiporter plays a secondary role in transporting cytosolic Ca^{2+} across the basolateral membrane and is not regulated by vitamin D. The transport capacity of this exchanger is about 20% of that of the Ca^{2+}-ATPase. However, this transport capacity is constant along the length of the small intestine, and in the ileum both systems are of equal effect (Ghijsen *et al.*, 1983).

The vesicular transport model

Norman's research group (Nemere *et al.*, 1986) proposed an alternative model for transcellular absorption in which Ca^{2+} is recognized at the brush-border membrane by a specific receptor and internalized by endocytosis. The endocytotic vesicles are conveyed along microtubules to lysosomes where fusion of the membrane-bounded organelles occurs. The lysosomes, in turn, move along microtubules to the basolateral membrane where exocytosis of Ca^{2+} and receptor completes the transport process. Disruption of the microtubules by colchicine completely inhibited the rapid effect of $1\alpha,25(OH)_2D_3$ on calcium transport from lumen to blood supply; there was no such inhibition in response to lumicolchicine, a light-inactivated analogue of colchicine (Nemere *et al.*, 1984). deBoland & Norman (1990) considered it conceivable that activation of PKA and PKC by $1\alpha,25(OH)_2D_3$ might stimulate basolateral entry of Ca^{2+} into the enterocyte (transcaltachia) through activation of calcium channels. The transient increase of intracellular Ca^{2+}, in turn, may activate exocytosis of calcium-containing vesicles as well as Ca^{2+} efflux by the calcium pump and the Na^+:Ca^{2+} antiporter, resulting in a net increase of intestinal calcium transport.

Paracellular route

The paracellular movement of calcium occurs largely by diffusion and is independent of vitamin D status and age. Even in total vitamin D deficiency, Ca^{2+} absorption is ensured by the paracellular route (Bronner, 1990). The rate of movement is essentially the same along the entire length of the small intestine. In the rat, some 16% of the luminal content of soluble calcium is absorbed by the paracellular route in 1 hour, regardless of the calcium concentration of the chyme (Bronner *et al.*, 1986). Paracellular calcium movement is dominant under conditions when transcellular transport is down-regulated, as in old age (Armbrecht *et al.*, 1979) or when the food content of calcium is abundant (Pansu *et al.*, 1981).

8.6.3   Renal calcium reabsorption

The kidney plays a crucial role in calcium homeostasis. To maintain a net calcium balance, more than 98% of the filtered load of calcium must be reabsorbed along the nephron. Tubular reabsorption of calcium can take place via the transcellular and paracellular routes by mechanisms similar to those described for calcium transport in the intestine.

Paracellular, diffusional movement predominates in the proximal convoluted tubule and thick ascending limb of Henle's loop, in which the epithelium has a low electrical resistance and hence high permeability. Transcellular, active transport takes place in the distal nephron where the epithelia are less permeable. The rate of active calcium reabsorption is controlled by PTH and $1\alpha,25(OH)_2D_3$. The involvement of calbindin-D_{28k} in active calcium transport is suggested by its exclusive presence in the distal nephron and its increased production in response to $1\alpha,25(OH)_2D_3$ treatment of collecting duct cells (Bindels, 1993).

8.6.4 Na^+/Pi co-transporters

Three families of vertebrate Na^+/Pi co-transporter have been identified: type I, type II (IIa and IIb isoforms) and type III. Type I proteins have been found in the apical membrane of renal proximal tubules, but their function is not yet clearly established. Type II proteins are also located in apical membranes – type IIa in renal proximal tubules and type IIb in small intestinal enterocytes. Type III co-transporters are found in many tissues and appear to be located at the basolateral membrane. Type II (IIa and IIb) Na^+/Pi co-transporters mediate secondary active phosphate transport in which the immediate energy source is the downhill concentration gradient for Na^+ maintained by the action of the sodium pump at the basolateral membrane. The parallel operation of other sodium-coupled transport systems will indirectly affect the Na^+/Pi co-transport rate due to competition for driving forces (Danisi & Murer, 1991). Type II co-transporters operate with a $3Na^+$ to $1Pi$ stoichiometry (Murer *et al.*, 2001). In the presence of divalent phosphate, these transporters interact with the substrate (Pi) followed by the loading of two Na^+ ions. Thus the translocation of the fully loaded transporter is an electroneutral process. The observed negative charge

Vitamin D 213

transfer within the transport cycle is the result of the reorientation of the unloaded transporter (Murer *et al.*, 2002).

8.6.5 Intestinal phosphate absorption

Dietary phosphorus is a mixture of inorganic phosphate and organic phosphorus. The phosphorus in meat and fish exists largely in the form of phosphoproteins and phospholipids; over 80% of the phosphorus in grains such as wheat, rice and maize is found as phytic acid (hexaphosphoinositol); about 33% of the phosphorus in milk exists as inorganic phosphate; milk protein (casein) is particularly highly phosphorylated. Regardless of its dietary form, most phosphorus is absorbed in inorganic form. Organically bound phosphorus is hydrolysed enzymatically in the lumen of the small intestine. The phosphorus within phytic acid has poor bioavailability owing to incomplete hydrolysis.

Phosphate absorption takes place mainly in the jejunum by an energy-dependent transcellular route that is regulatable and a passive paracellular route that is not regulatable. The transcellular pathway involves secondary active transport at the brush-border membrane mediated by the type IIb Na^+/Pi co-transporter. Both the monovalent and divalent forms of phosphate are transported (Quamme, 1985). The capacity (V_{max}) of the transport system is significantly greater at pH 6.1 than at 7.4, thus the acidic environment of the unstirred layer favours Pi uptake (Borowitz & Ghishan, 1989). The basolateral membrane also contains a Na^+/Pi co-transporter, which has a lower capacity and a higher affinity compared to the brush-border co-transporter (Kikuchi & Ghishan, 1987).

A low-phosphorus diet leads to a rapid decrease of plasma Pi concentration and activation of the renal 25(OH)D-1α-hydroxylase. The resultant increase in circulating 1α,25(OH)$_2$D$_3$ induces an increased capacity of the type IIb Na^+/Pi co-transporter in the brush border of the intestinal epithelium. The hormonal response requires several hours and involves protein synthesis. The rapid adaptive response observed in the kidney (see below) does not take place in the intestine (Hattenhauer *et al.*, 1999).

8.6.6 Renal phosphate reabsorption

Renal reabsorption of phosphate takes place in the proximal convoluted tubule and, under normal physi-

ological conditions, ~80% of phosphate contained in the glomerular filtrate is reabsorbed. The brush-border uptake, which is mediated by the type IIa Na^+/Pi co-transporter, is rate-limiting in most situations and the target of physiological control mechanisms. Basolateral exit is ill-defined, but may involve another Na^+/Pi co-transporter (Schwab *et al.*, 1984). Transport of phosphate in the opposite direction (from the peritubular interstitium into the tubular cell) can take place across the basolateral membrane if apical entry is insufficient to satisfy the cell's metabolic requirements.

The existence of multiple systems for transporting phosphate across the brush-border membrane of the tubular epithelium has been recognized since 1977. Walker *et al.* (1987) demonstrated two sodium-dependent systems in the early segments of the proximal tubule: a high-capacity, low-affinity system and a low-capacity, high-affinity system. A third transport system in the late proximal segments was found by the same group to be independent of sodium and mediated by an hydroxyl ion/Pi exchanger or a proton/Pi co-transport system (Yan *et al.*, 1988). The renal control of acid–base balance requires secretion of hydrogen ions into the tubular lumen by the tubular epithelial cells, causing a progressive decrease in luminal pH from 7.4 to 6.8 along the length of the proximal tubule. Such a decline in pH results in a fall of the divalent to monovalent phosphate ratio from 4:1 to 1:1 at any given Pi concentration (Quamme & Wong, 1984). It has been demonstrated that the two sodium-dependent systems mentioned above transport the divalent form of phosphate, whereas the sodium-independent system located in the late proximal tubule has a preference for the monovalent form (Yan *et al.*, 1988). Accordingly, the multiple transport systems act in concert to reclaim filtered phosphate along the proximal tubule.

The rate of renal phosphate reabsorption is adjusted in response to deviations in plasma Pi concentration to achieve a correct phosphate homeostasis. A low-phosphorus diet induces a rapid (2–4 hour) nongenomic response followed by a long-term genomic response if phosphorus deprivation persists. Both types of response involve stimulation of sodium-dependent phosphate transport by 1α,25(OH)$_2$D$_3$. The rapid response may be mediated by a microtubule-dependent translocation of the Na^+/Pi co-transporter protein from intracellular compartments to the brush-border membrane (Lötscher *et al.*, 1996). Rapid down-regulation of the co-transporter in response to acute administration of a large dose of phosphate is probably mediated by endocytosis of the protein (Lötscher *et al.*, 1996). The long-term response involves transactivation of the Na⁺/Pi co-transporter gene (Taketani *et al.*, 1997).

8.6.7 Calcium movement in bone

Bone contains a fluid compartment that is separated from the extracellular fluid by the lining cells on the surface of bone. As shown in Fig. 8.9, the bone fluid compartment comprises the fluid-filled space between the lining cells and bone matrix, around the protoplasmic extensions in the canaliculi, and around osteocytes in their lacunae. The bone fluid is therefore in direct contact with bone crystals or amorphous calcium phosphate deposits (Talmage, 1970).

The Ca^{2+} concentration in the bone fluid compartment is normally about one-third that in the extracellular fluid. The lining cells exert the primary control on extracellular calcium homeostasis. These cells have open channels between them, permitting paracellular entry of Ca^{2+} into the bone fluid compartment down the concentration gradient. The uphill movement of Ca^{2+} from the bone fluid compartment to the extracellular fluid involves active pump-driven transport through the lining cells.

In the presence of vitamin D, parathyroid hormone (PTH) increases the calcium permeability of the lining cell plasma membrane facing the bone fluid, allowing Ca^{2+} to diffuse into the cells from the bone fluid. The increase in intracellular Ca^{2+} then activates the calcium pump on the opposite membrane. This action of PTH results in the rapid removal of Ca^{2+}, accompanied by Pi, from amorphous calcium phosphate deposits in the vicinity of the lining cells and transference of these ions to the extracellular fluid.

8.6.8 Vitamin D action on bone

It is well documented that $1\alpha,25(OH)_2D_3$ is required for normal development and mineralization of bone, and for bone remodelling. The results of some studies suggest that the effect of $1\alpha,25(OH)_2D_3$ on bone is indirect, being attributable to the increased availability of calcium and phosphate for incorporation into bone that results from the increased intestinal absorption of these minerals. Rickets can be cured in

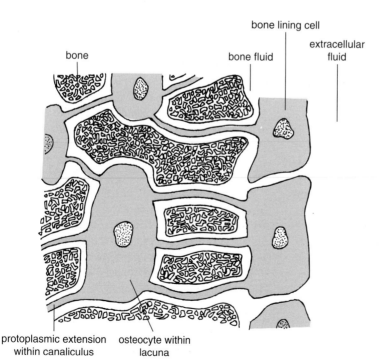

bone lining cell

bone   bone fluid   extracellular fluid

protoplasmic extension   osteocyte within
within canaliculus   lacuna

Fig. 8.9 The extracellular fluid and bone fluid compartments.

vitamin D-deficient rats by increasing the calcium and phosphorus content of the diet (Holtrop et al., 1986; Clark et al., 1987) or by maintaining normal circulating concentrations of these minerals through infusion (Underwood & DeLuca, 1984; Weinstein et al., 1984). The use of intravenous (Balsan et al., 1986) and combined intravenous and oral (Al-Alqel et al., 1993) calcium is also effective for the treatment of hereditary vitamin D resistant rickets, a childhood disease arising from a lack of responsiveness of target tissues to $1\alpha,25(OH)_2D_3$. In VDR-ablated mice, skeletal defects were evident in the hypocalcaemic state, but similar mice fed a calcium/phosphorus/lactose-enriched diet to normalize their mineral ion homeostasis did not develop skeletal defects (Amling et al., 1999).

A major physiological function of $1\alpha,25(OH)_2D_3$ in calcium homeostasis is stimulation of bone resorption, which refers to localized bone dissolution by osteoclasts with resultant net calcium movement from bone to blood. The hormone acts by increasing the expression of proteins essential to the resorptive process, proteins such as carbonic anhydrase. The hormone also inhibits bone formation by decreasing alkaline phosphatase activity (Manolagas et al., 1981) and collagen synthesis (Rowe & Kream, 1982) in osteoblasts and increasing the synthesis of osteocalcin, a potent inhibitor of mineralization (Price, 1985).

Three events are essential in osteoclastic bone resorption: (1) differentiation of osteoclast progenitors into mature osteoclasts (2) attachment of osteoclasts to the bone matrix and (3) activation of quiescent osteoclasts.

Differentiation of osteoclast progenitors into mature osteoclasts

$1\alpha,25$-Dihydroxyvitamin D_3 enhances bone resorption by stimulating differentiation and fusion of mononuclear osteoclast progenitors into mature multinucleated osteoclasts (Clohisy et al., 1987; Takahashi et al., 1988). This process, osteoclastogenesis, involves a complex interaction of osteoclast progenitors, osteoblasts and bone marrow-derived stromal cells (Suda et al., 1992a). Studies using VDR-ablated mice showed that stimulation of osteoclast formation by $1\alpha,25(OH)_2D_3$ requires the presence of VDR in osteoblast-like cells but not in osteoclast precursor cells; however, if VDR is absent in the osteoblastic cells, PTH or interleukin-1α can stimulate osteoclast formation (Takeda et al., 1999).

Stromal cells of the bone marrow control osteoclastogenesis through the production of cytokines capable of promoting the proliferation and differentiation of osteoclast progenitors. One particular cytokine, interleukin-11 (IL-11), is a rather specific product of the mesenchymal cell lineage, which includes bone marrow stromal cells and osteoblasts (Paul et al., 1990). IL-11 is a potent inducer of osteoclast development (Girasole et al., 1994) and its production by primary osteoblasts can be stimulated by $1\alpha,25(OH)_2D_3$ among other osteoclastogenic factors (Romas et al., 1996). The addition of anti-IL-11 antibody to bone marrow cell cultures suppresses the ability of $1\alpha,25(OH)_2D_3$ to induce osteoclast development (Girasole et al., 1994), suggesting that IL-11 is an essential factor for the osteoclastogenic effect of $1\alpha,25(OH)_2D_3$. Another soluble factor, macrophage-colony stimulating factor (M-CSF), is essential for osteoclast differentiation from progenitors, but its production by osteoblasts/stromal cells does not appear to be regulated by $1\alpha,25(OH)_2D_3$ (Suda et al., 1992a).

In 1997, two independent research groups reported the discovery of novel cytokines which inhibited the differentiation of osteoclast progenitors into mature osteoclasts. These secreted proteins were named osteoclastogenesis inhibitory factor (OCIF) and osteoprotegerin (OPG) by the respective groups (Tsuda et al., 1997; Simonet et al., 1997). Yasuda et al. (1998a) found these two proteins to be identical, hence the present term, OPG/OCIF. Transgenic mice with over-expressed OPG/OCIF and mice injected with OPG/OCIF exhibited profound yet non-lethal osteopetrosis, coincident with arrested osteoclast development in the later stages (Simonet et al., 1997). Yasuda et al. (1998a) reported that the expression of the OPG/OCIF gene in stromal cells is down-regulated by $1\alpha,25(OH)_2D_3$ and up-regulated by calcium ions. These results imply that OPG/OCIF regulates osteoclastogenesis in response to stimulators of bone resorption and calcium ions released at bone-resorbing sites.

$1\alpha,25$-Dihydroxyvitamin D_3, along with PTH and a number of other factors, stimulate osteoclastogenesis through signal transduction pathways mediated by an osteoclast differentiation factor (ODF) on the membrane of osteoblasts/stromal cells (Suda et al., 1992b). OPG/OCIF inhibits in vitro osteoclastogenesis by directly binding to the ODF, thereby interrupting ODF-mediated signalling from osteoblast/stromal cells to osteoclast progenitors for their differentiation into mature osteoclasts (Tsuda *et al.*, 1997). $1\alpha,25$-Dihydroxyvitamin D_3, by down-regulating OPG/OCIF, permits osteoclastic bone resorption.

Yasuda *et al.* (1998b) showed that ODF is identical to a regulator of T lymphocyte cells and dendritic cells designated TRANCE or RANKL. Expression of the TRANCE/RANKL/ODF gene was up-regulated by osteotropic factors, including $1\alpha,25(OH)_2D_3$.

Sato *et al.* (1991) reported that mouse bone marrow-derived stromal cells and primary osteoblastic cells *in vitro* produce the third component of complement (C3) in response to $1\alpha,25(OH)_2D_3$. This appears to be a bone-specific effect as C3 production by hepatocytes is not dependent on $1\alpha,25(OH)_2D_3$. Bone C3 is also induced tissue-specifically by $1\alpha,25(OH)_2D_3$ *in vivo* (Jin *et al.*, 1992). Actinomycin D completely inhibits the effect of $1\alpha,25(OH)_2D_3$ on both mRNA expression and protein production of C3, indicating that the hormone acts at the transcriptional level (Hong *et al.*, 1991). The addition of anti-C3 antibody to mouse bone marrow cultures completely inhibits the $1\alpha,25(OH)_2D_3$-induced formation of osteoclast-like cells, suggesting that the C3 produced by stromal cells in response to $1\alpha,25(OH)_2D_3$ is somehow involved in osteoclast formation (Sato *et al.*, 1991). The production of C3 in stromal cells and osteoblastic cells is also stimulated by local bone-resorbing agents, such as interleukin-1, tumour necrosis factor-α and lipopolysaccharides (Hong *et al.*, 1991). Sato *et al.* (1993) concluded that the bone C3, acting in concert with other factors induced by $1\alpha,25(OH)_2D_3$, potentiates proliferation of bone marrow cells and induces differentiation of these cells into osteoclasts.

Attachment of osteoclasts to the bone matrix
1,25-Dihydroxyvitamin D_3 activates the transcription of integrin α_v and β_3 subunit genes, resulting in an increased number of integrin $\alpha_v\beta_3$ receptors on the surface of osteoclast progenitors (Medhora *et al.*, 1993; Mimura *et al.*, 1994). These receptors recognize and bind to the bone matrix proteins osteopontin and bone sialoprotein. Expression of integrin $\alpha_v\beta_3$ coincides with the differentiation of progenitors into osteoclasts and is essential to the resorptive process.

Activation of quiescent osteoclasts
$1\alpha,25$-Dihydroxyvitamin D_3 stimulates osteoclastic bone resorption in tissue culture (Raisz *et al.*, 1972)

and in rat bones *in vivo* (Holtrop *et al.*, 1981). Mc-Sheehy & Chambers (1987) reported that isolated osteoclasts do not respond to $1\alpha,25(OH)_2D_3$ if incubated alone, but they do so if incubated in the presence of osteoblastic-like cells. Incubation of osteoblastic cells in the presence of $1\alpha,25(OH)_2D_3$ produced a soluble factor that stimulated osteoclastic bone resorption. Jimi *et al.* (1996) demonstrated that cell-to-cell contact between osteoblastic cells and osteoclast-like cells was required to promote pit-forming activity. Mee *et al.* (1996) were the first to show that active human osteoclasts *in vivo* possess mRNA for the VDR. It seems, therefore, $1\alpha,25(OH)_2D_3$ can act directly on osteoclasts to stimulate bone resorption as well as indirectly through its effects on osteoblasts.

8.6.9   Calcium homeostasis

The control of calcium homeostasis involves three major sites: bone, the kidneys and the intestine. Bone is the major reservoir of calcium in the body, storing around 99% of the total. The role of bone in calcium homeostasis is to 'buffer' blood calcium level, releasing Ca^{2+} to the blood when the blood level decreases and taking Ca^{2+} back when the level rises. Calcium homeostasis is coordinately regulated by $1\alpha,25(OH)_2D_3$ and parathyroid hormone (PTH), with calcitonin playing an important supporting role. PTH is a peptide hormone produced by the parathyroid glands in response to low plasma calcium levels. Its action is mediated by PKA via the second messenger cyclic AMP (cAMP) (Horiuchi *et al.*, 1977). In the kidney, PTH activates the 25(OH)D_3-1α-hydroxylase by increasing the enzyme's mRNA through effects on gene transcription (Brenza *et al.*, 1998; Murayama *et al.*, 1998). Simultaneously, PTH suppresses the renal 24R-hydroxylase (Shinki *et al.*, 1992), the enzyme responsible for catalysing the C-24 oxidation pathway. This reciprocal regulation by PTH in the kidney allows for $1\alpha,25(OH)_2D_3$ production with minimal concomitant catabolism. The effect of $1\alpha,25(OH)_2D_3$ is to restore plasma calcium levels to normal. PTH has no effect on intestinal 24R-hydroxylase activity (Shinki *et al.*, 1992), which is not surprising as the intestine lacks PTH receptors. In osteoblasts, PTH acts synergistically with $1\alpha,25(OH)_2D_3$ to increase transcription of the 24R-hydroxylase gene (Armbrecht *et al.*, 1998). Thus PTH exerts opposite effects in kidney and bone with respect to 24R-hydroxylase regulation.

Activation of the 24R-hydroxylase in bone is a means of regulating the resorptive action of 1α,25(OH)$_2$D$_3$. Cycloheximide has no effect on the capacity of PTH to increase 24R-hydroxylase mRNA levels in osteoblasts, showing that the action of PTH does not require new protein synthesis. One possible mechanism by which PTH could increase 24R-hydroxylase promoter activity in conjunction with 1α,25(OH)$_2$D$_3$ is phosphorylation of the cAMP-response element binding protein (CREB) by PKA and consequent binding of the CREB to a cAMP-response element (CRE). Interaction between CREB/CRE and VDR/VDRE complexes would synergistically increase 24R-hydroxylase promoter activity.

PTH and 1α,25(OH)$_2$D$_3$ mutually regulate each other's synthesis and/or secretion. PTH down-regulates VDR abundance in the kidney (Reinhardt & Horst, 1990), while 1α,25(OH)$_2$D$_3$ lowers pre-proPTH mRNA levels in the parathyroids (Silver *et al.*, 1985, 1986) with a subsequent reduction in PTH secretion (Cantley *et al.*, 1985). In osteoblastic cells, 1α,25(OH)$_2$D$_3$ reduces PTH-stimulated cAMP production (Pols *et al.*, 1986), while PTH up-regulates VDR abundance (Krishnan *et al.*, 1995).

The homeostatic control of calcium is represented schematically in Fig. 8.10. In response to a lowered concentration of serum Ca^{2+}, the parathyroid glands are stimulated, within minutes, to secrete PTH. This hormone stimulates, within hours, the activity of renal 25(OH)D-1α-hydroxylase. The 1α,25(OH)$_2$D$_3$ thus produced acts by itself to initiate active calcium transport in the intestine. In bone, 1α,25(OH)$_2$D$_3$ acts synergistically with PTH to mobilize Ca^{2+} (accompanied by Pi) from the bone fluid compartment into the bloodstream. The presence of both PTH and the vitamin D hormone are required for this system to operate *in vivo* (Jones *et al.*, 1998). In the kidney, PTH and 1α,25(OH)$_2$D$_3$ act in concert to cause the reabsorption of the last 1% of the filtered load of calcium into the plasma compartment. The resultant increase in the concentration of circulating Ca^{2+} provides a powerful negative feedback signal to the parathyroids, suppressing the secretion of PTH and ultimately stopping the renal production of 1α,25(OH)$_2$D$_3$.

Calcitonin, a known inhibitor of osteoclastic bone resorption, is secreted by parafollicular cells of the thyroid gland in response to elevated serum Ca^{2+}. Total thyroidectomy without calcitonin replacement does not result in any demonstrable derangement of calcium or phosphate homeostasis, therefore the hormone does not seem to be important in 'normal' bone metabolism. It has been suggested that calcitonin may be important during periods of heightened calcaemic challenge, such as growth, pregnancy and lactation.

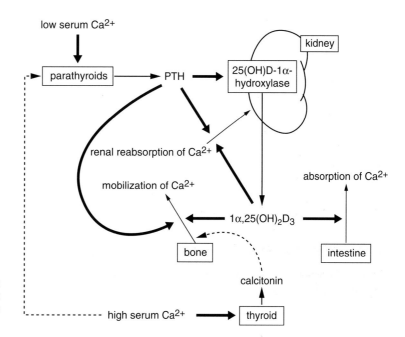

Fig. 8.10 Simplified diagram of calcium homeostasis. The heavy solid lines represent stimulatory effects and the dotted lines represent inhibitory effects.

PTH-related peptide shares a common receptor with PTH and binds to this receptor with equal affinity. Consequently, the peptide elicits a similar range of biological activities to PTH. The peptide normally circulates at considerably lower concentration than PTH and probably has no major role in the day-to-day maintenance of calcium and phosphate. However, the related peptide may be important in certain special processes, such as placental calcium transport, possibly as an autocrine or paracrine agent (Lobaugh, 1996).

8.6.10   Phosphate homeostasis

Plasma phosphate levels are maintained within a concentration range of 1.12–1.45 mM. The restoration of the normal plasma calcium level in response to hypocalcaemia is not accompanied by a rise in plasma phosphate because PTH independently causes a phosphate diuresis. Unlike calcium, dietary phosphate usually exceeds the body's nutritional requirement, therefore a major component of phosphate homeostasis is renal excretion. A diet that is low in phosphorus is likely to be low also in calcium, which complicates the picture of phosphate homeostasis. Let us consider a hypothetical situation of a normal plasma calcium level during hypophosphataemia. A lowering of plasma phosphate will stimulate the kidney to release $1\alpha,25(OH)_2D_3$, which elicits both the previously mentioned rapid (nongenomic) and long-term (genomic) responses in the kidney, leading to increased renal reabsorption of phosphate. The $1\alpha,25(OH)_2D_3$ will also increase the intestinal absorption of phosphate and calcium. The parathyroids will not be stimulated to produce PTH. In the absence of PTH, mobilization of phosphate from the bone will be retarded and there will be no phosphate diuresis. The net effect will be an elevation of plasma phosphate. Hyperphosphataemia is countered through phosphate excretion, governed by the fact that the blood phosphate concentration is maintained at or near the renal transport maximum for the ion.

8.6.11   Effects of vitamin D deficiency

Vitamin D deficiency can arise from lack of sunlight exposure, lack of dietary vitamin D intake, or im-

paired intestinal absorption of the vitamin. At the onset of deficiency, there is a decreased efficiency of intestinal calcium absorption and a consequent fall in the plasma calcium level. In response to the hypocalcaemia, the plasma Ca^{2+} concentration is restored to normal, but the Pi concentration falls. The rise in Ca^{2+} concentration is caused principally by two effects. Firstly, PTH, acting with whatever $1\alpha,25(OH)_2D$ is still present at the onset of deficiency, elicits the mobilization of Ca^{2+} and Pi from bone; secondly, PTH, acting alone, causes an increase in the renal reabsorption of calcium. The decline in plasma Pi concentration is caused by a very strong effect of PTH on the kidney in causing excessive phosphate excretion, an effect that is usually great enough to override increased phosphate mobilization from the bone.

During prolonged vitamin D deficiency, the increase in PTH secretion necessary to maintain calcium homeostasis causes extreme osteoclastic resorption of bone. This in turn causes the bone to become progressively weaker and imposes marked physical stress on the bone, resulting in rapid osteoblastic activity. The osteoblasts lay down large quantities of osteoid but, because of insufficient Ca^{2+} and Pi, calcification does not occur. Thus failure to calcify newly formed bone matrix leads ultimately to rickets or osteomalacia.

8.7   Immunoregulatory properties

Background information can be found in Chapter 5.

8.7.1   Presence of the vitamin D receptor in cells of the immune system

The VDR has been identified in almost all nucleated cell types in the body, including malignant and non-malignant cells of haemopoietic origin. Peripheral blood monocytes express the VDR constitutively. Resting T and B lymphocytes do not express the VDR: only when activated by mitogens and antigens do these cells express the receptor. Interaction of T-cell receptors with the peptide–MHC complex of antigen-presenting tissue cells and cells of the immune system leads to T-cell activation and subsequent gene expression events (Manolagas et al., 1990).

8.7.2   In vitro effects of 1α,25-dihydroxy-vitamin D₃ on cells of the immune system

Monocytes/macrophages

1α,25-Dihydroxyvitamin D_3 inhibits proliferation and promotes differentiation of bone marrow-derived macrophage precursors and specifically promotes expression of the differentiation-associated cell membrane receptor (mannose receptor) (Clohisy et al., 1987). The relatively quiescent resident macrophages are activated by immunogenic stimuli to become activated macrophages, now with a greatly enhanced ability to phagocytose and destroy pathogens.

1α,25-Dihydroxyvitamin D_3 appears to be essential for macrophage activation. Gavison & Bar-Shavit (1989) reported that macrophages from vitamin D-deficient mice injected with activating or eliciting agents had defective anti-tumour activity and an impaired respiratory burst (low production of hydrogen peroxide and superoxide). Activity of the lysosomal enzyme acid phosphatase was unaffected by vitamin D deficiency. Incubation of the vitamin D-deficient macrophages with 1α,25$(OH)_2D_3$ markedly enhanced their anti-tumour activity, but did not affect the cells' capacity to produce hydrogen peroxide and superoxide, or acid phosphatase. Abe et al. (1984) reported that 1α,25$(OH)_2D_3$ increases the number of Fc receptors on the surface of macrophages and induces cytotoxicity.

In cultured monocytes, 1α,25$(OH)_2D_3$ enhances by two- to three-fold the IFN-γ-induced expression of major histocompatibility complex (MHC) class II molecules that mediate antigen presentation to T lymphocytes (Morel et al., 1986). Pre-treatment of normal human monocytes with 1,25$(OH)_2D_3$ enhances their responsiveness to various chemoattractants (Girasole et al., 1990). Augmented monocyte chemotaxis to FMLP is associated with an increased number of high-affinity binding sites for this chemoattractant. The hormone is also able to stimulate the migratory capacity of monocytes obtained from patients with acquired immune deficiency syndrome (AIDS), a condition associated with impaired monocyte chemotaxis. 1α,25$(OH)_2D_3$ increased production of IL-1 by human peripheral blood monocytes (Bhalla et al., 1986) and also enhanced these cells' capacity for lipopolysaccharide-triggered release of tumour necrosis factor (Rook et al., 1987). Incubation of monocytes with 1α,25$(OH)_2D_3$ at 45°C led

to an increased synthesis of heat shock proteins accompanied by a relative preservation of total protein synthesis (Polla et al., 1986).

It has been postulated that vitamin D may have a protective role in tuberculosis infection (Davies, 1985). The bacterium responsible for tuberculosis is a bacillus, Mycobacterium tuberculosis. Monocytes, although phagocytic, have only a limited capacity to kill M. tuberculosis and can become infected with the bacillus in vitro. However, any bacilli released by dying monocytes are rapidly phagocytosed by other cells, especially macrophages, and destroyed. Rook et al. (1986) reported that 1α,25$(OH)_2D_3$ inhibited the growth of M. tuberculosis in cultured human monocytes and IFN-γ enhanced this inhibition. They also showed that incubation of monocytes with IFN-γ led to increased ability to metabolize 25$(OH)D_3$ to 1α,25$(OH)_2D_3$. This ability has also been demonstrated in normal human macrophages (Koeffler et al., 1985). Based on these observations, a possible scenario is that infected monocytes produce IFN-γ which induces these cells to synthesize 1α,25$(OH)_2D_3$ from circulating 25$(OH)D_3$. The locally produced hormone stimulates monocytes to differentiate into macrophages, which are better equipped to deal with the infection.

Natural killer cells

Merino et al. (1989) showed that 1,25$(OH)_2D_3$ inhibits the generation of cytotoxic activity from cultured natural killer cells. The hormone was, however, unable to interfere with the cytotoxic function of cells already established, placing the inhibition at the level of natural killer cell activation.

Lymphocytes

In contrast to the stimulatory effects of 1α,25$(OH)_2D_3$ on the innate arm of the immune response, the principal action of the hormone on the acquired immune response, mediated by lymphocytes, is immunosuppression. 1α,25$(OH)_2D_3$ inhibits T-lymphocyte proliferation after these cells have been activated and the VDR is expressed. The hormone prevents entry of the cells into the S phase of the cell cycle by blocking the RNA synthesis required for the transition of cells from early G1 to late G1 (Rigby et al., 1985). 1α,25-Dihydroxyvitamin D_3 also inhibits the growth-promoting interleukin-2 (IL-2) (Tsoukas et al., 1984). Inhibitors of IL-2 synthesis block the cell cycle at the same point as $1\alpha,25(OH)_2D_3$ blocks the cycle, suggesting that the inhibitory effect of $1\alpha,25(OH)_2D_3$ on T-cell proliferation is mediated by IL-2. Alroy *et al.* (1995) demonstrated that $1\alpha,25(OH)_2D_3$ represses IL-2 gene transcription by a direct, VDR-dependent effect. In the absence of intracellular $1\alpha,25(OH)_2D_3$, the IL-2 gene in T lymphocytes is activated by the binding of a T-cell-specific transcription factor, NFATp, to an NF-AT-1 element and subsequent recruitment of the ubiquitous transcription factors Jun and Fos (AP-1). VDR–RXR heterodimers, which would form in response to the intracellular presence of $1\alpha,25(OH)_2D_3$, directly inhibit the interaction between AP-1 and NFATp. Moreover, the stable binding of VDR–RXR to the NF-AT-1 element blocks the binding of any NFATp–AP-1 that may subsequently be formed; however, prebound NFATp–AP-1 cannot be destabilized by VDR–RXR. The suppressive effect of $1\alpha,25(OH)_2D_3$ on lymphocyte proliferation is countered indirectly by IL-1 produced by monocytes in response to stimulation by $1\alpha,25(OH)_2D_3$ (Bhalla *et al.*, 1986). IL-1 potentiates the release of IL-2 from activated T cells and the IL-2 stimulates lymphocyte proliferation. These differential effects of $1\alpha,25(OH)_2D_3$ provide a finely tuned mechanism for regulating T-cell proliferation.

Lemire *et al.* (1984) demonstrated an inhibitory role of $1\alpha,25(OH)_2D_3$ on proliferation and immunoglobulin production by normal activated human peripheral blood mononuclear cells *in vitro*. Further studies revealed the T helper cell to be particularly suppressed by $1\alpha,25(OH)_2D_3$ (Lemire *et al.*, 1985). T helper cells are divided into Th1 and Th2 subsets on the basis of their pattern of cytokine secretion. Th1 cells secrete interleukin (IL-2) and interferon (IFN-γ) and induce B cells to produce immunoglobulin IgG_{2a}, while Th2 cells secrete IL-4 and IL-10 and induce the production of IgG_1 and IgE by B cells. IL-12 that is produced by macrophages and B cells induces IFN-γ secretion by natural killer cells and Th1 cells and promotes the differentiation of Th1 cells from their uncommitted precursors.

Pre-incubation of T helper cells with $1\alpha,25(OH)_2D_3$ prevents these cells from inducing B cells to synthesize immunoglobulin. The hormone also reduces mRNA levels for IL-2 and IFN-γ in T helper cells. These observations are consistent with a selective suppressive effect of $1\alpha,25(OH)_2D_3$ on Th1 cells. $1\alpha,25(OH)_2D_3$ also inhibits the secretion of IL-12 by macrophages

and B cells, thereby preventing the differentiation of precursor cells to Th1 cells (Lemire *et al.*, 1995). Thus, the immunosuppressive activity of $1\alpha,25(OH)_2D_3$ that takes place *in vitro* is aimed specifically at Th1 cells, preventing their expression both directly or indirectly through inhibition of macrophage-derived IL-12.

Meehan *et al.* (1992) studied the effects of $1\alpha,25(OH)_2D_3$ on the human mixed lymphocyte reaction (MLR), the *in vitro* model of transplant compatibility. The hormone stimulated suppressor T-cell activity and prevented the generation of cytotoxic T-cell activity. A significant reduction in expression of MHC class II molecules (but not class I molecules) was also observed in the presence of the hormone. The suppression of IFN-γ production by $1\alpha,25(OH)_2D_3$ could explain the latter effect. The effects of $1\alpha,25(OH)_2D_3$ on the MLR are similar to those of the potent immunosuppressive drug, cyclosporin A (Hess & Tutschka, 1980).

8.7.3   Immunomodulatory role of $1\alpha,25$-dihydroxyvitamin D_3 in vivo

A beneficial role for vitamin D in the human immune system is suggested by the increase in susceptibility to infection of vitamin D-deficient children (El-Radi *et al.*, 1982). There are many laboratory reports that vitamin D deficiency impairs an animal's ability to mount an acute inflammatory response. Macrophages from vitamin D-deficient mice exhibited decreased migration and phagocytosis, which were both corrected when vitamin D was restored to the diet (Bar-Shavit *et al.*, 1981). The impaired phagocytic response could be corrected by incubating the macrophages with $1\alpha,25(OH)_2D_3$, but other vitamin D metabolites were without effect. Macrophages from vitamin D-deficient mice also had a defective capacity to produce cytokines (Kankova *et al.*, 1991). Yang *et al.* (1993a) showed that vitamin D deficiency suppresses cell-mediated immunity *in vivo*. The provision of a vitamin D-sufficient diet for 8 weeks (but not 3 weeks) corrected the impaired immunity in mice.

At pharmacological doses, $1\alpha,25(OH)_2D_3$ can act as an immunosuppressant *in vivo*. Daily injections of the hormone markedly suppressed immunoglobulin production and thymic lymphocyte proliferation in mice (Yang *et al.*, 1993b). The immunosuppressive properties of $1\alpha,25(OH)_2D_3$ have extended the therapeutic potential of vitamin D analogues in the treatment of autoimmune diseases and graft rejection. $1\alpha,25$-Dihydroxyvitamin D_3 itself cannot be used therapeutically at above physiological concentrations because of its toxicity (hypercalcaemic activity). Various analogues display reduced hypercalcaemic activity compared to the hormone, but their immunosuppressive activity is enhanced 10–100-fold. In experimental autoimmune encephalomyelitis, a mouse model of human multiple sclerosis, intraperitoneal injection of $1\alpha,25(OH)_2D_3$ prevents the disease entirely or arrests its development (Lemire, 1992). In another murine model of autoimmunity, the experimental autoimmune thyroiditis, Fournier *et al.* (1990) demonstrated a beneficial effect of combined treatment with $1\alpha,25(OH)_2D_3$ and cyclosporin A. Johnsson *et al.* (1995) reported enhanced cardiac allograft survival with a combination of a vitamin D analogue (MC 1288) and cyclosporin A.

Lymphocytes from rheumatoid arthritis patients, but not from normal subjects, spontaneously express the VDR (Manolagas *et al.*, 1989). Exposure of T lymphocytes from rheumatoid arthritis patients to a combination of cyclosporin A and $1\alpha,25(OH)_2D_3$ resulted in a synergistic inhibition of both IL-2 production and the proliferation of cells (Gepner *et al.*, 1989). This *in vitro* synergism occurred at a concentration of cyclosporin A (1 ng mL^{-1}) that was 100 times lower than the optimal dose *per se*. The potentiating concentration of $1\alpha,25(OH)_2D_3$ was in the physiological, non-toxic range. Boissier *et al.* (1992) found that a combination of cyclosporin A and $1\alpha,25(OH)_2D_3$ was additively beneficial in the treatment of adjuvant arthritis, an animal model of rheumatoid arthritis.

8.7.4 Summary

In its capacity as an immunoregulator, $1\alpha,25(OH)_2D_3$ functions as a paracrine hormone. Activation of macrophages by IFN-γ at the site of infection or tissue inflammation induces 1α-hydroxylase activity and localized generation of $1\alpha,25(OH)_2D_3$ from $25(OH)D_3$. The $1\alpha,25(OH)_2D_3$ thus produced enhances the immune response in many ways. As discussed above, it activates resident macrophages; promotes macrophage precursor cell differentiation; recruits monocytes to the affected site by chemotaxis and induction of adhesion molecules in capillary endothelial cells; and activates T lymphocytes via antigen presentation

and cytokine secretion. These stimulatory effects of $1\alpha,25(OH)_2D_3$ are countered by its suppressive effect upon lymphocytes, which represents part of the feedback control of the immune response.

8.8 Effects of vitamin D on insulin secretion

$1\alpha,25$-Dihydroxyvitamin D_3 is considered to be a modulator of insulin secretion because vitamin D deficiency in rats is associated with marked impairment of insulin secretion (Chertow *et al.*, 1983) and the insulin-secreting β-cells of the pancreas contain the vitamin D-regulated protein calbindin-D_{28k} (Buffa *et al.*, 1989) as well as the VDR (Clark *et al.*, 1980). Lee *et al.* (1994) speculated that $1\alpha,25(OH)_2D_3$ may primarily affect intracellular calcium mobilization, resulting in an inhibition or stimulation of insulin secretion depending on the vitamin D status and other biochemical variables.

8.9 Vitamin D-related diseases

8.9.1 Rickets and osteomalacia

Rickets
Rickets, a word from the Anglo-Saxon *wrikken* (to twist) is the classic vitamin D deficiency disease in children. The disease is characterized by bow legs or knock knees, curvature of the spine, and pelvic and thoracic bone deformities. These deformities result from the mechanical stresses of body weight and muscular activity applied to the soft uncalcified bone.

Without vitamin D, the cartilaginous growth plate of the growing child fails to calcify. With this defect, the cartilage cannot be replaced by bone on the diaphyseal side and the growth plate becomes progressively thicker. This results in enlargement of the joints in the knees, wrists and ankles.

The prevalence of rickets among city-dwelling children during the industrial revolution was attributable to a limited exposure to sunlight and a lack of sufficient vitamin D in the diet. The narrow streets and alleys in which the children lived and the smoke-polluted atmosphere were responsible for the lack of sunlight. During the 1930s, the practice of adding provitamin D to milk followed by UV irradiation drastically reduced the incidence of rickets in the

United States and some European countries. Later, the commercial production of crystalline vitamin D_2 led to its use in the fortification of foods. Nowadays, rickets is a rare disease among the indigenous populations of the United States and Europe, but it is still evident among the children of immigrants, particularly Asians in Europe.

Osteomalacia

In adults, when the skeleton is fully developed, vitamin D is still necessary for the continuous remodelling of bone. During prolonged vitamin D deficiency, the newly formed, uncalcified bone tissue gradually takes the place of the older bone tissue and the weakened bone structure is easily prone to fracture. This condition, osteomalacia, should not be confused with osteoporosis in which the ratio of mineral to osteoid is unchanged. In osteomalacia, the epiphyses do not swell, as they do in rickets, because the epiphyseal growth plates no longer exist. Patients with osteomalacia frequently suffer from muscle weakness and bone tenderness or pain in the spine, shoulder, ribs or pelvis. Pelvic deformation can occur causing potential problems with childbirth. Women with low vitamin D status may develop osteomalacia after several pregnancies because they are unable to replace the calcium lost from their bone reserves to the fetus *in utero* and in lactation.

8.9.2 Vitamin D-dependent rickets

Vitamin D-dependent rickets is a rare inherited disorder in which clinical and biochemical features of rickets are evident despite an adequate intake of vitamin D. This disorder is classified into type I and type II disease states, both of which appear to follow an autosomal recessive pattern of inheritance (Brown *et al.*, 2000).

Type I

Type I vitamin D-dependent rickets arises from impaired renal synthesis of $1\alpha,25(OH)_2D_3$, which may be due to a mutation in the gene encoding 25(OH)D-1α-hydroxylase. The disease is diagnosed by normal blood levels of 25(OH)D and profoundly decreased levels of $1\alpha,25(OH)_2D_3$. At birth, affected children appear healthy, but during the first year or two of life severe hypocalcaemia with tetany becomes evident. The hypocalcaemia leads to secondary hyperparathyroidism with elevated PTH levels and hypophos-

phataemia. The calcium and phosphate deficiencies result in impaired mineralization of newly forming bone, producing the classical symptoms of rickets. The treatment of type I vitamin D-dependent rickets is long-term administration of physiological doses of $1\alpha,25(OH)_2D_3$.

Type II

Type II vitamin D-dependent rickets, now more commonly called hereditary vitamin D-resistant rickets (HVDRR), arises from a lack of responsiveness of target tissues to $1\alpha,25(OH)_2D_3$ and in almost all cases is due to a mutation in the gene encoding the VDR. Some mutations lead to defective ligand binding, while others lead to defective binding of the hormone–receptor complex to the DNA. Hewison *et al.* (1993) described an exceptional case attributable not to a mutation of the VDR gene, but to a defect in VDR translocation to the nucleus. Whereas the type I disease state is characterized by depressed levels of $1\alpha,25(OH)_2D_3$, this metabolite is elevated in the type II state. Impaired hormonal function at the intestine and bone causes deficiencies in calcium and phosphate, leading to rickets within months of birth. Afflicted children are often growth retarded and suffer convulsions due to tetany. Some children have total scalp and body alopecia, including eyebrows and, in some cases, eyelashes. The treatment of type II vitamin D-deficient rickets is supra-physiological doses of $1\alpha,25(OH)_2D_3$ (Malloy *et al.*, 1999).

8.9.3 Vitamin D-resistant rickets

Vitamin D-resistant rickets is a group of hereditable abnormalities of renal phosphate transport, the most common of which is X-linked hypophosphataemia. The rickets cannot be explained solely by the severe hypophosphataemia that is present and the undefined pathological mechanism may involve both abnormal phosphate transport and renal 1-hydroxylase function. Treatment entails a combination of oral phosphate and $1\alpha,25(OH)_2D_3$ (Brown *et al.*, 2000).

8.10 Therapeutic applications of vitamin D analogues

There have been several trials to assess the efficacy of vitamin D compounds in the treatment of postmenopausal osteoporosis. The most critical parameter for successful treatment, a decrease in fracture rate, was observed in some, but not all, studies (Brown *et al.*, 2000). In one Japanese study (Shiraki *et al.*, 1996), new fracture occurrence in the group treated with $1\alpha(OH)D_3$ was around one-third of that in the placebo group. The ideal vitamin D analogue would be one which promotes bone formation and slow resorption, yet has less tendency than $1\alpha,25(OH)_2D_3$ to produce hypercalcaemia.

When cultured human epidermal keratinocytes are exposed to physiological concentrations of $1\alpha,25(OH)_2D_3$, the cells cease to proliferate and start to differentiate (Smith *et al.*, 1986). The inhibition of proliferation has been utilized in the treatment of hyperproliferative diseases of the skin. Psoriasis, for example, can be effectively treated by topical application of the vitamin D analogue calcipotriol, which is about 200 times less potent than $1\alpha,25(OH)_2D_3$ in its effects on calcium metabolism, although similar in receptor affinity (Kragballe, 1992). Non-toxic derivatives of $1\alpha,25(OH)_2D_3$ also have potential for the treatment of some cancers and a variety of autoimmune disorders (Holick, 1995a).

8.11   Toxicity

An excessive chronic intake of vitamin D can result in toxicity with a fatal outcome. As in vitamin A toxicity, hypervitaminosis D results from the excessive consumption of vitamin D supplements, and not from the consumption of usual diets. Toxic concentrations of vitamin D have not resulted from unlimited exposure to sunshine. Vitamin D intoxication can be a concern in patients with specific diseases being treated with unusual amounts of vitamin D or analogues of the vitamin. In Great Britain, during the 1940s and early 1950s, an epidemic of 'idiopathic hypercalcaemia' broke out in newborn infants, who failed to thrive and exhibited symptoms of toxicity. This epidemic was eventually traced to over-supplementation of commercial infant milk formulas with vitamin D. The government policy was to supplement milk with up to 2000 IU (50 µg) of vitamin D to compensate for nutritional deprivation that British children had suffered during World War II. To allow for anticipated degradation of vitamin D during processing and storage, some manufacturers put 1.5 to 2 times the correct amount of vitamin D into the pre-processed milk.

Vitamin D toxicity is due primarily to the hypercalcaemia caused by the increased intestinal absorption of calcium, together with increased resorption of bone. The cause of the hypercalcaemia is therefore a drastic exaggeration of the normal physiological action of vitamin D. The increased serum calcium level can lead to a variety of non-specific symptoms, such as anorexia, nausea, vomiting, muscle weakness and constipation. Polyuria and polydipsia result from the failure of the kidney to concentrate the urine. The hypercalciuria that accompanies hypercalcaemia encourages the formation of kidney stones in the renal tubules. Chronic hypercalcaemia results in irreversible calcification of the kidneys (nephrocalcinosis), causing permanent damage to the glomeruli and renal tubules. Calcium salts may be deposited in other extra-skeletal tissues as well, such as the heart, blood vessels and lungs. The renal damage results in a decrease in the glomerular filtration rate and severe hypertension. In long-term hypervitaminosis D, the excessive bone resorption results in part of the bone being replaced by fibrous tissue. Where hypervitaminosis D is fatal, the usual cause of death is renal insufficiency.

High amounts of $25(OH)D_3$ can promote calcium translocation in intestine and bone *in vitro*, suggesting that overwhelming concentrations of $25(OH)D_3$ can displace $1\alpha,25(OH)_2D_3$ from the VDR and directly elicit the biological responses. Brumbaugh & Haussler (1973) predicted from their data that $25(OH)D_3$ must be present in 150 times the concentration of $1\alpha,25(OH)_2D_3$ to displace the physiological hormone. Hypervitaminosis D patients typically exhibit a 15-fold increase in plasma $25(OH)D$ concentrations compared to normal individuals, but their $1\alpha,25(OH)_2D$ levels are not substantially altered (Hughes *et al.*, 1976). These observations have led to the general conclusion that $25(OH)D$, rather than $1\alpha,25(OH)_2D$, is responsible for vitamin D toxicity.

An alternative hypothesis, presented by Vieth (1990), is that $1\alpha,25(OH)_2D$ is, in fact, the agent causing toxicity. This hypothesis is based on the differential binding affinities of the various vitamin D metabolites for the DBP in the plasma. The $25(OH)D$ metabolite binds much more tightly to the DBP than does $1\alpha,25(OH)_2D$. Therefore, when the plasma concentration of $25(OH)D$ increases many-fold, a certain fraction of the circulating 1α,25(OH)$_2$D will be displaced from the DBP by 25(OH)D, thereby increasing the concentration of free 1α,25(OH)$_2$D. The liberated hormone is now able to interact with a greater than normal number of VDRs in target cells and elicit an exaggerated response.

Hypercalcaemia resulting from excessive intake of the parent vitamin D can persist for weeks or months after intake has ceased, because of the accumulation of this vitamin in adipose tissue and its gradual release into the circulation. Treatment must therefore be continued for a long time to counteract the hypercalcaemic response. The treatment includes drugs to enhance urinary excretion of calcium and drugs to diminish the calcium efflux from bone and absorption of calcium from the intestine. The duration of the patient's toxic episode is brief if the administered agent is 1α,25(OH)$_2$D, because the half-life of this hormone is only 4–6 h.

8.12   Dietary requirement

The dietary requirement for vitamin D depends upon the amount of vitamin synthesized by solar irradiation of the skin. This in turn is dependent on age and degree of skin pigmentation, among other factors. It has been estimated that for white adults living in Boston, USA, exposing hands, arms and face on a clear summer day for 10–15 min, two to three times a week, should yield sufficient cutaneous production of vitamin D to meet daily needs (Holick, 1987). To maintain satisfactory plasma 25(OH)D levels without any input from skin irradiation, an oral input in the region of 10–15 µg of vitamin D per day would be required (Holick, 1995b).

The variable exposure to sunlight makes it impracticable to establish an Estimated Average Requirement for vitamin D from which a Recommended Dietary Allowance could be calculated, hence an Adequate Intake has to suffice. In the United States, the recommended Adequate Intake of vitamin D, assuming no exposure to sunlight, is 5 µg per day up to the age of 51 years for both genders. For the age ranges of 51–70 and above 70, the levels are set at 10 and 15 µg per day, respectively (Institute of Medicine, 1997). As a serving of food containing only natural sources of vitamin D and no egg or fish probably supplies less than 1 µg of the vitamin (Parrish, 1979), these intakes can only be realized by the consumption of fortified foods or supplements.

Further reading

Armbrecht, H. J. (1998) Age-related changes in calcium homeostasis and bone loss. In: *Principles and Practice of Geriatric Medicine*, 3rd edn. (Ed. M. S. J. Pathy), pp. 1195–1201. John Wiley & Sons Ltd, New York.

Carlberg, C. (1996) The vitamin D$_3$ receptor in the context of the nuclear receptor superfamily. *Endocrine*, **4**, 91–105.

Casteels, K., Bouillon, R., Waer, M. & Mathieu, C. (1995) Immunomodulatory effects of 1,25-dihydroxyvitamin D$_3$. *Current Opinion in Nephrology and Hypertension*, **4**, 313–18.

Christakos, S., Raval-Pandya, M., Wernyj, R. P. & Yang, W. (1996) Genomic mechanisms involved in the pleiotropic actions of 1,25-dihydroxyvitamin D$_3$. *Biochemical Journal*, **316**, 361–71.

Haussler, M. R., Whitfield, G. K., Haussler, C. A., Hsieh, J.-C., Thompson, P. D., Selznick, S. H., Dominguez, C. E. & Jurutka, P. W. (1998) The nuclear vitamin D receptor: biological and molecular regulatory properties revealed. *Journal of Bone and Mineral Research*, **13**, 325–49.

van Leeuwen, J. P. T. M., van den Bemd, G.-J. C. M., van Driel, M., Buurman, C. J. & Pols, H. A. P. (2001) 24,25-Dihydroxyvitamin D$_3$ and bone metabolism. *Steroids*, **66**, 375–80.

References

Abe, E., Shiina, Y., Miyaura, C., Tanaka, H., Hayashi, T., Kanegasaki, S., Saito, M., Nishii, Y., DeLuca, H. F. & Suda, T. (1984) Activation and fusion induced by 1α, 25-dihydroxyvitamin D$_3$ and their relation in alveolar macrophages. *Proceedings of the National Academy of Sciences of the U.S.A.*, **81**, 7112–16.

Adams, J. S., Clemens, T. L. Parrish, J. A. & Holick, M. F. (1982) Vitamin-D synthesis and metabolism after ultraviolet irradiation of normal and vitamin D-deficient subjects. *New England Journal of Medicine*, **306**, 722–5.

Al-Aqeel, A., Ozand, P., Sobki, S., Sewairi, W. & Marx, S. (1993) The combined use of intravenous and oral calcium for the treatment of vitamin D dependent rickets type II (VDDRII). *Clinical Endocrinology*, **39**, 229–37.

Alroy, I., Towers, T. L. & Freedman, L. P. (1995) Transcriptional repression of the interleukin-2 gene by vitamin D$_3$: direct inhibition of NFATp/AP-1 complex formation by a nuclear hormone receptor. *Molecular and Cellular Biology*, **15**, 5789–99.

Amling, M., Priemel, M., Holzmann, T., Chapin, K., Rueger, J. M., Baron, R. & Demay, M. B. (1999) Rescue of the skeletal phenotype of vitamin D receptor-ablated mice in the setting of normal mineral ion homeostasis: formal histomorphometric and biomechanical analyses. *Endocrinology*, **140**, 4982–7.

Armbrecht, H. J. & Hodam, T. L. (1994) Parathyroid hormone and 1,25-dihydoxyvitamin D synergistically induce the 1,25-dihydroxyvitamin D-24-hydroxylase in rat UMR-106 osteoblast-like cells. *Biochemical and Biophysical Research Communications*, **205**, 674–9.

Armbrecht, H. J., Zenser, T. V., Bruns, M. E. H. & Davis, B. B. (1979) Effect of age on intestinal calcium absorption and adaptation to dietary calcium. *American Journal of Physiology*, **236**, E769–74.

Armbrecht, H. J., Boltz, M. A. & Wongsurawat, N. (1992) Expression of plasma membrane calcium pump mRNA in rat intestine

– effect of age and 1,25-dihydroxyvitamin D. *Journal of Bone and Mineral Research*, 7 (Suppl. 1), S166.

Armbrecht, H. J., Hodam, T. L., Boltz, M. A. & Chen, M. L. (1993) Phorbol ester markedly increases the sensitivity of intestinal epithelial cells to 1,25-dihydroxyvitamin D_3. *FEBS Letters*, **327**, 13–16.

Armbrecht, H. J., Chen, M. L., Hodam, T. L. & Boltz, M. A. (1997) Induction of 24-hydroxylase cytochrome P450 mRNA by 1,25-dihydroxyvitamin D and phorbol esters in normal rat kidney (NRK-52E) cells. *Journal of Endocrinology*, **153**, 199–205.

Armbrecht, H. J., Hodam, T. L., Boltz, M. A., Partridge, N. C., Brown, A. J. & Kumar, V. B. (1998) Induction of the vitamin D 24-hydroxylase (CYP24) by 1,25-dihydroxyvitamin D_3 is regulated by parathyroid hormone in UMR106 osteoblastic cells. *Endocrinology*, **139**, 3375–81.

Arnaud, S. B., Goldsmith, R. S., Lambert, P. W. & Go, V. L. W. (1975) 25-Hydroxyvitamin D_3: evidence of an enterohepatic circulation in man. *Proceedings of the Society for Experimental Biology and Medicine*, **149**, 570–2.

Balsan, S., Garabédian, M., Larchet, M., Gorski, A.-M., Cournot, G., Tau,, C., Bourdeau, A., Silve, C. & Ricour, C. (1986) Long-term nocturnal calcium infusions can cure rickets and promote normal mineralization in hereditary resistance to 1,25-dihydroxyvitamin D. *Journal of Clinical Investigation*, **77**, 1661–7.

Baran, D. T. & Sorensen, A. M. (1994) Rapid actions of 1α-25-dihydroxyvitamin D_3 physiologic role. *Proceedings of the Society of Experimental Biology and Medicine*, **207**, 175–9.

Baran, D. T., Sorensen, A. M. & Honeyman, T. W. (1988) Rapid action of 1,25-dihydroxyvitamin D_3 on hepatocyte phospholipids. *Journal of Bone and Mineral Research*, **3**, 593–600.

Baran, D. T., Sorensen, A. M., Shalhoub, V., Owen, T., Oberdorf, A., Stein, G. & Lian, J. (1991) 1α,25-Dihydroxyvitamin D_3 rapidly increases cytosolic calcium in clonal rat osteosarcoma cells lacking the vitamin D receptor. *Journal of Bone and Mineral Research*, **6**, 1269–75.

Baran, D. T., Sorensen, A. M., Shalhoub, V., Owen, T., Stein, G. & Lian, J. (1992) The rapid nongenomic actions of 1α,25-dihydroxyvitamin D_3 modulate the hormone-induced increments in osteocalcin gene transcription in osteoblast-like cells. *Journal of Cellular Biochemistry*, **50**, 124–9.

Baran, D. T., Quail, J. M., Ray, R., Leszyk, J. & Honeyman, T. (2000) Annexin II is the membrane receptor that mediates the rapid actions of 1α,25-dihydroxyvitamin D_3. *Journal of Cellular Biochemistry*, **78**, 34–46.

Bar-Shavit, Z., Noff, D., Edelstein, S., Meyer, M., Shibolet, S. & Goldman, R. (1981) 1,25-Dihydroxyvitamin D_3 and the regulation of macrophage function. *Calcified Tissue International*, **33**, 673–6.

Baudino, T. A., Kraichely, D. M., Jefcoat, S. C. Jr., Winchester, S. K., Partridge, N. C. & MacDonald, P. N. (1998) Isolation and characterization of a novel coactivator protein, NCoA-62, involved in vitamin D-mediated transcription. *Journal of Biological Chemistry*, **273**(26), 16 434–41.

Bedo, G., Sanstisteban, P. & Aranda, A. (1989) Retinoic acid regulates growth hormone gene expression. *Nature*, **339**, 231–4.

Bhalla, A. K., Amento, E. P. & Krane, S. M. (1986) Differential effects of 1,25-dihydroxyvitamin D_3 on human lymphocytes and monocyte/macrophages: inhibition of interleukin-2 and augmentation of interleukin-1 production. *Cellular Immunology*, **98**, 311–22.

Bindels, R. J. M. (1993) Calcium handling by the mammalian kidney. *Journal of Experimental Biology*, **184**, 89–104.

Blanco, J. C. G., Wang, I.-M., Tsai, S. Y., Tsai, M.-J., O'Malley, B. W., Jurutka, P. W., Haussler, M. R. & Ozato, K. (1995) Transcription factor TFIIB and the vitamin D receptor cooperatively activate ligand-dependent transcription. *Proceedings of the National Academy of Sciences of the U.S.A.*, **92**, 1535–9.

Boissier, M.-C., Chiocchia, G. & Fournier, C. (1992) Combination of cyclosporin A and calcitriol in the treatment of adjuvant arthritis. *Journal of Rheumatology*, **19**, 754–7.

Borowitz, S. M. & Ghishan, F. K. (1989) Phosphate transport in human jejunal brush-border membrane vesicles. *Gastroenterology*, **96**, 4–10.

Bourdeau, A., Atmani, F., Grosse, B. & Lieberherr, M. (1990) Rapid effects of 1,25-dihydroxyvitamin D_3 and extracellular Ca^{2+} on phospholipid metabolism in dispersed porcine parathyroid cells. *Endocrinology*, **127**, 2738–43.

Boyan, B. D., Dean, D. D., Sylvia, V. L. & Schwartz, Z. (1994) Nongenomic regulation of extracellular matrix events by vitamin D metabolites. *Journal of Cellular Biochemistry*, **56**, 331–9.

Boyan, B. D., Sylvia, V. L., Dean, D. D. & Schwartz, Z. (2001) 24,25-$(OH)_2D_3$ regulates cartilage and bone via autocrine and endocrine mechanisms. *Steroids*, **66**, 363–74.

Brasitus, T. A., Dudeja, P. K., Eby, B. & Lau, K. (1986) Correction by 1,25-dihydroxycholecalciferol of the abnormal fluidity and lipid composition of enterocyte brush border membranes in vitamin D-deprived rats. *Journal of Biological Chemistry*, **261**(35), 16 404–9.

Brenza, H. L., Kimmel-jehan, C., Jehan, F., Shinki, T., Wakino, S., Anazawa, H., Suda, T. & DeLuca, H. F. (1998) Parathyroid hormone activation of the 25-hydroxyvitamin D_3-1α-hydroxylase gene promoter. *Proceedings of the National Academy of Sciences of the U.S.A.*, **95**, 1387–91.

Bronner, F. (1990) Intestinal calcium transport: the cellular pathway. *Mineral and Electrolyte Metabolism*, **16**, 94–100.

Bronner, F. (1991) Calcium transport across epithelia. *International Review of Cytology*, **131**, 169–212.

Bronner, F., Pansu, D. & Stein, W. D. (1986) An analysis of intestinal calcium transport across the rat intestine. *American Journal of Physiology*, **250**, G561–9.

Brown, A. J., Dusso, A. & Slatopolsky, E. (1999) Vitamin D. *American Journal of Physiology*, **277**, F157–75.

Brown, A., Dusso, A. & Slatopolsky, E. (2000) Vitamin D. In: *The Kidney*, 3rd edn, Vol. 1. (Ed. D. W. Seldin & G. Giebisch), pp. 1047–90. Lippincott, Williams & Wilkins, Philadelphia.

Brown, T. A. & DeLuca, H. F. (1990) Phosphorylation of the 1,25-dihydroxyvitamin D_3 receptor. A primary event in 1,25-dihydroxyvitamin D_3 action. *Journal of Biological Chemistry*, **265**(17), 10 025–9.

Brumbaugh, P. F. & Haussler, M. R. (1973) 1α,25-Dihydroxyvitamin D_3 receptor: competitive binding of vitamin D analogs. *Life Sciences*, **13**, 1737–46.

Buffa, R., Mare, P., Salvadore, M., Solcia, M., Furness, J. B. & Lawson, D. E. M. (1989) Calbindin 28 kDa in endocrine cells of known or putative calcium regulating function. *Histochemistry*, **91**, 107–13.

Caffrey, J. M. & Farach-Carson, M. C. (1989) Vitamin D_3 metabolites modulate dihydropyridine-sensitive calcium currents in clonal rat osteosarcoma cells. *Journal of Biological Chemistry*, **264**(34), 20 265–74.

Cai, Q., Chandler, J. S., Wasserman, R. H., Kumar, R. & Penniston, J. T. (1993) Vitamin D and adaptation to dietary calcium and phosphate deficiencies increase intestinal plasma membrane calcium pump gene expression. *Proceedings of the National Academy of Sciences of the U.S.A.*, **90**, 1345–9.

Cantley, L. K., Russell, J., Lettieri, D. & Sherwood, L. M. (1985) 1,25-Dihydroxyvitamin D_3 suppresses parathyroid hormone secretion from bovine parathyroid cells in tissue culture. *Endocrinology*, **117**, 2114–19.

Cao, X., Ross, P., Zhang, L., MacDonald, P. N., Chappel, J. & Teitelbaum, S. L. (1993) Cloning of the promoter for the avian integrin β_3 subunit gene and its regulation by 1,25-dihydroxy-vitamin D_3. *Journal of Biological Chemistry*, **268**(36), 27 371–80.

Chandra, S., Fullmer, C. S., Smith, C. A., Wasserman, R. H. & Morrison, G. H. (1990) Ion microscopic imaging of calcium transport in the intestinal tissue of vitamin D-deficient and vitamin D-replete chickens: a ^{44}Ca stable isotope study. *Proceedings of the National Academy of Sciences of the U.S.A.*, **87**, 5715–19.

Chen, K.-S. & DeLuca, H. F. (1995) Cloning of the human 1α,25-dihydroxyvitamin D-3 24-hydroxylase gene promoter and identification of two vitamin D-responsive elements. *Biochimica et Biophysica Acta*, **1263**, 1–9.

Chen, M. L., Boltz, M. A. & Armbrecht, H. J. (1993) Effects of 1,25-dihydroxyvitamin D_3 and phorbol ester on 25-hydroxyvitamin D_3 24-hydroxylase cytochrome P_{450} messenger ribonucleic acid levels in primary cultures of rat renal cells. *Endocrinology*, **132**, 1782–8.

Chen, M. L., Heinrich, G., Ohyama, Y.-I., Okuda, K., Omdahl, J. L., Chen, T. C. & Holick, M. F. (1994) Expression of 25-hydroxyvitamin D_3-24-hydroxylase mRNA in cultured human keratinocytes. *Proceedings of the Society of Experimental Biology and Medicine*, **207**, 57–61.

Chertow, B. S., Sivitz, W. I., Baranetsky, N. G., Clark, S. A., Waite, A. & DeLuca, H. F. (1983) Cellular mechanisms of insulin release: the effects of vitamin D deficiency and repletion on rat insulin secretion. *Endocrinology*, **113**, 1511–18.

Civitelli, R., Kim, Y. S., Gunsten, S. L., Fujimori, A., Huskey, M., Avioli, L. V. & Hruska, K. A. (1990) Nongenomic activation of the calcium message system by vitamin D metabolites in osteoblast-like cells. *Endocrinology*, **127**, 2253–62.

Clark, S. A., Stumpf, W. E., Sar, M., DeLuca, H. F. & Tanaka, Y. (1980) Target cells for 1,25-dihydroxyvitamin D_3 in the pancreas. *Cell and Tissue Research*, **209**, 515–20.

Clark, S. A., Boass, A. & Toverud, S. U. (1987) Effects of high dietary contents of calcium and phosphorus on mineral metabolism and growth of vitamin D-deficient suckling and weaned rats. *Bone and Mineral*, **2**, 257–70.

Clemens, T. L., Henderson, S. L., Adams, J. S. & Holick, M. F. (1982) Increased skin pigment reduces the capacity of skin to synthesize vitamin D_3. *Lancet*, **I**(8263), 74–6.

Clements, M. R., Chalmers, T. M. & Fraser, D. R. (1984) Enterohepatic circulation of vitamin D: a reappraisal of the hypothesis. *Lancet*, **I**(8391), 1376–9.

Clohisy, D. R., Bar-Shavit, Z., Chappel, J. C. & Teitelbaum, S. L. (1987) 1,25-Dihydroxyvitamin D_3 modulates bone marrow macrophage precursor proliferation and differentiation. Upregulation of the mannose receptor. *Journal of Biological Chemistry*, **262**(33), 15 922–9.

Danisi, G. & Murer, H. (1991) Inorganic phosphate absorption in small intestine. In: *Handbook of Physiology*, Section 6: *The Gastrointestinal System*, Vol. IV, *Intestinal Absorption and Secretion*. (Ed. S. G. Schultz), pp. 323–36. American Physiological Society, Bethesda, MD.

Darwish, H. M. & DeLuca, H. F. (1992) Identification of a 1,25-dihydroxyvitamin D_3-response element in the 5′-flanking region of the rat calbindin D-9k gene. *Proceedings of the National Academy of Sciences of the U.S.A.*, **89**, 603–7.

Davies, M., Mawer, E. B. & Krawitt, E. L. (1980) Comparative absorption of vitamin D_3 and 25-hydroxyvitamin D_3 in intestinal disease. *Gut*, **21**, 287–92.

Davies, P. D. O. (1985) A possible link between vitamin D deficiency and impaired host defence to *Mycobacterium tuberculosis*. *Tubercle*, **66**, 301–6.

de Boland, A. R. & Norman, A. (1990) Evidence for involvement of protein kinase C and cyclic adenosine 3′,5′-monophosphate-dependent protein kinase in the 1,25-dihydroxy-vitamin D_3-mediated rapid stimulation of intestinal calcium transport, (transcaltachia). *Endocrinology*, **127**, 39–45.

de Boland, A. R., Nemere, I. & Norman, A. W. (1990) Ca^{2+}-channel agonist BAY K8644 mimics 1,25(OH)$_2$-vitamin D_3 rapid enhancement of Ca^{2+} transport in chick perfused duodenum. *Biochemical and Biophysical Research Communications*, **166**, 217–22.

Demay, M. B., Kiernan, M. S., DeLuca, H. F. & Kronenberg, H. M. (1992a) Characterization of 1,25-dihydroxyvitamin D_3 receptor interactions with target sequences in the rat osteocalcin gene. *Molecular Endocrinology*, **6**, 557–62.

Demay, M. B., Kiernan, M. S., DeLuca, H. F. & Kronenberg, H. M. (1992b) Sequences in the human parathyroid hormone gene that bind the 1,25-dihydroxyvitamin D_3 receptor and mediate transcriptional repression in response to 1,25-dihydroxyvitamin D_3. *Proceedings of the National Academy of Sciences of the U.S.A.*, **89**, 8097–8101.

Desai, R. K., van Wijnen, A. J., Stein, J. L., Stein, G. S. & Lian, J. B. (1995) Control of 1,25-dihydroxyvitamin D_3 receptor-mediated enhancement of osteocalcin gene transcription: effects of perturbing phosphorylation pathways by okadaic acid and staurosporine. *Endocrinology*, **136**, 5685–93.

Ducy, P., Desbois, C., Boyce, B., Pinero, G., Story, B., Dunstan, C., Smith, E., Bonadio, J., Goldstein, S., Gundberg, C., Bradley, A. & Karsenty, G. (1996) Increased bone formation in osteocalcin-deficient mice. *Nature*, **382**, 448–52.

Dueland, S., Pedersen, J. I., Helgerud, P. & Drevon, C. A. (1982) Transport of vitamin D_3 from rat intestine. *Journal of Biological Chemistry*, **257**(1), 146–50.

Dueland, S., Helgerud, P., Pedersen, J. I., Berg, T. & Drevon, C. A. (1983a) Plasma clearance, transfer, and distribution of vitamin D_3 from intestinal lymph. *American Journal of Physiology*, **245**, E326–31.

Dueland, S., Pedersen, J. I., Helgerud, P. & Drevon, C. A. (1983b) Absorption, distribution, and transport of vitamin D_3 and 25-hydroxyvitamin D_3 in the rat. *American Journal of Physiology*, **245**, E463–7.

El-Radhi, A. S., Mansor, N., Majeed, M. & Ibrahim, M. (1982) High incidence of rickets in children with wheezy bronchitis in a developing country. *Journal of the Royal Society of Medicine*, **75**, 884–7.

Falzon, M. (1996) DNA sequences in the rat parathyroid hormone-related peptide gene responsible for 1,25-dihydroxyvitamin D_3-mediated transcriptional repression. *Molecular Endocrinology*, **10**, 672–81.

Farach-Carson, M. C., Sergeev, I. & Norman, A. W. (1991) Nongenomic actions of 1,25-dihydroxyvitamin D_3 in rat osteosarcoma cells: structure–function studies using ligand analogs. *Endocrinology*, **129**, 1876–84.

Favus, M. J. & Tembe, V. (1992) The use of pharmacologic agents to study mechanisms of intestinal calcium transport. *Journal of Nutrition*, **122**, 683–6.

Favus, M. V., Tembe, V., Ambrosic, K. A. & Nellans, H. N. (1989) Effects of 1,25(OH)$_2$D$_3$ on enterocyte basolateral membrane calcium transport in rats. *American Journal of Physiology*, **256**, G613–7.

Fleet, J. C. & Wood, R. J. (1999) Specific 1,25(OH)$_2$D$_3$-mediated regulation of transcellular calcium transport in Caco-2 cells. *American Journal of Physiology*, **276**, G958–64.

Fontaine, O., Matsumoto, T., Goodman, D. B. P. & Rasmussen, H. (1981) Liponomic control of Ca^{2+} transport: relationship to mechanism of action of 1,25-dihydroxyvitamin D_3. *Proceedings of the National Academy of Sciences of the U.S.A.*, **78**, 1751–4.

Fournier, C., Gepner, P., Sadouk, M. & Charreire, J. (1990) *In vivo* beneficial effects of cyclosporin A and 1,25-dihydroxyvitamin

D_3 on the induction of experimental autoimmune thyroiditis. *Clinical Immunology and Immunopathology*, **54**, 53–63.

Fraser, D. R. (1983) The physiological economy of vitamin D. *Lancet*, **I**(8331), 969–72.

Fullmer, C. S. (1992) Intestinal calcium absorption: calcium entry. *Journal of Nutrition*, **122**, 644–50.

García-Villalba, P., Au-Fliegner, M., Samuels, H. H. & Aranda, A. (1993) Interaction of thyroid hormone and retinoic acid receptors on the regulation of the rat growth hormone gene promoter. *Biochemical and Biophysical Research Communications*, **191**, 580–6.

García-Villalba, P., Jimenez-Lara, A.M. & Aranda, A. (1996) Vitamin D interferes with transactivation of the growth hormone gene by thyroid hormone and retinoic acid. *Molecular and Cellular Biology*, **16**, 318–27.

Gavison, R. & Bar-Shavit, Z. (1989) Impaired macrophage activation in vitamin D_3 deficiency: differential in vitro effects of 1,25-dihydroxyvitamin D_3 on mouse peritoneal macrophage functions. *Journal of Immunology*, **143**, 388–90.

Gepner, P., Amor, B. & Fournier, C. (1989) 1,25-Dihydroxyvitamin D_3 potentiates the in vitro inhibitory effects of cyclosporin A on T cells from rheumatoid arthritis patients. *Arthritis and Rheumatism*, **32**, 31–6.

Ghijsen, W. E. J. M. & van Os, C. H. (1982) 1α,25-Dihydroxyvitamin D-3 regulates ATP-dependent calcium transport in basolateral plasma membranes of rat enterocytes. *Biochimica et Biophysica Acta*, **689**, 170–2.

Ghijsen, W. E. J. M., De Jong, M. D. & van Os, C. H. (1982) ATP-dependent calcium transport and its correlation with Ca^{2+}-ATPase activity in basolateral plasma membranes of rat duodenum. *Biochimica et Biophysica Acta*, **689**, 327–36.

Ghijsen, W. E. J. M., De Jong, M. D. & van Os, C. H. (1983) Kinetic properties of Na^+/Ca^{2+} exchange in basolateral plasma membranes of rat small intestine. *Biochimica et Biophysica Acta*, **730**, 85–94.

Gill, R. K. & Christakos, S. (1993) Identification of sequence elements in mouse calbindin-D_{28k} gene that confer 1,25-dihydroxyvitamin D_3- and butyrate-inducible responses. *Proceedings of the National Academy of Sciences of the U.S.A.*, **90**, 2984–8.

Girasole, G., Wang, J. M., Pedrazzoni, M., Pioli, G., Balotta, C., Passeri, M., Lazzarin, A., Ridolfo, A. & Mantovani, A. (1990) Augmentation of monocyte chemotaxis by 1α,25-dihydroxyvitamin D_3. Stimulation of defective migration of AIDS patients. *Journal of Immunology*, **145**, 2459–64.

Girasole, G., Passeri, G., Jilka, R. L. & Manolagas, S. C. (1994) Interleukin-11: a new cytokine critical for osteoclast development. *Journal of Clinical Investigation*, **93**, 1516–24.

Gross, M. & Kumar, R. (1990) Physiology and biochemistry of vitamin D-dependent calcium binding proteins. *American Journal of Physiology*, **259**, F195–F209.

Grosse, B., Bourdeau, A. & Lieberherr, M. (1993) Oscillations in inositol 1,4,5-triphosphate and diacylglycerol induced by vitamin D_3 metabolites in confluent mouse osteoblasts. *Journal of Bone and Mineral Research*, **8**, 1059–69.

Guggino, S. E., Lajeunesse, D., Wagner, J. A. & Snyder, S. H. (1989) Bone remodeling signaled by a dihydropyridine- and phenylalkylamine-sensitive calcium channel. *Proceedings of the National Academy of Sciences of the U.S.A.*, **86**, 2957–60.

Guo, B., Aslam, F., van Wijnen, A. J., Roberts, S. G. E., Frenkel, B., Green, M. R., DeLuca, H. F., Lian, J. B., Stein, G. S. & Stein, J. L. (1997) YY1 regulates vitamin D receptor/retinoid X receptor mediated transactivation of the vitamin D responsive osteocalcin gene. *Proceedings of the National Academy of Sciences of the U.S.A.*, **94**, 121–6.

Hattenhauer, O., Traebert, M., Murer, H. & Biber, J. (1999) Regulation of small intestinal Na-Pi type IIb cotransporter by dietary phosphate intake. *American Journal of Physiology*, **277**, G756–62.

Haussler, M. R., Whitfield, G. K., Haussler, C. A., Hsieh, J.-C., Thompson, P. D., Selznik, S. H., Dominguez, C. E. & Jurutka, P. W. (1998) The nuclear vitamin D receptor: biological and molecular regulatory properties revealed. *Journal of Bone and Mineral Research*, **13**, 325–49.

Henry, H. L., Midgett, R. J. & Norman, A. W. (1974) Regulation of 25-hydroxyvitamin D_3-1-hydroxylase in vivo. *Journal of Biological Chemistry*, **249**(23), 7584–92.

Hess, A. D. & Tutschka, P. J. (1980) Effect of cyclosporin A on human lymphocyte reponses in vitro. I. CsA allows for the expression of alloantigen-activated suppressor cells while preferentially inhibiting the induction of cytolytic effector lymphocytes in MLR. *Journal of Immunology*, **124**, 2601–2608.

Hewison, M., Rut, A. R., Kristjansson, K., Walker, R. E., Dillon, M. J., Hughes, M. R. & O'Riordan, J. L. H. (1993) Tissue resistance to 1,25-dihydroxyvitamin D without a mutation of the vitamin D receptor gene. *Clinical Endocrinology*, **39**, 663–70.

Holick, M. F. (1987) Photosynthesis of vitamin D in the skin: effect of environmental and life-style variables. *Federation Proceedings*, **46**, 1876–82.

Holick, M. F. (1995a) Noncalcemic actions of 1,25-dihydroxyvitamin D_3 and clinical applications. *Bone*, **17**(2 suppl), 107S–111S.

Holick, M. F. (1995b) Environmental factors that influence the cutaneous production of vitamin D. *American Journal of Clinical Nutrition*, **61**, 638S–45S.

Holick, M. F., MacLaughlin, J. A. & Doppelt, S. H. (1981) Regulation of cutaneous previtamin D_3 photosynthesis in man: skin pigment is not an essential regulator. *Science*, **211**, 590–3.

Holick, M. F., Matsuoka, L. Y. & Wortsman, J. (1989) Age, vitamin D, and solar ultraviolet. *Lancet*, **II**(8671), 1104–5.

Hollander, D., Muralidhara, K. S. & Zimmerman, A. (1978) Vitamin D-3 intestinal absorption in vivo: influence of fatty acids, bile salts, and perfusate pH on absorption. *Gut*, **19**, 267–72.

Hollis, B. W., Iskersky, V. N. & Chang, M. K. (1989) In vitro metabolism of 25-hydroxyvitamin D_3 by human trophoblastic homogenates, mitochondria, and microsomes: lack of evidence for the presence of 25-hydroxyvitamin D_3-1 α- and 24R-hydroxylases. *Endocrinology*, **125**, 1224–30.

Holtrop, M. E., Cox, K. A., Clark, M. B., Holick, M. F. & Anast, C. S. (1981) 1,25-Dihydroxycholecalciferol stimulates osteoclasts in rat bones in the absence of parathyroid hormone. *Endocrinology*, **108**, 2293–2301.

Holtrop, M. E., Cox, K. A., Carnes, D. L. & Holick, M. F. (1986) Effects of serum calcium and phosphorus on skeletal mineralization in vitamin D-deficient rats. *American Journal of Physiology*, **251**, E234–40.

Homaiden, F. R., Donowitz, M., Weiland, G. A. & Sharp, G. W. G. (1989) Two calcium channels in basolateral membranes of rabbit ileal epithelial cells. *American Journal of Physiology*, **257**, G86–93.

Hong, M. H., Jin, C. H., Sato, T., Ishimi, Y., Abe, E. & Suda, T. (1991) Transcriptional regulation of the production of the third component of complement (C3) by 1α,25-dihydroxyvitamin D_3 in mouse marrow-derived stromal cells (ST2) and primary osteoblastic cells. *Endocrinology*, **129**, 2774–9.

Horiuchi, N., Suda, T., Takahashi, H., Shimazawa, E. & Ogata, E. (1977) In vivo evidence for the intermediary role of 3′,5′ cyclic AMP in parathyroid hormone-induced stimulation of 1α,25-dihydroxyvitamin D_3 synthesis in rats. *Endocrinology*, **101**, 969–74.

Hörlein, A. J., Näär, A. M., Heinzel, T., Torchia, J., Gloss, B., Kurokawa, R., Ryan, A., Kamei, Y., Söderström, M., Glass, C. K.

& Rosenfeld, M. G. (1995) Ligand-independent repression by the thyroid hormone receptor mediated by a nuclear receptor co-repressor. *Nature*, **377**, 397–404.

Horst, R. L., Napoli, J. L. & Littledike, E. T. (1982) Discrimination in the metabolism of orally dosed ergocalciferol and cholecalciferol by the pig, rat and chick. *Biochemical Journal,* **204**, 185–9.

Hsieh, J.-C., Jurutka, P. W., Galligan, M. A., Terpening, C. M., Haussler, C. A., Samuels, D. S., Shimizu, Y., Shimizu, N. & Haussler, M. R. (1991) Human vitamin D receptor is selectively phosphorylated by protein kinase C on serine 51, a residue crucial to its trans-activation function. *Proceedings of the National Academy of Sciences of the U.S.A.*, **88**, 9315–19.

Hsieh, J.-C., Jurutka, P. W., Nakajima, S., Galligan, M. A., Haussler, C. A., Shimizu, Y., Shimizu, N., Whitfield, G. K. & Haussler, M. R. (1993) Phosphorylation of the human vitamin D receptor by protein kinase C. Biochemical and functional evaluation of the serine 51 recognition site. *Journal of Biological Chemistry*, **268**(20), 15 118–26.

Hughes, M. R., Baylink, D. J., Jones, P. G. & Haussler, M. R. (1976) Radioligand receptor assay for 25-hydroxyvitamin D_2/D_3 and $1\alpha,25$-dihydroxyvitamin D_2/D_3. *Journal of Clinical Investigation*, **58**, 61–70.

Institute of Medicine (1997) *Dietary Reference Intakes for Calcium, Phosphorus, Magnesium, Vitamin D, and Fluoride.* National Academy Press, Washington, DC.

Jenis, L. G., Lian, J. B., Stein, G. S. & Baran, D. T. (1993) $1\alpha,25$-Dihydroxyvitamin D-induced changes in intracellular pH in osteoblast-like cells modulate gene expression. *Journal of Cellular Biochemistry*, **53**, 234–9.

Jimi, E., Nakamura, I., Amano, H., Taguchi, Y., Tsurukai, T., Tamura, M., Takahashi, N. & Suda, T. (1996) Osteoclast function is activated by osteoblastic cells through a mechanism involving cell-to-cell contact. *Endocrinology*, **137**, 2187–90.

Jin, C. H., Shinki, T., Hong, M. H., Sato, T., Yamaguchi, A., Ikeda, T., Yoshiki, S., Abe, E. & Suda, T. (1992) $1\alpha,25$-Dihydroxyvitamin D_3 regulates *in vivo* production of the third component of complement (C3) in bone. *Endocrinology*, **131**, 2468–75.

Johnsson, C., Binderup, L. & Tufveson, G. (1995) The effects of combined treatment with the novel vitamin D analogue MC 1288 and cyclosporine A on cardiac allograft survival. *Transplant Immunology*, **3**, 245–50.

Jones, G., Strugnell, S. A. & DeLuca, H. F. (1998) Current understanding of the molecular actions of vitamin D. *Physiological Reviews,*, **78**, 1193–231.

Jurutka, P. W., Hsieh, J.-C., Nakajima, S., Haussler, C. A., Whitfield, G. K. & Haussler, M. R. (1996) Human vitamin D receptor phosphorylation by casein kinase II at ser-208 potentiates transcriptional activation. *Proceedings of the National Academy of Sciences of the U.S.A.*, **93**, 3519–24.

Kahlen, J.-P. & Carlberg, C. (1996) Functional characterization of a 1,25-dihydroxyvitamin D_3 receptor binding site found in the rat atrial natriuretic factor promoter. *Biochemical and Biophysical Research Communications*, **218**, 882–6.

Kamimura, S., Gallieni, M., Zhong, M., Beron, W., Slatopolsky, E. & Dusso, A. (1995) Microtubules mediate cellular 25-hydroxyvitamin D_3 trafficking and the genomic response to 1,25-dihydroxyvitamin D_3 in normal human monocytes. *Journal of Biological Chemistry*, **270**(38), 22 160–6.

Kankova, M., Luini, W., Pedrazzoni, M., Riganti, F., Sironi, M., Bottazzi, B., Mantovani, A. & Vecchi, A. (1991) Impairment of cytokine production in mice fed a vitamin D3-deficient diet. *Immunology*, **73**, 466–71.

Kato, A., Seo, E.-G., Einhorn, T. A., Bishop, J. E. & Norman, A. W. (1998) Studies on 24R,25-dihydroxyvitamin D_3: evidence for a nonnuclear membrane receptor in the chick tibial fracture-heal-

ing callus. *Bone*, **23**, 141–6.

Kerry, D. M., Dwivedi,, P. P., Hahn, C. N., Morris, H. A., Omdahl, J. L. & May, B. K. (1996) Transcriptional synergism between vitamin D-responsive elements in the rat 25-hydroxyvitamin D_3 34-hydroxylase (*CYP24*) promoter. *Journal of Biological Chemistry*, **271**(47), 29 715–21.

Khoury, R., Ridall, A. L., Norman, A. W. & Farach-Carson, M. C. (1994) Target gene activation by 1,25-dihydroxyvitamin D_3 in osteosarcoma cells is independent of calcium influx. *Endocrinology*, **135**, 2446–53.

Kikuchi, K. & Ghishan, F. K. (1987) Phosphate transport by basolateral plasma membranes of human small intestine. *Gastroenterology*, **93**, 106–13.

Kim, R. H., Li, J. J., Ogata, Y., Yamuchi, M., Freedman, L. P. & Sodek, J. (1996) Identification of a vitamin D_3-response element that overlaps a unique inverted TATA box in the rat bone sialoprotein gene. *Biochemical Journal*, **318**, 219–26.

Koeffler, H. P., Reichel, H., Bishop, J. E. & Norman, A. W. (1985) γ-Interferon stimulates production of 1,25-dihydroxyvitamin D_3 by normal human macrophages. *Biochemical and Biophysical Research Communications*, **127**, 596–603.

Koyama, H., Inaba, M., Nishizawa, Y., Ohno, S. & Morii, H. (1994) Protein kinase C is involved in 24-hydroxylase gene expression induced by $1,25(OH)_2D_3$ in rat intestinal epithelial cells. *Journal of Cellular Biochemistry*, **55**, 230–40.

Kragballe, K. (1992) Vitamin D analogues in the treatment of psoriasis. *Journal of Cellular Biochemistry*, **49**, 46–52.

Kremer, R., Sebag, M., Champigny, C., Meerovitch, K., Hendy, G. N., White, J. & Goltzman, D. (1996) Identification and characterization of 1,25-dihydroxyvitamin D_3-responsive repressor sequences in the rat parathyroid hormone-related peptide gene. *Journal of Biological Chemistry*, **271**(27), 16 310–16.

Krishnan, A. V. & Feldman, D. (1991) Activation of protein kinase-C inhibits vitamin D receptor gene expression. *Molecular Endocrinology*, **5**, 605–12.

Krishnan, A. V. & Feldman, D. (1992) Cyclic adenosine 3′,5′-monophosphate up-regulates 1,25-dihydroxyvitamin D_3 receptor gene expression and enhances hormone action. *Molecular Endocrinology*, **6**, 198–206.

Krishnan, A. V., Cramer, S. D., Bringhurst, F. R. & Feldman, D. (1995) Regulation of 1,25-dihydroxyvitamin D_3 receptors by parathyroid hormone in osteoblastic cells: role of second messenger pathways. *Endocrinology*, **136**, 705–12.

Lawson, E. (1985) Vitamin D. In: *Fat-Soluble Vitamins. Their Biochemistry and Applications.* (Ed. A. T. Diplock), pp. 76–153. Heinemann, London.

Lee, S., Clark, S. A., Gill, R. K. & Christakos, S. (1994) 1,25-Dihydroxyvitamin D_3 and pancreatic β-cell function: vitamin D receptors, gene expression, and insulin secretion. *Endocrinology*, **134**, 1602–10.

Lemire, J. M. (1992) Immunomodulatory role of 1,25-dihydroxyvitamin D_3. *Journal of Cellular Biochemistry*, **49**, 26–31.

Lemire, J. M., Adams, J. S., Sakai, R. & Jordan, S. C. (1984) $1\alpha,25$-Dihydroxyvitamin D_3 suppresses proliferation and immunoglobulin production by normal human peripheral blood mononuclear cells. *Journal of Clinical Investigation*, **74**, 657–61.

Lemire, J. M., Adams, J. S., Kermani-Arab, V., Bakke, A. C., Sakai, R. & Jordan, S. C. (1985) 1,25-Dihydroxyvitamin D_3 suppresses human T helper-inducer lymphocyte activity *in vitro*. *Journal of Immunology*, **134**, 3032–5.

Lemire, J. M., Archer, D. C., Beck, L. & Spiegelberg, H. L. (1995) Immunosuppressive actions of 1,25-dihydroxyvitamin D_3: preferential inhibition of TH_1 functions. *Journal of Nutrition*, **125**, 1704S–1708S.

Li, B., Chik, C. L., Taniguchi, N., Ho, A. K. & Karpinski, E. (1996)

24,25(OH)$_2$ Vitamin D$_3$ modulates the L-type Ca^{2+} channel current in UMR 106 cells: involvement of protein kinase A and protein kinase C. *Cell Calcium*, **19**, 193–200.

Li, H., Gomes, P. J. & Chen, J. D. (1997) RAC3, a steroid/nuclear receptor-associated coactivator that is related to SRC-1 and TIF2. *Proceedings of the National Academy of Sciences of the U.S.A.*, **94**, 8479–84.

Lian, J. B. & Stein, G. S. (1992) Transcriptional control of vitamin D-regulated proteins. *Journal of Cellular Biochemistry*, **49**, 37–45.

Lidor, C., Atkin, I., Ornoy, A., Dekel, S. & Edelstein, S. (1987) Healing of rachitic lesions in chicks by 24R,25-dihydroxycholecalciferol administered locally into bone. *Journal of Bone and Mineral Research*, **2**, 91–8.

Lieberherr, M., Grosse, B., Duchambon, P. & Drücke, T. (1989) A functional cell surface type receptor is required for the early action of 1,25-dihydroxyvitamin D$_3$ on the phosphoinositide metabolism in rat enterocytes. *Journal of Biological Chemistry*, **264**(34), 20 403–6.

Liu, M., Lee, M.-H., Cohen, M., Bommakanti, M. & Freedman, L. P. (1996a) Transcriptional activation of the Cdk inhibitor p21 by vitamin D$_3$ leads to the induced differentiation of the myelomonocytic cell line U937. *Genes & Development*, **10**, 142–53.

Liu, S. M., Koszewski, N,., Lupez, M., Malluche, H. H., Olivera, A. & Russell, J. (1996b) Characterization of a response element in the 5′-flanking region of the avian (chicken) PTH gene that mediates negative regulation of gene transcription by 1,25-dihydroxyvitamin D$_3$ and binds the vitamin D$_3$ receptor. *Molecular Endocrinology*, **10**, 206–15.

Lobaugh, B. (1996) Blood calcium and phosphorus regulation. In: *Calcium and Phosphorus in Health and Disease*. (Ed. J. J. B. Anderson & S. C. Garner), pp. 27–43. CRC Press, Boca Raton, FL.

Lötscher, M., Wilson, P., Nguyen, S., Kaissling, B., Biber, J., Murer, H. & Levi, M. (1996) New aspects of adaptation of rat renal Na-Pi cotransporter to alterations in dietary phosphate. *Kidney International*, **49**, 1012–18.

Lowe, K. E., Maiyar, A. C. & Norman, A. W. (1992) Vitamin D-mediated gene expression. *Critical Reviews in Eukaryotic Gene Expression*, **2**, 65–109.

MacDonald, P. N., Dowd, D. R., Nakajima, S., Galligan, M. A., Reeder, M. C., Haussler, C. A., Ozato, K. & Haussler, M. R. (1993) Retinoid X receptors stimulate and 9-*cis* retinoic acid inhibits 1,25-dihydroxyvitamin D$_3$-activated expression of the rat osteocalcin gene. *Molecular and Cellular Biology*, **13**, 5907–17.

MacDonald, P. N., Sherman, D. R., Dowd, D. R., Jefcoat, S. C. Jr. & DeLisle, R. K. (1995) The vitamin D receptor interacts with general transcription factor IIB. *Journal of Biological Chemistry*, **270**(9), 4748–52.

MacDonald, P. N., Baudino, T. A., Tokumaru, H., Dowd, D. R. & Zhang, C. (2001) Vitamin D receptor and nuclear receptor coactivators: crucial interactions in vitamin D-mediated transcription. *Steroids*, **66**, 171–6.

MacLaughlin, J. & Holick, M. F. (1985) Aging decreases the capacity of human skin to produce vitamin D$_3$. *Journal of Clinical Investigation*, **76**, 1536–8.

MacLaughlin, J. A., Anderson, R. R. & Holick, M. F. (1982) Spectral character of sunlight modulates photosynthesis of previtamin D$_3$ and its photoisomers in human skin. *Science*, **216**, 1001–3.

MacLaughlin, J. A., Cantley, L. C. & Holick, M. F. (1990) 1,25(OH)$_2$D$_3$ increases calcium and phosphatidylinositol metabolism in differentiating cultured human keratinocytes. *Journal of Nutritional Biochemistry*, **1**, 81–7.

Malloy, P. J., Pike, J. W. & Feldman, D. (1999) The vitamin D receptor and the syndrome of hereditary 1,25-dihydroxyvitamin D-resistant rickets. *Endocrine Reviews*, **20**, 156–88.

Mangalam, H. J., Albert, V. R., Ingraham, H. A., Kapiloff, M.,

Wilson, L., Nelson, C., Elsholtz, H. & Rosenfeld, M. G. (1989) A pituitary POU domain protein, Pit-1, activates both growth hormone and prolactin promoters transcriptionally. *Genes & Development*, **3**, 946–58.

Manolagas, S. C., Burton, D. W. & Deftos, L. J. (1981) 1,25-Dihydroxyvitamin D$_3$ stimulates the alkaline phosphatase activity of osteoblast-like cells. *Journal of Biological Chemistry*, **256**(14), 7115–17.

Manolagas, S. C., Hustmyer, F. G. & Yu, X.-P. (1989) 1,25-Dihydroxyvitamin D$_3$ and the immune system. *Proceedings of the Society of Experimental Biology and Medicine*, **191**, 238–45.

Manolagas, S. C., Hustmyer, F. G. & Yu, X.-P. (1990) Immunomodulating properties of 1,25-dihydroxyvitamin D$_3$. *Kidney International*, **38** (Suppl. 29), S9–S16.

Martell, R. E., Simpson, R. U. & Taylor, J. M. (1987) 1,25-Dihydroxyvitamin D$_3$ regulation of phorbol ester receptors in HL-60 leukemia cells. *Journal of Biological Chemistry*, **262**(12), 5570–5.

Matsumoto, T., Fontaine, O. & Rasmussen, H. (1981) Effect of 1,25-dihydroxyvitamin D$_3$ on phospholipid metabolism in chick duodenal mucosal cell. Relationship to its mechanism of action. *Journal of Biological Chemistry*, **256**, 3354–60.

Matsuoka, L. Y., Ide, L., Wortsman, J., MacLaughlin, J. A. & Holick, M. F. (1987) Sunscreens suppress cutaneous vitamin D$_3$ synthesis. *Journal of Clinical Endocrinology and Metabolism*, **64**, 1165–8.

Mawer, E. B., Backhouse, J, Holman, C. A., Lumb, G. A. & Stanbury, S. W. (1972) The distribution and storage of vitamin D and its metabolites in human tissues. *Clinical Science*, **43**, 413–31.

McSheehy, P. M. J. & Chambers, T. J. (1987) 1,25-Dihydroxyvitamin D$_3$ stimulates rat osteoblastic cells to release a soluble factor that increases osteoclastic bone resorption. *Journal of Clinical Investigation*, **80**, 425–9.

Medhora, M. M., Teitelbaum, S., Chappel, J., Alvarez, J., Mimura, H., Ross, F. P. & Hruska, K. (1993) 1α,25-Dihydroxyvitamin D$_3$ up-regulates expression of the osteoclast integrin α$_v$β$_3$. *Journal of Biological Chemistry*, **268**(2), 1456–61.

Mee, A. P., Hoyland, J. A., Braidman, I. P., Freemont, A. J., Davies, M. & Mawer, E. B. (1996) Demonstration of vitamin D receptor transcripts in actively resorbing osteoclasts in bone sections. *Bone*, **18**, 295–9.

Meehan, M. A., Kerman, R. H. & Lemire, J. M. (1992) 1,25-Dihydroxyvitamin D$_3$ enhances the generation of nonspecific suppressor cells while inhibiting the induction of cytotoxic cells in a human MLR. *Cellular Immunology*, **140**, 400–9.

Merino, F., Alvarez-Mon, M., de la Hera, A., Alés, J. E., Bonilla, F. & Durantez, A. (1989) Regulation of natural killer cytotoxicity by 1,25-dihydroxyvitamin D$_3$. *Cellular Immunology*, **118**, 328–36.

Mimura, H., Cao, X., Ross, F. P., Chiba, M. & Teitelbaum, S. L. (1994) 1,25-Dihydroxyvitamin D$_3$ transcriptionally activates the β$_3$-integrin subunit gene in avian osteoclast precursors. *Endocrinology*, **134**, 1061–6.

Montagna, W. & Carlisle, K. (1979) Structural changes in aging human skin. *Journal of Investigative Dermatology*, **73**, 47–53.

Mooseker, M. S., Wolenski, J. S., Coleman, T. R., Hayden, S. M., Cheney, R. D., Espreafico, E., Heintzelman, M. B. & Peterson, M. D. (1991) Structural and functional dissection of a membrane-bound mechanoenzyme: brush-border myosin I. *Current Topics in Membranes*, **33**, 31–55.

Morel, P. A., Manolagas, S. C., Provvedini, D. M., Wegmann, D. R. & Chiller, J. M (1986) Interferon-γ-induced Ia expression in WEHI-3 cells is enhanced by the presence of 1,25-dihydroxyvitamin D$_3$. *Journal of Immunology*, **136**, 2181–6.

Morelli, S., de Boland, A. R. & Boland, R. L. (1993) Generation of inositol phosphates, diacylglycerol and calcium fluxes in myoblasts treated with 1,25-dihydroxyvitamin D$_3$. *Biochemical*

Journal, **289**, 675–9.

Murayama, A., Takeyama, K., Kitanaka, S., Kodera, Y., Hosoya, T. & Kato, S. (1998) The promoter of the human 25-hydroxyvitamin D₃ 1α-hydroxylase gene confers positive and negative responsiveness to PTH, calcitonin, and 1α25(OH)₂D₃. *Biochemical and Biophysical Research Communications*, **249**, 11–16.

Murer, H., Hernando, N., Forster, I. & Biber, J. (2001) Molecular aspects in the regulation of renal inorganic phosphate reabsorption: the type IIa sodium/inorganic phosphate co-transporter as the key player. *Current Opinion in Nephrology and Hypertension*, **10**, 555–61.

Murer, H., Köhler, K., Lambert, G., Stange, G., Biber, J. & Forster, I. (2002) The renal type II Na/Pi cotransporter. *Cell Biochemistry and Biophysics*, **36**, 215–20.

Need, A. G., Morris, H. A., Horowitz, M. & Nordin, B. E. C. (1993) Effects of skin thickness, age, body fat, and sunlight on serum 25-hydroxyvitamin D. *American Journal of Clinical Nutrition*, **58**, 882–5.

Nemere, I. (1999) 24,25-Dihydroxyvitamin D₃ suppresses the rapid actions of 1,25-dihydroxyvitamin D₃ and parathyroid hormone on calcium transport in chick intestine. *Journal of Bone and Mineral Research*, **14**, 1543–9.

Nemere, I., Leathers, V. & Norman, A. W. (1986) 1,25-Dihydroxyvitamin D₃-mediated intestinal calcium transport. *Journal of Biological Chemistry*, **261**(34), 16 106–14.

Nemere, I., Yoshimoto, Y. & Norman, A. W. (1984) Calcium transport in perfused duodena from normal chicks: enhancement within fourteen minutes of exposure to 1,25-dihydroxyvitamin D₃. *Endocrinology*, **115**, 1476–83.

Nemere, I., Dormanen, M. C., Hammond, M. W., Okamura, W. H. & Norman, A. W. (1994) Identification of a specific binding protein for 1α,25-dihydroxyvitamin D₃ in basal-lateral membranes of chick intestinal epithelium and relationship to transcaltachia. *Journal of Biological Chemistry*, **269**(38), 23 750–6.

Nemere, I., Schwartz, Z., Pedrozo, H., Sylvia, V. L., Dean, D. D. & Boyan, B. D. (1998) Identification of a membrane receptor for 1,25-dihydroxyvitamin D₃ which mediates rapid activation of protein kinase C. *Journal of Bone and Mineral Research*, **13**, 1353–9.

Nemere, I., Ray, R. & McManus, W. (2000) Immunochemical studies on the putative plasmalemmal receptor for 1,25(OH)₂D₃. I. Chick intestine. *American Journal of Physiology*, **278**, E1104–14.

Noda, M. & Denhardt, D. T. (2002) Osteopontin. In: *Principles of Bone Biology*, 2nd edn, Vol. I. (Ed. J. P. Bilezikien, L. G. Raisz & G. A. Rodan), pp. 239–50. Academic Press, San Diego.

Noda, M., Vogel, R. L., Craig, A. M., Prahl, J., DeLuca, H. F. & Denhardt, D. T. (1990) Identification of a DNA sequence responsible for binding of the 1,25-dihydroxyvitamin D₃ receptor and 1,25-dihydroxyvitamin D₃ enhancement of mouse secreted phosphoprotein 1 (*Spp-1* or osteopontin) gene expression. *Proceedings of the National Academy of Sciences of the U.S.A.*, **87**, 9995–9.

Norman, A. W. (1998) Receptors for 1α,25(OH)₂D₃: past, present, and future. *Journal of Bone and Mineral Research*, **13**, 1360–9.

Nykjaer, A., Dragun, D., Walther, D., Vorum, H., Jacobsen, C., Herz, J., Melsen, F., Christensen, E. I. & Willnow, T. E. (1999) An endocytic pathway essential for renal uptake and activation of the steroid 25-(OH) vitamin D₃. *Cell*, **96**, 507–15.

Owen, T. A., Aronow, M. S., Barone, L. M., Bettencourt, B., Stein, G. S. & Lian, J. B. (1991) Pleiotropic effects of vitamin D on osteoblast gene expression are related to the proliferative and differentiated state of the bone cell phenotype: dependency upon basal levels of gene expression, duration of exposure, and bone matrix competency in normal rat osteoblast cultures. *Endocrinology*, **128**, 1496–504.

Ozono, K., Liao, J., Kerner, S. A., Scott, R. A. & Pike, J. W. (1990) The vitamin D-responsive element in the human osteocalcin gene. Association with a nuclear proto-oncogene enhancer. *Journal of Biological Chemistry*, **265**(35), 21 881–8.

Pansu, D., Bellaton, C. & Bronner, F. (1981) Effect of Ca intake on saturable and nonsaturable components of duodenal Ca transport. *American Journal of Physiology*, **240**, G32–7.

Pansu, D., Bellaton, C., Roche, C. & Bronner, F. (1983) Duodenal and ileal calcium absorption in the rat and effects of vitamin D. *American Journal of Physiology*, **244**, G695–700.

Parrish, D. B. (1979) Determination of vitamin D in foods: a review. *CRC Critical Reviews in Food Science and Nutrition*, **12**, 29–57.

Paul, S. R., Bennett, F., Calvetti, J. A., Kelleher, K., Wood, C. R., O'Hara, R. M. Jr., Leary, A. C., Sibley, B., Clark, S. C., Williams, D. A. & Yang, Y.-C. (1990) Molecular cloning of a cDNA encoding interleukin 11, a stromal cell-derived lymphopoietic and hematopoietic cytokine. *Proceedings of the National Academy of Sciences of the U.S.A.*, **87**, 7512–16.

Pedrozo, H. A., Schwartz, Z., Rimes, S., Sylvia, V. L., Nemere, I., Posner, G. H., Dean, D. D. & Boyan, B. D. (1999) Physiological importance of the 1,25(OH)₂D₃ membrane receptor and evidence for a membrane receptor specific for 24,25(OH)₂D₃. *Journal of Bone and Mineral Research*, **14**, 856–67.

Polla, B. S., Healy, A. M., Amento, E. P. & Krane, S. M. (1986) 1,25-Dihydroxyvitamin D₃ maintains adherence of human monocytes and protects them from thermal injury. *Journal of Clinical Investigation*, **77**, 1332–9.

Polly, P., Carlberg, C., Eisman, J. A. & Morrison, N. A. (1996) Identification of a vitamin D response element in the fibronectin gene that is bound by a vitamin D₃ receptor homodimer. *Journal of Cellular Biochemistry*, **60**, 322–33.

Pols, H. A. P., Schilte, J. P., Herrmann-Erlee, M. P. M., Visser, T. J. & Birkenhäger, J. C. (1986) The effects of 1,25-dihydroxyvitamin D₃ on growth, alkaline phosphatase and adenylate cyclase of rat osteoblast-like cells. *Bone and Mineral*. **1**, 397–405.

Price, P. A. (1985) Vitamin K-dependent formation of bone Gla protein (osteocalcin) and its function. *Vitamins and Hormones*, **42**, 65–108.

Quamme, G. A. (1985) Phosphate transport in intestinal brush-border membrane vesicles: effect of pH and dietary phosphate. *American Journal of Physiology*, **249**, G168–76.

Quamme, G. A. & Wong, N. L. M. (1984) Phosphate transport in the proximal convoluted tubule: effect of intraluminal pH. *American Journal of Physiology*, **246**, F323–33.

Quélo, I., Kahlen, J.-P., Rascle, A., Jurdic, P. & Carlberg, C. (1994) Identification and characterization of a vitamin D₃ response element of chicken carbonic anhydrase II. *DNA and Cell Biology*, **13**, 1181–7.

Rachez, C., Suldan, Z., Ward, J., Chang, C.-P. B., Burakov, D., Erdjument-Bromage, H., Tempst, P. & Freedman, L. P. (1998) A novel protein complex that interacts with the vitamin D₃ receptor in a ligand-dependent manner and enhances VDR transactivation in a cell-free system. *Genes & Development*, **12**, 1787–800.

Rachez, C., Lemon, B. D., Suldan, Z., Bromleigh, V., Gamble, M., Näär, A. M., Erdjument-Bromage, H., Tempst, P. & Freedman, L. P. (1999) Ligand-dependent transcription activation by nuclear receptors requires the DRIP complex. *Nature*, **398**, 824–8.

Raisz, L. G., Trummel, C. L., Holik, M. F. & DeLuca, H. F. (1972) 1,25-Dihydroxycholecalciferol: a potent stimulator of bone resorption in tissue culture. *Science*, **175**, 768–9.

Reinhardt, T. A. & Horst, R. L. (1990) Parathyroid hormone downregulates 1,25-dihydroxyvitamin D receptors (VDR) and VDR messenger ribonucleic acid *in vitro* and blocks homologous upregulation of VDR *in vivo*. *Endocrinology*, **127**, 942–8.

Rhodes, S. J., Chen, R., DiMattia, G. E., Scully, K. M., Kalla, K. A., Lin, S.-C., Yu, V. C. & Rosenfeld, M. G. (1993) A tissue-specific enhancer confers Pit-1-dependent morphogen inducibility and autoregulation on the *pi-1* gene. *Genes & Development*, 7, 913–32.

Rigby, W. F. C., Noelle, R. J., Krause, K. & Fanger, M. W. (1985) The effects of 1,25-dihydroxyvitamin D₃ on human T lymphocyte activation and proliferation: a cell cycle analysis. *Journal of Immunology*, 135, 2279–86.

Roche, C., Bellaton, C., Pansu, D., Miller, A. III & Bronner, F. (1986) Localization of vitamin D-dependent active Ca²⁺ transport in rat duodenum and relation to CaBP. *American Journal of Physiology*, 251, G314–20.

Romas, E., Udagawa, N., Zhou, H., Tamura, T., Saito, M., Taga, T., Hilton, D. J., Suda, T., Ng, K. W. & Martin, T. J. (1996) The role of gp130-mediated signals in osteoclast development: regulation of interleukin 11 production by osteoblasts and distribution of its receptor in bone marrow cultures. *Journal of Experimental Medicine*, 183, 2581–91.

Rook, G. A. W., Steele, J., Fraher, L., Barker, S., Karmali, R., O'Riordan, J. & Stanford, J. (1986) Vitamin D₃, gamma interferon, and control of proliferation of *Mycobacterium tuberculosis* by human monocytes. *Immunology*, 57, 159–63.

Rook, G. A. W., Taverne, J., Leveton, C. & Steele, J. (1987) The role of gamma-interferon, vitamin D₃ metabolites and tumour necrosis factor in the pathogenesis of tuberculosis. *Immunology*, 62, 229–34.

Rowe, D. W. & Kream, B. E. (1982) Regulation of collagen synthesis in fetal rat calvaria by 1,25-dihydroxyvitamin D₃. *Journal of Biological Chemistry*, 257(14), 8009–15.

Sampson, H. W., Matthews, J. L., Martin, J. H. & Kunin, A. S. (1970) An electron microscopic localization of calcium in the small intestine of normal, rachitic, and vitamin D-treated rats. *Calcified Tissue Research*, 5, 305–16.

Sato, T., Hong, M. H., Jin, C. H., Ishimi, Y., Udagawa, N., Shinki, T., Abe, E. & Suda, T. (1991) The specific production of the third component of complement in osteoblastic cells treated with 1α,25-dihydroxyvitamin D₃. *FEBS Letters*, 285, 21–4.

Sato, T., Abe, E., Jin, C. H., Hong, M. H., Katagiri, T., Kinoshita, T., Amizuka, N., Ozawa, H. & Suda, T. (1993) The biological roles of the third component of complement in osteoclast formation. *Endocrinology*, 133, 397–404.

Schedl, H. P., Ronnenberg, W., Christensen, K. K. & Hollis, B. W. (1994) Vitamin D and enterocyte brush border membrane calcium transport and fluidity in the rat. *Metabolism*, 43, 1093–103.

Schräder, M., Müller, K. M., Nayeri, S., Kahlen, J.-P. & Carlberg, C. (1994) Vitamin D₃–thyroid hormone receptor heterodimer polarity directs ligand sensitivity of transactivation. *Nature*, 370, 382–6.

Schräder, M., Nayeri, S., Kahlen, J.-P., Müller, K. M. & Carlberg, C. (1995) Natural vitamin D₃ response elements formed by inverted palindromes: polarity-directed ligand sensitivity of vitamin D₃ receptor–retinoid X receptor heterodimer-mediated transactivation. *Molecular and Cellular Biology*, 15, 1154–61.

Schräder, M., Kahlen, J.-P. & Carlberg, C. (1997) Functional characterization of a novel type of 1α,25-dihydroxyvitamin D₃ response element identified in the mouse c-*fos* promoter. *Biochemical and Biophysical Research Communications*, 230, 646–51.

Schüle, R., Umesono, K., Mangelsdorf, D. J., Bolado, J., Pike, J. W. & Evans, R. M. (1990) Jun–Fos and receptors for vitamins A and D recognize a common response element in the human osteocalcin gene. *Cell*, 61, 497–504.

Schwab, S. J., Klahr, S. & Hammerman, M. R. (1984) Na⁺ gradient-dependent Pi uptake in basolateral membrane vesicles from dog kidney. *American Journal of Physiology*, 246, F663–9.

Seo, E.-G. & Norman, A. W. (1997) Three-fold induction of renal 25-hydroxyvitamin D₃-24-hydroxylase activity and increased serum 24,25-dihydroxyvitamin D₃ levels are correlated with the healing process after chick tibial fracture. *Journal of Bone and Mineral Research*, 12, 598–606.

Seo, E.-G., Schwartz, Z., Dean, D. D., Norman, A. W. & Boyan, B. D. (1996) Preferential accumulation *in vivo* of 24R,25-dihydroxyvitamin D₃ in growth plate cartilage of rats. *Endocrine*, 5, 147–55.

Seo, E.-G., Einhorn, T. A. & Norman, A. W. (1997) 24R,25-Dihydroxyvitamin D₃: an essential vitamin D₃ metabolite for both normal bone integrity and healing of tibial fracture in chicks. *Endocrinology*, 138, 3864–72.

Shinki, T., Jin, C. H., Nishimura, A., Nagai, Y., Ohyama, Y., Noshiro, M., Okuda, K. & Suda, T. (1992) Parathyroid hormone inhibits 25-hydroxyvitamin D₃–24-hydroxylase mRNA expression stimulated by 1α,25-dihydroxyvitamin D₃ in rat kidney but not in intestine. *Journal of Biological Chemistry*, 267(19), 13 757–62.

Shiraki, M., Kushida, K., Yamazaki, K., Nagai, T., Inoue, T. & Orimo, H. (1996) Effects of 2 year's treatment of osteoporosis with 1α-hydroxy vitamin D₃ on bone mineral density and incidence of fracture: a placebo-controlled, double-blind prospective study. *Endocrine Journal*, 43, 211–20.

Shrivastava, A. & Calame, K. (1994) An analysis of genes regulated by the multi-functional transcriptional regulator Yin Yang-1. *Nucleic Acids Research*, 22, 5151–5.

Silver, J., Russell, J. & Sherwood, L. M. (1985) Regulation by vitamin D metabolites of messenger ribonucleic acid for preproparathyroid hormone in isolated bovine parathyroid cells. *Proceedings of the National Academy of Sciences of the U.S.A.*, 82, 4270–3.

Silver, J., Naveh-Many, T., Mayer, H., Schmeizer, H. J. & Popvtzer, M. M. (1986) Regulation by vitamin D metabolites of parathyroid hormone gene transcription in vivo in the rat. *Journal of Clinical Investigation*, 78, 1296–301.

Simboli-Campbell, M., Gagnon, A. M., Franks, D. J. & Welsh, J. E. (1994) 1,25-Dihydroxyvitamin D₃ translocates protein kinase Cβ to nucleus and enhances plasma membrane association of protein kinase Cα in renal epithelial cells. *Journal of Biological Chemistry*, 269(5), 3257–64.

Simonet, W. S., Lacey, D. L., Dunstan, C. R., Kelley, M., Chang, M.-S., Lüthy, R., Nguyen, H. Q., Wooden, S., Bennett, L., Boone, T., Shimamoto, G., DeRose, M., Elliott, R., Colombero, A., Tan, H.-L., Trail, G., Sullivan, J., Davy, E., Bucay, N., Renshaw-Gegg, L., Hughes, T. M., Hill, D., Pattison, W., Campbell, P., Sander, S., Van, G., Tarpley, J., Derby, P., Lee, R., Amgen EST Program & Boyle, W. J. (1997) Osteoprotegerin: a novel secreted protein involved in the regulation of bone density. *Cell*, 89, 309–19.

Slater, S. J., Kelly, M. B., Taddeo, F. J., Larkin, J. D., Yeager, M. D., McLane, J. A., Ho, C. & Stubbs, C. D. (1995) Direct activation of protein kinase C by 1α,25-dihydroxyvitamin D₃. *Journal of Biological Chemistry*, 270(12), 6639–43.

Smith, E. L., Walworth, N. C. & Holick, M. F. (1986) Effect of 1α,25-dihydroxyvitamin D₃ on the morphologic and biochemical differentiation of cultured human epidermal keratinocytes grown in serum-free conditions. *Journal of Investigative Dermatology*, 86, 709–14.

Sneddon, W. B., Bogado, C. E., Kiernan, M. S. & Demay, M. B. (1997) DNA sequences downstream from the vitamin D response element of the rat osteocalcin gene are required for ligand-dependent transactivation. *Molecular Endocrinology*, 11, 210–17.

Sorensen, A. M. & Baran, D. T. (1993) 1α,25-Dihydroxyvitamin D₃ rapidly alters phospholipid metabolism in the nuclear envelope of osteoblasts. *Journal of Bone and Mineral Research*, 8, S127.

Sorensen, A. M., Bowman, D. & Baran, D. T. (1993) 1α,25-Dihydroxyvitamin D₃ rapidly increases nuclear calcium levels in rat osteosarcoma cells. *Journal of Cellular Biochemistry*, **52**, 237–42.

St-Arnaud, R. (1999) Targeted inactivation of vitamin D hydroxylases in mice. *Bone*, **25**, 127–9.

St-Arnaud, R., Arabian, A., Travers, R., Barletta, F., Raval-Pandya, M., Chapin, K., Depovere, J., Mathieu, C., Christakos, S., Demay, M. B. & Glorieux, F. H. (2000) Deficient mineralization of intramembranous bone in vitamin D-24-hydroxylase-ablated mice is due to elevated 1,25-dihydroxyvitamin D and not to the absence of 24,25-dihydroxyvitamin D. *Endocrinology*, **141**, 2658–66.

Stein, G. S. & Lian, J. B. (1993) Molecular mechanisms mediating proliferation/differentiation interrelationships during progressive development of the osteoblast phenotype. *Endocrine Reviews*, **14**, 424–42.

Suda, T., Takahashi, N. & Abe, E. (1992a) Role of vitamin D in bone resorption. *Journal of Cellular Biochemistry*, **49**, 53–8.

Suda, T., Takahashi, N. & Martin, T. J. (1992b) Modulation of osteoclast differentiation. *Endocrine Reviews*, **13**, 66–80.

Takahashi, N., Yamana, H., Yoshiki, S., Roodman, G. D., Mundy, G. M., Jones, S. J., Boyde, A. & Suda, T. (1988) Osteoclast-like cell formation and its regulation by osteotropic hormones in mouse bone marrow cultures. *Endocrinology*, **122**, 1373–82.

Takeda, S., Yoshizawa, T., Nagai, Y., Yamoto, H., Fukumoto, S., Sekine, K., Kato, S., Matsumoto, T. & Fujita, T. (1999) Stimulation of osteoclast formation by 1,25-dihydroxyvitamin D requires its binding to vitamin D receptor (VDR) in osteoblastic cells: studies using VDR knockout mice. *Endocrinology*, **140**, 1005–8.

Taketani, Y., Miyamoto, K., Tanaka, K., Katai, K., Chikamori, M., Tatsumi, S., Segawa, H., Yamamoto, H., Morita, K. & Takeda, E. (1997) Gene structure and functional analysis of the human Na$^+$/phosphate co-transporter. *Biochemical Journal*, **324**, 927–34.

Takito, J., Shinki, T., Sasaki, T. & Suda, T. (1990) Calcium uptake by brush-border and basolateral membrane vesicles in chick duodenum. *American Journal of Physiology*, **258**, G16–23.

Talmage, R. V. (1970) Morphological and physiological considerations in a new concept of calcium transport in bone. *American Journal of Anatomy*, **129**, 467–76.

Thompson, P. D., Jurutka, P. W., Haussler, C. A., Whitfield, G. K. & Hausler, M. R. (1998) Heterodimeric DNA binding by the vitamin D receptor and retinoid X receptors is enhanced by 1,25-dihydroxyvitamin D$_3$ and inhibited by 9-*cis*-retinoic acid. Evidence for allosteric receptor interactions. *Journal of Biological Chemistry*, **273**(14), 8483–91.

Thompson, P. D., Hsieh, J.-C., Whitfield, G. K., Haussler, C. A., Jurutka, P. W., Galligan, M. A., Tillman, J. B., Spindler, S. R. & Haussler, M. R. (1999) Vitamin D receptor displays DNA binding and transactivation as a heterodimer with the retinoid X receptor, but not with the thyroid hormone receptor. *Journal of Cellular Biochemistry*, **75**, 462–80.

Tian, X. Q., Chen, T. C., Matsuoka, L. Y., Wortsman, J. & Holick, M. F. (1993) Kinetic and thermodynamic studies of the conversion of previtamin D$_3$ to vitamin D$_3$ in human skin. *Journal of Biological Chemistry*, **268**(20), 14 888–92.

Tornquist, K. & Tashjian, A. H. Jr. (1989) Dual actions of 1,25-dihydroxycholecalciferol on intracellular Ca^{2+} in GH$_4$C$_1$ cells: evidence for effects on voltage-operated Ca^{2+} channels and Na$^+$/Ca^{2+} exchange. *Endocrinology*, **124**, 2765–76.

Tsoukas, C. D., Provvedini, D. M. & Manolagas, S. C. (1984) 1,25-Dihydroxyvitamin D$_3$: a novel immunoregulatory hormone. *Science*, **224**, 1438–40.

Tsuda, E., Goto, M., Mochizuki, S., Yano, K., Kobayashi, F., Morinaga, T. & Higashio, K. (1997) Isolation of a novel cytokine from human fibroblasts that specifically inhibits osteoclastogenesis. *Biochemical and Biophysical Research Communications*, **234**, 137–42.

Underwood, J. L. & DeLuca, H. F. (1984) Vitamin D is not directly necessary for bone growth and mineralization. *American Journal of Physiology*, **246**, E493–8.

van den Berg, H. (1997) Bioavailability of vitamin D. *European Journal of Clinical Nutrition*, **51**, Suppl. 1, S76–9.

Vieth, R. (1990) The mechanisms of vitamin D toxicity. *Bone and Mineral*, **11**, 267–72.

vom Baur, E., Zechel, C., Heery, D., Heine, M. J. S., Garnier, J. M., Vivat, V., Le Douarin, B., Gronemeyer, H., Chambon, P. & Losson, R. (1996) Differential ligand-dependent interactions between the AF-2 activating domain of nuclear receptors and the putative transcriptional intermediary factors mSUG1 and TIF1. *EMBO Journal*, **15**, 110–24.

Wali, R. K., Baum, C. L., Sitrin, M. D. & Brasitus, T. A. (1990) 1,25(OH)$_2$ vitamin D$_3$ stimulates membrane phosphoinositide turnover, activates protein kinase C, and increases cytosolic calcium in rat colonic epithelium. *Journal of Clinical Investigation*, **85**, 1296–1303.

Wali, R. K., Kong, J., Sitrin, M. D., Bissonnette, M. & Li, Y. C. (2003) Vitamin D receptor is not required for the rapid actions of 1,25-dihydroxyvitamin D$_3$ to increase intracellular calcium and activate protein kinase C in mouse osteoblasts. *Journal of Cellular Biochemistry*, **88**, 794–801.

Walker, J. J., Yan, T. S. & Quamme, G. A. (1987) Presence of multiple sodium-dependent phosphate transport processes in proximal brush-border membranes. *American Journal of Physiology*, **252**, F226–31.

Walters, J. R. F. (1989) Calbindin-D$_{9k}$ stimulates the calcium pump in rat enterocyte basolateral membranes. *American Journal of Physiology*, **256**, G124–8.

Walters, J. R. F. & Weiser, M. M. (1987) Calcium transport by rat duodenal villus and crypt basolateral membranes. *American Journal of Physiology*, **252**, G170–7.

Walters, S. N., Reinhardt, T. A., Dominick, M. A., Horst, R. L. & Littledike, E. T. (1986) Intracellular location of unoccupied 1,25-dihydroxyvitamin D receptors: a nuclear–cytoplasmic equilibrium. *Archives of Biochemistry and Biophysics*, **246**, 366–73.

Wasserman, R. H. & Fullmer, C. S. (1995) Vitamin D and intestinal calcium transport: facts, speculations and hypotheses. *Journal of Nutrition*, **125**, 1971S–9S.

Wasserman, R. H., Smith, C. A., Brindak, M. E., De Talamoni, N., Fullmer, C. S., Penniston, J. T. & Kumar, R. (1992) Vitamin D and mineral deficiencies increase the plasma membrane calcium pump of chicken intestine. *Gastroenterology*, **102**, 886–94.

Webb, A. R., Kline, L. & Holick, M. F. (1988) Influence of season and latitude on the cutaneous synthesis of vitamin D$_3$: exposure to winter sunlight in Boston and Edmonton will not promote vitamin D$_3$ synthesis in human skin. *Journal of Clinical Endocrinology and Metabolism*, **67**, 373–8.

Webb, A. R., deCosta, B. R. & Holick, M. F. (1989) Sunlight regulates the cutaneous production of vitamin D$_3$ by causing its photodegradation. *Journal of Clinical Endocrinology and Metabolism*, **68**, 882–7.

Weinstein, R. S., Underwood, J. L., Hutson, M. S. & DeLuca, H. F. (1984) Bone histomorphometry in vitamin D-deficient rats infused with calcium and phosphorus. *American Journal of Physiology*, **246**, E499–E505.

Wilson, H. D., Schedl, H. P. & Christensen, K. (1989) Calcium uptake by brush-border membrane vesicles from the rat intestine. *American Journal of Physiology*, **257**, F446–53.

Wolenski, J. S., Hayden, S. M., Forscher, P. & Mooseker, M. S. (1993) Calcium-calmodulin and regulation of brush border myosin-I MgATPase and mechanochemistry. *Journal of Cell Biology*, **122**, 613–21.

Xie, Z. & Bikle, D. D. (1997) Cloning of the human phospholipase C-γ1 promoter and identification of a DR6-type vitamin D-responsive element. *Journal of Biological Chemistry*, **272**(10), 6573–7.

Xiong, Y., Hannon, G. J., Zhang, H., Casso, D., Kobayashi, R. & Beach, D. (1993) p21 is a universal inhibitor of cyclin kinases. *Nature*, **366**, 701–4.

Yan, T., Walker, J. & Quamme, G. (1988) Sodium-independent phosphate transport in brush-border membrane vesicles prepared from the outer medulla of pig kidneys. *Progress in Clinical and Biological Research*, **252**, 81–6.

Yang, S., Smith, C. & DeLuca, H. F. (1993a) 1α,25-Dihydroxy-vitamin D_3 and 19-nor-1α,25-dihydroxyvitamin D_2 suppress immunoglobulin production and thymic lymphocyte proliferation in vivo. *Biochimica et Biophysica Acta*, **1158**, 279–86.

Yang, S., Smith, C., Prahl, J. M., Luo, X. & DeLuca, H. F. (1993b) Vitamin D deficiency suppresses cell-mediated immunity *in vivo*. *Archives of Biochemistry and Biophysics*, **303**, 98–106.

Yasuda, H., Shima, N., Nakagawa, N., Mochizuki, S., Yano, K., Fujise, N., Sato, Y., Goto, M., Yamaguchi, K., Kuriyama, M., Kanno, T., Murakami, A., Tsuda, E., Morinaga, T. & Higashio, K. (1998a) Identity of osteoclastogenesis inhibitory factor (OCIF) and osteoprotegerin (OPG): a mechanism by which OPG/OCIF inhibits osteoclastogenesis *in vitro*. *Endocrinology*, **139**, 1329–37.

Yasuda, H., Shima, N., Nakagawa, N., Yamaguchi, K., Kinosaki, M., Mochizuki, S., Tomoyasu, A., Yano, K., Goto, M., Murakami, A., Tsuda, E. Morinaga, T., Higashio, K., Udagawa, N., Takahashi, N. & Suda, T. (1998b) Osteoclast differentiation factor is a ligand for osteoprotegerin osteoclastogenesis-inhibitory factor and is identical to TRANCE/RANKL. *Proceedings of the National Academy of Sciences of the U.S.A.*, **95**, 3597–602.

Zelinski, J. M., Sykes, D. E. & Weiser, M. M. (1991) The effect of vitamin D on rat intestinal plasma membrane Ca-pump mRNA. *Biochemical and Biophysical Research Communications*, **179**, 749–55.

Zhang, Q., Wrana, J. L. & Sodek, J. (1992) Characterizaton of the promoter region of the porcine *opn* (osteopontin, secreted phosphoprotein 1) gene. Identificaton of positive and negative regulatory elements and a 'silent' second promoter. *European Journal of Biochemistry*, **207**, 649–59.

Zierold, C., Darwish, H. M. & DeLuca, H. F. (1995) Two vitamin D response elements function in the rat 1,25-dihydroxyvitamin D 24-hydroxylase promoter. *Journal of Biological Chemistry*, **270**(4), 1675–8.

9
Vitamin E

Key discussion topics

- α-Tocopherol is a potent lipophilic antioxidant that protects biomembranes from degenerative lipid peroxidation.
- α-Tocopherol plays an essential role in maintaining the structure and function of the human nervous system. A deficiency in the vitamin causes a severe neurological disorder.
- α-Tocopherol protects against atherosclerosis by decreasing the susceptibility of low-density lipoprotein to oxidation and preserving nitric oxide-mediated arterial relaxation.
- α-Tocopherol plays a role in signal transduction by desensitizing the protein kinase C signalling pathway.
- α-Tocopherol inhibits mitogen-induced cell proliferation.
- The hepatic α-tocopherol transfer protein has an essential role in maintaining plasma α-tocopherol concentrations.

9.1   Historical overview

In 1922, H. M. Evans and Katherine S. Bishop reported from the University of California that pregnant rats fed on formulated diets containing all of the then known nutritional factors did not reach term. Death and resorption of the fetuses were prevented by supplementation of the formulated diet with fresh lettuce, thus implying the existence of a hitherto unknown nutritional factor. By 1924, these initial studies had been independently verified by Sure, who recommended that the unknown factor be officially designated as vitamin E. The active fat-soluble substance was isolated from wheat germ by Evans in 1936. On recognition that more than one compound possessed vitamin E activity, the vitamin was given the generic name, tocopherol, which is derived from the Greek language meaning 'to bring forth in childbirth'. By 1944, it was found that a multiplicity of deficiency syndromes occurs in animals deprived of vitamin E. The structure of the vitamin was elucidated by Fernholz in 1937 and synthesis was accomplished by Karrer in the following year.

9.2   Chemistry, biopotency and units of activity

Vitamin E is represented by a family of structurally related compounds (vitamers) which show pronounced quantitative differences in biological activity. Eight of these vitamers are known to occur in nature, having been isolated from vegetable oils and other plant materials. The vitamers comprise four tocopherols and four tocotrienols, whose parent structures are tocol and tocotrienol, respectively. Tocotrienol differs from

tocol in having three double bonds in the phytyl side chain. The tocol molecule exhibits optical isomerism attributable to the three asymmetric carbon atoms at positions 2, 4′ and 8′, thus the tocopherols can exist as one of eight possible diastereoisomers. The tocotrienols possess only one centre of asymmetry at position 2, in addition to sites of geometrical isomerism at positions 3′ and 7′ in the unsaturated side chain. The RS system of asymmetric configuration is used to specify the chirality of vitamin E compounds. In nature, the tocopherols exist exclusively as their 2R,4′R,8′R stereoisomers (RRR-forms), while the tocotrienols exist exclusively in the 2R,3′-trans,7′-trans configuration. The stereochemical structures of tocol and tocotrienol are depicted in Fig. 9.1.

The vitamin E vitamers are designated as alpha- (α), beta- (β), gamma- (γ) and delta- (δ) according to the number and position of substituent methyl groups on the chromanol ring of tocol or tocotrienol (Table 9.1). The biopotencies of the various tocopherols and tocotrienols evaluated by the rat resorption–gestation assay are listed in Table 9.2. In this text the term 'vitamin E' is used as the generic descriptor for all tocol and tocotrienol derivatives that exhibit qualitatively the biological activity of α-tocopherol. The term 'tocopherol' refers specifically to the methyl-substituted derivatives of tocol and is not synonymous with the term 'vitamin E'. The tocopherols and tocotrienols may be referred to collectively as tocochromanols.

Vitamin E is available commercially for use as a dietary supplement in both its natural form, RRR-α-tocopherol, and synthetic form, all-racemic 2RS,4′RS,8′RS-α-tocopherol (all-rac-α-tocopherol). Both forms of α-tocopherol are usually sold as acetate esters (α-tocopheryl acetate) or, less frequently, as succinate esters because of their greater stability. The

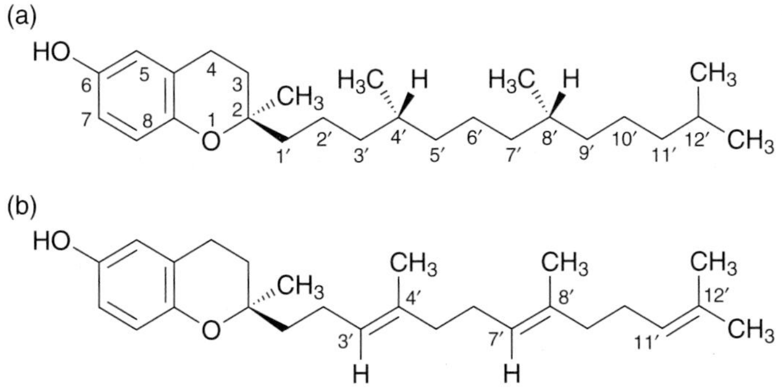

Fig. 9.1 Stereochemical structures of tocol and tocotrienol. (a) R,R,R-tocol, (b) 2R,3′-trans, 7′-trans-tocotrienol.

Table 9.1 Designation of tocopherols and tocotrienols.

Methyl substitution of tocol or tocotrienol molecule	Tocopherol (T)	Tocotrienol (T3)
5,7,8-Trimethyl	α-T	α-T3
5,8-Dimethyl	β-T	β-T3
7,8-Dimethyl	γ-T	γ-T3
8-Methyl	δ-T	δ-T3

Table 9.2 Relative percentage biopotencies of vitamin E compounds by the rat resorption–gestation assay.

Compound[a]	Relative biopotency (%)	Reference
α-Tocopherol	100	Joffe & Harris (1943)
β-Tocopherol	40	Joffe & Harris (1943)
γ-Tocopherol	8	Joffe & Harris (1943)
δ-Tocopherol	1	Stern et al. (1947)
α-Tocotrienol	21	Bunyan et al. (1961)
β-Tocotrienol	4	Bunyan et al. (1961)

[a] *RRR* forms.

bioavailability of *all-rac*-α-tocopherol in humans is roughly half that of *RRR*-α-tocopherol (Burton *et al.*, 1998).

In the early days of vitamin assays, when bioassays were the only methods for estimating the vitamin contents of foods, the vitamin activity of a food sample was expressed in international units (IU) and was determined by comparing the activity in the bioassay with the activity of an official international standard. In 1980, the designation of vitamin E activity was changed from IU to an expression of equivalents, based on biological activity. In this notation, all vitamin E activity is expressed relative to the naturally occurring, most active form of the vitamin, *RRR*-α-tocopherol. The total vitamin E activity in a food should be reported as α-tocopherol equivalents (α-TE).

α-TE = α-tocopherol (mg × 1.0) + β-tocopherol (mg × 0.5) + γ-tocopherol (mg × 0.1) + α-tocotrienol (mg × 0.3)

The remaining vitamers have negligible activity.

Although the IU is no longer officially recognized as a unit of vitamin activity, many fortified foods and supplements still retain this terminology. One IU of vitamin E is defined as the biological activity of 1 mg of *all-rac*-α-tocopheryl acetate. One milligram of *RRR*-α-tocopherol is equivalent to 1.49 IU of vitamin E.

9.3　Dietary sources

The important plant sources of vitamin E are the cereal grains and those nuts, beans and seeds that are also rich in high-potency oils. The vegetable oils extracted from these plant sources are the richest dietary sources of vitamin E. Cereal grain products, fish, meat, eggs, dairy products and green leafy vegetables also provide significant amounts. Major sources of vitamin E in the United States include margarine, mayonnaise and salad dressings, fortified breakfast cereals, vegetable shortenings and cooking oils, peanut butter, eggs, potato crisps, whole milk, tomato products and apples.

9.4　Absorption, transport and delivery to tissues

Background information can be found in Section 3.6.

9.4.1　Stable isotope labelling

Biokinetic studies of vitamin E have been radically improved by the application of stable isotope labelling and gas chromatography–mass spectrometry (GC–MS) to the measurement of absorption, transport, uptake and retention of tocopherols in humans and laboratory animals (Burton & Traber, 1990). Deuterated tocopherols containing three or six atoms of deuterium (^{2}H) per molecule may be ingested safely because deuterium is a stable isotope and has no deleterious effects. The deuterated tocopherols do not undergo any measurable exchange at the positions of substitution. Stable isotope labelling makes it possible to evaluate, within the same subject, the simultaneous competitive uptake of two (or even three) different forms of α-tocopherol labelled with different amounts of deuterium. This approach has the great advantage of eliminating the effects of variations in solute uptake between individual subjects. Furthermore, the deuterated tocopherol taken with a meal is easily distinguishable from the nondeuterated tocopherol already present in the subject.

9.4.2   Intestinal absorption

Absorption of vitamin E depends on the simultaneous digestion and absorption of dietary fat. Individuals with impaired fat absorption invariably exhibit low vitamin E utilization. Before absorption, any ingested supplemental α-tocopheryl acetate or succinate is hydrolysed in the lumen of the small intestine by pancreatic esterase, which requires bile salts as cofactors. The free α-tocopherol thus formed, together with vitamin E of natural origin, is solubilized within mixed micelles for passage across the unstirred water layer of the intestinal lumen. The micelles dissociate and the liberated vitamin E is absorbed by simple diffusion. The absorption efficiency of vitamin E in the rat is greater when the vitamin is solubilized in micelles containing medium-chain triglycerides as compared with long-chain triglycerides (Gallo-Torres et al., 1971). Within the enterocyte, vitamin E is incorporated into chylomicrons and the chylomicrons are secreted into the bloodstream via the lymphatic route.

Absorption studies have focused mainly on α-tocopherol; yet the dietary intake of γ-tocopherol is about twice that of α-tocopherol in the United States and γ-tocopherol contributes an estimated 20% of the total vitamin E activity in a typical United States diet (Bieri & Poukka Evarts, 1974). Despite this, the concentration of γ-tocopherol averages only 10–15% of the concentration of α-tocopherol in adult human plasma (Drevon, 1991). Studies in thoracic duct-cannulated rats have shown no significant difference in the rate of absorption of α- and γ-tocopherol and even a 50-fold excess of α-tocopherol did not affect the absorption of γ-tocopherol (Traber et al., 1986).

The few reported studies in normal human subjects have shown that the absorption of vitamin E is incomplete. Estimates of the absorption of physiological oral doses of tritiated all-rac-α-tocopherol based on the measurement of unabsorbed faecal radioactivity gave efficiencies ranging from 51 to 86% (mean 72%) (Kelleher & Losowsky, 1970) and from 55 to 79% (mean 69%) (MacMahon & Neale, 1970). Pharmacological doses of vitamin E are absorbed with progressively less efficiency as the dose is increased until eventually a limit is reached. Even if dosages exceed the daily requirement 100-fold, the plasma concentrations do not increase beyond 2 to 4-fold (Kayden & Traber, 1993). There is no compensatory increase

in absorption in the presence of vitamin E deficiency (Losowsky et al., 1972).

There have been many conflicting reports concerning the relative absorption efficiency of α-tocopherol and its acetate ester. The situation has been clarified by Burton et al. (1988) using deuterium-substitution and GC–MS in studies with rats and humans. In the human study, a capsule containing an equimolar mixture of RRR-α-tocopherol and RRR-α-tocopheryl acetate was taken with an evening meal on successive days. The amount of α-tocopherol from the free phenol form was found to be equal to that from the acetate in plasma and erythrocytes, signifying an equal efficiency of absorption. These two forms should therefore be accorded equal potency on a molar basis.

9.4.3   Transport and delivery to tissues

Major pathways of vitamin E transport are shown in Fig. 9.2. On entering the bloodstream, the chylomicrons are attacked by lipoprotein lipase located on the capillary walls of most tissues. Hydrolysis of the core triglycerides results in the formation of chylomicron remnants. During chylomicron lipolysis and erosion of the triglyceride core, the excess surface components, including some vitamin E, are transferred to circulating HDL (Havel, 1994). HDL can readily exchange surface components with other types of lipoprotein (Traber et al., 1992), this interchange being accelerated by the phospholipid transfer protein (Kostner et al., 1995). Thus the various tocochromanols that were consumed are distributed to all of the circulating lipoproteins.

The chylomicron remnants, still containing some vitamin E, are taken up by the liver by receptor-mediated endocytosis. The liver then secretes into the plasma the newly absorbed vitamin E within very-low-density lipoproteins (VLDL). These triglyceride-rich particles are also subject to lipolysis by lipoprotein lipase in extrahepatic tissues (particularly adipose tissue and skeletal muscle). When much of the triglyceride has been removed, the VLDL becomes intermediate-density lipoprotein (IDL). Some IDL particles are taken up by the liver, while the remainder are converted to low-density lipoproteins (LDL). The newly ingested vitamin E equilibrates between LDL and high-density lipoproteins (HDL), which are the principal carriers for transport in human plasma. Un-

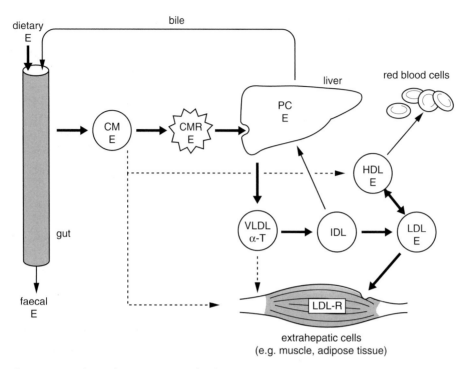

Fig. 9.2 Major pathways of vitamin E transport. After absorption, vitamin E enters the circulation incorporated into the outer layer of chylomicrons (CM). During chylomicron lipolysis, some vitamin E is transferred to high-density lipoproteins (HDL) and some to peripheral tissues. Interchange of vitamin E takes place between HDL and low-density lipoproteins (LDL). Chylomicron remnants (CMR) are taken up by hepatic parenchymal cells (PC). The hepatic α-tocopherol transfer protein selects *R,R,R*-α-tocopherol and facilitates its secretion into the bloodstream in very-low-density lipoproteins (VLDL). Non-α-tocopherol vitamers and excess α-tocopherol are returned to the intestine in the bile and excreted in the faeces. Lipolysis of the VLDL transforms these particles into intermediate-density lipoproteins (IDL). Some IDL particles are taken up by the liver; the remainder are converted to LDL. Cells expressing the LDL receptor (LDL-R) take up the vitamin E in LDL by receptor-mediated endocytosis. Erythrocytes and other cells take up the vitamin E in HDL. Reproduced with permission of Taylor & Francis from Drevon (1991), *Free Radical Research*, Vol. 14, pp. 229–46 (http://www.tandf.co.uk/journals/titles/10715762.html).

like vitamins A and D, there is no evidence of a specific plasma protein for transporting vitamin E.

The liver secretes α-tocopherol in the VLDL in preference to γ-tocopherol, the latter being preferentially excreted in the bile (Traber & Kayden, 1989). This discrimination explains why α-tocopherol is the predominant circulating form of vitamin E, despite γ-tocopherol being the predominant dietary form. The liver further discriminates between stereoisomers of α-tocopherol, secreting *RRR*-α-tocopherol in preference to *SRR*-α-tocopherol (Traber *et al.*, 1990). This discriminatory ability has been attributed to a hepatic tocopherol-binding protein known as the α-tocopherol transfer protein that is present exclusively in hepatocytes (Yoshida *et al.*, 1992) and has been identified in human liver (Kuhlenkamp *et al.*, 1993). The protein

seems to function by stimulating the secretion of cytosolic α-tocopherol into the sinusoidal space where it becomes associated with nascent VLDL. The secretion utilizes a novel non-Golgi-mediated pathway that may be linked to cellular cholesterol metabolism and/or transport (Arita *et al.*, 1997).

The α-tocopherol transfer protein salvages α-tocopherol that is returned to the liver during the course of normal lipoprotein metabolism and promotes its resecretion in VLDL. Thus α-tocopherol delivered to the liver is recycled rather than excreted in the bile. α-Tocopherol has the highest antioxidant activity (commensurate with biological activity) and the ability of the transfer protein to select this vitamer ensures that the most effective form of vitamin E reaches the tissues. The transfer protein may also play a supporting role to decreased fractional absorption in limiting plasma concentrations of α-tocopherol during oral vitamin E supplementation.

The α-tocopherol circulating in LDL is available for tissue uptake by receptor-mediated endocytosis via the cellular LDL receptor. The LDL receptor is found on essentially all cells, but is most prolific on liver cells. LDL is also taken up by an unregulated, receptor-independent process (Jones & Kubow, 1999). Circulating erythrocytes likely obtain their vitamin E by transfer of vitamers from lipoproteins, especially HDL (Traber, 1999). Kitabchi & Wimalasena (1982) showed that human erythrocyte plasma membranes have specific binding sites for α-tocopherol. HDL binding proteins have been identified on plasma membranes of hepatocytes and adipocytes (Jones & Kubow, 1999). Dutta-Roy et al. (1994) identified a protein in the cytosol of liver (rat) and heart (rat and rabbit) that binds α-tocopherol in preference to other tocopherols. The authors speculated that the binding protein may be involved in the cellular uptake of α-tocopherol and regulation of α-tocopherol levels in the subcellular membranes. Finally, lipoprotein lipase can mediate the transfer of some vitamin E from both chylomicrons and VLDL to the tissues (Traber et al., 1985).

9.4.4 Excretion

The major route of excretion of ingested vitamin E is faecal elimination. The non-*RRR*-α-tocopherol forms of vitamin E that are not preferentially secreted by the liver in VLDL, together with any excess α-tocopherol, are probably excreted unchanged in bile. Increasing doses of supplemental vitamin E in humans result in increasing urinary excretion of 2,5,7,8-tetramethyl-2-(2′-carboxyethyl)-6-hydroxychroman (α-CEHC), a metabolite that results from degradation of the phytyl tail. Urinary excretion of this metabolite may indicate excess vitamin E intake (Institute of Medicine, 2000). Sebaceous glands in the skin may secrete vitamin E to provide antioxidant protection for cutaneous lipids.

9.4.5 Deposition in tissues and turnover

No organ functions as a storage site for α-tocopherol, releasing it on demand. More than 90% of the human body pool of α-tocopherol is located in fat droplets within adipose tissue. The accumulation of vitamin E in adipose tissue is due simply to its lipid solubility. Some tissues, such as erythrocytes, liver and spleen, have rapid turnover times, quickly replacing 'old' with 'new' α-tocopherol. The brain has the slowest α-tocopherol turnover time by far. In general, the vitamin E content of the nervous system is spared during vitamin E depletion. Within the nervous system, the peripheral nerves are the most responsive to vitamin E concentrations in the diet (Traber, 1999).

9.5 Antioxidant role

Vitamin E is the major antioxidant in the lipid environment of cellular and subcellular membranes, and also in plasma lipoproteins, protecting the vital phospholipids from peroxidation. The relative susceptibility of microsomes from various tissues to lipid peroxidation correlates with vitamin E content. Notably, highly oxygenated heart and lung tissues have a high content of membranous vitamin E (Kornbrust & Mavis, 1980). The vitamin, chiefly α-tocopherol, is specifically and actively incorporated within biological membranes, where it stabilizes the lipoprotein structure. The tocopherol molecule is anchored in the phospholipid bilayer by means of its phytyl side chain with its polar head group located very close to the lipid–water interface. Protection by vitamin E against endothelial cell injury by hydroperoxides has been demonstrated (Hennig et al., 1987).

By scavenging peroxyl radicals that otherwise would propagate the chain reaction of lipid peroxidation, vitamin E acts as a chain-breaking antioxidant. It does this by donating a hydrogen atom from its phenolic hydroxyl group to a lipid peroxyl radical (LOO$^\bullet$), forming the tocopheroxyl radical (TO$^\bullet$) and a lipid hydroperoxide (LOOH) (reaction 9.1).

$$\text{LOO}^\bullet + \text{T–OH} \rightarrow \text{LOOH} + \text{T–O}^\bullet \qquad (9.1)$$

The tocopheroxyl radical, being relatively stable and unreactive, is unable to continue the chain reaction by attacking other species. Instead it may combine with another peroxyl radical to form inactive molecular products (reaction 9.2) or it may be reduced to tocopherol by reduced coenzyme Q (reaction 9.3) or by ascorbic acid (reaction 9.4).

$$\text{T–O}^\bullet + \text{LOO}^\bullet \rightarrow \text{molecular products} \qquad (9.2)$$

$$T–O^\bullet + CoQH_2 \rightarrow T–OH + CoQH^\bullet + H^+ \qquad (9.3)$$

$$T–O^\bullet + AH^- \text{ (ascorbate) } \rightarrow$$
$$T–OH + A^{-\bullet} \text{ (ascorbyl radical)} \qquad (9.4)$$

The semiquinone radical $CoQH^\bullet$ produced in reaction 9.3 can be converted back to $CoQH_2$ through the electron transport chain in the mitochondria. Regeneration of ascorbate is discussed in Section 19.9.

Whatever the fate of the tocopheroxyl radical, the result of vitamin E intervention is termination of the lipid peroxidation chain reaction. The relative antioxidant activity of tocopherols is the same as biological potency, i.e. $\alpha > \beta > \gamma > \delta$.

The diverse vitamin E deficiency signs observed in animals (Section 9.8.1) are attributable to secondary effects of the widespread damage caused to the membranes of muscle and nerve cells by lipid peroxidation. The prevention of encephalomalacia in chicks by adding low concentrations of synthetic antioxidants to vitamin E-deficient diets strongly suggests that, in preventing this particular disease, vitamin E acts solely as an antioxidant and that such action is non-specific. Vitamin E and selenium can act independently in preventing exudative diathesis and liver necrosis: synthetic antioxidants have little or no effect upon these diseases.

Selenium is implicated in certain vitamin E deficiency diseases because of its role as an essential cofactor for glutathione peroxidase, the enzyme which converts potentially harmful lipid peroxides to harmless hydroxy acids. A constant supply of dietary sodium selenate is essential to maintain the enzyme's activity.

The sulphur-containing amino acids, methionine and cystine, exert a sparing effect on both selenium and vitamin E as shown by their ability to delay the onset of necrotizing myopathy in the chick. This effect is presumably due to an increased *de novo* synthesis of glutathione.

9.6   Effect upon the ageing immune responses

Background information can be found in Chapter 5.

It is well established that human immune responsiveness declines with age and this decline is associated with an increased incidence of infections, tumours and autoimmune diseases (Makinodan *et al.*, 1984). Both the humoral and cellular limbs of the immune system show age-related functional changes, the most dramatic being a decline in T cell-mediated immunity, including decreases in mitogen-induced T-cell proliferation and interleukin (IL)-2 production (Gottesman, 1987). An impaired T cell-mediated immunity is indicated by a patient's inability to mount a delayed-type hypersensitivity (DTH) reaction.

It seems likely that increased production of suppressive factors or a decrease in support by another cell type may contribute to the decline in T cell-mediated immunity. Certainly, co-operation between T cells and macrophages is essential for proper functioning of the immune system (Unanue, 1980). Macrophages have a high concentration of arachidonic acid in their membrane phospholipids and, upon stimulation, up to 50% of this fatty acid can be released for conversion to prostaglandins and other eicosanoids (Meydani *et al.*, 1989). The pathway of prostaglandin synthesis is discussed in Section 5.3.2.

Macrophages from old mice produce more prostaglandin E_2 (PGE_2) than those from young mice (Hayek *et al.*, 1994). This age-associated increase in PGE_2 production is due to increased cyclooxygenase (COX) activity resulting from higher expression of COX mRNA and protein (Hayek *et al.*, 1997). At low concentrations, PGE_2 is believed to be necessary for certain aspects of cellular immunity, while at higher concentrations it suppresses T cell-mediated immunity, as demonstrated by decreases in mitogen-induced T-cell proliferation and IL-2 production. The inhibitory effects of PGE_2 result from the specific binding of PGE_2 to a receptor on the T-cell surface. Receptor binding stimulates the production of cyclic AMP, which mediates the PGE_2 effect by activating protein kinase A.

Goodwin & Messner (1979) showed that proliferation of cultured lymphocytes from human subjects aged over 70 is more sensitive to inhibition by PGE_2 compared to cells from younger subjects. This decreased responsiveness to PGE_2 was partially reversed by blocking endogenous production of PGE_2 with indomethacin, an inhibitor of prostaglandin synthesis.

The above observations suggest that the decline in immunoresponsiveness with advancing age could be at least partly explained by an increased production of immunosuppressive PGE_2.

Vitamin E supplementation has a stimulatory effect on both humoral and cellular immunity. Its effect is most pronounced in infectious diseases where phago-cytosis is the main defence mechanism; it is least effective where cell-mediated immunity is the main defence. Vitamin E deficiency predictably leads to impairment of immune function and reduced disease resistance. The effective dietary dose for optimal immune protection is about 4–6 times higher than vitamin E levels found in normal diets (Tengerdy, 1989).

The mechanism for the immune-enhancing effect of vitamin E has not yet been established. One hypothesis is that vitamin E, through its antioxidant function, could decrease the production of immunosuppressive PGE_2 by activated macrophages. Meydani et al. (1986) showed that increasing the vitamin E intake of aged (24-month-old) mice to almost 20 times their recommended daily allowances for 6 weeks enhanced the mitogenic response of splenocytes and improved the response to a delayed-type hypersensitivity skin test. The vitamin E-supplemented mice had significantly less PGE_2 than non-supplemented controls, suggesting that the immunostimulatory effect of the vitamin might have been due to its inhibition of PGE_2 synthesis.

Beharka et al. (1997) conducted experiments in which combinations of purified macrophages and T cells from young or old mice were cultured together. Key observations were: (1) macrophages from old mice suppressed proliferation and IL-2 secretion by T cells from young mice; (2) addition of vitamin E increased proliferation and IL-2 production by co-cultures containing cells from old mice; (3) addition of vitamin E to co-cultures containing cells from old mice significantly reduced PGE_2 production by mitogen-stimulated macrophages; there was no such effect in co-cultures containing cells from young mice; (4) addition of indomethacin produced similar effects to vitamin E; and (5) a synthetic fat-soluble antioxidant, DPPD, did not mimic the effects of vitamin E. These results demonstrate that increased production of PGE_2 by macrophages contributes to the age-associated decrease in T-cell function. The results support the idea that the immunostimulatory effect of vitamin E is attributable, at least partly, to inhibition of PGE_2 synthesis by macrophages.

Meydani et al. (1990) conducted a double-blind, placebo-controlled study in healthy elderly adults residing in a metabolic research unit to investigate the effect of vitamin E supplementation (800 mg dl-α-tocopheryl acetate/day for 30 days) on immune responses. The following significant changes were observed in the vitamin supplemented group and not in the placebo group: (1) improved DTH reaction; (2) enhanced mitogen-induced T cell proliferation and IL-2 production, the increase in IL-2 concentration being positively correlated with changes in plasma α-tocopherol concentration; and (3) reduction in PGE_2 production by peripheral blood mononuclear cells. The results closely paralleled the early study in aged mice (Meydani et al., 1986) and demonstrated that short-term supplementation of healthy elderly subjects with 800 mg dl-α-tocopheryl acetate improved immune responsiveness.

9.7   Vitamin E and atherosclerosis

Background information can be found in Section 4.5.

Vitamin E counteracts many of the atherogenic effects of oxidized LDL (listed in Section 4.5.3) by mechanisms that may be independent of its antioxidant properties. As discussed in this section, some mechanisms are attributable to an inhibitory effect of vitamin E on protein kinase C (PKC) activity.

9.7.1   Inhibition of protein kinase C activity

Physiological concentrations of α-tocopherol markedly inhibit PKC activity in vascular smooth muscle cells (Azzi & Stocker, 2000). Inhibition is obtained only at the cellular level; addition of α-tocopherol to recombinant PKC in vitro does not result in inhibition. β-Tocopherol, which possesses 89% of the antioxidant potency of α-tocopherol, is not inhibitory; however, it is able to reverse the inhibitory effect of α-tocopherol. Other tocochromanols (γ- and δ-tocopherols and α- and γ-tocotrienols) are also not inhibitory (Chatelain et al., 1993). Thus the inhibitory effect of vitamin E on PKC activity is specific to α-tocopherol and is apparently unrelated to its antioxidant activity. Although various isoforms of PKC (α, β, δ, ε, ζ and μ) have been shown to be present in rat aortic smooth muscle cells, only PKCα is inhibited by α-tocopherol (Ricciarelli et al., 1998). The inhibition is indirect and not attributable to a decreased synthesis of the enzyme. There is evidence that α-tocopherol induces the activity of a type 2A phosphatase (Ricciarelli et al., 1998), an enzyme which desensitizes the PKC signalling pathway by dephosphorylating PKCα (Hansra *et al.*, 1996). Whether or not the type 2A phosphatase is the only target of α-tocopherol is under investigation.

9.7.2 Protection of low-density lipoprotein from oxidation

Several reports indicate protection of LDL from oxidation following supplementation of human diets with α-tocopherol (Dieber-Rotheneder *et al.*, 1991; Jialal & Grundy, 1992; Princen *et al.*, 1992; Reaven *et al.*, 1993; Jialal *et al.*, 1995). Supplementation can increase the vitamin E content of LDL to about four times its basal level (Esterbauer *et al.*, 1990). In one report (Reaven *et al.*, 1993), dietary supplementation with 1600 mg *all-rac-*α-tocopherol per day (1760 IU per day) for 5 months resulted in a 2.5-fold increase in LDL vitamin E levels and a 50% decrease in LDL susceptibility to oxidation as measured by *in vitro* assays. Jialal *et al.* (1995) showed that the minimum dose of α-tocopherol needed to significantly decrease the susceptibility of LDL to oxidation was 400 IU per day.

The release of superoxide by phagocytic monocytes during the respiratory burst (Section 5.2.3) induces oxidation of LDL and renders it toxic to proliferating cells (Cathcart *et al.*, 1989). Monocytes from healthy human subjects taking oral vitamin E supplements (1200 IU per day) showed lower superoxide production and a reduced capacity to oxidize LDL (Devaraj *et al.*, 1996). This effect of vitamin E appeared to be mediated via inhibition of PKC. Vitamin E may therefore protect circulating LDL from oxidation induced by activated phagocytes. The enzyme responsible for superoxide production in phagocytes is NADPH-oxidase. Activation of this enzyme, elicited by appropriate stimulation of the phagocytic cell, requires translocation of several cytosolic enzyme components to the membrane. PKC is involved in the activation of NADPH-oxidase and can phosphorylate one of its cytosolic components, p47^{phox}. Cachia *et al.* (1998a) studied the effect of vitamin E on NADPH-oxidase activation elicited by phorbol myristate acetate in human monocytes. They found that α-tocopherol inhibited translocation and phosphorylation of p47^{phox}. The results suggested that the attenuating effect of α-tocopherol on the respiratory burst is due to inhibition of PKC activity.

The lysolecithin that accumulates in oxidized LDL increases production of superoxide anion in the walls of blood vessels, which may further enhance LDL oxidation (Ohara *et al.*, 1994). When human monocytes were stimulated by phorbol ester to produce superoxide *in vitro*, the addition of native LDL inhibited superoxide production in a manner highly sensitive to the increasing α-tocopherol content; the free form of α-tocopherol produced lower inhibition compared with the lipoprotein-associated form (Cachia *et al.*, 1998b). It was suggested that a vitamin E-induced decrease in monocyte superoxide production could lead to a decrease in lysolecithin production in LDL. Lysolecithin is responsible for many of the atherogenic properties of oxidized LDL and any means of reducing its production would promote an anti-atherogenic status of vessels.

9.7.3 Prevention of monocyte transmigration

Incubation of co-cultures of human aortic endothelial and smooth muscle cells with LDL in the presence of human serum resulted in an increased synthesis of monocyte chemotactic protein 1 (MCP-1) mRNA and protein. This was accompanied by an increase in the adhesion of monocytes (but not neutrophil-like cells) to the endothelial monolayer and an increased transmigration of monocytes into the subendothelial space. The increase in monocyte migration was most likely due to the increased levels of MCP-1, since it was completely blocked by a specific antibody to MCP-1. Pre-treatment of the co-cultures with α-tocopherol before the addition of LDL prevented the LDL-induced monocyte transmigration (Navab *et al.*, 1991).

9.7.4 Inhibition of monocyte–endothelial cell adhesion

The induced expression of the endothelial adhesion molecules, ICAM-1, VCAM-1 and E-selectin, is a key event in the pathogenesis of atherosclerosis. The genetic expression of protein molecules is regulated by transcription factors which, when activated, bind to specific regulatory elements on the DNA of target genes where they mediate gene transcription and synthesis of the encoded protein. Expression of genes involved in early defence reactions, such as the genes for cytokines and cytokine receptors, endothelial and leucocyte adhesion molecules, and some growth and differentiation factors, depends upon a particular transcription factor, nuclear factor-κB (NF-κB). NF-κB is found in many different cell types and tissues, but has been characterized best in cells of the immune system, such as lymphocytes, monocytes and macrophages.

In the absence of a stimulus, NF-κB resides in the cytoplasm as an inactive complex composed of three subunits – two DNA-binding subunits (p65 and p50) and an inhibitory subunit called 1κB. Various extracellular activators cause an alteration in 1κB, allowing it to be released from the complex. The NF-κB dimer then migrates to the nucleus where it binds to the DNA recognition site.

The cytoplasmic NF-κB–1κB complex is activated by a great variety of agents. These include the cytokines IL-1 and TNF-α, viruses, double-stranded RNA, bacterial lipopolysaccharide (LPS), endotoxins, T-cell mitogens, phorbol 12-myristate 13-acetate (PMA), protein synthesis inhibitors (e.g. cycloheximide) and UV radiation (Schreck et al., 1992).

Schreck et al. (1991) reported that treatment of T lymphocytes with micromolar concentrations of hydrogen peroxide activated NF-κB; that is, hydrogen peroxide induced the nuclear appearance and DNA-binding of the transcription factor. Hydrogen peroxide also induced the expression of the HIV-1 provirus, whose gene is controlled by NF-κB. The activation of NF-κB by hydrogen peroxide was inhibited by the antioxidant and free radical scavenger N-acetyl-L-cysteine (NAC). These experiments strongly supported the preconceived idea that oxygen free radicals were involved in the activation process. After its passive diffusion through the cell plasma membrane, the relatively innocuous hydrogen peroxide can be converted into the highly reactive hydroxyl radical (Section 4.3.1). Activation of NF-κB by cycloheximide, double-stranded RNA, IL-1 and LPS (Schreck et al., 1991) and TNF-α and PMA (Staal et al., 1990) was also inhibited by NAC.

Every type of cell produces oxygen radicals constitutively. It is well established that different cell types are stimulated to enhance the production of oxygen radicals by the binding of extracellular cytokines such as TNF-α and IL-1 to their respective cell surface receptors. Since these cytokines and other agents, and also hydrogen peroxide (a free radical precursor), are able to activate NF-κB, and all of these activators can be inhibited by a radical-scavenging antioxidant,

Schreck & Baeuerle (1991) postulated that oxygen radicals act as second messengers in relaying extracellular signals to the cytosolic NF-κB–1κB complex. Oxygen radicals are well suited for this purpose; they are small, diffusible and ubiquitous, and can be synthesized and destroyed rapidly. The oxygen radicals somehow activate NF-κB, which then migrates to the nucleus and binds to its transcription site on the DNA (Fig. 9.3).

Faruqi et al. (1994) observed that agonist-induced adhesion of monocytes to cultured human umbilical vein endothelial cells was inhibited by prior treatment with α-tocopherol. The inhibition correlated with a decrease in steady-state levels of E-selectin mRNA and cell surface expression of E-selectin. Probucol and NAC were also inhibitory, whereas other antioxidants had no significant effect. PKC did not appear to play a role in the α-tocopherol effect since no suppression of phosphorylation of PKC substrates was observed. Cominacini et al. (1997) showed that expression of ICAM-1 and VCAM-1 induced by oxidized LDL could be reduced by pre-treatment of either the oxLDL or the endothelial cells with vitamin E. Martin et al. (1997) demonstrated an inhibitory effect of α-tocopherol upon LDL-induced adhesion of monocytes to human aortic endothelial cells and an accompanying decrease in the release of ICAM-1. Devaraj et al. (1996) reported that monocytes isolated from healthy human subjects supplemented with 1200 IU per day of α-tocopherol over 8 weeks were less able, when activated, to adhere to activated endothelial cells compared with monocytes isolated from placebo controls. The vitamin E-enriched monocytes also showed a 90% decrease in the release of interleukin 1β (IL-1β) when activated. IL-1β is a proatherogenic, proinflammatory cytokine that promotes monocyte–endothelial cell adhesion; it also augments smooth muscle cell proliferation via induction of platelet-derived growth factor. Enrichment of monocytes with α-tocopherol resulted in a reduced expression of the monocyte adhesion molecules MAC-1 and VLA-4 (Islam et al., 1998). Furthermore, pre-treatment of monocytes with α-tocopherol significantly decreased the LPS-induced activation of NF-κB. The results of these and other experiments suggest that α-tocopherol inhibits transcription of adhesion molecule genes by preventing the activation of NF-κB by oxygen radicals generated within the cell.

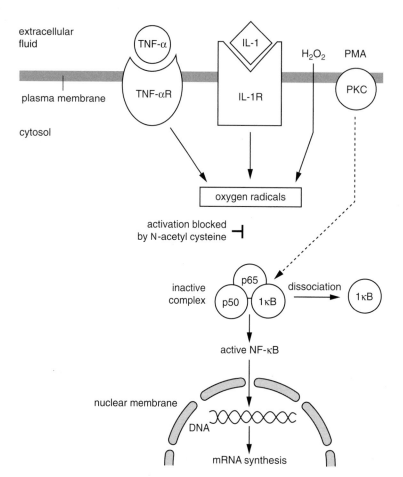

Fig. 9.3 The postulated involvement of oxygen radicals in the activation of NF-κB. TNF-α, tumour necrosis factor-α; IL-1, interleukin-1; PMA, phorbol ester (phorbol 12-myristate 13-acetate); TNF-αR and IL-1R, cell surface receptors; PKC, protein kinase C. Reproduced from Schreck, R., Rieber, P. & Baeuerle, P. A. (1991) Reactive oxygen intermediates as apparently widely used messengers in the activation of the NF-κB transcription factor and HIV-1. *EMBO Journal*, Vol. 10, pp. 2247–58, by permission of Oxford University Press.

9.7.5   Inhibition of vascular smooth muscle cell proliferation

Vascular smooth muscle cell proliferation represents a significant central event in the formation of the fibrous atherosclerotic plaque. α-Tocopherol at physiological concentrations specifically inhibits mitogen-induced proliferation of vascular smooth muscle cells and certain other cell types in a parallel manner to the inhibition of PKC activity (Boscoboinik *et al.*, 1991a,b; Chatelain *et al*, 1993). The degree of inhibition of cell proliferation depends on the mitogen responsible for stimulating growth. Proliferation induced by platelet-derived growth factor (PDGF), endothelin and unmodified LDL was almost completely inhibited by α-tocopherol, whereas proliferation produced by other mitogens, such as bombesin and lysophosphatidic acid, was only moderately or slightly inhibited (Azzi *et al.*, 1993). In cultured smooth mus-

cle cells, α-tocopherol activated the cellular release of the growth-inhibiting transforming growth factor-β (TGF-β) (Özer *et al.*, 1995). Calphostin C, a specific PKC inhibitor, also inhibits smooth muscle cell proliferation, supporting the notion that the antiproliferative effect of α-tocopherol is mediated through the inhibition of PKC activity (Tasinato *et al.*, 1995).

9.7.6   Protection of prostacyclin generation in arteries

Prostacyclin (PGI$_2$), a member of the prostaglandin family, is a product of arachidonic acid metabolism (see Fig. 5.3). Prostacyclin is a potent stimulator of adenylyl cyclase, the enzyme which converts ATP to cyclic AMP. Because platelet aggregation is inhibited by cyclic AMP, prostacyclin acts as a platelet anti-aggregating agent. This effect upon platelets is opposed by another product of arachidonic metabolism, thromboxane A$_2$, which inhibits adenylyl cyclase. Prostacyclin is also a strong vasodilator; moreover, it inhibits polymorphonuclear leucocyte adhesion to endothelial cells *in vitro* (Boxer *et al.*, 1980).

In experimental atherosclerosis the capacity of arterial endothelial cells to generate prostacyclin at the site of plaque formation is considerably impaired (Gryglewski *et al.*, 1978). This decrease in prostacyclin production may be caused by oxidative stress. Prostacyclin synthesis in cultured aortic endothelial cells was depressed by the presence of high glucose concentration in the medium and synthesis could be restored by the simultaneous addition of vitamin E (Kunisaki *et al.*, 1992). Vitamin E probably acted as an antioxidant by preventing the build-up of lipid hydroperoxides which are inhibitory to prostacyclin synthesis. The results suggested that vitamin E may restore depressed prostacyclin production by the vascular wall in hyperglycaemic conditions such as those seen in patients with diabetes mellitus. Szczeklik *et al.* (1985) reported that feeding an atherogenic diet to rabbits for a week resulted in elevation of plasma lipid hydroperoxides and a 90% decrease in arterial generation of prostacyclin. Enrichment of the atherogenic diet with 100 mg of vitamin E daily prevented the increase in lipid hydroperoxides and protected the prostacyclin generating system in arteries.

Chan & Leith (1981) showed that prostacyclin synthesis in dissected rabbit aorta is decreased when the tissue is depleted of vitamin E. Enrichment of cultured human endothelial cells with vitamin E caused an increase in arachidonic acid release and spontaneous prostacyclin synthesis (Tran & Chan, 1988, 1990). A potentiating effect of vitamin E on arachidonic acid release in megakaryocytes was attributed to an up-regulation of phospholipase A$_2$ (Chan *et al.*, 1998).

The above findings suggest that a defect in the local production of prostacyclin may be an underlying factor in the pathogenesis of atherosclerosis in terms of platelet aggregation and monocyte adhesion to endothelial cells. An increased dietary intake of vitamin E can overcome this defect.

9.7.7 Preservation of nitric oxide-mediated arterial relaxation

Background information can be found in Section 4.5.9.

Nitric oxide, an important relaxant of arterial smooth muscle, is released from vascular endothe-

lial cells in response to acetylcholine (Furchgott & Zawadzki, 1980) and other agents. Exposure of the vascular wall to oxidized LDL (oxLDL) inhibits the release of nitric oxide, thereby preventing relaxation (Kugiyama *et al.*, 1990). This dysfunction has, in part, been attributed to PKC stimulation (Ohgushi *et al.*, 1993).

Keaney *et al.* (1996) fed rabbits diets deficient in or supplemented with α-tocopherol and examined the effects of the vitamin on oxLDL-induced endothelial dysfunction. Exposure of thoracic aorta segments from vitamin-deficient animals to ox-LDL produced dose-dependent inhibition of acetylcholine-mediated relaxation, while similarly treated segments from animals consuming α-tocopherol showed no such inhibition. Vessel resistance to endothelial dysfunction in the vitamin-replete animals was strongly correlated with the vascular content of α-tocopherol. Incorporation of α-tocopherol into the vasculature limited endothelial dysfunction induced by phorbol ester, a direct activator of PKC. Using cultured human aortic endothelial cells, Keaney *et al.* (1996) confirmed that oxLDL stimulates endothelial PKC and that cellular incorporation of α-tocopherol inhibits this stimulation. Desrumaux *et al.* (1999) showed that plasma phospholipid transfer protein, by supplying vascular endothelial cells with α-tocopherol, plays a distinct role in the prevention of endothelial dysfunction.

9.7.8 Inhibition of platelet aggregation

α-Tocopherol has long been known to inhibit platelet aggregation *in vitro*, an effect that was initially attributed to the inhibition of lipid peroxidation. However, α-tocopheryl quinone (which is not an antioxidant) also inhibits platelet aggregation (Cox *et al.*, 1980), making this theory unlikely. Freedman *et al.* (1996) found that inhibition of platelet aggregation by α-tocopherol was closely linked to its incorporation into platelets. Incorporation of α-tocopherol inhibited phorbol ester-induced stimulation of platelet PKC, thus implicating this enzyme in the inhibition of aggregation.

Platelet-rich plasma from healthy individuals receiving varying doses of supplemental vitamin E showed a marked decrease in platelet adhesion compared to pre-supplementation adhesiveness. A daily supplement of 400 IU was near the optimum to reduce platelet adhesivity (Jandak *et al.*, 1988). Vitamin E supplementation

(727 mg per day) of healthy humans with low antioxidant status over a 5-week period showed no effects on the capacity of platelets to aggregate *in vitro* (Stampfer *et al.*, 1988). Over a 5-month period, supplementation of human diets with a combination of 300 mg vitamin E, 600 mg ascorbic acid, 27 mg β-carotene and 75 µg selenium in yeast significantly reduced platelet aggregability (Salonen *et al.*, 1991).

9.7.9 Protection against oxLDL-mediated cytotoxicity

Marchant *et al.* (1995) incubated LDL with copper ions for varying periods in the presence or absence of α-tocopherol. They then incubated these LDL preparations with human monocyte-macrophages and measured the toxicity produced in the cells. Toxicity increased with increasing duration of copper-catalysed oxidation in the absence of α-tocopherol. The presence of α-tocopherol protected the LDL from oxidation and the cells from toxicity. Martin *et al.* (1998) reported that enrichment of human aortic endothelial cells with α-tocopherol *in vitro* dose-dependently increased their resistance to cytotoxic injury from oxLDL.

9.7.10 Effects of vitamin E supplementation on experimentally induced atherosclerosis

Verlangieri & Bush (1992) studied the effects of α-tocopherol supplementation on experimentally induced atherosclerosis in monkeys using duplex ultrasound scanning and B-mode imaging to monitor lesion formation and progression. The animals were randomly assigned to one of four groups and atherosclerosis was monitored over a 36-month period. One group was fed a basal diet, while three other groups consumed an atherogenic diet (basal diet plus 0.4% cholesterol, w/w). Two of the latter groups also received α-tocopherol, one at the onset of the study (prevention group) and the other after atherosclerosis was established (regression group). The dosage of α-tocopherol was approximately eight times the daily requirement for primates. A steady initial rise in percent stenosis was detected in the three groups fed an atherogenic diet. However, stenosis in the unsupplemented animals progressed more rapidly and to greater extent than stenosis in the prevention group. In the regression group, stenosis reached a plateau at 4 months post-supplementation, while that of the unsupplemented group continued to rise. The data indicated that, while α-tocopherol does not totally prevent atherosclerosis, it appears to lessen the severity and reduce the rate of disease progression. Moreover, supplemental vitamin E may regress well-established lesions.

9.7.11 Epidemiological studies and clinical trials

Epidemiological studies have shown increased protection against coronary artery disease in subjects consuming vitamin E in daily doses >100 mg taken for more than 2 years (Rimm *et al.*, 1993; Stampfer *et al.*, 1993).

The CHAOS clinical trial (Stephens *et al.*, 1996) was designed to study the effects of α-tocopherol at doses of 400 IU or 800 IU daily on the risk of cardiovascular death and nonfatal myocardial infarction in patients with established coronary atherosclerosis at recruitment. The results showed that α-tocopherol, compared to placebo, reduced the risk of non-fatal myocardial infarction by 77%; there was no difference in deaths due to cardiovascular causes. The results of more recent clinical trials have not agreed with the results of the CHAOS trial. HOPE Study Investigators (2000) reported that 400 IU of vitamin E administered daily for 4 to 6 years had no beneficial effects on cardiovascular outcomes in a high-risk population of patients who were 55 years or older. In an Italian trial (GISSI-Prevenzione Investigators, 1999), the number of patients with nonfatal myocardial infarction was slightly higher in patients receiving 300 IU of vitamin E per day than those receiving placebo, and the number of deaths from coronary heart disease was slightly smaller. Neither difference was statistically significant.

The lack of agreement between CHAOS and GSSI has been discussed by Pryor (2000) in his extensive review of the effects of vitamin E on heart disease, Pryor concluded that in view of the difficulty in obtaining more than about 30 IU per day from a balanced diet, vitamin E supplementation (100 to 400 IU per day) should be part of a general programme of heart-healthy behaviour that includes a fruit- and vegetable-rich diet and regular exercise.

9.8 Vitamin E deficiency

9.8.1 Deficiency in animals

Vitamin E deficiency in animals is readily demonstrable and results in a variety of pathological conditions that affect the muscular, cardiovascular, reproductive and central nervous systems as well as the liver, kidney and erythrocytes. There is a marked difference between animal species in their susceptibility to different deficiency disorders. A complex biochemical interrelationship exists between vitamin E and the trace element selenium. Unsaturated fat, sulphur-containing amino acids and synthetic fat-soluble antioxidants are also implicated in some disorders. Consequently, in order to experimentally induce a particular deficiency syndrome in a given species, it is usually necessary to adjust the balance of these nutrients in the diet. The most extensively studied deficiency syndromes are listed in Table 9.3.

Fetal resorption

In female rats deprived of vitamin E all reproductive events are normal up to implantation of the fertilized ova. Several days later, however, the developing fetus shows abnormalities followed by intra-uterine death, rapid autolysis and resorption. A defect in the fetal blood vessels may be the primary event leading to death of the fetus (Nelson, 1980). This disease can be prevented by administering an adequate dose of vitamin E as late as the tenth day of pregnancy. The synthetic antioxidant DPPD is at least as effective as α-tocopherol in preventing fetal resorption, but ethoxyquin, which readily prevents encephalomalacia in chicks, is inactive (Draper et al., 1964). Selenium compounds have no effect on fetal resorption in rats.

Erythrocyte haemolysis

Erythrocyte plasma membranes are particularly vulnerable to lipid peroxidation because of their direct exposure to molecular oxygen and the presence of haemoproteins which are catalysts of peroxidation. Erythrocytes isolated from blood samples of vitamin E-depleted rats exhibit spontaneous haemolysis when added to dilute solutions of dialuric acid, whereas erythrocytes of rats receiving vitamin E are resistant to this haemolysis. This early manifestation of vitamin E deficiency can be prevented by certain synthetic antioxidants administered to the animal or added to the cell suspension in vitro as well as by vitamin E. Selenium compounds have no effect on erythrocyte haemolysis.

Encephalomalacia

This nutritional disorder occurs in growing chicks fed vitamin E-deficient diets containing adequate amounts of selenium for the prevention of exudative diathesis and sufficient methionine or cystine for the prevention of necrotizing myopathy. Encephalomalacia is manifested by lesions of the cerebellum, the part of the brain concerned with coordination of movement. The cerebellum is softened, swollen and oedematous with minute haemorrhages on the surface and

Table 9.3 Some vitamin E deficiency diseases (from Scott, 1980).

Disease	Experimental animal	Tissue affected	Severity dependent upon dietary PUFA	Prevented by:			
				Vitamin E	Se	Synthetic antioxidants	Sulphur amino acids
Fetal resorption	Female rat	Vascular system of fetus	Yes	Yes	No	Yes	No
Erythrocyte haemolysis	Rat, chick, man (premature infant)	Erythrocytes	Yes	Yes	No	Yes	No
Encephalomalacia	Chick	Cerebellum	Yes	Yes	No	Yes	No
Exudative diathesis	Chick	Vascular system	No	Yes	Yes	No	No
Liver necrosis	Rat, pig	Liver	No	Yes	Yes	No	No
Testicular atrophy	Male rat	Testes	No	Yes	No	No	No
Necrotizing myopathy	Rabbit	Skeletal muscle	No	Yes	No	?	No
Necrotizing myopathy	Chick	Skeletal muscle	—[a]	Yes	No	No	Yes

[a] A low level (0.5%) of linoleic acid was necessary to produce dystrophy; higher levels did not increase the amount of vitamin E required for prevention.

greenish-yellow necrotic areas. The necrosis may be the result of thrombosis in the capillaries. Once established, the lesions are irreversible. The main symptoms are ataxia of gait and stance, backward or downward retraction of the head, tremors, spasms of the limb muscles, and eventually prostration, stupor and death within a few hours. The incidence and severity of the disease are markedly increased with increasing levels of linoleic acid in the diet. Low concentrations of synthetic antioxidants such as DPPD and ethoxyquin in the diet readily prevent encephalomalacia, but selenium has no effect.

Exudative diathesis

This is a vascular disease of chicks which develops as a result of feeding diets that are low in both vitamin E and selenium. The disease can be induced for experimental purposes by feeding diets based on Torula yeast, which is low in both micronutrients and contains substantial amounts of unsaturated fatty acids. The most obvious manifestation is a massive accumulation of a greenish fluid under the skin of the breast and abdomen. Internally, the oedema extends to the muscles and many organs, including the heart and lungs. The oedema is the result of a leakage of plasma from the capillaries caused by an increased permeability of the capillary walls. The disease can be prevented by administration of either vitamin E or selenium, provided that the selenium deficiency is not too severe (Thompson & Scott, 1969). A severe deficiency of selenium causes degeneration of the exocrine component of the pancreas and consequent impairment of dietary lipid absorption, which will affect the absorption of vitamin E (Thompson & Scott, 1970). In this event, extremely high doses of vitamin E are required to prevent exudative diathesis. Some synthetic antioxidants, including DPPD and ethoxyquin, are also effective, but only at concentrations distinctly greater than those required to prevent encephalomalacia.

Liver necrosis

Necrotic liver degeneration develops in weanling rats after commencement of a diet based on Torula yeast, which is deficient in both vitamin E and selenium and low in sulphur-containing amino acids. Necrosis is preceded by degeneration of the sinusoidal cellular plasma membrane and lipid peroxidation has been detected late in the progress of the disease. The onset of necrosis is delayed by cystine, which appears to have a sparing action on the amount of vitamin E or selenium required to prevent the disease.

Testicular atrophy

In male rats depleted of vitamin E from early life there is no testicular injury until the onset of sexual maturity, when a progressive degeneration of the germinal epithelium of the seminiferous tubules occurs and the testes atrophy. The resultant sterility does not respond to vitamin E and is truly permanent.

Necrotizing myopathy

This disease is manifested as a progressive muscular weakness which affects the skeletal muscles of many vertebrate species. It was originally called nutritional muscular dystrophy, but this term suggests an aetiological relationship between the myopathy of vitamin E deficiency and human muscular dystrophy. Although many of the pathological lesions are similar in these two diseases, human muscular dystrophy is genetically determined and does not respond to vitamin E treatment.

Necrotizing myopathy is characterized histologically by marked variation in the cross-sectional diameter of the muscle fibres, segmental fragmentation with interstitial oedema and necrosis and, in the later stages, extensive replacement of muscle tissue by connective tissue. The disease can be detected in its early stages by an increased excretion of creatine in the urine (creatinuria), which is the result of a loss of creatine from the affected muscles. Creatine excretion is often expressed as the creatine:creatinine ratio, the excretion of creatinine being relatively constant on a body weight basis.

Necrotizing myopathy in rabbits, guinea pigs, rats and monkeys responds primarily to vitamin E. Selenium is not capable of completely replacing vitamin E in these species, although it does reduce the vitamin requirement. The myopathy, as studied in the chick, does not respond to dietary synthetic antioxidants at levels several times those needed to prevent encephalomalacia. The disease is induced in the chick when the dietary vitamin E is accompanied by a deficiency in the sulphur-containing amino acids, methionine and cystine. Approximately 0.5% of dietary linoleic acid (but not linolenic acid) is necessary to produce myopathy. Concentrations above 0.5% do not increase the amount of vitamin E required for prevention. The chick appears to be unique in that the myopathy can be prevented in the absence of vitamin E by supplementing the diet with cystine or methionine. Cystine is about twice as effective as methionine on an equal sulphur basis (Scott, 1970).

9.8.2 Deficiency in humans

Apart from haemolytic anaemia in premature infants, vitamin E, in the context of human nutrition, has long been considered 'a vitamin looking for a disease'. It is now recognized that vitamin E is responsible for the neurological abnormalities that had been described in patients with long-term disorders of fat absorption.

Haemolytic anaemia
Newborn infants generally have low serum vitamin E levels because of the vitamin's limited transfer through the placenta. A haemolytic anaemia associated with vitamin E deficiency in premature infants 6 to 10 weeks after birth was first reported by Oski & Barness (1967). This deficiency syndrome was further investigated in infants fed commercial milk formulas that were high in PUFA and relatively low in vitamin E (Hassan et al., 1966; Ritchie et al., 1968). Control infants were fed identical formulas supplemented with vitamin E. The syndrome consisted of haemolytic anaemia, oedema and skin lesions. The erythrocytes lysed when treated in vitro with dilute hydrogen peroxide (i.e. the cell contents leaked out of the damaged cell membrane) and the blood film showed abnormal red cell morphology, such as spiky and fragmented cells. Erythrocyte survival was shortened and an increase in the number of reticulocytes (erythrocyte precursors newly arrived in the blood from the bone marrow) indicated a response to increased erythrocyte destruction. Erythroid hyperplasia was observed in the bone marrow and an increased platelet count was indicative of a general increase in bone-marrow activity. The infants were restless, breathing was noisy and there was a watery nasal discharge. Oedema appeared and slowly progressed until it involved the entire face, lower limbs and genitalia. The oedema is analogous to the exudative diathesis observed in vitamin E-deficient chicks. The skin lesions began on the sides of the face extending into the neck and adjacent parts of the scalp. All of the symptoms were associated with low serum vitamin E levels; the symptoms

were not observed in the controls, which had higher serum vitamin E levels. The symptoms disappeared in response to oral vitamin E therapy; there was no response to iron or vitamin B_{12}. The lengthening of erythrocyte survival coincident with the rise in serum vitamin E was direct in vivo evidence that vitamin E prevented haemolytic anaemia. The therapeutic effect of vitamin E in these experiments is presumably attributable to its ability to protect the vital phospholipids in cell membranes from peroxidative degeneration. Nowadays, infant milk formulas contain added vitamin E and an adequate ratio of vitamin E to PUFA; this has almost completely eradicated haemolytic anaemia.

It is well documented that a diet rich in polyunsaturated fat, but which does not contain a correspondingly high amount of vitamin E, induces deficiency signs in animals. This also applies to humans as shown by the above experiments with premature infants. In a long-term human study (the Elgin project), adult male volunteers received a diet in which about half of the fat content was composed of vitamin E-stripped lard. After 30 months this fraction of the fat content was replaced by stripped corn oil and 9 months later the amount of stripped corn oil was doubled. No manifestations of anaemia were observed and it was not until the 72nd month that a well-controlled study of erythrocyte survival was performed. The data obtained showed that the erythrocytes of the vitamin E-depleted subjects were being destroyed at a rate about 8–10% faster than in the subjects in the control groups. The experiment was terminated soon after these observations, but it is logical to assume that if the diet had been made more deficient, the pathology would have been more severe (Horwitt, 1976).

Fat malabsorption
Because of the intimate association between intestinal absorption of dietary fat and vitamin E, any condition causing the prolonged malabsorption of fat (steatorrhoea) will lead to a secondary deficiency of vitamin E. Thus, patients with a variety of chronic fat malabsorption conditions exhibit low plasma vitamin E concentrations. The major nongenetic causes of steatorrhoea associated with a symptomatic vitamin E deficiency state are chronic cholestatic hepatobiliary disorders, cystic fibrosis and short bowel syndrome. Abetalipoproteinaemia and homozygous hypobetalipoproteinaemia are genetic causes of steatorrhoea.

Chronic cholestatic hepatobiliary disorders

These disorders include diseases of the liver and of the intrahepatic and extrahepatic bile ducts. The impaired bile flow leads to an insufficient concentration of bile constituents in the intestinal lumen and a consequent failure to produce micelles. The result is malabsorption of dietary fat-soluble substances. Because of their low vitamin E body stores, infants with cholestatic liver disease show symptoms of neuropathy as early as the second year of life, the neurological damage becoming irreversible if the vitamin E deficiency is not corrected. Correction of the deficiency by oral administration requires very high doses of vitamin E (100–200 IU per kg per day) or the use of a water-soluble form (α-tocopheryl polyethylene glycol-1000 succinate) which forms micelles. Alternatively, vitamin E can be administered by intramuscular injection.

Cystic fibrosis

In cystic fibrosis, increased viscosity of pancreatic secretions causes obstruction of pancreatic ducts leading ultimately to destruction and fibrosis of the exocrine pancreas. The resultant failure to secrete pancreatic digestive enzymes causes steatorrhoea and vitamin E deficiency. Despite the common observation of neuroaxonal lesions in the posterior column of the spinal cord at autopsy, overt neurological dysfunction is rare in vitamin E-deficient cystic fibrosis patients. Most patients who do exhibit neurological dysfunction also have fibrotic livers.

Short bowel syndrome

Short bowel syndrome is a collection of signs and symptoms used to describe the nutritional consequences of major surgical resections of the small intestine. Resections are carried out for treatment of Crohn's disease and mesenteric vascular thrombosis, among other disorders. The causes of vitamin E deficiency in these conditions are a reduced intestinal absorptive surface area and excessive faecal bile acid losses. Although low plasma vitamin E concentrations may be present within several years of surgical resection, 10 to 20 years of severe malabsorption are generally required before the manifestation of neurological symptoms. This is because of the prior accumulation of vitamin E in most tissues and its relatively slow release from nervous tissues.

Abetalipoproteinaemia

Chylomicrons contain apoB-48, among other apoproteins, while VLDL and LDL contain apoB-100. These two apoB proteins are encoded by the same gene, apoB-48 being synthesized in the intestinal mucosa and apoB-100 in the liver. Abetalipoproteinaemia is a rare inborn error of lipoprotein production and transport characterized by undetectable or very small amounts of apoB-containing lipoproteins (chylomicrons, VLDL and LDL) in the circulation. The underlying genetic defect in abetalipoproteinaemia is a mutation in the gene coding for the microsomal triglyceride-transfer protein. This protein is essential for lipoprotein assembly in the Golgi apparatus; without it the lipoproteins are not secreted by the intestine or liver. Abetalipoproteinaemia patients become vitamin E deficient because the steatorrhoea caused by the absence of chylomicrons severely impairs absorption of the vitamin. Furthermore, the lack of VLDL secretion by the liver means that no LDL can be formed, and so any vitamin E that might have been absorbed cannot be transported in the usual manner. The treatment of abetalipoproteinaemic patients with massive oral doses of vitamin E (100 IU per kg per day) allows a small proportion to be absorbed, resulting in detectable plasma levels and correction of in vitro erythrocyte haemolysis (Traber et al., 1993). Normal plasma levels are rarely, if ever, attained. Interestingly, the enterocytes of abetalipoproteinaemic patients are able to synthesize HDL, which do not require apoB for their formation (Deckelbaum et al., 1982). It is possible that this abnormally produced enteric HDL facilitates the intestinal secretion and plasma transport of vitamin E in the absence of the apoB-containing lipoproteins. The principal clinical features of abetalipoproteinaemia are steatorrhoea and spiky erythrocytes (both congenital), pigmented retinopathy and a chronic progressive neurological disorder. The characteristic neurological and retinal symptoms manifest in the first decade of life, evolving into a crippling ataxia with visual impairment by the second or third decades (Sokol, 1989).

Homozygous hypobetalipoproteinaemia

Patients with this condition have a defect in the apoB gene and secrete lipoproteins containing truncated forms of apoB. These defective lipoproteins can transport minor amounts of vitamin E but they have a rapid turnover and constitute only a tiny fraction of the circulating lipoproteins in these patients.

Ataxia with vitamin E deficiency (AVED)

Ataxia with vitamin E deficiency (AVED) uniquely represents a primary vitamin E-deficient state. Originally called 'isolated vitamin E deficiency syndrome', and later 'familial isolated vitamin E' (FIVE) deficiency, AVED is the result of a mutation in the gene for α-tocopherol transfer protein (α-TTP) on chromosome 8. Infants born with this syndrome have normal gastrointestinal function and yet their plasma vitamin E levels are only 1% of normal. There is either a complete absence of α-TTP or a defect in the α-tocopherol-binding region of the protein (Traber, 1994); in either case, there is impaired hepatic secretion of α-tocopherol in VLDL. The dramatic fall in the plasma level of vitamin E is due to the rapid removal of α-tocopherol from the plasma to the liver and excretion in the bile, with no α-TTP to salvage it. The ataxia and other neurological symptoms appear between the ages of 4 and 18 years. They are manifestations of the neurological damage that arises from the impaired delivery of vitamin E to the nervous tissues, which are especially sensitive to variations in plasma vitamin E. When given vitamin E supplements (about 1 g per day), patients maintain normal plasma α-tocopherol concentrations and progression of the neurological damage is halted. If patients stop taking the supplements, their plasma concentrations fall to deficiency levels within days and the damage progresses.

Clinical features and histopathology of vitamin E deficiency

Sokol (1988) compared the clinical features found in abetalipoproteinaemia, chronic childhood cholestasis, other fat malabsorption disorders and isolated vitamin E deficiency (now known as AVED). The most common findings include loss of deep tendon reflexes, truncal and limb ataxia, loss of positional and vibratory sensation, muscle weakness and dysarthria. Ophthalmoplegia (impairment of eye movements) and pigmented retinopathy are common features in abetalipoproteinaemia, cholestasis and other fat malabsorption disorders, but they are not seen in AVED. A possible explanation is the fact that the first three disorders represent secondary deficiency states, malabsorption being the primary cause. In contrast, AVED, with no evidence of fat malabsorption or of other

nutritional deficiencies, represents a primary deficiency state. A concomitant deficiency of vitamin A is probably required to produce the ocular symptoms present in cases of secondary vitamin E deficiency, the two vitamins acting synergistically.

Sokol (1988) also described the histopathology of vitamin E deficiency in humans. Axonal degeneration and demyelination of large-calibre neurons are universal in both primary and secondary advanced deficiency. Disturbance in function of the posterior columns of the spinal cord, sensory nerves and spinocerebellar tracts account for the loss of vibratory and positional sensation and truncal and limb ataxia. The nerve degeneration presumably originates from peroxidation of constituent phospholipids. Peroxidative injury and the formation of lipopigments is the cause of pigmented retinopathy commonly seen in older patients with abetalipoproteinaemia.

9.9   Dietary intake

9.9.1   Human requirement

For the 19- to 50-year age group, an EAR of 12 mg of α-tocopherol is derived from studies in men based on the criterion of vitamin E intakes sufficient to prevent hydrogen peroxide-induced haemolysis. The RDA is 120% of the EAR which, after rounding up, is 15 mg per day of α-tocopherol. There is no increase for pregnancy, but for lactation the RDA is increased to 19 mg per day (Institute of Medicine, 2000).

9.9.2   Effects of high intake

Vitamin E is regarded to be non-toxic. There is no evidence of adverse effects from the consumption of vitamin E naturally occurring in foods. The question of toxicity arises when vitamin E is used in pharmacological amounts for 'therapeutic' purposes. Animal studies have shown that α-tocopherol is not mutagenic, carcinogenic or teratogenic. In human studies with double-blind protocols and in large population studies, oral vitamin E supplementation resulted in few side effects even at doses as high as 3200 IU per day (Bendich & Machlin, 1988). However, most human studies have been conducted over periods of a few weeks to a few months, so the possible chronic effects of multiyear ingestion of high doses of α-tocopherol are unknown. In view of the known inhibitory effect of high doses of vitamin E on platelet aggregation and two reported cases of post-surgery bleeding associated with intakes of 800–1200 IU of vitamin E per day, it is advisable to discourage vitamin E supplementation two weeks before and following surgery (Bendich & Machlin, 1993). In addition, vitamin supplements should not be taken by individuals receiving anticoagulant therapy. The tolerance and safety of vitamin E has been reviewed (Kappus & Diplock, 1992) and a Hazard Identification compiled (Institute of Medicine, 2000).

9.9.3   Assessment of vitamin E status

The functional adequacy of vitamin E intake can be assessed by *in vitro* measurement of erythrocyte haemolysis induced by dilute hydrogen peroxide.

Further reading

Devaraj, S. & Jialal, I. (1998) The effects of alpha-tocopherol on critical cells in atherogenesis. *Current Opinion in Lipidology*, **9**, 11–15.

Keaney, J. F. Jr., Simon, D. I. & Freedman, J. E. (1999) Vitamin E and vascular homeostasis: implications for atherosclerosis. *FASEB Journal*, **13**, 965–76.

Stocker, R. (1999) The ambivalence of vitamin E in atherogenesis. *Trends in Biochemical Sciences*, **24**, 219–23.

Traber, M. (1997) Regulation of human plasma vitamin E. In: *Antioxidants in Disease Mechanisms and Therapy*. (Ed. H. Sies), pp. 49–63. Academic Press, San Diego.

Traber, M. G. & Packer, L. (1995) Vitamin E: beyond antioxidant function. *American Journal of Clinical Nutrition*, **62**, 1501S–9S.

References

Arita, M., Nomura, K., Arai, H. & Inoue, K. (1997) α-Tocopherol transfer protein stimulates the secretion of α-tocopherol from a cultured liver cell line through a brefeldin A-insensitive pathway. *Proceedings of the National Academy of Sciences of the U.S.A.*, **94**, 12 437–41.

Azzi, A. & Stocker, A. (2000) Vitamin E: non-antioxidant roles. *Progress in Lipid Research*, **39**, 231–55.

Azzi, A., Boscoboinik, D., Chatelain, E., Özer, N. K. & Stäuble, B. (1993) d-α-Tocopherol control of cell proliferation. *Molecular Aspects of Medicine*, **14**, 265–71.

Beharka, A. A., Wu, D., Han, S. N. & Meydani, S. N. (1997) Macrophage prostaglandin production contributes to the age-associated decrease in T cell function which is reversed by the dietary antioxidant vitamin E. *Mechanisms of Ageing and Development*, **93**, 59–77.

Bendich, A. & Machlin, L. J. (1988) Safety of oral intake of vitamin E. *American Journal of Clinical Nutrition*, **48**, 612–19.

Bendich, A. & Machlin, L. J. (1993) The safety of oral intake of vitamin E: data from clinical studies from 1986 to 1991. In: *Vitamin E in Health and Disease*. (Ed. L. Packer & J. Fuchs), pp. 411–16. Marcel Dekker, Inc., New York.

Bieri, J. G. & Poukka Evarts, R. (1974) Gamma tocopherol: metabolism, biological activity and significance in human vitamin E nutrition. *American Journal of Clinical Nutrition*, **27**, 980–6.

Boscoboinik, D., Szewczyk, A. & Azzi, A. (1991a) α-Tocopherol (vitamin E) regulates vascular smooth muscle cell proliferation and protein kinase C activity. *Archives of Biochemistry and Biophysics*, **286**, 264–9.

Boscoboinik, D., Szewczyk, A., Hensey, C. & Azzi, A. (1991b) Inhibition of cell proliferation by α-tocopherol. Role of protein kinase C. *Journal of Biological Chemistry*, **266**(10), 6188–94.

Boxer, L. A., Allen, J. M., Schmidt, M., Yoder, M. & Baehner, R. L. (1980) Inhibition of polymorphonuclear leukocyte adherence by prostacyclin. *Journal of Laboratory and Clinical Medicine*, **95**, 672–8.

Bunyan, J., McHale, D., Green, J. & Marcinkiewicz, S. (1961) Biological potencies of ε- and ζ-tocopherol and 5-methyltocol. *British Journal of Nutrition*, **15**, 253–7.

Burton, G. W. & Traber, M. G. (1990) Vitamin E: antioxidant activity, biokinetics, and bioavailability. *Annual Review of Nutrition*, **10**, 357–82.

Burton, G. W., Ingold, K. U., Foster, D. O., Cheng, S. C., Webb, A., Hughes, L. & Lusztyk, E. (1988) Comparison of free α-tocopherol and α-tocopheryl acetate as sources of vitamin E in rats and humans. *Lipids*, **23**, 834–40.

Burton, G. W., Traber, M. G., Acuff, R. V., Walters, D. N., Kayden, H., Hughes, L. & Ingold, K. U. (1998) Human plasma and tissue α-tocopherol concentrations in response to supplementation with deuterated natural and synthetic vitamin E. *American Journal of Clinical Nutrition*, **67**, 669–84.

Cachia, O., El Benna, J., Pedruzzi, E., Descomps, B., Gougerot-Pocidalo, M.-A. & Leger, C.-L. (1998a) α-Tocopherol inhibits the respiratory burst in human monocytes. *Journal of Biological Chemistry*, **273**(49), 32 801–5.

Cachia, O., Léger, C. L. & Descomps, B. (1998b) Monocyte superoxide production is inversely related to normal content of α-tocopherol in low-density lipoprotein. *Atherosclerosis*, **138**, 263–9.

Cathcart, M. K., McNally, A. K., Morel, D. W. & Chisolm, G. M. III (1989) Superoxide anion participation in human monocyte-mediated oxidation of low-density lipoprotein and conversion of low-density lipoprotein to a cytotoxin. *Journal of Immunology*, **142**, 1963–9.

Chan, A. C. & Leith, M. K. (1981) Decreased prostacyclin synthesis in vitamin E-deficient rabbit aorta. *American Journal of Clinical Nutrition*, **34**, 2341–7.

Chan, A. C., Wagner, M., Kennedy, C., Chen, E., Lanuville, O., Mezl, V. A., Tran, K. & Choy, P. C. (1998) Vitamin E up-regulates arachidonic acid release and phospholipase A$_2$ in megakaryocytes. *Molecular and Cellular Biochemistry*, **189**, 153–9.

Chatelain, E., Boscoboinik, D. O., Bartoli, G.-M., Kagan, V. E., Gey, F. K., Packer, L. & Azzi, A. (1993) Inhibition of smooth muscle cell proliferation and protein kinase C activity by tocopherols and tocotrienols. *Biochimica et Biophysica Acta*, **1176**, 83–9.

Cominacini, L., Garbin, U., Pasini, A. F., Davoli, A., Campagnola, M., Contessi, G. B., Pastorino, A. M., & Cascio, V. L. (1997) Antioxidants inhibit the expression of intercellular cell adhesion molecule-1 and vascular cell adhesion molecule-1 induced by oxidized LDL on human umbilical vein endothelial cells. *Free Radical Biology and Medicine*, **22**, 117–27.

Cox, A. C., Rao, G. H. R., Gerrard, J. M. & White, J. G. (1980) The influence of vitamin E quinone on platelet structure, function, and biochemistry. *Blood*, **55**, 907–14.

Deckelbaum, R. J., Eisenberg, S., Oschry, Y., Cooper, M. & Blum, C. (1982) Abnormal high density lipoproteins of abetalipoproteinemia: relevance to normal HDL metabolism. *Journal of Lipid Research*, **23**, 1274–82.

Desrumaux, C., Deckert, V., Athias, A., Masson, D., Lizard, G., Palleau, V., Gambert, P. & Lagrost, L. (1999) Plasma phospholipid transfer protein prevents vascular endothelium dysfunction by delivering α-tocopherol to endothelial cells. *FASEB Journal*, **13**, 883–92.

Devaraj, S., Li, D. & Jialal, I. (1996) The effects of alpha tocopherol supplementation on monocyte function. Decreased lipid oxidation, interleukin-1β secretion, and monocyte adhesion to endothelium. *Journal of Clinical Investigation*, **98**, 756–63.

Dieber-Rotheneder, M., Puhl, H., Waeg, G., Striegl, G. & Esterbauer, H. (1991) Effect of oral supplementation with D-α-tocopherol on the vitamin E content of human low density lipoproteins and resistance to oxidation. *Journal of Lipid Research*, **32**, 1325–32.

Draper, H. H., Bergan, J. G., Chiu, M., Csallany, A. S. & Boaro, A. V. (1964) A further study of the specificity of the vitamin E requirement for reproduction. *Journal of Nutrition*, **84**, 395–400.

Drevon, C. A. (1991) Absorption, transport and metabolism of vitamin E. *Free Radical Research Communications*, **14**, 229–46.

Dutta-Roy, A. K., Gordon, M. J., Campbell, F. M., Duthie, G. G. & James, W. P. T. (1994) Vitamin E requirements, transport, and metabolism: role of α-tocopherol-binding proteins. *Journal of Nutritional Biochemistry*, **5**, 562–70.

Esterbauer, H., Dieber-Rotheneder, M., Waeg, G., Striegl, G. & Jürgens, G. (1990) Biochemical, structural, and functional properties of oxidized low-density lipoprotein. *Chemical Research in Toxicology*, **3**, 77–92.

Faruqi, R., de la Motte, C. & DiCorleto, P. E. (1994) α-Tocopherol inhibits agonist-induced monocyte cell adhesion to cultured human endothelial cells. *Journal of Clinical Investigation*, **94**, 592–600.

Freedman, J. E., Farhat, J. H., Loscalzo, J. & Keaney, J. F. Jr. (1996) α-Tocopherol inhibits aggregation of human platelets by a protein kinase C-dependent mechanism. *Circulation*, **94**, 2434–40.

Furchgott, R. F. & Zawadzki, J. V. (1980) The obligatory role of endothelial cells in the relaxation of arterial smooth muscle by acetylcholine. *Nature*, **288**, 373–6.

Gallo-Torres, H. E., Weber, F. & Wiss, O. (1971) The effect of different dietary lipids on the lymphatic appearance of vitamin E. *International Journal for Vitamin and Nutrition Research*, **41**, 504–15.

GISSI-Prevenzione Investigators (1999) Dietary supplementation with n-3 polyunsaturated fatty acids and vitamin E after myocardial infarction: results of the GSSI-Prevenzione trial. *Lancet*, **354**, 447–55.

Goodwin, J. S. & Messner, R. P. (1979) Sensitivity of lymphocytes to prostaglandin E_2 increases in subjects over age 70. *Journal of Clinical Investigation*, **64**, 434–9.

Gottesman, S. R. S. (1987) Changes in T-cell-mediated immunity with age: an update. *Review of Biological Research in Aging*, **3**, 95–127.

Gryglewski, R. J., Dembinska-Kiec, A., Chytkowski, A. & Gryglewska, T. (1978) Prostacyclin and thromboxane biosynthetic capacities of the heart, arteries and platelets at various stages of experimental atherosclerosis in rabbits. *Atherosclerosis*, **31**, 385–94.

Hansra, G., Bornancin, F., Whelan, R., Hemmings, B. A. & Parker, P. J. (1996) 12-O-tetradecanoylphorbol-13-acetate-induced dephosphorylation of protein kinase Cα correlates with the presence of a membrane-associated protein phosphatase 2A heterotrimer. *Journal of Biological Chemistry*, **271**(51), 32 785–8.

Hassan, H., Hashim, S. A., Van Itallie, T. B. & Sebrell, W. H. (1966) Syndrome in premature infants associated with low plasma vitamin E levels and high polyunsaturated fatty acid diet. *American Journal of Clinical Nutrition*, **19**, 147–57.

Havel, R. (1994) McCollum award lecture, 1993: triglyceride-rich lipoproteins and atherosclerosis – new perspectives. *American Journal of Clinical Nutrition*, **59**, 795–9.

Hayek, M. G., Meydani, S. N., Meydani, M. & Blumberg, J. B. (1994) Age differences in eicosanoid production of mouse splenocytes: effects on mitogen-induced T-cell proliferation. *Journal of Gerontology*, **49**, B197–B207.

Hayek, M. G., Mura, C., Wu, D., Beharka, A. A., Han, S. N., Paulson, K. E., Hwang, D. & Meydani, S. N. (1997) Enhanced expression of inducible cyclooxygenase with age in murine macrophages. *Journal of Immunology*, **159**, 2445–51.

Hennig, B., Enoch, C. & Chow, C. K. (1987) Protection by vitamin E against endothelial cell injury by linoleic acid hydroperoxides. *Nutrition Research*, **7**, 1253–9.

HOPE (Heart Outcomes Prevention Evaluation) Study Investigators (2000) Vitamin E supplementation and cardiovascular events in high-risk patients. *New England Journal of Medicine*, **342**, 154–60.

Horwitt, M. K. (1976) Vitamin E; a reexamination. *American Journal of Clinical Nutrition*, **29**, 569–78.

Institute of Medicine (2000) *Dietary Reference Intakes for Vitamin C, Vitamin E, Selenium, and Carotenoids*. National Academy Press, Washington, DC.

Islam, K. N., Devaraj, S. & Jialal, I. (1998) α-Tocopherol enrichment of monocytes decreases agonist-induced adhesion to human endothelial cells. *Circulation*, **98**, 2255–61.

Jandak, J., Steiner, M. & Richardson, P. D. (1988) Reduction of platelet adhesiveness by vitamin E supplementation in humans. *Thrombosis Research*, **49**, 393–404.

Jialal, I. & Grundy, S. M. (1992) Effect of dietary supplementation with alpha-tocopherol on the oxidative modification of low density lipoprotein. *Journal of Lipid Research*, **33**, 899–906.

Jialal, I., Fuller, C. J. & Huet, B. A. (1995) The effect of α-tocopherol supplementation on LDL oxidation. A dose–response study. *Arteriosclerosis, Thrombosis, and Vascular Biology*, **15**, 190–8.

Joffe, M. & Harris, P. L. (1943) The biological potency of the natural tocopherols and certain derivatives. *Journal of the American Chemical Society*, **65**, 925–7.

Jones, P. J. H. & Kubow, S. (1999) Lipids, sterols, and their metabolites. In: *Modern Nutrition in Health and Disease*, 9th edn. (Ed. M. E. Shils, J. A. Olson, M. Shike & A. C. Ross), pp. 67–94. Lippincott Williams & Wilkins, Philadelphia.

Kappus, H. & Diplock, A. T. (1992) Tolerance and safety of vitamin E: a toxicological position report. *Free Radical Biology & Medicine*, **13**, 55–74.

Kayden, H. J. & Traber, M. G. (1993) Absorption, lipoprotein transport, and regulation of plasma concentrations of vitamin E in humans. *Journal of Lipid Research*, **34**, 343–58.

Keaney, J. F. Jr., Guo, Y., Cunningham, D., Shwaery, G. T., Xu, A. & Vita, J. A. (1996) Vascular incorporation of α-tocopherol prevents endothelial dysfunction due to oxidized LDL by inhibiting protein kinase C stimulation. *Journal of Clinical Investigation*, **98**, 386–94.

Kelleher, J. & Losowsky, M. S. (1970) The absorption of α-tocopherol in man. *British Journal of Nutrition*, **24**, 1033–47.

Kitabchi, A. E. & Wimalasena, J. (1982) Demonstration of specific binding sites for ^{3}H-*RRR*-α-tocopherol on human erythrocytes. *Annals of the New York Academy of Sciences*, **393**, 300–15.

Kornbrust, D. J. & Mavis, R. D. (1980) Relative susceptibility of microsomes from lung, heart, liver, kidney, brain and testes to lipid peroxidation: correlation with vitamin E content. *Lipids*, **15**, 315–22.

Kostner, G. M., Oettl, K., Jauhiainen, M., Enholm, C., Esterbauer, H. & Dieplinger, H. (1995) Human plasma phospholipid transfer protein accelerates exchange/transfer of α-tocopherol between lipoproteins and cells. *Biochemical Journal*, **305**, 659–67.

Kugiyama, K., Kerns, S. A., Morrisett, J. D., Roberts, R. & Henry, P. D. (1990) Impairment of endothelium-dependent arterial relaxation by lysolecithin in modified low-density lipoproteins. *Nature*, **344**, 160–2.

Kuhlenkamp, J., Ronk, M., Yusin, M., Stolz, A. & Kaplowitz, N. (1993) Identification and purification of a human liver cytosolic tocopherol binding protein. *Protein Expression and Purification*, **4**, 382–9.

Kunisaki, M., Umeda, F., Inoguchi, T. & Nawata, H. (1992) Vitamin E restores reduced prostacyclin synthesis in aortic endothelial cells cultured with a high concentration of glucose. *Metabolism*, **41**, 613–21.

Losowsky, M. S., Kelleher, J., Walker, B. E., Davies, T. & Smith, C. L. (1972) Intake and absorption of tocopherol. *Annals of the New York Academy of Sciences*, **203**, 212–22.

MacMahon, M. T. & Neale, G. (1970) The absorption of α-tocopherol in control subjects and in patients with intestinal malabsorption. *Clinical Science*, **38**, 197–210.

Makinodan, T., James, S. J., Inamizu, T. & Chang, M.-P. (1984) Immunologic basis for susceptibility to infection in the aged. *Gerontology*, **30**, 279–89.

Marchant, C. E., Law, N. S., van der Veen, C., Hardwick, S. J., Carpenter, K. L. H. & Mitchinson, M. J. (1995) Oxidized low-density lipoprotein is cytotoxic to human monocyte-macrophages: protection with lipophilic antioxidants. *FEBS Letters*, **358**, 175–8.

Martin, A., Foxall, T., Blumberg, J. B. & Meydani, M. (1997) Vitamin E inhibits low-density lipoprotein-induced adhesion of monocytes to human aortic endothelial cells in vitro. *Arteriosclerosis, Thrombosis, and Vascular Biology*, **17**, 429–36.

Martin, A., Wu, D., Meydani, S. N., Blumberg, J. B. & Meydani, M. (1998) Vitamin E protects human aortic endothelial cells from cytotoxic injury induced by oxidized LDL in vitro. *Journal of Nutritional Biochemistry*, **9**, 18–41.

Meydani, S. N., Meydani, M., Verdon, C. P., Shapiro, A. A., Blumberg, J. B. & Hayes, K. C. (1986) Vitamin E supplementation suppresses prostaglandin E_2 synthesis and enhances the immune response of aged mice. *Mechanisms of Ageing and Development*, **34**, 191–201.

Meydani, S. N., Meydani, M., Barklund, P. M., Liu, S., Miller, R. A., Cannon, J. G., Rocklin, R. & Blumberg, J. B. (1989) Effect of vitamin E supplementation on immune responsiveness of the aged. *Annals of the New York Academy of Sciences*, **570**, 283–90.

Meydani, S. N., Barklund, M. P., Liu, S., Meydani, M., Miller, R. A., Cannon, J. G., Morrow, F. D., Rocklin, R. & Blumberg, J. B. (1990) Vitamin E supplementation enhances cell-mediated immunity in healthy elderly subjects. *American Journal of Clinical Nutrition*, **52**, 557–63.

Navab, M., Imes, S. S., Hama, S. Y., Hough, G. P., Ross, L. A., Bork, R. W., Valente, A. J., Berliner, J. A., Drinkwater, D. C., Laks, H. & Fogelman, A. M. (1991) Monocyte transmigration induced by modification of low density lipoprotein in cocultures of human aortic wall cells is due to induction of monocyte chemotactic protein 1 synthesis and is abolished by high density lipoprotein. *Journal of Clinical Investigation*, **88**, 2039–46.

Nelson, J. S. (1980) Pathology of vitamin E deficiency. In: *Vitamin E. A Comprehensive Treatise*. (Ed. L. J. Machlin), pp. 397–428. Marcel Dekker, Inc., New York.

Ohara, Y., Peterson, T. E., Zheng, B., Kuo, J. F. & Harrison, D. G. (1994) Lysophosphatidylcholine increases vascular superoxide anion production via protein kinase C activation. *Arteriosclerosis and Thrombosis*, **14**, 1007–13.

Ohgushi, M., Kugiyama, K., Fukunaga, K., Murohara, T., Sugiyama, S., Miyamoto, E. & Yasue, H. (1993) Protein kinase C inhibitors

prevent impairment of endothelium-dependent relaxation by oxidatively modified LDL. *Arteriosclerosis and Thrombosis*, **13**, 1525–32.

Oski, F. A. & Barness, L. A. (1967) Vitamin E deficiency: a previously unrecognized cause of hemolytic anemia in the premature infant. *Journal of Pediatrics*, **70**, 211–20.

Özer, N. K., Boscoboinik, D. & Azzi, A. (1995) New roles of low density lipoproteins and vitamin E in the pathogenesis of atherosclerosis. *Biochemistry and Molecular Biology International*, **35**, 117–24.

Princen, H. M. G., van Poppel, G., Vogelezang, C., Buytenhek, R. & Kok, F. J. (1992) Supplementation with vitamin E but not with β-carotene in vivo protects low density lipoprotein from lipid peroxidation in vitro. Effect of cigarette smoking. *Arteriosclerosis and Thrombosis*, **12**, 554–62.

Pryor, W. A. (2000) Vitamin E and heart disease: basic science to clinical intervention trials. *Free Radical Biology & Medicine*, **28**, 141–64.

Reaven, P. D., Khouw, A., Beltz, W. F., Parthasarathy, S. P. & Witztum, J. L. (1993) Effect of dietary antioxidant combinations in humans. Protection of LDL by vitamin E but not by β-carotene. *Arteriosclerosis and Thrombosis*, **13**, 590–600.

Ricciarelli, R., Tasinato, A., Clément, S., Özer, N. K., Boscoboinik, D. & Azzi, A. (1998) α-Tocopherol specifically inactivates cellular protein kinase C α by changing its phosphorylation state. *Biochemical Journal*, **334**, 243–9.

Rimm, E. B., Stampfer, M. J., Ascherio, A., Giovannucci, E., Colditz, G. A. & Willett, W. C. (1993) Vitamin E consumption and the risk of coronary heart disease in men. *New England Journal of Medicine*, **328**, 1450–6.

Ritchie, J. H., Fish, M. B., McMasters, V. & Grossman, M. (1968) Edema and hemolytic anemia in premature infants. A vitamin E deficiency syndrome. *New England Journal of Medicine*, **279**, 1185–90.

Salonen, J. T., Salonen, R., Seppänen, K., Rinta-Kiikka, S., Kuukka, M., Korpela, H., Alfthan, G., Kantola, M. & Schalch, W. (1991) Effects of antioxidant supplementation on platelet function: a randomized pair-matched, placebo-controlled, double-blind trial in men with low antioxidant status. *American Journal of Clinical Nutrition*, **53**, 1222–9.

Schreck, R. & Baeuerle, P. A. (1991) A role for oxygen radicals as second messengers. *Trends in Cell Biology*, **1**, 39–42.

Schreck, R., Rieber, P. & Baeuerle, P. A. (1991) Reactive oxygen intermediates as apparently widely used messengers in the activation of the NF-κB transcription factor and HIV-1. *EMBO Journal*, **10**, 2247–58.

Schreck, R., Albermann, K. & Baeuerle, P. A. (1992) Nuclear factor κB: an oxidative stress-responsive transcription factor of eukaryotic cells (a review). *Free Radical Research Communications*, **17**, 221–37.

Scott, M. L. (1970) Studies on vitamin E and related factors in nutrition and metabolism. In: *The Fat-Soluble Vitamins*. (Ed. H. F. DeLuca & J. W. Suttie), pp. 355–68. The University of Wisconsin Press, Madison.

Scott, M. L. (1980) Advances in our understanding of vitamin E. *Federation Proceedings*, **39**, 2736–9.

Sokol, R. J. (1988) Vitamin E deficiency and neurologic disease. *Annual Review of Nutrition*, **8**, 351–73.

Sokol, R. J. (1989) Vitamin E and neurologic function in man. *Free Radical Biology and Medicine*, **6**, 189–207.

Staal, F. J. T., Roederer, M., Herzenberg, L. A. & Herzenberg, L. A. (1990) Intracellular thiols regulate activation of nuclear factor κB and transcription of human immunodeficiency virus. *Proceedings of the National Academy of Sciences of the U.S.A.*, **87**, 9943–7.

Stampfer, M. J., Jakubowski, J. A., Faigel, D., Vaillancourt, R. & Deykin, D. (1988) Vitamin E supplementation effect on human platelet function, arachidonic acid metabolism, and plasma prostacyclin levels. *American Journal of Clinical Nutrition*, **47**, 700–6.

Stampfer, M. J., Hennekens, C. H, Manson, J. E., Colditz, G. A., Rosner, B. & Willett, W. C. (1993) Vitamin E consumption and the risk of coronary disease in women. *New England Journal of Medicine*, **328**, 1444–9.

Stephens, N. G., Parsons, A., Schofield, P. M., Kelly, F., Cheeseman, K., Mitchinson, M. J. & Brown, M. J. (1996) Randomised controlled trial of vitamin E in patients with coronary disease: Cambridge Heart Antioxidant Study (CHAOS). *Lancet*, **347**, 781–6.

Stern, M. H., Robeson, C. D., Weisler, L. & Baxter, J. G. (1947) δ-Tocopherol. I. Isolation from soybean oil and properties. *Journal of the American Chemical Society*, **69**, 869–74.

Szczeklik, A., Gryglewski, R. J., Domagala, B., Dworski, R. & Basista, M. (1985) Dietary supplementation with vitamin E in hyperlipoproteinemias: effects on plasma lipid peroxides, antioxidant activity, prostacyclin generation and platelet aggregability. *Thrombosis and Haemostasis*, **54**, 425–30.

Tasinato, A., Boscoboinik, D., Bartoli, G.-M., Maroni, P. & Azzi, A. (1995) d-α-Tocopherol inhibition of vascular smooth muscle cell proliferation occurs at physiological concentrations, correlates with protein kinase C inhibition, and is independent of its antioxidant properties. *Proceedings of the National Academy of Sciences of the U.S.A.*, **92**, 12 190–4.

Tengerdy, R. P. (1989) Vitamin E, immune response, and disease resistance. *Annals of the New York Academy of Sciences*, **570**, 335–44.

Thompson, J. N. & Scott, M. L. (1969) Role of selenium in the nutrition of the chick. *Journal of Nutrition*, **97**, 335–42.

Thompson, J. N. & Scott, M. L. (1970) Impaired lipid and vitamin E absorption related to atrophy of the pancreas in selenium-deficient chicks. *Journal of Nutrition*, **100**, 797–809.

Traber, M. G. (1994) Determinants of plasma vitamin E concentrations. *Free Radical Biology & Medicine*, **16**, 229–39.

Traber, M. G. (1999) Vitamin E. In: *Modern Nutrition in Health and Disease*, 9th edn. (Ed. M. E. Shils, J. A. Olson, M. Shike & A. C. Ross), pp. 347–62. Lippincott Williams & Wilkins, Philadelphia.

Traber, M. G. & Kayden, H. J. (1989) Preferential incorporation of α-tocopherol vs γ-tocopherol in human lipoproteins. *American Journal of Clinical Nutrition*, **49**, 517–26.

Traber, M. G., Olivecrona, T. & Kayden, H. J. (1985) Bovine milk lipoprotein lipase transfers tocopherol to human fibroblasts during triglyceride hydrolysis in vitro. *Journal of Clinical Investigation*, **75**, 1729–34.

Traber, M. G., Kayden, H. J., Green, J. B. & Green, M. H. (1986) Absorption of water-miscible forms of vitamin E in a patient with cholestasis and in thoracic duct-cannulated rats. *American Journal of Clinical Nutrition*, **44**, 914–23.

Traber, M. G., Burton, G. W., Ingold, K. U. & Kayden, H. J. (1990) *RRR*- and *SRR*-γ-tocopherols are secreted without discrimination in human chylomicrons, but *RRR*-α-tocopherol is preferentially secreted in very low density lipoproteins. *Journal of Lipid Research*, **31**, 675–85.

Traber, M. G., Lane, J. C., Lagmay, N. & Kayden, H. J. (1992) Studies on the transfer of tocopherol between lipoproteins. *Lipids*, **27**, 657–63.

Traber, M. G., Cohn, W. & Muller, D. P. R. (1993) Absorption, transport and delivery to tissues. In: *Vitamin E in Health and Disease*. (Ed. L. Packer & J. Fuchs), pp. 35–51. Marcel Dekker, Inc., New York.

Tran, K. & Chan, A. C. (1988) Effect of vitamin E enrichment on arachidonic acid release and cellular phospholipids in cultured human endothelial cells. *Biochimica et Biophysica Acta*, **963**, 468–75.

Tran, K. & Chan, A. C. (1990) *R,R,R*-tocopherol potentiates prostacyclin release in human endothelial cells. Evidence for structural specificity of the tocopherol molecule. *Biochimica et Biophysica Acta*, **1043**, 189–97.

Unanue, E. R. (1980) Cooperation between mononuclear phagocytes and lymphocytes in immunity. *New England Journal of Medicine*, **303**, 977–85.

Verlangieri, A. J. & Bush, M. J. (1992) Effects of d-α-tocopherol supplementation on experimentally induced primate atherosclerosis. *Journal of the American College of Nutrition*, **11**, 131–8.

Yoshida, H., Yusin, M., Ren, I., Kuhlenkamp, J., Hirano, T., Stolz, A. & Kaplowitz, N. (1992) Identification, purification, and immunochemical characterization of a tocopherol-binding protein in rat liver cytosol. *Journal of Lipid Research*, **33**, 343–50.

10
Vitamin K

Key discussion topics

- The biochemical role of vitamin K is the post-trans-lational conversion of a number of glutamic acids in precursor proteins to γ-carboxyglutamic acids in the mature proteins.
- Vitamin K-dependent proteins include four blood clotting factors, two anticoagulation factors and two proteins in skeletal tissues.
- Vitamin K stimulates bone formation and inhibits bone resorption, thereby reducing the bone loss that occurs in elderly people.
- A low vitamin K status is associated with the develop-ment of atherosclerotic calcifications.

10.1 Historical overview

The first indication of the existence of vitamin K oc-curred in 1929 whilst Henrik Dam was investigating the possible essentiality of cholesterol in the diet of the chick. When the chicks were fed diets which had been extracted with nonpolar solvents to remove the ster-ols, they developed internal haemorrhages and blood taken from these chicks clotted slowly. In 1935, Dam proposed that the curative factor present in vegetable and animal sources was a new fat-soluble vitamin which he called vitamin K. Another rich source of the vitamin was bran or fishmeal which had become putrefied by bacterial action. In 1939, Doisy's group isolated an active compound designated vitamin K_1 from alfalfa and another, vitamin K_2, from putrefied fishmeal. The laboratory synthesis of phylloquinone was accomplished independently by Karrer and Fieser in 1939.

10.2 Chemistry

The term 'vitamin K' is a generic term used for all compounds possessing cofactor activity for γ-glutamylcarboxylase. Two forms of vitamin K exist in nature: vitamin K_1 and vitamin K_2.

Vitamin K_1, known as phylloquinone, is synthesized by green plants and possesses unequivocal biological activity in humans. Phylloquinone is a component of the photosynthetic electron transport system and it occurs exclusively in the thylakoid membranes of the chloroplasts. The phylloquinone molecule comprises a methyl-substituted naphthoquinone ring structure attached at C-3 to a phytyl side chain composed of three saturated and one unsaturated isoprene units,

each unit having five carbon atoms. The structure of phylloquinone, together with that of phytol, is shown in Fig. 10.1. Phylloquinone, having a 20-carbon side chain, may be designated $K_{1(20)}$ to distinguish it from structural analogues such as $K_{1(25)}$, a synthetic compound with an extra isoprene unit. The natural form of phylloquinone is the *trans* isomer, whose stereochemistry is 2′-*trans*,7′R,11′R. Synthetic phylloquinone usually contain both the *trans* and the *cis* isomers, but only the *trans* isomer is essentially responsible for the vitamin's cofactor activity.

Vitamin K_2 refers to a family of structural analogues called menaquinones that are synthesized exclusively by bacteria. There is no certain evidence for utilization of menaquinones by humans, but they are generally assumed to contribute to vitamin K nutriture. Menaquinones have a common ring structure that is identical to that of phylloquinone and side chains composed of a number of unsaturated isoprene units. They are designated MK_n (where n is the number of isoprene units) e.g. menaquinone-4 (MK-4). The predominant menaquinones in nature range from MK-4 to MK-13; those with more than 8 isoprene units (i.e. MK-9 and upwards) are referred to arbitrarily as long-chain menaquinones. The geranylgeranyl side chain of MK-4 confers unique

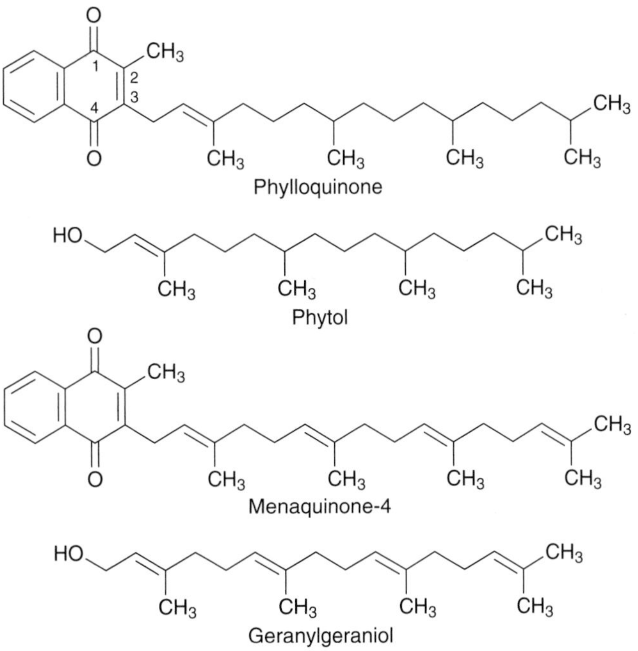

Fig. 10.1 Chemical structures of phylloquinone, phytol, menaquinone-4 and geranylgeraniol.

properties among menaquinones with regard to bone metabolism. The structure of MK-4 is shown in Fig. 10.1 together with the parent of its side chain, geranylgeraniol.

10.3 Dietary sources

The highest concentrations of vitamin K (in the form of phylloquinone) are found in green leafy vegetables, e.g. cabbage, broccoli, Brussels sprouts and spinach. Such vegetables are the top contributors to vitamin K intake in the American diet. Other types of vegetables (roots, bulbs and tubers), cereal grains and their milled products, fruits and fruit juices are poor sources of vitamin K. Animal products (meat, fish, milk products and eggs) contain low concentrations of phylloquinone, but appreciable amounts of menaquinones are present in liver.

Some vegetable oils, including canola (rapeseed), soybean and olive oils, are rich sources of phylloquinone, whereas peanut and corn (maize) are not. Soybean oil is the most commonly consumed vegetable oil in the American diet. The addition of phylloquinone-rich vegetable oils in the processing and cooking of foods that are otherwise poor sources of vitamin K makes them potentially important dietary sources of the vitamin. This is particularly evident, for example, when chicken, eggs and potatoes are fried in certain vegetable oils. Those margarines, mayonnaises and regular-calorie salad dressings that are derived from phylloquinone-rich vegetable oils are second to green leafy vegetables in their phylloquinone content. The addition of these fats and oils to mixed dishes and desserts has an important impact on the amount of vitamin K in the American diet.

Various menaquinones have been found in fermented foods (Sakano et al., 1988), salmon, shellfish, beef, pork, chicken, egg yolk, cheese and butter (Hirauchi et al., 1989a) but the amounts may not be nutritionally significant in some of these foods. Livers of ruminant species (e.g. cow) contain significant concentrations (10–20 μg per 100 g) of some menaquinones (Hirauchi et al., 1989b), while cheese contains significant quantities of MK-8 (5–10 μg per 100 g) and MK-9 (10–20 μg per 100 g) (Shearer et al., 1996).

10.4 Absorption, transport and metabolism

10.4.1 Absorption of dietary vitamin K

Phylloquinone, the major form of vitamin K in the diet, is absorbed in the jejunum, and less efficiently in the ileum, in a process that is dependent on the normal flow of bile and pancreatic juice (Shearer et al., 1974). Both long- and short-chain menaquinones are readily absorbed by rats after oral ingestion (Groenen-van Dooren et al., 1995) and therefore dietary menaquinones are likely to be incorporated into mixed micelles through the action of bile salts and absorbed along with phylloquinone.

The efficiency of vitamin K absorption varies widely depending on the source of the vitamin and the amount of fat in the meal. Pure phylloquinone is absorbed with an efficiency of 80% (Shearer et al., 1974). The phylloquinone present in cooked spinach was only 4% as bioavailable as that from a commercial detergent suspension of phylloquinone. Adding butter to the spinach increased this to 13% (Gijsbers et al., 1996). The absorption of phylloquinone was six times higher after the ingestion of a 500-μg phylloquinone tablet than after the ingestion of 150 g of raw spinach containing 495 μg phylloquinone (Garber et al., 1999). The phylloquinone from a phylloquinone-fortified oil was absorbed better than that from an equivalent amount from cooked broccoli, regardless of adjustment to triglyceride concentrations (Booth et al., 2002). The tight binding of phylloquinone to the thylakoid membranes of chloroplasts explains the poor bioavailability of the vitamin in green plants. The free phylloquinone in vegetable oils, margarines and dairy products is well absorbed owing to the stimulating effect of fat.

10.4.2 Bacterially synthesized menaquinones as a possible endogenous source of vitamin K

The large intestine of healthy adult humans contains a microflora of bacteria, many species of which synthesize menaquinones ranging mainly from MK-6 to MK-12. The menaquinones are incorporated into the bacterium's cytoplasmic membrane where they function under reduced (anaerobic) conditions as redox compounds in bacterial respiration. The most prevalent menaquinone-producing bacteria in the intestine are *Bacteroides* species which synthesize MK-10, MK-11 and MK-12. Among other prevalent species, *Escherichia coli* synthesizes mainly MK-8 (Ramotar *et al.*, 1984).

Conly & Stein (1992a) reported quantitative and qualitative measurements of phylloquinone and menaquinones at different sites within the human intestinal tract. Overall, long-chain menaquinones (MK-9, -10 and -11) predominated. Menaquinones were found mostly in the distal colon (10 faecal samples) and totalled 19.85 ± 0.36 µg per g dry weight. Menaquinones in two samples of terminal ileal contents taken during appendectomy totalled 8.85 µg per g dry weight. Little menaquinone was found in samples of proximal jejunal contents collected by means of a nasojejunal tube (total, 0.03 µg per g dry weight).

The menaquinones incorporated into membranes of viable bacteria are not available for absorption. However, Conly & Stein (1992b) described *in vitro* experiments showing that significant amounts of biologically active menaquinones can be secreted or liberated from bacteria. For example, when a dialysis bag containing *Staphylococcus aureus* (a known producer of menaquinones) was immersed into 100 mL of media, 0.18% of total menaquinone was recovered from the surrounding media, representing a concentration of 0.6 nmol L^{-1}. Inoculation of the media with *Bacteroides levii* (a vitamin K-requiring organism) before dialysis resulted in a luxurious growth of this organism, but not in controls containing no *Staphylococcus aureus*.

Being strongly lipophilic, the bacterially synthesized menaquinones require the presence of bile salts and the formation of mixed micelles for absorption to take place. Because bile salts are reabsorbed in the distal ileum and the amounts remaining are degraded by colonic bacteria, there is no opportunity for absorption of menaquinones to take place in the colon. Indeed, colonic absorption of MK-9 in rats is extremely poor (Ichihashi *et al.*, 1992; Groenen-van Dooren *et al.*, 1995). However, bearing in mind the appreciable amounts of menaquinones found in the terminal ileum of two subjects (Conly & Stein, 1992a), and considering the possibility that contents from the caecum (where large amounts of bacteria reside) may backwash past the ileocaecal valve into the ileum, one can envisage some degree of bile salt-mediated

absorption taking place in this region. In addition, Hollander *et al.* (1977) demonstrated ileal absorption of MK-9 in the conscious rat and showed that the absorption rate increased with increasing bile salt concentration.

Direct evidence to support absorption of menaquinones from the distal human intestinal tract, where intestinal microflora are most prevalent, is lacking. Indirect evidence that enteric menaquinones are absorbed is the fact that about 90% of liver stores of vitamin K is in the form of menaquinones (Shearer, 1992) despite phylloquinone predominating in the diet. Moreover, the various menaquinones found in liver are remarkably consistent with the menaquinone profile of human intestinal content. However, it has not been possible to prove that the hepatic menaquinones do not originate from the diet. Studies performed on human volunteers placed on a vitamin K-deficient diet have consistently failed to demonstrate any significant changes in prothrombin time. However, bleeding episodes associated with a prolonged prothrombin time have been reported in vitamin K-deprived volunteers receiving broad-spectrum antibiotics (Allison *et al.*, 1987). The data from the latter study did not support the hypothesis discussed by Lipsky (1988) that *N*-methylthiotetrazole-containing antibiotics suppress vitamin K-dependent clotting factor biosynthesis. Collectively, these data imply that enteric menaquinones are absorbed and utilized to some extent.

Conly *et al.* (1994) demonstrated that menaquinones can be absorbed directly from the human ileum and be functionally active. Their study consisted of an experimental phase followed by a control phase, using the same four volunteers. The volunteers were started on a vitamin K-deficient diet and then given adjusted doses of warfarin to maintain a stable elevated prothrombin time. A 1.5-mg dose of mixed menaquinones (MK-4 to MK-9) extracted from harvested *Staphylococcus aureus* was then placed directly into the ileum by means of a nasoileal tube after an overnight fast. Within 24 hours of menaquinone administration, the prothrombin time decreased significantly and the factor VII level increased significantly, indicating that the menaquinones had been absorbed and utilized. The results of this study provide an explanation as to why starvation or a complete lack of dietary intake of vitamin K alone cannot induce a clinically manifest vitamin K deficiency.

In conclusion, a report by Ferland *et al.* (1993) that subclinical vitamin K deficiency can be induced in healthy adults by dietary deprivation of the vitamin suggests that absorption of bacterially synthesized menaquinones may not be sufficient to sustain adequate vitamin K status.

10.4.3 Plasma transport of absorbed phylloquinone

Absorbed phylloquinone enters the systemic circulation chemically unchanged via the lymphatic route in association with chylomicrons. Following lipolysis of the chylomicrons in the bloodstream, the chylomicron remnants containing the phylloquinone are taken up by the liver, where the vitamin can be utilized for the synthesis of clotting factors. Bone marrow may also take up chylomicron remnants (see Section 10.4.4). It is not known how or if phylloquinone is secreted from the liver and distributed to extrahepatic tissues. One might assume that phylloquinone would behave like vitamin E, since, in the absence of specific carrier proteins, both of these fat-soluble vitamins depend on lipoproteins for their transport in the bloodstream. Newly absorbed vitamin E is secreted from the liver within VLDLs, which, on losing much of their triglyceride content, are converted to LDL. The vitamin E equilibrates between LDL and HDL, which are the principal carriers for transport in plasma. However, the situation with vitamin K is different. In serum obtained after an overnight fast from healthy subjects, approximately half of the phylloquinone was recovered from the triglyceride-rich lipoprotein (TRL) density fraction, and only a quarter was associated with the major lipoprotein in serum, LDL (Table 10.1) (Kohlmeier *et al.*, 1996). The TRL fraction comprises chylomicrons and VLDL, which are poorly resolved with current techniques. Earlier observations (Shearer *et al.*, 1974) that absorbed radiolabelled phylloqui-

none contained within chylomicrons disappears from the circulation at the same rate as chylomicrons are consistent with the assumption that chylomicrons and chylomicron remnants are the main carriers of phylloquinone in blood. The phylloquinone found in LDL and HDL can be explained by the interchange of lipoprotein constituents among lipoproteins that is known to occur.

Lamon-Fava *et al.* (1998) reported that the TRL fraction accounted for 91% of plasma phylloquinone 3 hours after a meal and for 70% 12 hours after a meal. The proportion of plasma phylloquinone carried by LDLs and HDLs during the post-prandial phase increased progressively from 3% and 4% at 3 hours to 14% and 11% at 12 hours, respectively. The transport of phylloquinone in mainly triglyceride-rich lipoproteins rather than LDL explains the strong positive correlation between plasma phylloquinone and triglycerides reported by Sadowsky *et al.* (1989).

Effect of apolipoprotein E polymorphism on plasma phylloquinone concentrations

Apolipoprotein E (apoE) is a surface constituent of chylomicron remnants as well as other plasma lipoproteins (VLDL, IDL, and HDL). It acts as a recognition site for the binding of chylomicron remnants to receptors on liver cells (hepatocytes), which internalize the remnants by receptor-mediated endocytosis. ApoE is therefore necessary for normal clearance of chylomicron remnants from the circulation.

In humans, the single gene locus for apoE is polymorphic, giving rise to three common alleles which encode the three major isoforms of the apoE protein, E2, E3 and E4 (Zannis & Breslow, 1981). The isoforms differ by cysteine–arginine interchanges at residues 112 and 158; the latter site is within the receptor binding region between residues 140 and 160. The most common allele gene product, apoE3, contains a cysteine at residue 112 and an arginine at residue 158.

	Total serum	TRL	LDL	HDL
Phylloquinone (nmol L^{-1})	0.85 ± 0.52	0.45 ± 0.29	0.16 ± 0.14	0.16 ± 0.08
Phylloquinone, % of total	100	51.4 ± 17.0	25.2 ± 7.6	23.3 ± 10.9
Cholesterol (mmol L^{-1})	5.3 ± 1.4	0.9 ± 0.5	3.2 ± 1.3	1.1 ± 0.2
Triglycerides (mmol L^{-1})	2.1 ± 1.1	1.7 ± 1.1	n.d.	n.d.

Values are means ± SD; $n = 10$; n.d., not determined.
TRL, triglyceride-rich lipoproteins; LDL, low density lipoproteins; HDL, high density lipoproteins.

Table 10.1 Phylloquinone in the main lipoprotein fractions of fasting healthy subjects. From Kohlmeier *et al.* (1996).

apoE2 has a cysteine at both sites, while apoE4 has an arginine at both sites (Rall *et al.*, 1982). These subtle molecular changes have marked effects on lipoprotein metabolism. Since humans have two copies of each chromosome (one from each parent) and both alleles are expressed, six phenotypes are possible. These are (with frequencies in parentheses) E3/E3 (60%), E3/E2 (15%), E3/E4 (20%), E4/E2 (2%), E4/E4 (2%) and E2/E2 (1%) (Semenkovich, 1999).

apoE2 is defective in its ability to bind to lipoprotein receptors, owing to the loss of a positive charge at residue 158 that results from the amino acid interchange (Weisgraber *et al.*, 1982). The binding activity is <2% of normal apoE3 (Rall *et al.*, 1983). The reduced binding capacity of apoE2 impairs uptake of chylomicron remnants by the liver and results in an accumulation of remnants in the bloodstream. Individuals who are homozygous for the apoE2 genotype (E2/2) can develop type III hyperlipoproteinaemia, which is characterized by the presence of chylomicron remnants in the bloodstream after fasting. Individuals with the heterozygous E3/E2 genotype also exhibit delayed post-prandial clearance of chylomicron remnants, but in a milder form to what is seen in E2/E2 individuals (Weintraub *et al.*, 1987). apoE4, although a metabolically abnormal isoform of apoE (Gregg *et al.*, 1986), has essentially the same binding capacity to the LDL receptor as apoE3 (Weisgraber *et al.*, 1982). Despite this, individuals with the E3/E4 genotype clear chylomicron remnants into the liver more rapidly than E3/E3 individuals and twice as fast as E3/E2 individuals (Weintraub *et al.*, 1987). This greater uptake by the liver may be explained by the increased binding of apoE4 to the glycocalyx of hepatocytes, specifically to heparan sulphate proteoglycans (Newman *et al.*, 2002).

Patients with end-stage renal failure who are on haemodialysis have a much greater range of plasma phylloquinone concentrations than healthy subjects (Saupe *et al.*, 1993) and hence have been selected for studying the relationship between apoE phenotype and plasma phylloquinone concentration. This relationship corresponds to that between apoE phenotype and the clearance rate of chylomicron remnants. Thus patients with the E3/E2 and E2/E2 genotypes tend to have higher plasma phylloquinone concentrations than average (E3/E3), while those with E3/E4 and E4/E4 genotypes have lower than average concentrations (Table 10.2).

10.4.4 Transport of phylloquinone to bone and uptake by osteoblasts

Unlike most tissues, which are separated from the bloodstream by the capillary endothelial cells, receptor-bearing cells in liver, spleen and bone marrow have direct access to blood and can thus bind and acquire circulating lipoproteins preferentially. Among the bone marrow cells, stem cells migrate to sites of bone resorption where they line the activated bone surface and form osteoid tissue. These cells will carry whatever amounts of circulating vitamin K they extracted when in the marrow and thus act as vehicles for transporting vitamin K from blood to bone (Kohlmeier *et al.*, 1996).

Saupe *et al.* (1993) demonstrated that apoE polymorphism influences the uptake of circulating phylloquinone by osteoblasts, which is evidence for receptor-mediated uptake. Despite an enhanced plasma concentration of phylloquinone in haemodialysis patients with the E2 variant, less vitamin was actually taken up by the bone because of the reduced binding capacity of apoE2. The delivery of phylloquinone to bone was also impaired in patients with the apoE4 variant. In this case, the enhanced uptake of chylomicron remnants by the liver results in a low circulating concentration of phylloquinone and hence a lower proportion of the vitamin is able to reach the bone.

Table 10.2 Relationship between apoE phenotype and serum phylloquinone concentrations in patients on chronic maintenance haemodialysis. From Kohlmeier *et al.* (1995).

	apoE phenotype				
	Total	E2/E2	E3/E2	E3/E3	E3/E4 + E4/E4
Phylloquinone (nmol L^{-1})	1.08	1.52[a]	1.43[a]	1.07	0.59
(SEM)	(0.36)	(0.64)	(1.07)	(0.74)	(0.16)
Number of patients	28	7	7	7	6 + 1

[a]Significantly different ($p < 0.05$) from values for apoE phenotypes E3/E4 and E4/E4.

Saupe *et al.* (1993) also showed that transport of phylloquinone to the bone is closely linked to the sustained concentration of TRLs in the bloodstream. A highly active catabolism of TRLs produces remnants that are more avidly taken up by the liver than by bone.

In bone marrow, perisinusoidal macrophages take up chylomicron remnants (Mahley & Hussain, 1991). Cultured osteoblasts can also take up lipoprotein-borne phylloquinone by a mechanism that involves the glycocalyx (specifically heparan sulphate proteoglycans) and apoE (Newman *et al.*, 2002). apoE-enriched TRLs bind avidly to heparan sulphate proteoglycans on the surface of osteoblasts as well as on hepatocytes (see Section 3.6.3). Exogenous apoE4 increased uptake of TRL-phylloquinone more than either apoE2 or apoE3, which both had a roughly equal effect. This greater uptake may be explained partly by the increased binding of apoE4 to the glycocalyx.

10.4.5 Maternal to fetal transfer of phylloquinone

The transfer of phylloquinone from the maternal to fetal circulation is poor. Despite a 500-fold increase in maternal plasma phylloquinone concentration following the intravenous administration of 1 mg of phylloquinone to pregnant women at term, the corresponding increase in cord plasma was only about five-fold. The levels attained in cord plasma (0.10–0.14 ng mL^{-1}) after injection were at most near the lower end of the normal fasting adult range (0.10–0.66 ng mL^{-1}) (Shearer *et al.*, 1982). When pregnant women were given daily oral doses of 20 mg phylloquinone for at least 3 days, cord plasma levels of phylloquinone were boosted 30-fold at mid-trimester and 60-fold at term. Again, these levels were substantially lower than corresponding supplemented maternal levels (Mandelbrot *et al.*, 1988). The large concentration gradient of phylloquinone between maternal and neonatal plasma suggests that phylloquinone does not cross the placenta readily. Alternatively, uptake by fetal plasma is low, perhaps because of low levels of transporting lipoproteins.

The cord plasma of premature infants increased by an average of 2.3-fold after their mothers received 5 mg of phylloquinone intramuscularly several hours to 35 min before delivery (Yang *et al.*, 1989). Thus supplemental phylloquinone given to the mother antenatally can be transferred to premature infants, but to a lesser degree than to term babies.

10.4.6 Storage and catabolism in the liver

Storage
The liver has a limited capacity for long-term storage of vitamin K compared to vitamin A. Surprisingly, phylloquinone comprises only about 10% of the total liver stores of vitamin K. Menaquinones ranging from MK-4 to MK-13 make up the bulk of stores with the long-chain forms (MK-9 to MK-13), constituting 73% of total vitamin K (Usui *et al.*, 1990). Unlike phylloquinone, which undergoes rapid turnover, the hepatic turnover of long-chain menaquinones is low, presumably because of their high affinity for membranes (Shearer, 1992). The contrasting turnovers of phylloquinone and menaquinones may account for the predominance of the latter in liver. Whether the menaquinones originate from the diet or from bacterial synthesis, their strong retention relative to phylloquinone would enable concentrations to gradually build up while phylloquinone is being constantly utilized and metabolized. In support of this concept, hepatic stores of phylloquinone are rapidly depleted during dietary restriction of vitamin K, but hepatic stores of menaquinones are not (Usui *et al.*, 1990). Also, the common hepatic menaquinones (MK-9 to MK-13) are not detectable in plasma, suggesting that they are not easily mobilized. It appears, therefore, that the large hepatic pool of menaquinones does not contribute significantly to vitamin K nutriture but represents a very slow turnover of the extremely lipophilic long-chain menaquinones. Further work is needed to establish the origin of hepatic menaquinones and their nutritional relevance.

In the liver of the human fetus, phylloquinone is detectable as early as 10 weeks gestation, and at term the concentration is about one-fifth the value in adults. Hepatic concentrations of menaquinones are usually undetectable at birth and in the first week of life. The gradual build-up of hepatic stores of menaquinones is consistent with the colonization of the neonatal gut by enteric bacteria.

Catabolism and excretion
Phylloquinone is extensively catabolized by the liver, which explains the rapid turnover of hepatic reserves and depletion during dietary deprivation. The catabolic products are excreted partly in the urine and partly in the faeces via the bile. Based on tracer experiments with labelled phylloquinone, it appears that

60–70% of the amounts of phylloquinone absorbed from each meal will ultimately be excreted (Shearer *et al.*, 1996).

10.4.7   Conversion of phylloquinone to menaquinone-4

When chicks are fed phylloquinone as a sole source of vitamin K, their livers contain more MK-4 than phylloquinone (Will *et al.*, 1992). In the rat, the addition of phylloquinone to a vitamin K-free diet leads to low liver and plasma MK-4 concentrations, but in brain, pancreas, salivary gland and sternum the concentration of MK-4 exceeds that of phylloquinone (Thijssen & Drittij-Reijnders, 1994). These observations indicate that the tissues of chicks and rats can convert phylloquinone to MK-4. The absence of MK-3, MK-5 and MK-6 in the rat experiments indicates that the MK-4 synthesis is specific (Thijssen *et al.*, 1996). Humans show tissue-specific accumulation of phylloquinone and MK-4 with distribution patterns comparable to those in the rat (Thijssen & Drittij-Reijnders, 1996). Previous investigators have attributed this conversion of oral phylloquinone to bacterial action in the gut rather than tissue metabolism. However, faecal analysis in the chick experiments did not indicate appreciable amounts of enterically produced MK-4 (Will *et al.*, 1992) and this vitamer is not even a minor isoprenalogue among the menaquinones produced by the normal human intestinal flora (Ramotar *et al.*, 1984). Evidence that the host tissues do in fact convert phylloquinone to MK-4 is the formation of MK-4 when phylloquinone is administered intravenously to vitamin K-deprived chicks (Will *et al.*, 1992) or rats (Thijssen & Drittij-Reijnders, 1994). Furthermore, phylloquinone is converted readily to MK-4 in both gnotobiotic (germ-free) rats and in aseptic mammalian cell cultures (Davidson *et al.*, 1998), clearly demonstrating that bacterial action is not required for the conversion.

10.5   Biochemical and physiological functions

10.5.1   The vitamin K-dependent glutamate γ-carboxylation reaction

Vitamin K functions as a cofactor for γ-glutamyl carboxylase, a microsomal enzyme which catalyses a unique post-translational conversion of protein-bound glutamate (Glu) residues into γ-carboxyglutamate (Gla) residues at well-defined sites in a limited number of proteins (Fig. 10.2). Therefore, vitamin K-dependent proteins are also referred to as Gla proteins. Because Glu is only a weak Ca^{2+} chelator and Gla a much stronger one, the vitamin K-dependent step subsequently increases the Ca^{2+}-binding capacity of a protein (Vermeer, 1990). The binding of Ca^{2+} to the Gla residue of a protein leads to a conformational change required for its biological activity.

10.5.2   The vitamin K epoxide cycle

In the liver, γ-glutamyl carboxylation is linked to the vitamin K epoxide cycle – a metabolic cycle which serves to conserve the pool of vitamin K available to the carboxylase (Fig. 10.3). The vitamin K must be in the reduced (hydroquinone) form for carboxylation to take place. The carboxylation reaction is catalysed by γ-glutamyl carboxylase (E_1) coupled to a vitamin K epoxidase (E_2) which simultaneously converts vitamin K hydroquinone to vitamin K 2,3-epoxide. The epoxide is reduced to the quinone by vitamin K epoxide reductase (E_3). The cycle is completed by the reduction of the recycled quinone by a vitamin K reductase (E_4). The reductase enzymes E_3 and E_4 are dithiol-dependent and are inhibited by coumarin vitamin K antagonists such as warfarin. It is probable that E_3 and E_4 are one and the same enzyme. Exogenous vitamin K from the diet may enter the cycle via

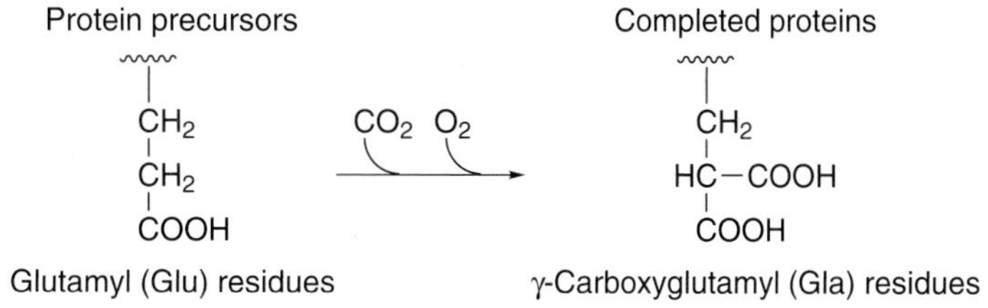

Fig. 10.2 The vitamin K-dependent glutamate γ-carboxylation reaction.

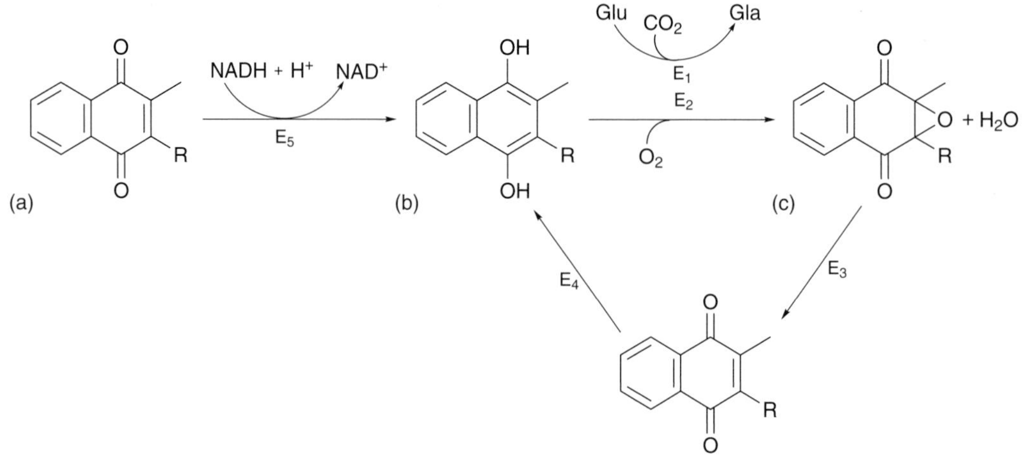

Fig. 10.3 The vitamin K epoxide cycle. (a) Vitamin K quinone; (b) vitamin K hydroquinone; (c) vitamin K 2,3-epoxide. The enzymes E_1 to E_5 are identified in the text. Reproduced with permission from C. Vermeer (1990) *Biochemical Journal*, **266**, 625–36.© the Biochemical Society.

an NAD(P)H-dependent vitamin K reductase (E_5), which is not inhibited by warfarin (Shearer, 1992).

10.5.3   Markers of vitamin K status

Coagulation assays such as prothrombin time lack the sensitivity to detect subclinical vitamin K deficiency. More sensitive tests are based on the detection in plasma of undercarboxylated species of vitamin K-dependent proteins that are the product of protein synthesis when either vitamin K is in low supply or its action is blocked by antagonists. These species are sometimes called PIVKA (proteins induced by vitamin K absence or antagonism). Assays to measure undercarboxylated species in plasma have been developed for two vitamin K-dependent proteins, prothrombin and osteocalcin, allowing independent assessment of two different functional roles of vitamin K (Shearer, 1995a).

Sokoll & Sadowski (1996) evaluated biochemical markers for assessing vitamin K nutritional status in healthy adult humans and found that undercarboxylated serum osteocalcin is the most sensitive marker. Both serum native osteocalcin and undercarboxylated osteocalcin can be quantitated by radioimmunoassay using a rabbit polyclonal antibody raised against purified bovine bone osteocalcin (Sokoll et al., 1995). The degree of γ-carboxylation of osteocalcin can also be assessed by determining the in vitro binding capacity of serum osteocalcin to hydroxyapatite (Jie et al. 1992).

10.5.4   Role of vitamin K in blood coagulation

Background information can be found in Section 4.4.3.

The liver synthesizes a group of Gla proteins that have a regulatory function in blood coagulation: factor II (prothrombin) and factors VII, IX and X have a coagulant function, while proteins C and S have an anticoagulant function.

The chick bioassay for vitamin K is based upon the degree of lowering of elevated blood clotting times in vitamin K-depleted chicks. Blood clotting measurements (actually prothrombin times) are rapidly determined following the addition of a clotting agent (thromboplastin) and calcium chloride solution to oxalated or citrated blood. The chick is the animal of choice because its vitamin K requirement is five-fold that of the rat, it is readily depleted of vitamin K, and coprophagy (faecal recycling) is easier to control. The chick's higher requirement for vitamin K compared with the rat is at least partly attributable to the short length of its colon and rapid transit time.

Matschiner & Doisy (1966) determined the molar activities of several forms of vitamin K using the chick bioassay. Compared to phylloquinone, which was arbitrarily assigned an activity of 100, MK-4 had the highest activity (156) followed by MK-7 (122) and MK-5 (116).

10.5.5   Role of vitamin K in bone metabolism

Gla proteins occurring in bone

Three Gla proteins are found in bone tissue: osteocalcin (also known as bone Gla protein), matrix Gla protein and protein S. Osteocalcin is a relatively small molecule (5.5 kDa) containing three Gla residues. It is synthesized exclusively by osteoblasts and odontoblasts and comprises about 15% to 20% of non-collagen protein in bone. Approximately 20% of the newly synthesized osteocalcin is not bound to the hydroxyapatite matrix in bone, but is set free in the bloodstream (Vermeer *et al.*, 1995). Matrix Gla protein is a larger molecule of 9.6 kDa containing five Gla residues. This protein is synthesized by chondrocytes and is present in every cartilaginous structure; it is expressed in developing bone prior to ossification. Little or nothing is known about the precise functions of the Gla proteins. Osteocalcin has been proposed as a specific regulator of the size of the hydroxyapatite crystals in bone; it is also involved in osteoclast recruitment (Robey & Boskey, 1996). Matrix Gla protein inhibits inappropriate calcification of the epiphyseal (growth) plate (Olson, 1999). Protein S has been identified as a ligand of tyrosine kinase-type receptors that modulate cell proliferation (Kohlmeier *et al.*, 1996). Children with inherited protein S deficiency not only suffer from recurrent thrombosis, but also have severely reduced bone mass (osteopenia) (Pan *et al.*, 1990).

Vitamin K status and osteoporosis

Individuals carrying the E4 allele of apoE experience a higher incidence of bone fractures during their lifetimes than do individuals without the E4 allele (Kohlmeier *et al.*, 1998). The increased risk of hip and wrist fracture in women with the apoE4 allele is not explained by bone density, impaired cognitive function or falling (Cauley *et al.*, 1999). This predisposition toward bone fracture is consistent with E3/E4 and E4/E4 phenotypes having lower plasma phylloquinone levels than normal.

Vitamin K sufficiency of the bone is related to the degree of γ-carboxylation of osteocalcin and this in turn is related to the plasma phylloquinone concentration. As vitamin K intake decreases, circulating osteocalcin seems to be the first Gla protein to occur in an undercarboxylated form (Vermeer *et al.*, 1995).

Circulating osteocalcin is about 92% γ-carboxylated in healthy young adults on a normal diet. Daily supplementation with 250 µg of phylloquinone increases osteocalcin carboxylation to 96%, while 1000-µg supplements are required to achieve 100% carboxylation (Binkley *et al.*, 2002). These observations reveal that a diet sufficient to maintain normal clotting would not be able to maximize γ-carboxylation of osteocalcin and probably other vitamin K-dependent proteins. It remains unknown whether maximal osteocalcin carboxylation is necessary for optimal bone health.

Most studies have shown that the circulating levels of total osteocalcin increase with ageing in normal women, especially after the menopause. This increase is likely to reflect an increase in bone turnover, which is associated with low bone mass in all skeletal regions (Ravn *et al.*, 1996). The γ-carboxylation of circulating osteocalcin is significantly impaired in women over 80 years of age (Plantalech *et al.*, 1991). Also in elderly women, high concentrations of circulating undercarboxylated osteocalcin is associated with low hip bone mineral density (BMD) (Szulc *et al.*, 1994) and increased risk of hip fracture (Szulc *et al.*, 1993, 1996; Vergnaud *et al.*, 1997). Plasma levels of phylloquinone and of the menaquinones MK-7 and MK-8 are depressed in elderly women within a few hours of hip fracture, suggesting that vitamin K is sequestered from the circulation for use at the fracture site (Hodges *et al.*, 1993). Vitamin K_1 supplementation (1000 µg per day) corrected undercarboxylation of osteocalcin in postmenopausal women (Knapen *et al.*, 1989; Douglas *et al.*, 1995) and decreased two markers of bone resorption, urinary calcium and hydroxyproline excretion (Knapen *et al.*, 1989, 1993). Booth *et al.* (1999) reported that 15 days of dietary vitamin K depletion led to increased bone turnover as measured by serum osteocalcin and urinary NTx (*N*-telopeptides of type I collagen) concentration. These markers were subsequently normalized by 10 days of phylloquinone repletion (200 µg per day). As elevated bone turnover is associated with rapid bone loss, vitamin K insufficiency would be expected to contribute to the development of osteoporosis. However, associations do not necessarily imply causation and no direct evidence for the participation of decreased plasma vitamin K in osteopenia in the elderly has been reported.

In a prospective study involving 72 327 women (Feskanich *et al.*, 1999), dietary vitamin K intakes less than 109 μg per day were associated with an increased risk of hip fracture. Booth *et al.* (2003) assessed dietary vitamin K intake with a food-frequency questionnaire in 1112 men and 1479 women (mean ± SD age: 59 ± 9 years) and measured BMD of the hip and spine. Women in the lowest quartile of vitamin K intake (mean: 70.2 μg per day) had significantly lower BMD at the hip and spine than did those in the highest quartile of intake (mean: 309 μg per day). No significant association was found between dietary vitamin K intake and BMD in men.

Tamatani *et al.* (1998) evaluated the possible participation of circulating levels of testosterone, vitamin D metabolites and vitamin K in osteopenia in elderly men. No significant correlation between plasma testosterone and BMD was observed, despite the age-related decrease in plasma testosterone. However, elderly men with decreased BMD showed significant decreases in the circulating levels of 25-hydroxyvitamin D, phylloquinone and MK-7 compared with elderly men with normal BMD.

Effects of menaquinone-4 on bone metabolism

Akedo *et al.* (1992) reported that MK-4 suppresses the proliferation of osteoblastic cells *in vitro*. Warfarin reversed this effect, implicating the γ-carboxylation system in the modulation of proliferation. Koshihara *et al.* (1996) reported that MK-4 enhanced 1,25-dihydroxyvitamin D_3-induced mineralization by human osteoblasts *in vitro*. This was due to enhanced γ-carboxylation of the osteocalcin induced by 1,25-dihydroxyvitamin D_3, and accumulation of carboxylated osteocalcin in the extracellular matrix, causing mineralization (Koshihara & Hoshi, 1997). Hara *et al.* (1993) reported that MK-4 inhibited the bone resorption induced by interleukin-1α, prostaglandin E_2, parathyroid hormone and 1,25-dihydroxyvitamin D_3 in a dose-dependent manner *in vitro*. MK-4 also inhibited the prostaglandin E_2 production stimulated by interleukin-1α. Koshihara *et al.* (1993) showed that MK-4-induced inhibition of prostaglandin synthesis in cultured human osteoblast-like periosteal cells was reduced by cycloheximide, indicating that newly synthesized protein participates in the inhibitory effect.

Akiyama *et al.* (1994) examined the effects of MK-4 on osteoclast-like multinucleated cell formation in bone marrow cell cultures. MK-4 showed the most potent inhibitory effect on cell formation when present in cultures during the last 3 days, suggesting that the vitamin blocks cell differentiation and/or cell fusion. MK-4 did not influence 1,25-dihydroxyvitamin D_3-induced osteoclast-like cell formation when present in the culture during the first 4 days, indicating that it does not affect proliferation of osteoclast precursor cells. MK-4 did not affect the proliferation of many other cell types in the bone marrow culture, suggesting that the observed inhibitory effect of MK-4 on osteoclast-like cells was not a result of cytotoxicity.

Hara *et al.* (1995) compared the effects of phylloquinone and MK-4 on bone resorption *in vitro*. Calcium concentration in the medium was used as a parameter of bone resorption. MK-4 inhibited the calcium release from mouse calvaria organ cultures induced by 1,25-dihydroxyvitamin D_3 or prostaglandin E_2, and it also inhibited osteoclast-like cell formation induced by 1,25-dihydroxyvitamin D_3 in co-culture of spleen cells and stromal cells at the same concentrations. In contrast, the same doses of phylloquinone had no effects on bone resorption and osteoclast-like cell formation in these *in vitro* systems. The inhibitory effect of MK-4 on the calcium release from calvaria was not affected by the addition of warfarin, suggesting that the effect of MK-4 is not due to γ-carboxylation coupling with the vitamin K epoxide cycle. The structures of MK-4 and phylloquinone differ only in their side chains (see Fig. 10.1), therefore whether the difference in their effects is related to the differences in side chain structure was evaluated in the co-culture system. Geranylgeraniol inhibited osteoclast-like cell formation to almost the same degree as MK-4, whereas the effect of phytol was weak. Moreover, multi-isoprenyl alcohols of two to seven units, except the four-unit geranylgeraniol, did not affect osteoclast-like cell formation. Thus the specific inhibitory effect of MK-4 is attributable to the geranylgeranyl side chain.

Kameda *et al.* (1996) demonstrated that MK-4, but not phylloquinone, inhibits bone resorption by targeting osteoclasts to undergo programmed cell death (apoptosis). MK-4 did not induce apoptosis in other cell types in unfractionated bone cells. Calcitonin, which strongly inhibits osteoclastic bone resorption via calcitonin receptors, did not cause osteoclast apoptosis. MK-4 might be an appropriate therapeutic drug against bone diseases with excess bone resorption, because of its selective and direct induction of osteoclast apoptosis.

Clinical use of menaquinone-4 in osteoporosis

A number of Japanese studies have claimed beneficial results using synthetic MK-4 (menatetranone) in the treatment of osteoporosis. The rationale includes the possibility that MK-4 may have different effects on bone metabolism than phylloquinone. The dosage currently used (45 mg per day) is far in excess of daily vitamin K requirements and any effect must be regarded as pharmacological rather than a dietary correction of a nutritional deficiency. MK-4 was shown to be effective in increasing bone mineral density of cortical bone in osteoporotic patients (Orimo et al., 1998) as well as preventing the occurrence of new fractures and sustaining lumbar bone mineral density (Shiraki et al., 2000). In the latter study, MK-4 treatment enhanced γ-carboxylation of the osteocalcin molecule. There were no significant changes in bone resorption markers, therefore the prevention of bone fractures by MK-4 may not be caused entirely by inhibition of bone resorption.

10.5.6   Vitamin K and atherosclerosis

Background information can be found in Section 4.5.8.

The mRNA of matrix Gla protein (MGP) is expressed by a wide variety of soft tissues, as well as in developing bone (Fraser & Price, 1988). However, the protein itself has been found only in bone and calcified cartilage (Price et al., 2000). This observation suggests that the protein may accumulate at sites of calcification owing to its strong binding affinity to hydroxyapatite. Indeed, MGP, synthesized in the arterial intima by macrophages and to a lesser extent by vascular smooth muscle cells, accumulates in calcified atherosclerotic plaques. MGP is also synthesized by vascular smooth muscle cells directly abutting calcified regions in the arterial media (Shanahan et al., 2000).

Solid evidence confirming that MGP is a potent inhibitor of calcification in vivo comes from mice that lack MGP (Luo et al., 1997). Targeted deletion of the MGP gene causes rapid calcification of the elastic lamellae in the tunica media of the arteries, but not of the arterioles, capillaries or veins. The entire media is replaced by chondrocytes, producing a typical cartilage that starts to progressively calcify at birth. By 3 to 6 weeks of age, calcification is so extensive that the arteries become rigid tubes and, within 8 weeks of age, death occurs due to rupture of the thoracic or abdominal aorta. There is also inappropriate calcification of proliferating chondrocytes at the epiphyseal plate of growing long bones, resulting in stunted bone growth and osteopenia. The vascular phenotype of the MGP-deficient mouse suggests that MGP is an essential inhibitor of arterial calcification. Furthermore, it indicates that vascular calcification occurs spontaneously if not actively inhibited. In humans, mutations in the MGP gene are responsible for Keutel syndrome, a rare inherited disease characterized by multiple peripheral pulmonary stenoses, neural hearing loss, short terminal phalanges, midfacial hypoplasia, and abnormal calcification of the cartilage of the auricles, nose, larynx, trachea and ribs (Munroe et al., 1999).

Contrary to expectations, Shanahan et al. (1994) found that MGP mRNA is up-regulated in association with vascular calcification. However, this does not necessarily mean that the protein product is functional: function is crucially dependent on vitamin K-dependent post-translational conversion of Glu residues to Gla residues. Although γ-carboxylase activity has been demonstrated in the vessel wall (de Boer-van den Berg et al., 1986), advancing age and environmental factors such as diet and medication may lead to reduced levels of functional MGP. Jie et al. (1995) reported that post-menopausal women with calcified atherosclerotic lesions had higher levels of undercarboxylated osteocalcin and a lower dietary vitamin K intake than women without calcifications. This study demonstrated that aortic calcification is associated with a reduced vitamin K status. Furthermore, the presence of atherosclerotic calcifications was associated with a lower bone mass (Jie et al., 1996). On the basis that MGP is produced by the vessel wall as a defence mechanism against calcification, an insufficiency of vitamin K will lead to the production of nonfunctional MGP, and hence inappropriate calcification.

Another Gla protein has been isolated from calcified human atherosclerotic plaques and partly characterized (Gijsbers et al., 1990). This protein, named plaque Gla protein (PGP), has a mass of 23 kDa, contains five Gla residues per molecule, and is structurally dissimilar from any of the known Gla proteins. *In vitro*, PGP is extremely potent in inhibiting the precipitation of various calcium salts, but its role *in vivo* has yet to be demonstrated.

10.5.7   Possible role of vitamin K in the nervous system

A more recently discovered Gla protein encoded by a growth arrest-specific gene and known as Gas6 has a wide tissue distribution, including the nervous system. Gas6 is a ligand for a class of tyrosine kinase receptors and as such is involved in cell cycle regulation and cell–cell adhesion. In the nervous system, Gas6 is a growth factor for Schwann cells and is implicated in neuronal survival (Tsaioun, 1999).

10.6   Vitamin K deficiency

10.6.1   Deficiency in adults

In adult humans, clinical vitamin K deficiency manifests as occult bleeding. Abnormal blood coagulation is more likely to arise from secondary causes such as malabsorption syndromes or biliary obstruction than from a dietary inadequacy of vitamin K. However, subclinical deficiency, manifested as decreased urinary γ-carboxyglutamic acid excretion, has been induced in healthy adults by dietary deprivation of the vitamin (Ferland *et al.*, 1993).

In a placebo-controlled study involving healthy young and elderly adults, Binkley *et al.* (2000) reported that vitamin K supplementation (1000 µg of synthetic phylloquinone per day) resulted in a 10-fold increase in serum phylloquinone concentration. The mean percentage undercarboxylated osteocalcin decreased from 7.6% to 3.4% without significant differences by age or sex. The results showed that the usual dietary practices in the population studied did not provide adequate vitamin K for maximal osteocalcin carboxylation. Further research is needed to establish whether maximal osteocalcin γ-carboxylation is important for optimum bone mass density and whether submaximal osteocalcin γ-carboxylation should be used as a marker of vitamin K nutritional status.

10.6.2   Deficiency in infants

Plasma concentrations of the Gla-containing blood-clotting factors (factors II, VII, IX and X) in normal newborns range between 30 and 60% of adult values (Vermeer & Hamulyák, 1991). These relatively low values are not due to vitamin K deficiency as raising cord blood levels of phylloquinone to the endogenous maternal range by maternal oral supplementation does not improve coagulation in the fetus or neonate (Mandelbrot *et al.*, 1988). Also, there is no detectable difference in coagulation between breast-fed and formula-fed infants in the first month of life, despite the marked differences in serum phylloquinone concentrations (Pietersma-de Bruyn *et al.*, 1990). The likely explanation for the low neonatal concentrations of vitamin K-dependent clotting factors is reduced synthesis of their precursor proteins. In the mouse, gestational factor IX mRNA levels are <5% of adult levels up to 2 days before birth, when levels begin to rise steeply, reaching 43% of adult levels at birth. This is followed by a gradual increase until adult levels are reached at about 24 days of age (Yao *et al.*, 1991).

About 30% of full-term infants have low vitamin K status as indicated by the presence of des-γ-carboxyprothrombin (also known as PIVKA-II) in their plasma during the first week of life (Motohara *et al.*, 1985). Des-γ-carboxyprothrombin represents undercarboxylated prothrombin and is a sensitive haemostatic marker of subclinical vitamin K deficiency. The low vitamin K status, coupled with the low concentrations of vitamin K-dependent clotting factor precursor proteins, makes infants at birth and in early life susceptible to a syndrome referred to nowadays as vitamin K deficiency bleeding (VKDB) of early infancy. This disease, formerly known as haemorrhagic disease of the newborn, has a reported incidence of between 2 and 10 cases per 100 000 births (Shearer, 1995a). Three syndromes have been identified according to their time of presentation: early, classic and late VKDB. Early VKDB presents within 24 hours of birth and is commonly manifested as bleeding within the gut and around the genitalia. Classic VKDB presents 1 to 7 days after birth and the bleeding is usually gastrointestinal, dermal, nasal or from circumcision. Late VKDB, which presents 2 to 12 weeks after birth, is the most serious syndrome and is frequently associated with some abnormality of liver function. It has a 50% incidence of intracranial haemorrhage, resulting in death or severe and permanent brain damage (Shearer, 1995b).

Owing to limited placental transfer of maternal phylloquinone to the fetus, babies are born with low liver reserves of vitamin K. After birth, it takes several weeks before the liver stores of menaquinones attain adult levels. The absence of an intestinal microflora during the first few days of life may be significant in this regard. The newborn is entirely dependent on milk for its supply of vitamin K and hence any delay in the establishment of lactation may be a risk factor for classic VKDB. The vitamin K content of mature human milk ranges from 0.85 to 9.2 µg L^{-1} with a mean concentration of 2.5 µg L^{-1}, but can be increased by maternal intakes of pharmacological doses of the vitamin. By comparison, cow's milk contains 5 µg L^{-1} and infant formulas contain 50–100 µg L^{-1} (Institute of Medicine, 2001). Two major risk factors for VKDB are exclusive breast feeding and not giving vitamin K prophylaxis at birth. Premature babies now routinely receive intramuscular or (less effectively) oral doses of vitamin K as a prophylactic measure against VKDB.

Further reading

Ferland, G. (1998) The vitamin K-dependent proteins: an update. *Nutrition Reviews*, **56**, 223–30.

Newman, P. & Shearer, M. J. (1998) Vitamin K metabolism. In: *Subcellular Biochemistry, Vol. 30: Fat-Soluble Vitamins*. (Ed. P. J. Quinn & V. E. Kagan), pp. 455–88. Plenum Press, New York.

Olson, R. E. (1999) Vitamin K. In: *Modern Nutrition in Health and Disease*, 9th edn. (Ed. M. E. Shils, J. A. Olson, M. Shike & A. C. Ross), pp. 363–80. Lippincott Williams & Wilkins, Philadelphia.

Shearer, M. J. (1992) Vitamin K metabolism and nutriture. *Blood Reviews*, **6**, 92–104.

Shearer, M. J. (2000) Role of vitamin K and Gla proteins in the pathophysiology of osteoporosis and vascular calcification. *Current Opinion in Clinical Nutrition and Metabolic Care*, **3**, 433–8.

Vermeer, C., Gijsbers, B. L. M. G., Craciun, A. M., Groenen-van Dooren, M. C. L. & Knapen, M. H. J. (1996) Effects of vitamin K on bone mass and bone metabolism. *Journal of Nutrition*, **126**, 1187S–91S.

References

Akedo, Y., Hosoi, T., Inoue, S., Ikegami, A., Mizuno, Y., Kaneki, M., Nakamura, T., Ouchi, Y. & Orimo, H. (1992) Vitamin K_2 modulates proliferation and function of osteoblastic cells *in vitro*. *Biochemical and Biophysical Research Communications*, **187**, 814–20.

Akiyama, Y., Hara, K., Tajima, T., Murota, S. & Morita, I. (1994) Effect of vitamin K_2 (menatetrenone) on osteoclast-like cell formation in mouse bone marrow cultures. *European Journal of Pharmacology*, **263**, 181–5.

Allison, P. M., Mummah-Schendel, L. L., Kindberg, C. G., Harms, C. S., Bang, N. U. & Suttie, J. W. (1987) Effects of a vitamin K-deficient diet and antibiotics in normal human volunteers. *Journal of Laboratory and Clinical Medicine*, **110**, 180–8.

Binkley, N. C., Krueger, D. C., Engelke, J. A., Foley, A. L. & Suttie, J. W. (2000) Vitamin K supplementation reduces serum concentrations of under-γ-carboxylated osteocalcin in healthy young and elderly adults. *American Journal of Clinical Nutrition*, **72**, 1523–8.

Binkley, N. C., Krueger, D. C., Kawahara, T. N., Engelke, J. A., Chappell, R. J. & Suttie, J. W. (2002) A high phylloquinone intake is required to achieve maximal osteocalcin γ-carboxylation. *American Journal of Clinical Nutrition*, **76**, 1055–60.

Booth, S. L., Gundberg, C. M., McKeown, N. M., Morse, M. O. & Wood, R. J. (1999) Vitamin K depletion increases bone turnover. *Journal of Bone and Mineral Research*, **14** (suppl 1), S393 (abstr).

Booth, S. L., Lichtenstein, A. H. & Dallal, G. E. (2002) Phylloquinone absorption from phylloquinone-fortified oil is greater than from a vegetable in younger and older men and women. *Journal of Nutrition*, **132**, 2609–12.

Booth, S. L., Broe, K. E., Gagnon, D. R., Tucker, K. L., Hannan, M. T., McClean, R. R., Dawson-Hughes, B., Wilson, P. W. F., Cupples, L. A. & Kiel, D. P. (2003) Vitamin K intake and bone mineral density in women and men. *American Journal of Clinical Nutrition*, **77**, 512–6.

Cauley, J. A., Zmuda, J. M., Yaffe, K., Kuller, L. H., Ferrell, R. E., Wisniewski, S. R. & Cummings, S. R. (1999) Apolipoprotein E polymorphism: a new genetic marker of hip fracture risk – the study of osteoporotic fractures. *Journal of Bone and Mineral Research*, **14**, 1175–81.

Conly, J. M. & Stein, K. (1992a) Quantitative and qualitative measurements of K vitamins in human intestinal contents. *American Journal of Gastroenterology*, **87**, 311–6.

Conly, J. M. & Stein, K. (1992b) The production of menaquinones (vitamin K_2) by intestinal bacteria and their role in maintaining coagulation homeostasis. *Progress in Food and Nutrition Science*, **16**, 307–43.

Conly, J. M., Stein, K., Worobetz, L. & Rutledge-Harding, S. (1994) The contribution of vitamin K_2 (menaquinones) produced by the intestinal microflora to human nutritional requirements for vitamin K. *American Journal of Gastroenterology*, **89**, 915–23.

Davidson, R. T., Foley, A. L., Engelke, J. A. & Suttie, J. W. (1998) Conversion of dietary phylloquinone to tissue menaquinone-4 in rats is not dependent on gut bacteria. *Journal of Nutrition*, **128**, 220–3.

de Boer-van den Berg, M. A. G., van Haarlem, L. J. M. & Vermeer, C. (1986) Vitamin K-dependent carboxylase in human vessel wall. *Thrombosis Research*, (suppl. VI), 134.

Douglas, A. S., Robins, S. P., Hutchison, J. D., Porter, R. W., Stewart, A. & Reid, D. M. (1995) Carboxylation of osteocalcin in postmenopausal osteoporotic women following vitamin K and D supplementation. *Bone*, **17**, 15–20.

Ferland, G., Sadowski, J. A. & O'Brien, M. E. (1993) Dietary induced subclinical vitamin K deficiency in normal human subjects. *Journal of Clinical Investigation*, **91**, 1761–8.

Feskanich, D., Weber, P., Willett, W. C., Rockett, H., Booth, S. L. & Colditz, G. A. (1999) Vitamin K intake and hip fractures in women: a prospective study. *American Journal of Clinical Nutrition*, **69**, 74–9.

Fraser, J. D. & Price, P. A. (1988) Lung, heart, and kidney express high levels of mRNA for the vitamin K-dependent matrix Gla protein. *Journal of Biological Chemistry*, **263**(23), 11 033–6.

Garber, A. K., Binkley, N. C., Krueger, D. C. & Suttie, J. W. (1999) Comparison of phylloquinone bioavailability from food sources or a supplement in human subjects. *Journal of Nutrition*, **129**, 1201–3.

Gijsbers, B. L. M. G., van Haarlem, L. J. M., Soute, B. A. M., Ebberink, R. H. M. & Vermeer, C. (1990) Characterization of a Gla-containing protein from calcified human atherosclerotic plaques. *Arteriosclerosis*, **10**, 991–5.

Gijsbers, B. L. M. G., Jie, K.-S. G. & Vermeer, C. (1996) Effect of food composition on vitamin K absorption in human volunteers. *British Journal of Nutrition*, **76**, 223–9.

Gregg, R. E., Zech, L. A., Schaefer, E. J., Stark, D., Wilson, D. & Brewer, H. B. Jr. (1986) Abnormal in vivo metabolism of apolipoprotein E₄ in humans. *Journal of Clinical Investigation*, **78**, 815–21.

Groenen-van Dooren, M. M. C. L., Ronden, J. E., Soute, B. A. M. & Vermeer, C. (1995) Bioavailability of phylloquinone and menaquinones after oral and colorectal administration in vitamin K-deficient rats. *Biochemical Pharmacology*, **50**, 797–801.

Hara, K., Akiyama, Y., Tajima, T. & Shiraki, M. (1993) Menatetrenone inhibits bone resorption partly through inhibition of PGE₂ synthesis in vitro. *Journal of Bone and Mineral Research*, **8**, 535–42.

Hara, K., Akiyama, Y., Nakamura, T., Murota, S. & Morita, I. (1995) The inhibitory effect of vitamin K₂ (menatetrenone) on bone resorption may be related to its side chain. *Bone*, **16**, 179–84.

Hirauchi, K., Sakano, T., Notsumoto, S., Nagaoka, T., Morimoto, A., Fujimoto, K., Masuda, S. & Suzuki, Y. (1989a) Measurement of K vitamins in foods by high-performance liquid chromatography with fluorometric detection. *Vitamins (Japan)*, **63**, 147–51 (in Japanese).

Hirauchi, K., Sakano, T., Notsumoto, S., Nagaoka, T., Morimoto, A., Fujimoto, K., Masuda, S. & Suzuki, Y. (1989b) Measurement of K vitamins in animal tissues by high-performance liquid chromatography with fluorimetric detection. *Journal of Chromatography, Biomedical Applications*, **497**, 131–7.

Hodges, S. J., Akesson, K., Vergnaud, P., Obrant, K. & Delmas, P. D. (1993) Circulating levels of vitamin K₁ and K₂ decreased in elderly women with hip fractures. *Journal of Bone and Mineral Research*, **8**, 1241–5.

Hollander, D., Rim, E. & Ruble, P. E. Jr. (1977) Vitamin K₂ colonic and ileal in vivo absorption: bile, fatty acids, and pH effects on transport. *American Journal of Physiology*, **233**, E124–9.

Ichihashi, T., Takagishi, Y., Uchida, K. & Yamada, H. (1992) Colonic absorption of menaquinone-4 and menaquinone-9 in rats. *Journal of Nutrition*, **122**, 506–12.

Institute of Medicine (2001) Vitamin K. In: *Dietary Reference Intakes for vitamin A, vitamin K, arsenic, boron, chromium, copper, iodine, iron, manganese, molybdenum, nickel, silicon, vanadium, and zinc*, pp. 162–96. National Academy Press, Washington, D.C.

Jie, K.-S. G., Hamulyák, K., Gijsbers, B. L. M. G., Roumen, F. J. M. E. & Vermeer, C. (1992) Serum osteocalcin as a marker for vitamin K-status in pregnant women and their newborn babies. *Thrombosis and Haemostasis*, **68**, 388–91.

Jie, K.-S. G., Bots, M. L., Vermeer, C., Witteman, J. C. M. & Grobbee, D. E. (1995) Vitamin K intake and osteocalcin levels in women with and without aortic atherosclerosis: a population-based study. *Atherosclerosis*, **116**, 117–23.

Jie, K.-S. G., Bots, M. L., Vermeer, C., Witteman, J. C. M. & Grobbee, D. E. (1996) Vitamin K status and bone mass in women with and without aortic atherosclerosis: a population-based study. *Calcified Tissue International*, **59**, 352–6.

Kameda, T., Miyazawa, K., Mori, Y., Yuasa, T., Shiokawa, M., Nakamaru, Y., Mano, H., Hakeda, Y., Kameda, A. & Kumegawa,

M. (1996) Vitamin K₂ inhibits osteoclastic bone resorption by inducing osteoclast apoptosis. *Biochemical and Biophysical Research Communications*, **220**, 515–19.

Knapen, M. H. J., Hamulyák, K. & Vermeer, C. (1989) The effect of vitamin K supplementation on circulating osteocalcin (bone Gla protein) and urinary calcium excretion. *Annals of Internal Medicine*, **111**, 1001–5.

Knapen, M. H. J., Jie, K.-S. G., Hamulyák, K. & Vermeer, C. (1993) Vitamin K-induced changes in markers for osteoblast activity and urinary calcium loss. *Calcified Tissue International*, **53**, 81–5.

Kohlmeier, M., Saupe, J. Drossel, H.-J. & Shearer, M. J. (1995) Variation in phylloquinone (vitamin K₁) concentration in hemodialysis patients. *Thrombosis and Haemostasis*, **74**, 1252–4.

Kohlmeier, M., Salomon, A., Saupe, J. & Shearer, M. J. (1996) Transport of vitamin K to bone in humans. *Journal of Nutrition*, **126**, 1192S–6S.

Kohlmeier, M., Saupe, J. Schaefer, K. & Asmus, G. (1998) Bone fracture history and prospective bone fracture risk of hemodialysis patients are related to apolipoprotein E genotype. *Calcified Tissue International*, **62**, 278–81.

Koshihara, Y. & Hoshi, K. (1997) Vitamin K₂ enhances osteocalcin accumulation in the extracellular matrix of human osteoblasts in vitro. *Journal of Bone and Mineral Research*, **12**, 431–8.

Koshihara, Y., Hoshi, K. & Shiraki, M. (1993) Vitamin K₂ (menatetrenone) inhibits prostaglandin synthesis in cultured human osteoblast-like periosteal cells by inhibiting prostaglandin H synthase activity. *Biochemical Pharmacology*, **46**, 1355–62.

Koshihara, Y., Hoshi, K., Ishibashi, H. & Shiraki, M. (1996) Vitamin K₂ promotes 1α,25(OH)₂ vitamin D₃-induced mineralization in human periosteal osteoblasts. *Calcified Tissue International*, **59**, 466–73.

Lamon-Fava, S., Sadowski, J. A., Davidson, K. W., O'Brien, M. E., McNamara, J. R. & Schaefer, E. J. (1998) Plasma lipoproteins as carriers of phylloquinone (vitamin K₁) in humans. *American Journal of Clinical Nutrition*, **67**, 1226–31.

Lipsky, J. J. (1988) Antibiotic-associated hypoprothrombinaemia. *Journal of Antimicrobial Chemotherapy*, **21**, 281–300.

Luo, G., Ducy, P., McKee, M. D., Pinero, G. J., Loyer, E., Behringer, R. R. & Karsenty, G. (1997) Spontaneous calcification of arteries and cartilage in mice lacking matrix GLA protein. *Nature*, **386**, 78–81.

Mahley, R. W. & Hussain, M. M. (1991) Chylomicron and chylomicron remnant catabolism. *Current Opinion in Lipidology*, **2**, 170–6.

Mandelbrot, L., Guillaumont, M., Leclercq, M., Lefrère, J. J., Gozin, D., Daffos, F. & Forestier, F. (1988) Placental transfer of vitamin K₁ and its implications in fetal hemostasis. *Thrombosis and Haemostasis*, **60**, 39–43.

Matschiner, J. T. & Doisy, E. A. Jr. (1966) Bioassay of vitamin K in chicks. *Journal of Nutrition*, **90**, 97–100.

Motohara, K., Endo, F. & Matsuda, J. (1985) Effect of vitamin K administration on acarboxy prothrombin (PIVKA-II) levels in newborns. *Lancet*, **II**(8449), 242–4.

Munroe, P. B., Olgunturk, R. O., Fryns, J.-P., Van Maldergem, L., Ziereisen, F., Yuksel, B., Gardiner, R. M. & Chung, E. (1999) Mutations in the gene encoding the human matrix Gla protein cause Keutel syndrome. *Nature Genetics*, **21**, 142–4.

Newman, P., Bonello, F., Wierzbicki, A. S., Lumb, P., Savidge, G. F. & Shearer, M. J. (2002) The uptake of lipoprotein-borne phylloquinone (vitamin K₁) by osteoblasts and osteoblast-like cells: role of heparan sulfate proteoglycans and apolipoprotein E. *Journal of Bone and Mineral Research*, **17**, 426–33.

Olson, R. E. (1999) Vitamin K. In: *Modern Nutrition in Health and Disease*, 9th edn. (Ed. M. E. Shils, J. A. Olson, M. Shike & A. C.

Ross), pp. 363–80. Lippincott Williams & Wilkins, Philadelphia.

Orimo, H., Shiraki, M., Tomita, A., Morii, H., Fujita, T. & Ohata, M. (1998) Effects of menatetrenone on the bone and calcium metabolism in osteoporosis: a double-blind placebo-controlled study. *Journal of Bone and Mineral Metabolism*, 16, 106–12.

Pan, E. Y., Gomperts, E. D., Millen, R. & Gilsanz, V. (1990) Bone mineral density and its association with inherited protein S deficiency. *Thrombosis Research*, 58, 221–31.

Pietersma-de Bruyn, A. L. J. M., van Haard, P. M. M., Beunis, M. H., Hamulyák, K. & Kuijpers, J. C. (1990) Vitamin K_1 levels and coagulation factors in healthy full term newborns till 4 weeks after birth. *Haemostasis*, 20, 8–14.

Plantalech, L., Guillaumont, M., Vergnaud, P., Leclercq, M. & Delmas, P. D. (1991) Impairment of gamma carboxylation of circulating osteocalcin (bone gla protein) in elderly women. *Journal of Bone and Mineral Research*, 6, 1211–16.

Price, P. A., Faus, S. A. & Williamson, M. K. (2000) Warfarin-induced artery calcification is accelerated by growth and vitamin D. *Arteriosclerosis, Thrombosis, and Vascular Biology*, 20, 317–27.

Rall, S. C. Jr., Weisgraber, K. H. & Mahley, R. W. (1982) Human apolipoprotein E. The complete amino acid sequence. *Journal of Biological Chemistry*, 257(8), 4171–8.

Rall, S. C. Jr., Weisgraber, K H., Innerarity, T. L. & Mahley, R. W. (1983) Identical structural and receptor binding defects in apolipoprotein E2 in hypo-, normo-, and hypercholesterolemic dysbetalipoproteinemia. *Journal of Clinical Investigation*, 71, 1023–31.

Ramotar, K., Conly, J. M., Chubb, H. & Louie, T. J. (1984) Production of menaquinones by intestinal anaerobes. *Journal of Infectious Diseases*, 150, 213–18.

Ravn, P., Fledelius, C., Rosenquist, C., Overgaard, K. & Christiansen, C. (1996) High bone turnover is associated with low bone mass in both pre- and postmenopausal women. *Bone*, 19, 291–8.

Robey, P. G. & Boskey, A. L. (1996) The biochemistry of bone. In: *Osteoporosis*. (Ed. R. Marcus, D. Feldman & J. Kelsey), pp. 95–183. Academic Press, San Diego.

Sadowski, J. A., Hood, S. J., Dallal, G. E. & Garry, P. J. (1989) Phylloquinone in plasma from elderly and young adults: factors influencing its concentration. *American Journal of Clinical Nutrition*, 50, 100–8.

Sakano, T., Notsumoto, S., Nagaoka, T., Morimoto, A., Fujimoto, K., Masuda, S., Suzuki, Y. & Hirauchi, K. (1988) Measurement of K vitamins in food by high-performance liquid chromatography with fluorometric detection. *Vitamins (Japan)*, 62, 393–8 (in Japanese).

Saupe, J., Shearer, M. J. & Kohlmeier, M. (1993) Phylloquinone transport and its influence on γ-carboxyglutamate residues of osteocalcin in patients on maintenance hemodialysis. *American Journal of Clinical Nutrition*, 58, 204–8.

Semenkovich, C. F. (1999) Nutrient and genetic regulation of lipoprotein metabolism. In: *Modern Nutrition in Health and Disease*, 9th edn. (Ed. M. E. Shils, J. A. Olson, M. Shike & A. C. Ross), pp. 1191–7. Lippincott Williams & Wilkins, Philadelphia.

Shanahan, C. M., Cary, N. R. B., Metcalfe, J. C. & Weissberg, P. L. (1994) High expression of genes for calcification-regulating proteins in human atherosclerotic plaques. *Journal of Clinical Investigation*, 93, 2393–402.

Shanahan, C. M., Proudfoot, D., Tyson, K. L., Cary, N. R. B., Edmonds, M. & Weissberg, P. L. (2000) Expression of mineralization-regulating proteins in association with human vascular calcification. *Zeitschrift für Kardiologie*, 89 (suppl. 2), II/63–8.

Shearer, M. J. (1992) Vitamin K metabolism and nutriture. *Blood Reviews*, 6, 92–104.

Shearer, M. J. (1995a) Vitamin K: its physiological role and the assessment of clinical and subclinical states. *Journal of the International Federation of Clinical Chemistry*, 7, 88–95.

Shearer, M. J. (1995b) Vitamin K. *Lancet*, 345, 229–34.

Shearer, M. J., McBurney, A. & Barkhan, P. (1974) Studies on the absorption and metabolism of phylloquinone (vitamin K_1) in man. *Vitamins and Hormones*, 32, 513–42.

Shearer, M. J., Rahim, S., Barkhan, P. & Stimmler, L. (1982) Plasma vitamin K_1 in mothers and their newborn babies. *Lancet*, II(8296), 460–3.

Shearer, M. J., Bach, A. & Kohlmeier, M. (1996) Chemistry, nutritional sources, tissue distribution and metabolism of vitamin K with special reference to bone health. *Journal of Nutrition*, 126, 1181S–6S.

Shiraki, M., Shiraki, Y., Aoki, C. & Miura, M. (2000) Vitamin K_2 (menatetrenone) effectively prevents fractures and sustains lumbar bone mineral density in osteoporosis. *Journal of Bone and Mineral Research*, 15, 515–21.

Sokoll, L. J. & Sadowski, J. A. (1996) Comparison of biochemical indexes for assessing vitamin K nutritional status in a healthy population. *American Journal of Clinical Nutrition*, 63, 566–73.

Sokoll, L. J., O'Brien, M. E., Camilo, M. E. & Sadowski, J. (1995) Undercarboxylated osteocalcin and development of a method to determine vitamin K status. *Clinical Chemistry*, 41, 1121–8.

Szulc, P., Chapuy, M.-C., Meunier, P. J. & Delmas, P. D. (1993) Serum undercarboxylated osteocalcin is a marker of the risk of hip fracture in elderly women. *Journal of Clinical Investigation*, 91, 1769–74.

Szulc, P., Arlot, M., Chapuy, M.-C., Duboeuf, F., Meunier, P. J. & Delmas, P. D. (1994) Serum undercarboxylated osteocalcin correlates with hip bone mineral density in elderly women. *Journal of Bone and Mineral Research*, 9, 1591–5.

Szulc, P., Chapuy, M.-C., Meunier, P. J. & Delmas, P. D. (1996) Serum undercarboxylated osteocalcin is a marker of the risk of hip fracture: a three year follow-up study. *Bone*, 18, 487–8.

Tamatani, M., Morimoto, S., Nakajima, M., Fukuo, K., Onishi, T., Kitano, S., Niinobu, T. & Ogihara, T. (1998) Decreased circulating levels of vitamin K and 25-hydroxyvitamin D in osteopenic elderly men. *Metabolism*, 47, 195–9.

Thijssen, H. H. W. & Drittij-Reijnders, M. J. (1994) Vitamin K distribution in rat tissues: dietary phylloquinone is a source of tissue menaquinone-4. *British Journal of Nutrition*, 72, 415–25.

Thijssen, H. H. W. & Drittij-Reijnders, M. J. (1996) Vitamin K status in human tissues: tissue-specific accumulation of phylloquinone and menaquinone-4. *British Journal of Nutrition*, 75, 121–7.

Thijssen, H. H. W. & Drittij-Reijnders, M. J. & Fischer, M. A. J. G. (1996) Phylloquinone and menaquinone-4 distribution in rats: synthesis rather than uptake determines menaquinone-4 organ concentrations. *Journal of Nutrition*, 126, 537–43.

Tsaioun, K. I. (1999) Vitamin K-dependent proteins in the developing and aging nervous system. *Nutrition Reviews*, 57, 231–40.

Usui, Y., Tanimura, H., Nishimura, N., Kobayashi, N., Okanoue, T. & Ozawa, K. (1990) Vitamin K concentrations in the plasma and liver of surgical patients. *American Journal of Clinical Nutrition*, 51, 846–52.

Vergnaud, P., Garnero, P., Meunier, P. J., Bréart, G., Kamihagi, K. & Delmas, P. D. (1997) Undercarboxylated osteocalcin measured with a specific immunoassay predicts hip fracture in elderly women: the EPIDOS study. *Journal of Clinical Endocrinology and Metabolism*, 82, 719–24.

Vermeer, C. (1990) γ-Carboxyglutamate-containing proteins and the vitamin K-dependent carboxylase. *Biochemical Journal*, 266, 625–36.

Vermeer, C. & Hamulyák, K. (1991) Pathophysiology of vitamin K deficiency and oral anticoagulants. *Thrombosis and Haemostasis*, 66, 153–9.

Vermeer, C., Jie, K.-S. G. & Knapen, M. J. H. (1995) Role of vitamin K in bone metabolism. *Annual Review of Nutrition*, **15**, 1–22.

Weintraub, M. S., Eisenberg, S. & Breslow, J. L. (1987) Dietary fat clearance in normal subjects is regulated by genetic variation in apolipoprotein E. *Journal of Clinical Investigation*, **80**, 1571–7.

Weisgraber, K. H., Innerarity, T. L. & Mahley, R. W. (1982) Abnormal lipoprotein receptor-binding activity of the human E apoprotein due to cysteine-arginine interchange at a single site. *Journal of Biological Chemistry*, **257**(5), 2518–21.

Will, B. H., Usui, Y. & Suttie, J. W. (1992) Comparative metabolism and requirement of vitamin K in chicks and rats. *Journal of Nutrition*, **122**, 2354–60.

Yang, Y.-M., Simon, N., Maertens, P., Brigham, S. & Liu, P. (1989) Maternal–fetal transport of vitamin K_1 and its effects on coagulation in premature infants. *Journal of Pediatrics*, **115**, 1009–13.

Yao, S.-N., DeSilva, A. H., Kurachi, S., Samuelson, L. C. & Kurachi, K. (1991) Characterization of a mouse factor IX cDNA and developmental regulation of the factor IX gene expression in liver. *Thrombosis and Haemostasis*, **65**, 52–8.

Zannis, V. I. & Breslow, J. L. (1981) Human very low density lipoprotein apolipoprotein E isoprotein polymorphism is explained by genetic variation and posttranslational modification. *Biochemistry*, **20**, 1033–41.

11
Thiamin (Vitamin B$_1$)

Key discussion topics

- Thiamin pyrophosphate is a coenzyme for three dehydrogenases which are directly or indirectly involved with the tricarboxylic acid cycle, and for a transketolase involved in the pentose phosphate pathway.

- Thiamin triphosphate is involved in nerve membrane function.
- A deficiency of vitamin B$_1$ gives rise to the neurological and cardiovascular symptoms of beriberi.
- The Wernicke–Korsakoff syndrome, a form of beriberi that affects the brain, is related to chronic alcoholism.

11.1   Historical overview

At one time, the disease beriberi was believed to be caused by a microorganism or toxin. The first indication of a nutritional aetiology was the virtual elimination of beriberi in the Japanese Navy in 1885, brought about by increasing the proportion of meat and vegetables in the staple rice diet. In 1890, Eijkman, a Dutch medical officer stationed in Java, discovered that feeding chickens on polished rice induced a polyneuritis closely resembling human beriberi, which could be prevented by the addition of rice bran to the avian diet. A few years later, Grijns extracted a water-soluble 'polyneuritis preventive factor' from rice bran and correctly concluded that beriberi is the result of a dietary lack of an essential nutrient. By 1926, two Dutch chemists, Jansen and Donath, had succeeded in isolating the factor (by now called vitamin B_1) in crystalline form from rice bran extracts. By 1936, Robert R. Williams had elucidated the structure of vitamin B_1, which he named 'thiamine', and accomplished its synthesis. The failure of thiamin-deficient pigeons to metabolize pyruvate led Sir Rudolph Peters and his colleagues in the early 1930s to establish the essential role of thiamin in pyruvate metabolism. Lohmann and Schuster then discovered that the active coenzyme form of the vitamin was the diphosphate ester.

(In this text, 'thiamin', rather than 'thiamine', is used in accordance with the nomenclature policy of the International Union of Nutritional Sciences Committee on Nomenclature.)

11.2   Chemistry and biological activity

The thiamin molecule comprises substituted pyrimidine and thiazole moieties linked by a methylene bridge (Fig. 11.1). It is a quaternary amine, which exists as a monovalent or divalent cation depending on the pH of the solution. Three phosphorylated forms of thiamin occur in nature. In living tissues the predominant form is the diphosphate, usually referred to as thiamin pyrophosphate (TPP) (Fig. 11.1), which serves as a coenzyme in several metabolic pathways. Small amounts of the monophosphate and triphosphate esters also occur in animal tissues. Thiamin

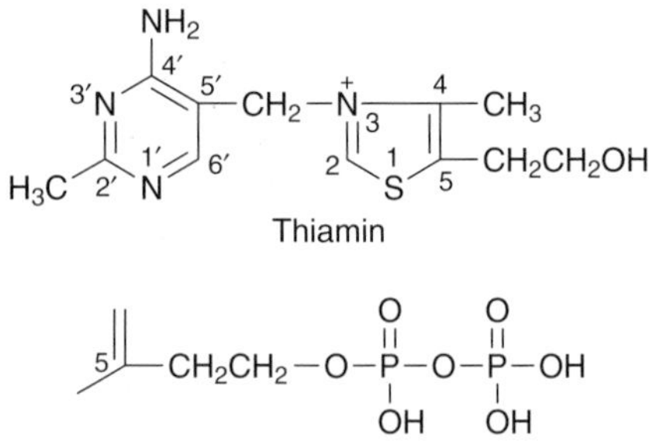

Fig. 11.1 Structures of thiamin and thiamin pyrophosphate.

triphosphate has no coenzyme function, but it has a role (not yet completely understood) in nerve transmission. Thiamin monophosphate appears to be biologically inactive.

The name thiamin and the individual phosphates of thiamin will be used as specific terms; total thiamin means the sum of thiamin and its phosphates, and vitamin B_1 is a non-specific generic term.

11.3   Dietary sources and bioavailability

11.3.1   Dietary sources

All plant and animal tissues contain vitamin B_1, and so the vitamin is present in all natural unprocessed foods. Rich sources of vitamin B_1 include yeast and yeast extract, wheat bran, oatmeal, whole-grain cereals, pulses, nuts, lean pork, heart, kidney and liver. Beef, lamb, chicken, eggs, vegetables and fruits contain intermediate amounts, while milk contains a relatively low amount. The milling of cereals removes most of the vitamin B_1, so white flour, breakfast cereals and, in certain countries, polished rice are enriched by addition of the vitamin.

In most animal tissues, over 90% of the thiamin is phosphorylated, with TPP predominating. Exceptions are pig skeletal muscle (Egi *et al.*, 1986) and chicken skeletal white muscle (Miyoshi *et al.*, 1990), in which the triphosphate constitutes 70–80% of the total thiamin present. The natural vitamin B_1 content of most cereals and cereal products, including white flour made from wheat, is present almost entirely in the form of non-phosphorylated thiamin.

11.3.2 Bioavailability

Few studies have been conducted on the bioavailability of vitamin B$_1$ present naturally in foods, but it is generally considered to be high. The presence of thermostable polyphenols possessing anti-thiamin activity has been demonstrated in a wide variety of fruits and vegetables as well as in tea and coffee (Hilker & Somogyi, 1982). These include hydroxylated derivatives of cinnamic acid, flavonoids and tannins. Vitamin C was found to counteract the anti-thiamin activity of tannic acid (Kositawattanakul *et al.*, 1977). A thiaminase has been found in shellfish and the viscera of freshwater fish (Murata, 1982; Vimokesant *et al.*, 1982). Habitual intakes of raw freshwater fish (with or without fermentation) and raw shellfish are risk factors for the development of vitamin B$_1$ deficiency. Since thiaminase is inactivated by heat, the cooking of such foods destroys the enzyme completely.

11.4 Absorption, transport and metabolism

Humans cannot synthesize vitamin B$_1$ and so must obtain this vitamin from the diet. Vitamin B$_1$ is synthesized by the microflora that normally inhabit the large intestine, but this exogenous vitamin does not appear to be available to the human host. Absorptive tissues such as placenta, kidney and intestine are known to express specific organic cation/H$^+$ antiport systems that are capable of transporting both endogenous as well as exogenous organic cations. There is evidence that such a system, with substrate specificity for thiamin, transports thiamin into intestine, liver and placenta.

11.4.1 Digestion and absorption of dietary vitamin B$_1$

Dietary sources of phosphorylated thiamin, mainly TPP, are completely hydrolysed to free thiamin in the intestinal lumen by different phosphatases, including alkaline phosphatase. Absorption of thiamin then takes place in the duodenum and proximal jejunum by a dual mechanism that is predominantly saturable at low, physiological concentrations of the vitamin (<2.5 µmol L^{-1}) and largely nonsaturable (diffusive) at higher concentrations (Laforenza *et al.*, 1997). A significant amount of the thiamin that is taken up by the enterocyte is phosphorylated, mainly to TPP, thereby trapping the transported thiamin inside the absorptive cell (Ricci & Rindi, 1992). Intracellular TPP is dephosphorylated by microsomal phosphatases to free thiamin before exit (Rindi, 1984).

Said *et al.* (1999) examined the uptake of radioactive [^{3}H]thiamin by an *in vitro* cell culture system comprising confluent monolayers of the human-derived Caco-2 intestinal epithelial cells. At the confluent stage, Caco-2 cells differentiate spontaneously to become enterocyte-like absorptive cells, having well-defined brush-border and basolateral membranes and intercellular junctional complexes. Thiamin uptake was found to be (1) dependent on temperature and metabolic energy, (2) pH-sensitive, (3) Na$^+$-independent, (4) saturable as a function of concentration and (5) competitively inhibited by structural analogues of thiamin. The saturability and competitive inhibition indicate a carrier-mediated transport process. Inhibition of the Ca^{2+}/calmodulin second messenger system (see Section 3.7.6) resulted in a significant inhibition of thiamin uptake, implicating this system in the regulation of thiamin absorption. The effect of one such inhibitor, trifluoperazine, was to decrease V_{max} (maximal transport rate) but not the K_m (half-saturation concentration) of the thiamin uptake process. This indicates that the inhibitory effect of trifluoperazine is mediated via down-regulation of thiamin carriers at the brush-border membrane, with no effect on carrier affinity.

The use of purified intestinal membrane vesicles permits transport mechanisms in brush-border and basolateral membranes to be studied separately, with no interference from intracellular metabolism. Laforenza *et al.* (1998) reported the existence of a thiamin/H$^+$ antiport mechanism for thiamin entry into brush-border membrane vesicles from rat small intestine. In the absence of H$^+$ gradient, changes in transmembrane electrical potential did not affect thiamin uptake. Studies using basolateral membrane vesicles showed that exit of thiamin from the enterocyte took place by primary active transport mediated by the basolateral membrane's Na$^+$–K$^+$-ATPase (Laforenza *et al.*, 1993).

Adaptive regulation of thiamin absorption
Laforenzo *et al.* (1997) used biopsy specimens of human gastrointestinal mucosa for their studies on thiamin absorption. One unusual patient showed

signs of acute vitamin B_1 deficiency that was not attributable to malabsorption. When biopsy samples from this patient were studied, the saturable component of thiamin uptake was found to be higher than in samples from non-deficient patients. The higher rate of uptake was reflected by an increased V_{max}, signifying up-regulation of thiamin carriers. The results from this one patient suggest that vitamin B_1 deficiency in humans may enhance the capacity of thiamin absorption, an adaptive mechanism which has been reported in rats (Patrini et al., 1981).

Effects of alcohol

Acute and chronic effects of alcohol on thiamin absorption in rats have been summarized by Hoyumpa (1986). The acute effect of single doses of ethanol in rats is to significantly reduce the absorption of thiamin by inhibiting in a reversible manner the low concentration, saturable component of the dual transport process. More specifically, ethanol appears to allow the initial uptake of thiamin across the apical membrane of the enterocyte but impairs the subsequent movement of the vitamin across the basolateral membrane into the serosa. The fall in the rate of cellular thiamin exit is associated with inhibition of the basolateral Na^+–K^+-ATPase activity. In contrast, chronic ethanol feeding for 6–8 weeks fails to alter thiamin absorption or Na^+–K^+-ATPase activity in rats. These data suggest that inhibition of thiamin absorption is dependent more on the concentration of ethanol bathing the basolateral membrane of the enterocyte rather than on the duration of exposure. Thiamin malabsorption may, therefore, be intermittent, depending on the ethanol concentration.

11.4.2   Absorption of bacterially synthesized thiamin in the large intestine

Instillation of thiamin directly into the colonic lumen of human subjects did not result in increased plasma concentrations of thiamin in blood samples taken 1, 2 and 4 hours after administration (Sorrell et al., 1971). Based on this observation, it appears that bacterially synthesized thiamin is not absorbed in the large intestine. Kasper (1970) pointed out that the intestinal flora destroys or utilizes a large part of the thiamin injected into the large intestine, and so the true capacity of the colon to absorb B vitamins can be determined only after eliminating the intestinal flora.

11.4.3   Post-absorptive metabolism

Following absorption, vitamin B_1 is carried by the portal blood to the liver. Both non-phosphorylated thiamin and thiamin monophosphate circulate in the bloodstream, the former bound to plasma proteins. In normal adults, 20–30% of total thiamin in the plasma is protein-bound (Davis et al., 1984).

Transport of thiamin at the membrane level in rat liver has been studied using basolateral (sinusoidal) plasma membrane vesicles (Moseley et al., 1992). A high-affinity, low-capacity thiamin/H^+ antiport mechanism was shown to be present with a narrow substrate specificity that was distinct from N^1-methylnicotinamide/H^+ exchange.

Within the liver and in other tissues, thiamin is converted to its coenzyme form, TPP, by the catalytic action of thiamin pyrophosphokinase:

$$\text{Thiamin} + \text{ATP} \rightarrow \text{TPP} + \text{AMP} \qquad (11.1)$$

In the brain and other nervous tissue, some of the TPP is converted to thiamin triphosphate (TTP) by thiamin pyrophosphate-ATP phosphoryltransferase:

$$\text{TPP} + \text{ATP} \rightarrow \text{TTP} + \text{ADP} \qquad (11.2)$$

Nervous tissue also contains thiamin pyrophosphatase which converts small amounts of TPP to thiamin monophosphate (TMP) and inorganic phosphate:

$$\text{TPP} \rightarrow \text{TMP} + \text{PPi} \qquad (11.3)$$

Also in nervous tissue, TTP may be hydrolysed by thiamin triphosphatase to yield TPP and inorganic phosphate.

$$\text{TTP} \rightarrow \text{TPP} + \text{PPi} \qquad (11.4)$$

Similarly, in nervous tissue, TMP may hydrolysed to thiamin by thiamin monophosphatase.

$$\text{TMP} \rightarrow \text{thiamin} + \text{PPi} \qquad (11.5)$$

The human body contains approximately 30 mg of total thiamin, of which about 80% is TPP, 10% is thiamin triphosphate, and the remainder is thiamin monophosphate and free thiamin. About half of the body content of total thiamin is found in skeletal muscles, the remainder being distributed mainly in the liver, heart, kidney and brain. The biological half-life of [^{14}C] thiamin in the body is 9 to 18 days. Because of this relatively high turnover rate and low storage capacity, a continuous dietary intake of vitamin B$_1$ is necessary. During deprivation there is a rather rapid loss of the vitamin from all tissues except the brain.

11.4.4 Brain homeostasis

Brain cells need a continuous supply of thiamin to replace that used in cerebral metabolism in the form of the TPP; moreover, thiamin triphosphate has been implicated in nerve cell function (see Section 11.6). The turnover of cerebrospinal fluid (CSF) also creates a need for continuing transfer of thiamin from blood to brain. Experimental depletion of thiamin from the brain causes neuromuscular disturbances, especially ataxia and convulsions.

Greenwood *et al.* (1982) used an *in vivo* technique to study thiamin transport across the blood–brain barrier of rats and found that the normal rate of thiamin entry into the brain was of a similar order of magnitude to the rate of thiamin turnover in different brain regions. This comparison shows that, although blood–brain transport is normally adequate to meet the needs of the brain for thiamin and to replace the obligatory losses, there is little margin of spare capacity. The transport of thiamin was evidently carrier-mediated and could be saturated by increasing the concentration of vitamin in the bloodstream. Less than 10% of the total flux was provided by a non-saturable process.

Thiamin monophosphate, which accompanies thiamin in plasma and CSF, is also transported across the blood–brain barrier by a saturable mechanism. The half-saturation concentration (K_m) ranged between 2.6 and 5.0 μM, depending on the cerebral region (Patrini *et al.*, 1988). This compares with K_m values of 1.9–2.6 μM for saturable thiamin transport across the blood–brain barrier (Reggiani *et al.*, 1984).

The entry of thiamin from blood into CSF via the choroid plexus and from the extracellular space of brain into brain cells themselves are both saturable processes (Spector, 1976). In brain slices from rabbits and rats, the uptake system for thiamin is half-saturated at ~0.3 μM, which is similar to the normal concentration of total thiamin in the CSF of these species (Spector, 1982). This means that the entry of excessive amounts of the vitamin into the brain is prohibited. Indeed, it has been shown that after the intravenous injection of large doses of thiamin, CSF and brain total thiamin levels are little changed.

11.4.5 Placental transport

Schenker *et al.* (1990) studied the transfer of physiological concentrations of thiamin across human placenta using an *in vitro* perfusion system which eliminated the confounding variables of maternal or fetal metabolism. A unidirectional maternal-to-fetal transfer of thiamin took place against a concentration gradient, implying active transport. There was no evidence of phosphorylation of thiamin during its transfer. Saturation kinetics and inhibition of transport by structural analogues of thiamin were indicative of a carrier-mediated process. The involvement of a thiamin-binding protein was ruled out because the concentration of albumin was identical on both sides of the placenta. The results of this study indicate the existence of a carrier-mediated, active transport mechanism for thiamin transport across the microvillous membrane of the syncytiotrophoblast.

Grassl (1998) demonstrated the existence of a thiamin/H⁺ antiport mechanism in human placental brush-border membrane vesicles. Substrate specificity studies suggested that the amine at position four of the pyrimidine ring, but not the hydroxyethyl side chain or an unmodified thiazolium ring, is an important chemical determinant for interaction with the transporter substrate binding site(s). Dutta *et al.* (1999) described the molecular cloning of a cDNA from human placenta which, when expressed in mammalian cells, induced the uptake of thiamin. This thiamin transporter shared significant homology (40% identity) with the reduced folate carrier previously cloned from human placenta.

11.4.6 Excretion

Thiamin in excess of binding and storage capacity is rapidly excreted in the urine together with small amounts of its metabolites. No direct evidence of reabsorption by the kidney has been reported. Only negligible amounts of thiamin are excreted in the bile. In very hot countries a significant loss of thiamin may occur through sweating (Bender & Bender, 1997).

11.5 Biochemical functions

Background information can be found in Section 4.1.

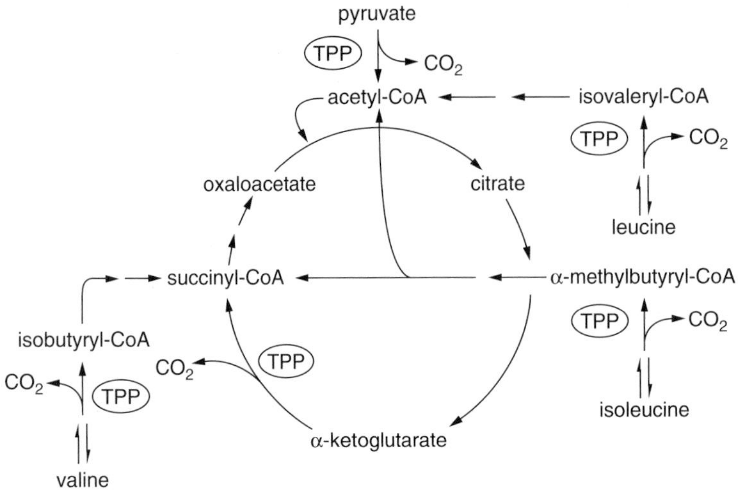

Fig. 11.2 Involvement of thiamin pyrophosphate (TPP) in the tricarboxylic acid cycle.

In mammalian tissues, TPP is a coenzyme for three mitochondrial enzymes involved in the oxidative decarboxylation of α-keto acids; these enzymes are the pyruvate dehydrogenase complex (EC 1.2.4.1), α-ketoglutarate dehydrogenase (EC 1.2.4.2) and branched-chain α-keto acid dehydrogenase (EC 1.2.4.4). The involvement of these dehydrogenases in the tricarboxylic acid cycle is shown in Fig. 11.2. In addition, TPP is a coenzyme for transketolase (EC 2.2.1.1), which is found in the cytosol.

11.5.1   *Oxidative decarboxylation of α-keto acids*

Pyruvate dehydrogenase is a multi-enzyme complex which catalyses the conversion of pyruvate to acetyl-CoA at a central point between glycolysis, lipid metabolism and the tricarboxylic acid cycle. The enzyme complex is composed of three subunit proteins that require TPP, Mg^{2+}, NAD^+, FAD, lipoic acid and coenzyme A (CoA–SH) as cofactors. The overall reaction (Fig. 11.3) is the sum of the individual reactions.

α-Ketoglutarate dehydrogenase, which is also composed of three subunits, catalyses the conversion of α-ketoglutarate to succinyl-CoA in the tricarboxylic acid cycle. The overall reaction is shown in Fig. 11.4. The composition of the multi-enzyme complex, the cofactor requirements and the steps in the formation of succinyl-CoA are similar to the oxidative decarboxylation of pyruvate.

Branched-chain α-keto acid dehydrogenase catalyses the oxidative decarboxylation of the branched-chain α-keto acids, α-ketoisocaproic acid, α-keto-β-methylvaleric acid and α-ketoisovaleric acid, which

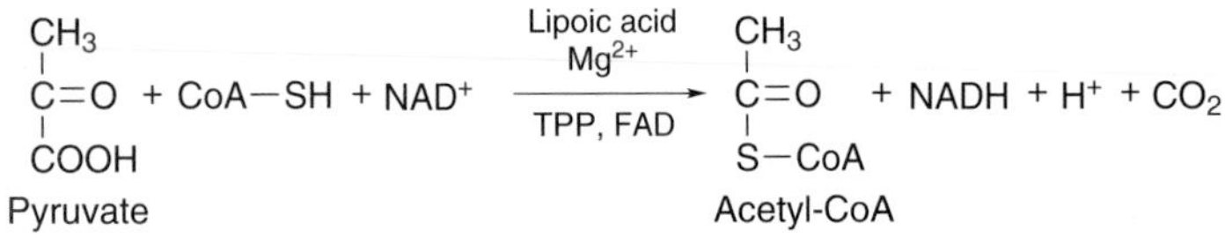

Fig. 11.3 Conversion of pyruvate to acetyl-CoA.

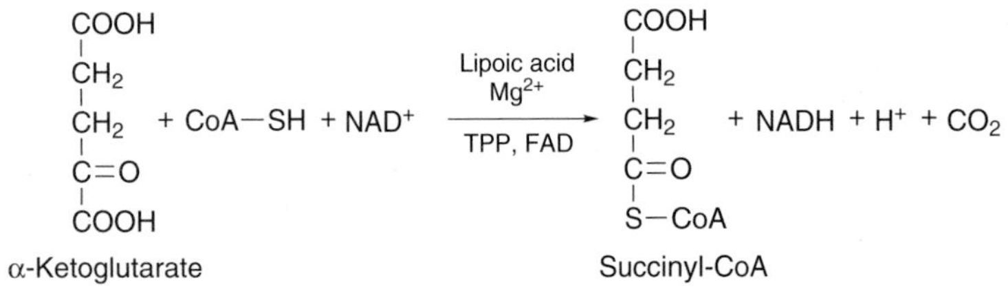

Fig. 11.4 Conversion of α-ketoglutarate to succinyl-CoA.

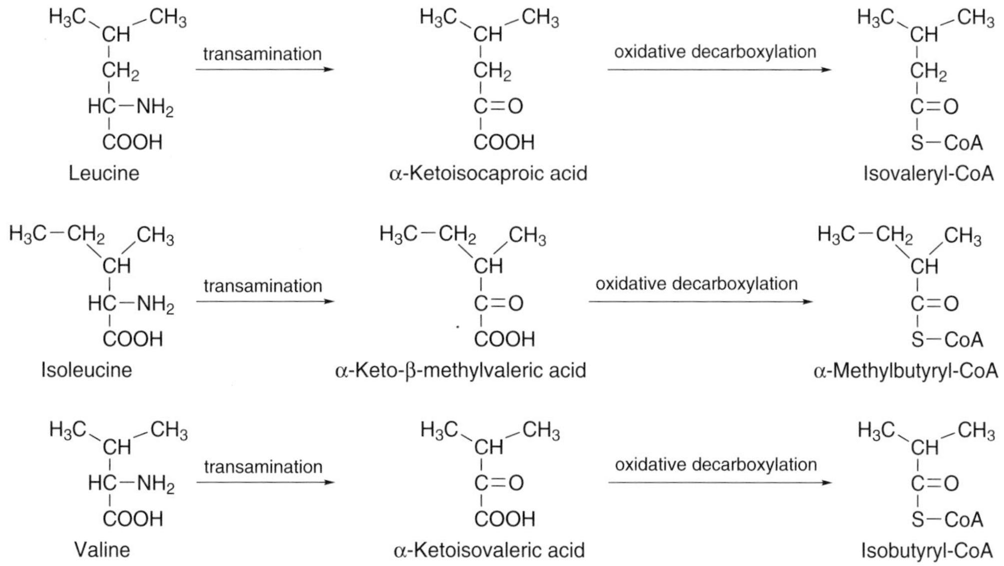

Fig. 11.5 Oxidative decarboxylation of branched-chain α-keto acids.

are formed after deamination of leucine, isoleucine, and valine, respectively (Fig. 11.5). The oxidative decarboxylation reactions are similar to those for pyruvate and α-ketoglutarate and require the same cofactors. The decarboxylation products, isovaleryl-CoA, α-methylbutyryl-CoA and isobutyryl-CoA, are indirectly involved with the tricarboxylic acid cycle, as shown in Fig. 11.2.

Maple syrup urine disease

A genetic mutation causing a defect in one of the components of the branched-chain α-keto acid de-hydrogenase complex impairs the metabolism of leucine, isoleucine and valine by blocking the oxidative decarboxylation of the corresponding keto acid to its acyl coenzyme A derivative. The inherited metabolic disease associated with this defect is branched-chain α-ketoaciduria, otherwise known as maple syrup urine disease. The frequency of this disease among newborn infants is approximately 1 in 250 000 worldwide. Signs of neurological dysfunction in the newborn, such as poor sucking, irregular respiration, periodic rigidity and seizures, appear after infants receive a protein-containing feed. A characteristic symptom is the production of urine with the odour of burnt sugar (caramel) or maple syrup. The disease can be diagnosed by elevated concentrations of leucine,

isoleucine and valine in plasma, and of branched-chain keto acids in urine. Early diagnosis and therapy lead to normal growth and development. Untreated cases who survive beyond early infancy have retarded physical and mental development. Treatment necessitates a dietary restriction of leucine, isoleucine and valine, which is met by a combination of medical and natural foods. In most instances, maple syrup urine disease is due to a complete lack of activity of the branched-chain α-keto acid dehydrogenase complex – an inborn error of metabolism. In cases where there is some, even slight, activity of the branched-chain α-keto acid dehydrogenase complex, daily oral doses of 100 to 1000 mg of thiamin can be beneficial (Elsas & Acosta, 1999).

11.5.2   Transketolation

In the pentose phosphate pathway, TPP is the coenzyme for two reversible transketolase reactions involving the transfer of a two-carbon ketol unit from a donor molecule to an acceptor molecule. In the first reaction (Fig. 11.6) the ketol group from xylulose-5-phosphate is donated to ribose-5-phosphate to form sedo-heptulose-7-phosphate and glyceraldehyde-3-phosphate. In the second reaction (Fig. 11.6) the ketol group from xylose-5-phosphate is donated to

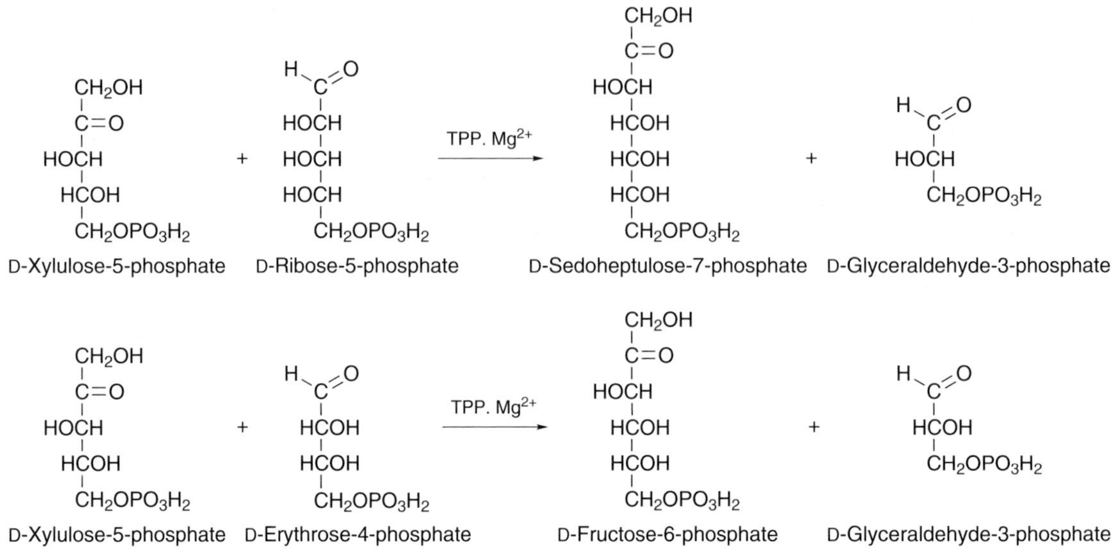

D-Xylulose-5-phosphate:
CH_2OH
$C=O$
$HOCH$
$HCOH$
$CH_2OPO_3H_2$

$+$

D-Ribose-5-phosphate:
$H{-}C{=}O$
$HOCH$
$HOCH$
$HOCH$
$CH_2OPO_3H_2$

$\xrightarrow{\text{TPP. Mg}^{2+}}$

D-Sedoheptulose-7-phosphate:
CH_2OH
$C=O$
$HOCH$
$HCOH$
$HCOH$
$HCOH$
$CH_2OPO_3H_2$

$+$

D-Glyceraldehyde-3-phosphate:
$H{-}C{=}O$
$HOCH$
$CH_2OPO_3H_2$

D-Xylulose-5-phosphate:
CH_2OH
$C=O$
$HOCH$
$HCOH$
$CH_2OPO_3H_2$

$+$

D-Erythrose-4-phosphate:
$H{-}C{=}O$
$HCOH$
$HCOH$
$CH_2OPO_3H_2$

$\xrightarrow{\text{TPP. Mg}^{2+}}$

D-Fructose-6-phosphate:
CH_2OH
$C=O$
$HOCH$
$HCOH$
$HCOH$
$CH_2OPO_3H_2$

$+$

D-Glyceraldehyde-3-phosphate:
$H{-}C{=}O$
$HCOH$
$CH_2OPO_3H_2$

Fig. 11.6 Two transketolation reactions in the pentose phosphate pathway.

erythrose-4-phosphate to form fructose-6-phosphate and glyceraldehyde-3-phosphate.

11.6　Neurophysiological functions

Background information can be found in Sections 3.7.2 and 3.7.3.

11.6.1　Introduction

There is increasing evidence that vitamin B_1, specifically thiamin triphosphate, is somehow involved in nerve membrane function. This property appears to be independent of the known coenzyme role of TPP. The evidence is substantiated by the finding that thiamin triphosphate, which accounts for 1% of total thiamin in rat brain, makes up 90% of total thiamin in the electric organ of the electric eel (Bettendorff *et al.*, 1987). In the lamb, vitamin B_1 deprivation for 4 weeks led to a 20% depletion of total thiamin in the brain, with a similar percentage loss of free thiamin, thiamin monophosphate and TPP. There was, however, no appreciable fall in thiamin triphosphate (Thornber *et al.*, 1980).

Most of the vitamin B_1 present in the brain and peripheral nerves is in the coenzyme form, TPP. The 1% or so of thiamin triphosphate present in whole brain is largely concentrated in the membrane fraction (Matsuda & Cooper, 1981). Fluorescence microscopy shows that the vitamin is localized in the membranes of peripheral nerves rather than in the axoplasm (Tanaka & Cooper, 1968). A complete set of enzymes catalysing the interconversion of thiamin and its phosphate esters has been isolated and purified from nervous tissue (Fox & Duppel, 1975).

As discussed in the following, vitamin B_1 may play a direct role in nerve conduction or it may be implicated in nerve transmission.

11.6.2　Nerve conduction

When Eichenbaum & Cooper (1971) UV-irradiated electrically stimulated vagus nerves dissected from a rabbit, action potentials were completely abolished after 2 hours and never spontaneously reappeared when the irradiated nerve was immersed in physiological solution. The irradiation almost completely destroyed endogenous thiamin in the nerve, as expected. Immersion of the irradiated nerve in physiological solution containing 1 mM thiamin restored the action potentials after about 1 hour. Thiamin is known to be rapidly taken up by the vagus nerve, so the delay may be explained by the two enzymatic steps required to convert thiamin to its triphosphate ester.

Sasa *et al.* (1976) studied the effects of thiamin, thiamin triphosphate and pyrithiamin on the excitability of the perfused giant axon of the crayfish. A stimulating current was delivered to the axon every 2 s. The following treatments were performed sequentially. Addition of thiamin to the perfusate produced an increase in the rising rate (dV/dt) of the action potential as early as 5 min; there was no accompanying effect on either the resting membrane potential or the threshold potential. Perfusing the axon with physiological solution restored dV/dt to control rates in 40 min. Addition of pyrithiamin elicited a decrease of dV/dt and prolongation of the duration of the action potential in 60 to 90 min; again the resting membrane potential and threshold potential were unaffected. Perfusing with physiological solution did not restore the action potential within 30 min, but addition of thiamin did so in 30 min. Addition of thiamin triphosphate produced a similar effect to thiamin. The additional finding that protein-binding thiamin was reduced in axons treated with pyrithiamin indicates a replacement of thiamin located in the membrane. Since dV/dt of the action potential reflects the sodium conductance, the finding that thiamin and thiamin triphosphate increased dV/dt could be construed as an increase in sodium conductance. Conversely, the finding that pyrithiamin decreased dV/dt could mean an impairment of sodium conductance. It was inferred from these experiments that thiamin plays an essential role in the membrane excitability of the crayfish giant axon.

In a series of experiments summarized by Itokawa (1977), treatment of perfused spinal cords or sciatic nerves with a variety of neuroactive agents released free thiamin and thiamin monophosphate. The nerve preparations were obtained from either bullfrogs or rats made deficient in thiamin by dietary restriction and injected with radioactive thiamin. The neuroactive agents also released free thiamin and thiamin monophosphate from the membrane-myelin fraction obtained from homogenized rat brain, spinal cord and sciatic nerves. As the bulk of thiamin in the membrane fraction consisted of TPP and thiamin triphosphate, the release phenomenon presumably involved dephosphorylation. One of the neuroactive agents, tetrodotoxin, acts as a nerve poison by inhibiting the early inward current of sodium. Itokawa (1976) postulated that the propagation of an action

potential involves the shift of TPP or thiamin triphosphate through dephosphorylation from a specific site in the sodium channel to allow the early inward current of sodium. Tetrodotoxin, by displacing these phosphate esters, would occupy the site and prevent the flow of current.

Goldberg *et al.* (1975), using voltage-clamped squid giant axons, showed that the magnitudes of both sodium and potassium conductance were decreased by treatment with thiamin antimetabolites. However, there was no appreciable change in the kinetics of the conductance changes, hinting that the mechanism of ion channel operation was unaffected. Most probably, the antimetabolites prevented the operation of a certain percentage of channels: those channels that remained open during perfusion with the antimetabolites functioned normally.

Fox & Duppel (1975) showed that B$_1$ vitamers (thiamin triphosphate > TPP thiamin) applied internally to the cut internodes of frog sciatic nerve preparations prevented the exponential decline of sodium and potassium currents in the node of Ranvier. Neither thiamin triphosphate nor TPP was active when applied to the node externally. Tetrodotoxin did not alter this property of the thiamin compounds, implying that the tetrodotoxin-induced release of thiamin from nerve membranes (shown by other investigators) is not related to the mechanism by which tetrodotoxin blocks the sodium channels. Fox and Duppel reasoned that the thiamin dephosphorylation and rephosphorylation process is probably not directly coupled to the excitation process. They suggested that the thiamin phosphates control the number of functioning voltage-gated ion channels by stabilizing the density of negative surface charges at the inner side of the nerve membrane.

Further evidence for a role of thiamin triphosphate as a membrane electrical field stabilizer was provided by Bettendorff *et al.* (1990). These authors reported that thiamin triphosphate (1 μM) increased the uptake of radioactive chloride (^{36}Cl$^-$) by rat brain membrane vesicles, while TPP, thiamin monophosphate and thiamin had no significant effect. The opening of chloride channels to allow an influx of negatively charged chloride ions into the postsynaptic neuron contributes to neuronal inhibition. Thus, if thiamin triphosphate controls the opening of chloride channels, it could act as a membrane stabilizer.

11.6.3   Nerve transmission

One of the characteristics of thiamin-deficiency encephalopathy is its predilection for specific brain structures with sparing of neighbouring ones. This selective vulnerability of certain brain regions to thiamin deficiency has been suggested to have a metabolic basis.

Butterworth (1982) reviewed evidence that the neurological signs of thiamin deficiency may involve a defect in synaptic transmission. Changes in the concentration or metabolism of catecholamines (noradrenaline and adrenaline), serotonin (5-hydroxytryptamine), γ-aminobutyric acid (GABA) and acetylcholine were reported in certain regions of the brain of pyrithiamin-treated animals. In addition to these recognized neurotransmitters, changes were also observed in the dicarboxylic amino acids glutamic acid and aspartic acid. These amino acids act like neurotransmitters in that they open sodium and potassium ionic channels and cause a rapid, powerful, excitatory response.

The synthesis of GABA, acetylcholine, glutamic acid and aspartic acid is directly associated with the metabolism of glucose in the brain. There is evidence to suggest that a decreased activity of TPP-dependent pyruvate and α-ketoglutarate dehydrogenases and transketolase due to vitamin B_1 deficiency may be ultimately responsible for a block in the synthesis of one or more of these neurotransmitters.

11.6.4   Subacute necrotizing encephalomyelopathy

Subacute necrotizing encephalomyelopathy (Leigh's disease) is a rare recessively inherited degenerative disease of the central nervous system which generally becomes symptomatic in the first year of life and is fatal. Diagnosis is complicated by the wide variety of symptoms, which include swallowing difficulties, abnormal respiration, ataxia, ophthalmoplegia, hypotonia, convulsions and progressive mental deterioration. The neuropathology at autopsy shows characteristic lesions of the brain stem and spinal cord, notable features being capillary infiltration and demyelination of axons. Dietary vitamin B_1 deficiency is not a factor in the aetiology of Leigh's disease. Early reports describing encouraging responses to large

doses of thiamin or thiamin derivatives have not been borne out by further experience (Blass, 1981).

Infants with Leigh's disease exhibit a deficiency of thiamin triphosphate in the brain. A substance, possibly a lipoprotein, that inhibits the synthesis of thiamin triphosphate from TPP via the thiamin pyrophosphate-ATP phosphotransferase has been detected in the blood, urine and cerebrospinal fluid of these patients (Cooper & Pincus, 1979). This substance only inhibits the brain enzyme; the phosphotransferase that catalyses the formation of thiamin triphosphate in the liver is unaffected. Leigh's disease appears therefore to be the result of disordered brain metabolism, possibly caused by the genetic lack of some enzyme. The resultant deficiency of thiamin triphosphate explains the neurological symptoms and neuropathological changes.

11.7   Vitamin B_1 deficiency

11.7.1   Causes and effects

A deficiency of vitamin B_1 may occur in situations of poor diet, chronic alcoholism, excessive diarrhoea or vomiting, malabsorption and genetic metabolic defects. Overloading the tissues with glucose without adequate thiamin coverage can precipitate deficiency, as can the use of diuretics. Diseases in which the metabolic rate is elevated (e.g. hyperthyroidism) can also lead to deficiency. Some researchers have demonstrated that secondary deficiency of a particular B-group vitamin can be induced by excessive dosing with another vitamin of this group. On the other hand, deficiencies in vitamins B_6 and B_{12} induced vitamin B_1 deficiency in rats, even when dietary thiamin levels were normal (Nishino & Itokawa, 1977). Howard et al. (1974) confirmed that folate deficiency in rats impairs thiamin absorption.

In humans, a lack of vitamin B_1 has widespread effects, causing anorexia and associated weight loss, gastrointestinal disturbances, peripheral and central neuropathy, muscle weakness, and cardiovascular irregularities. With severe vitamin B_1 deprivation, mental changes develop such as loss of emotional control, paranoid trends, manic or depressive episodes and confusion. The classic disease resulting from a gross deficiency of vitamin B_1 in humans is beriberi, which is prevalent in Far Eastern populations where polished rice is the staple diet. Not only is this diet deficient in vitamin B₁, but the high carbohydrate intake increases the requirement for the vitamin, and the consumption of antithiamin factors will exacerbate the deficiency. In other parts of the world where such a diet is not consumed, chronic alcoholism gives rise to the Wernicke–Korsakoff syndrome, a form of beriberi that affects the brain. Subclinical vitamin B₁ deficiencies are characterized by mental disturbances, fatigue, and loss of weight resulting from anorexia and digestive problems.

Note: The term 'polyneuritis' applies to the involvement of the peripheral nervous system only, while the symptoms of central nervous system dysfunction are more appropriately called 'encephalopathy' (Dreyfus, 1976).

11.7.2 *Metabolic consequences of vitamin B₁ deficiency*

Proper functioning of the nervous and cardiovascular systems relies upon normal carbohydrate metabolism, and this in turn depends upon a dietary supply of vitamin B₁ for conversion to TPP. The pyruvate dehydrogenase complex and α-ketoglutarate dehydrogenase, which require TPP as a coenzyme, are important in the main energy-yielding pathway of carbohydrate metabolism, the tricarboxylic acid cycle. The activities of these enzymes are decreased in selective regions of the brain that are reversibly damaged as a result of vitamin B₁ deprivation (Butterworth *et al.*, 1985, 1986). The decreased enzyme activities are due not only to a decrease in the level of coenzyme, but also of apoenzyme. It is logical to suppose that impairment of these dehydrogenases due to vitamin B₁ deficiency will lead to loss of energy production in the form of ATP. Actually, this does not happen – at least not in the brain. The brain finds alternative metabolic pathways to bypass the TPP-dependent steps, thereby maintaining and even increasing energy production. One possible pathway is the GABA shunt, which bypasses α-ketoglutarate dehydrogenase (Page *et al.*, 1989) (Fig. 11.7). Thus energy deprivation is not believed to be the direct cause of brain lesions resulting from vitamin B₁ deficiency, although the compensatory metabolic changes necessary for maintaining energy may affect biosynthetic processes.

Preventing the synthesis of acetylcholine through lack of conversion of pyruvate to acetyl-CoA will impair nerve impulse transmission at synapses, and blocking the pentose phosphate pathway through impaired transketolase activity will lead to a reduced synthesis of DNA through lack of ribose. Dreyfus & Hauser (1965) showed that transketolase is more severely affected by vitamin B₁ deficiency than is pyruvate dehydrogenase, and the reduction of transketolase activity is anatomically correlated to brain lesions.

11.7.3 *Experimental vitamin B₁ deficiency*

Rat studies

When rats are given a vitamin B₁-deficient diet, they show abnormalities of posture and equilibrium after several weeks. These neurological signs can be

Fig. 11.7 The GABA shunt and tricarboxylic acid cycle. α-Ketoglutarate is aminated to glutamate, which is decarboxylated to GABA. GABA is inactivated by transamination to succinic semi-aldehyde, which is oxidized to succinate, an intermediate in the tricarboxylic acid cycle. Enzymes: (1) α-Ketoglutarate dehydrogenase, (2) GABA aminotransferase and other aminotransferases, (3) glutamate decarboxylase, (4) succinic semi-aldehyde dehydrogenase. Reproduced with permission of the Nutrition Society from Page *et al.* (1989), *British Journal of Nutrition*, Vol. 62, pp. 245–53.

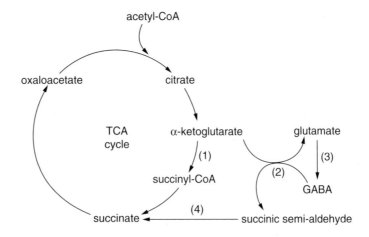

promptly reversed by the administration of 5–10 µg of thiamin. If no more thiamin is given, severe signs reappear in 3–6 days. Pathological examination of the nervous systems of rats which experienced several bouts of deficiency disclosed anatomical lesions of certain parts of the brain. The lesions consisted of areas of tissue destruction and a marked proliferation of glial cells. Within the centre of lesions all medullated nerve fibres were destroyed (Dreyfus & Victor, 1961). Experimental vitamin B_1 deficiency is produced more rapidly (12–16 days) and more effectively by the use of pyrithiamin, a direct antagonist of TPP that also crosses the blood–brain barrier.

When [^{14}C]glutamate was injected into the brains of vitamin B_1-deficient rats, the specific radioactivity of GABA in the brains rose by 45–50%, suggesting a considerable increase in GABA shunt activity (Page et al., 1989). This increase in brain GABA level may explain the anorexia observed in vitamin B_1-deficient rats. GABA aminotransferase, the enzyme principally responsible for GABA catabolism, is selectively inhibited by 1-(n-decyl)-3-pyrazolidinone. When this inhibitor was administered to rats, brain GABA levels were increased three-fold and anorexia was observed in the absence of other symptoms (White et al., 1982). This finding is consistent with speculations that GABA is implicated in appetite-controlling mechanisms (Kimura & Kuriyama, 1975).

Human studies

The combined results from several human studies have shown that inducement of vitamin B_1 deficiency in adults produces a wide range of disorders involving the gastrointestinal tract, central and peripheral nervous systems, and cardiovascular system. Anorexia is a constant finding. Indigestion results from hypochlorhydria. Gastric atony results in severe constipation through lack of gut motility. Thus, when a barium meal is given, there is incomplete emptying of the stomach and pooling of the barium in segments of the small intestine, producing the so-called stepladder pattern. Changes in mood are an outstanding finding. There are paresthesias with a stocking or glove type distribution, and impairment in perception of light, touch, pin prick, temperature and vibratory sensation. Subjects experience difficulty in rising from a squatting position owing to weakness of the calf muscles. The deep tendon reflexes (patella and Achilles) disappear after a while. Electrocardiograms show

irregularities, and subjects complain of shortness of breath, consciousness of the heartbeat, irregularities in heart rhythm and discomfort in the chest after exertion.

Biochemical changes include increased concentrations of pyruvate and lactate in the blood, particularly after exercise or the administration of glucose. Severe lactic acidosis can be life-threatening.

11.7.4 Beriberi

The development of beriberi, its symptoms and its pathology are extremely variable, making it difficult to describe a clinical picture or sequence of development. Many of the early writers described three forms of beriberi in adult humans: dry (wasting) and wet (oedematous) beriberi, which are chronic forms, and acute, fulminating (cardiac) beriberi. Which of these forms predominates depends on the circumstances. Vitamin B_1 deprivation accompanied by malnutrition and low physical activity tends to favour beriberi presenting in the dry form, whereas high carbohydrate intake and high physical activity during vitamin B_1 deprivation predispose to wet beriberi. It should be emphasized that any one of these forms may merge into another.

Dry beriberi is a disease of the peripheral nervous system involving bilateral impairment of sensory, motor and reflex functions. The pathological findings are segmental thinning of myelin in peripheral nerves, progressing to degeneration of fibre tracts. The neuropathy begins in the feet and legs and then extends up the body. Early signs of dry beriberi often include sensations of pins and needles and numbness in the feet. The legs, especially the calves, feel heavy and weak so that walking becomes uncomfortable. As the disease progresses, there is a marked wasting of the leg muscles and even slight pressure applied to the calves elicits severe pain. The characteristic foot and wrist drop develop and there may be complete flaccid paralysis of the lower, and occasionally upper, extremities.

In wet beriberi, vitamin B_1 deficiency affects the cardiovascular system by causing arteriolar dilation throughout the circulatory system and by weakening the heart muscle. The vasodilation causes a two-fold increase in the venous return of blood to the heart. Physical signs of wet beriberi are indicative of high-output cardiac failure; they include tachycardia, rapid circulation time, elevated peripheral venous pressure and widespread oedema. Pathological changes are an enlarged heart, swollen liver, and the presence of fluid in the pericardial, pleural and abdominal cavities. Microscopically, the cardiac muscle fibres show fragmentation and hydropic degeneration with interstitial oedema.

The acute form of beriberi, known in Japan as 'shoshin', usually results in sudden death from heart failure. The sufferer experiences severe dyspnoea, violent palpitation of the heart and intense precordial pain. The heart and liver become enlarged and there is neck vein distension, cyanosis and extreme tachycardia. Oedema is variable in this form of beriberi.

Infantile beriberi occurs in breast-fed babies between the second and fifth month of life. The mother may display no signs of beriberi although obviously her milk must be of low vitamin B$_1$ content through poor diet. As in adults, several clinical syndromes may occur and the condition may be chronic or acute. Vomiting is one of the most important early signs of infantile beriberi. In severe cases the child appears to be crying but no sound is heard or only a thin whine. This characteristic feature, aphonia, is due either to paralysis of the laryngeal nerve or to oedema of the vocal cords. A chronic, pseudomeningeal form of beriberi which affects the central nervous system and may cause convulsions occurs in older infants aged 7 to 9 months.

11.7.5 Wernicke–Korsakoff syndrome

The Wernicke–Korsakoff syndrome is a vitamin B$_1$ deficiency disease particularly associated with chronic alcoholics who derive more than half their daily calories from ethanol every day. Binge drinkers who eat normally between bouts and who are in a reasonable state of health are not prone to the disease. Alcoholic beverages contain water, ethanol, variable amounts of carbohydrate, and little else of nutritive value. Apart from beers, protein and vitamin content of these beverages is extremely low. Vitamin B$_1$ deficiency in the alcoholic is a combination of several factors. The main factor is reduced food intake due to depressed consciousness during inebriation and hangover. Suppression of appetite by alcohol has been postulated, but not studied much. Gastritis and diarrhoea caused by alcohol will impair digestion and absorption, and alcoholic pancreatitis results in decreased secretion of

digestive enzymes. Impairment of thiamin absorption has been reported in severely alcoholic patients (Tomasulo *et al.*, 1968). In cases of alcoholic cirrhosis of the liver, there may be a decreased conversion of thiamin to TPP and a decreased capacity of the liver to store vitamin B$_1$ (Leevy & Baker, 1968). The mortality of the Wernicke–Korsakoff syndrome is 90% without therapy, heart failure being the usual cause of death.

The Wernicke–Korsakoff syndrome has two components, Wernicke's encephalopathy (or Wernicke's disease) and Korsakoff's psychosis. The former is specific to vitamin B$_1$ deficiency, whereas the latter may be seen in association with other disorders of the nervous system.

Wernicke's disease is characterized by a triad of clinical signs: eye abnormalities, incoordination and altered state of consciousness. They occur simultaneously, or one may precede the other by days or weeks. The eye signs are caused by paralysis of one or more of the eye muscles (ophthalmoplegia). Typical signs are photophobia, nystagmus (oscillation of the eyeballs), strabismus (crossed eyes) and diplopia (double vision). In advanced cases, there may be complete loss of eye movement and the pupils may become non-reactive. The disorder of coordination is seen as a broad-based stance and ataxia (staggering gait). Common mental signs are listlessness, inattentiveness, apathy and confusion. There is sometimes delirium and, in extreme cases, stupor and coma.

Following the administration of thiamin, the symptoms of Wernicke's disease are alleviated and the features of Korsakoff's psychosis become evident. The most notable features are a form of amnesia in which events of ordinary daily life are forgotten as quickly as they occur but events in the distant past are well remembered. The patient is alert and can converse, think and solve problems, but is unable to memorize new information. The symptom of confabulation (story-telling) is an attempt by the patient to hide the amnesia.

Neuropathological changes are seen as brain lesions distributed in a bilaterally symmetrical fashion in the mammillary bodies, superior vermis of the cerebellum, hypothalamic nuclei and other diencephalic structures (Reuler *et al.*, 1985). Histology shows necrosis of neurons and glial cells. There is also capillary damage with endothelial proliferation and pin-point haemorrhages. Damage to specific regions of the brain can account for the clinical features of

Wernicke–Korsakoff syndrome. Thus, for example, the nystagmus is due to damage of the sixth cranial nerve; the ataxia is related to loss of neurons in the superior vermis of the cerebellum; and the amnesia is associated with atrophy of the mammillary bodies.

Although the Wernicke–Korsakoff syndrome results from a lack of dietary vitamin B_1, two clinical observations suggest that genetic factors are important in its pathogenesis: it develops in only a small majority of alcoholics and other chronically malnourished persons, and it occurs much more frequently among Europeans than among Asians. The possibility of a genetic effect was investigated by Blass & Gibson (1977) who found that transketolase in tissue-cultured cells from patients with Wernicke–Korsakoff syndrome was abnormal in that the binding of TPP to the apoenzyme was diminished. The abnormality persisted through more than 20 generations of culture in medium containing excess thiamin and no ethanol, and therefore appeared to be genetic rather than dietary. Thus the abnormal enzyme appears to be a structural mutant. Persistent aberrations had previously been found in erythrocyte transketolase from these patients, even after they had been treated with thiamin for months while in hospital. The abnormality appeared to be specific for transketolase as pyruvate dehydrogenase and α-ketoglutarate dehydrogenase were unaffected.

Because the symptoms of Wernicke's disease can be alleviated following the administration of thiamin, the abnormal transketolase is presumably clinically unimportant if the diet is adequate. This type of genetic abnormality is an example of an inborn predisposition to metabolic disorders. Unlike inborn errors of metabolism, inborn predispositions are likely to be clinically silent unless the person with the predisposition faces an appropriate stress. In cases of Wernicke–Korsakoff syndrome, the stress is a deficiency of vitamin B_1. Nixon et al. (1984) demonstrated a highly significant association between a particular variant of erythrocyte transketolase and the Wernicke–Korsakoff syndrome, supporting the concept that the syndrome has a genetic as well as a dietary origin.

11.7.6 Treatment of beriberi

Beriberi is treated with a proprietary thiamin preparation, the dosage and route depending on the patient's condition. To prevent further recurrences, a good diet containing all of the B-group vitamins should be instituted. Severe cardiac (shoshin) beriberi and Wernicke–Korsakoff syndrome constitute medical emergencies requiring immediate treatment with thiamin, given intravenously. Treatment of Wernicke–Korsakoff syndrome will eradicate the symptoms of encephalopathy (with abstinence of alcohol), but the psychosis is irreversible.

11.8 Nutritional aspects

11.8.1 Human requirement

Because TPP is essential as a coenzyme for the release of energy from carbohydrates, the requirement for vitamin B_1 varies with the proportion of carbohydrate in the diet. The requirement is also increased under conditions that elevate the metabolic rate, e.g. during high muscular activity, pregnancy and lactation, and also during protracted fever and hyperthyroidism. In practice, the requirement for vitamin B_1 is expressed in terms of total caloric intake.

11.8.2 Effects of high intake

Thiamin is non-toxic by the oral route because excess amounts of ingested thiamin are rapidly excreted in the urine. Large parenteral doses of thiamin administered over a long period have been reported to produce clinical manifestations and, in some cases, even death (Cumming et al., 1981).

11.8.3 Assessment of nutritional status

The most commonly used procedure for assessing vitamin B_1 nutritional status in humans has been the measurement of erythrocyte transketolase activity (ETKA) and its stimulation in vitro by the addition of TPP (TPP effect) (Sauberlich, 1984). The TPP effect reflects a decrease in dietary intake of vitamin B_1 before any other signs of vitamin B_1 inadequacy are detectable. It is calculated as the difference between basal and stimulation values expressed as a percentage of the basal value. As vitamin B_1 deficiency progresses, ETKA becomes lower and the TPP effect increases. A TPP effect >20% indicates vitamin B_1 deficiency, 15–20% indicates marginal deficiency, and <15% indicates sufficiency. However, in chronic deficiency, the TPP added in vitro cannot restore ETKA fully; under such conditions, the TPP effect may be in the normal range of 0–15%. Thus both ETKA and the TPP effect must be considered in assessing the adequacy of vitamin B$_1$ status (Tanphaichitr, 1999).

Further reading

Goldsmith, G. A. (1975) Vitamin B complex. Thiamine, riboflavin, niacin, folic acid (folacin), vitamin B$_{12}$, biotin. *Progress in Food & Nutrition Science*, **1**, 559–609.
Sauberlich, H. E. (1967) Biochemical alterations in thiamine deficiency – their interpretation. *American Journal of Clinical Nutrition*, **20**, 528–42.

References

Bender, D. A. & Bender, A. E. (1997) *Nutrition. A Reference Handbook*. Oxford University Press, Oxford.
Bettendorff, L., Michel-Cahay, C., Grandfils, C., De Rycker, C. & Schoffeniels, E. (1987) Thiamine triphosphate and membrane-associated thiamine triphosphatases in the electric organ of *Electrophorus electricus*. *Journal of Neurochemistry*, **49**, 495–502.
Bettendorff, L., Wins, P. & Schoffeniels, E. (1990) Regulation of ion uptake in membrane vesicles from rat brain by thiamine compounds. *Biochemical and Biophysical Research Communications*, **171**, 1137–44.
Blass, J. P. (1981) Thiamin and the Wernicke–Korsakoff syndrome. In: *Vitamins in Human Biology and Medicine*. (Ed. M. H. Briggs), pp. 107–35. CRC Press, Inc., Boca Raton, Florida.
Blass, J. P. & Gibson, G. E. (1977) Abnormality of a thiamine-requiring enzyme in patients with Wernicke–Korsakoff syndrome. *New England Journal of Medicine*, **297**, 1367–70.
Butterworth, R. F. (1982) Neurotransmitter function in thiamine-deficiency encephalopathy. *Neurochemistry International*, **4**, 449–64.
Butterworth, R. F., Giguère, J.-F. & Besnard, A.-M. (1985) Activities of thiamine-dependent enzymes in two experimental models of thiamine-deficiency encephalopathy. 1. The pyruvate dehydrogenase complex. *Neurochemical Research*, **10**, 1417–28.
Butterworth, R. F., Giguère, J.-F. & Besnard, A.-M. (1986) Activities of thiamine-dependent enzymes in two experimental models of thiamine-deficiency encephalopathy. 2. α-Ketoglutarate dehydrogenase. *Neurochemical Research*, **11**, 567–77.
Cooper, J. R. & Pincus, J. H. (1979) The role of thiamine in nervous tissue. *Neurochemical Research*, **4**, 223–39.
Cumming, F., Briggs, M. & Briggs, M. (1981) Clinical toxicology of vitamin supplements. In *Vitamins in Human Biology and Medicine*. (Ed. M. H. Briggs), pp. 187–243. CRC Press, Inc., Boca Raton, Florida.
Davis, R. E., Icke, G. C., Thom, J. & Riley, W. J. (1984) Intestinal absorption of thiamin in man compared with folate and pyridoxal and its subsequent urinary excretion. *Journal of Nutritional Science and Vitaminology*, **30**, 475–82.
Dreyfus, P. M. (1976) Thiamine and the nervous system: an overview. *Journal of Nutritional Science and Vitaminology*, **22** (Suppl.), 13–16.
Dreyfus, P. M. & Hauser, G. (1965) The effect of thiamine deficiency on the pyruvate decarboxylase system of the central nervous system. *Biochimica et Biophysica Acta*, **104**, 7–84.
Dreyfus, P. M. & Victor, M. (1961) Effects of thiamine deficiency on the central nervous system. *American Journal of Clinical Nutrition*, **9**, 414–25.
Dutta, B., Huang, W., Molero, M., Kekuda, R., Leibach, F. H., Devoe, L. D., Ganapathy, V. & Prasad, P. D. (1999) Cloning of the human thiamine transporter, a member of the folate transporter family. *Journal of Biological Chemistry*, **274**(45), 31 925–9.
Egi, Y., Koyama, S., Shikata, H., Yamada, K. & Kawasaki, T. (1986) Content of thiamin phosphate esters in mammalian tissues – an extremely high concentration of thiamin triphosphate in pig skeletal muscle. *Biochemistry International*, **12**, 385–90.
Eichenbaum, J. W. & Cooper, J. R. (1971) Restoration by thiamine of the action potential in ultraviolet irradiated nerves. *Brain Research*, **32**, 258–60.
Elsas, L. J. II & Acosta, P. B. (1999) Nutritional support of inherited metabolic disease. In: *Modern Nutrition in Health and Disease*, 9th edn. (Ed. M. E. Shils, J. A. Olson, M. Shike & A. C. Ross), pp. 1003–56. Lippincott Williams & Wilkins, Philadelphia.
Fox, J. M. & Duppel, W. (1975) The action of thiamine and its di- and triphosphates on the slow exponential decline of the ionic currents in the node of Ranvier. *Brain Research*, **89**, 287–302.
Goldberg, D. J., Begenisich, T. B. & Cooper, J. R. (1975) Effects of thiamine antagonists on nerve conduction. II. Voltage clamp experiments with antimetabolites. *Journal of Neurobiology*, **6**, 453–62.
Grassl, S. M. (1998) Thiamine transport in human placental brush border membrane vesicles. *Biochimica et Biophysica Acta*, **1371**, 213–22.
Greenwood, J., Love, E. R. & Pratt, O. E. (1982) Kinetics of thiamine transport across the blood–brain barrier in the rat. *Journal of Physiology*, **327**, 95–103.
Hilker, D. M. & Somogyi, J. C. (1982) Antithiamins of plant origin: their chemical nature and mode of action. *Annals of the New York Academy of Sciences*, **378**, 137–45.
Howard, L., Wagner, C. & Schenker, S. (1974) Malabsorption of thiamin in folate-deficient rats. *Journal of Nutrition*, **104**, 1024–32.
Hoyumpa, A. M. (1986) Mechanisms of vitamin deficiencies in alcoholism. *Alcoholism: Clinical and Experimental Research*, **10**, 573–81.
Itokawa, Y. (1976) Thiamine and nerve membrane. *Journal of Nutritional Science and Vitaminology*, **22** (Suppl.), 17–19.
Itokawa, Y. (1977) Thiamine (vitamin B$_1$) and diseases related to vitamin B$_1$ deficiencies. *Journal of Applied Nutrition*, **29**, 5–16.
Kasper, H. (1970) Vitamin absorption in the colon. *American Journal of Proctology*, **21**, 341–5.
Kimura, H. & Kuriyama, K. (1975) Distribution of gamma-aminobutyric acid (GABA) in the rat hypothalamus: functional correlates of GABA with activities of appetite controlling mechanisms. *Journal of Neurochemistry*, **24**, 903–7.
Kositawattanakul, T., Tosukhowong, P., Vimokesant, S. L. & Panijpan, B. (1977) Chemical interactions between thiamin and tannic acid. II. Separation of products. *American Journal of Clinical Nutrition*, **30**, 1686–91.
Laforenza, U., Gastaldi, G. & Rindi, G. (1993) Thiamine outflow from the enterocyte: a study using basolateral membrane vesicles from rat small intestine. *Journal of Physiology*, **468**, 401–12.
Laforenza, U., Patrini, C., Alvisi, C., Faelli, A., Licandro, A. & Rindi, G. (1997) Thiamine uptake in human intestinal biopsy specimens, including observations from a patient with acute thiamine deficiency. *American Journal of Clinical Nutrition*, **66**, 320–6.
Laforenza, U., Orsenigo, M. N., & Rindi, G. (1998) A thiamine/H$^+$ antiport mechanism for thiamine entry into brush border membrane vesicles from rat small intestine. *Journal of Membrane Biology*, **161**, 151–61.

Leevy, C. H. & Baker, H. (1968) Vitamins and alcoholism. Introduction. *American Journal of Clinical Nutrition*, **21**, 1325–8.

Matsuda, T. & Cooper, J. R. (1981) The separation and determination of thiamin and its phosphate esters in brain. *Analytical Biochemistry*, **117**, 203–7.

Miyoshi, K., Egi, Y., Shioda, T. & Kawasaki, T. (1990) Evidence for *in vivo* synthesis of thiamin triphosphate by cytosolic adenylate kinase in chicken skeletal muscle. *Journal of Biochemistry*, **108**, 267–70.

Moseley, R. H., Vashi, P. G., Jarose, S. M., Dickinson, C. J. & Permoad, P. A. (1992) Thiamine transport by basolateral rat liver plasma membrane vesicles. *Gastroenterology*, **103**, 1056–65.

Murata, K. (1982) Actions of two types of thiaminases on thiamin and its analogues. *Annals of the New York Academy of Sciences*, **378**, 146–56.

Nishino, K. & Itokawa, Y. (1977) Thiamin metabolism in vitamin B_6 or vitamin B_{12} deficient rats. *Journal of Nutrition*, **107**, 775–82.

Nixon, P. F., Kaczmarek, M. J., Tate, J., Kerr, R. A. & Price, J. (1984) An erythrocyte transketolase isoenzyme pattern associated with the Wernicke–Korsakoff syndrome. *European Journal of Clinical Investigation*, **14**, 278–81.

Page, M. G., Ankoma-Sey, V., Coulson, W. F. & Bender, D. A. (1989) Brain glutamate and γ-aminobutyrate (GABA) metabolism in thiamin-deficient rats. *British Journal of Nutrition*, **62**, 245–53.

Patrini, C., Cusaro, G., Ferrari, G. & Rindi, G. (1981) Thiamine transport by rat small intestine 'in vitro': influence of endogenous thiamine content of jejunal tissue. *Acta Vitaminologica et Enzymologica*, **3** n.s., 17–26.

Patrini, C., Reggiani, C., Laforenza, U. & Rindi, G. (1988) Blood–brain transport of thiamine monophosphate in the rat: a kinetic study in vivo. *Journal of Neurochemistry*, **50**, 90–3.

Reggiani, C., Patrini, C. & Rindi, G. (1984) Nervous tissue thiamine metabolism in vivo. I. Transport of thiamine and thiamine monophosphate from plasma to different brain regions of the rat. *Brain Research*, **293**, 319–27.

Reuler, J. B., Girard, D. E. & Cooney, T. G. (1985) Wernicke's encephalopathy. *New England Journal of Medicine*, **312**, 1035–9.

Ricci, V. & Rindi, G. (1992) Thiamin uptake by rat isolated enterocytes: relationship between transport and phosphorylation. *Archives Internationales de Physiologie, de Biochimie et de Biophysique*, **100**, 275–9.

Rindi, G. (1984) Thiamin absorption by small intestine. *Acta Vitaminologica et Enzymologica*, **6**, 47–55.

Said, H. M., Ortiz, A., Kumar, C. K., Chatterjee, N., Dudeja, P. K. & Rubin, S. (1999) Transport of thiamine in human intestine: mechanism and regulation in intestinal epithelial cell model Caco-2. *American Journal of Physiology*, **277**, C645–51.

Sasa, M., Takemoto, I., Nishino, K. & Itokawa, Y. (1976) The role of thiamine on excitable membrane of crayfish giant axon. *Journal of Nutritional Science and Vitaminology*, **22** (Suppl.), 21–46.

Sauberlich, H. E. (1984) Newer laboratory methods for assessing nutriture of selected B-complex vitamins. *Annual Review of Nutrition*, **4**, 377–407.

Schenker, S., Johnson, R. F., Hoyumpa, A. M. & Henderson, G. I. (1990) Thiamine-transfer by human placenta: normal transport and effects of ethanol. *Journal of Laboratory and Clinical Medicine*, **116**, 106–15.

Sorrell, M. F., Frank, O., Thomson, A. D., Aquino, H. & Baker, H. (1971) Absorption of vitamins from the large intestine *in vivo*. *Nutrition Reports International*, **3**, 143–8.

Spector, R. (1976) Thiamine transport in the central nervous system. *American Journal of Physiology*, **230**, 1101–7.

Spector, R. (1982) Thiamin homeostasis in the central nervous system. *Annals of the New York Academy of Sciences*, **378**, 344–54.

Tanaka, C. & Cooper, J. R. (1968) The fluorescent microscopic localization of thiamine in nervous tissue. *Journal of Histochemistry and Cytochemistry*, **16**, 362–5.

Tanphaichitr, V. (1999) Thiamin. In: *Modern Nutrition in Health and Disease*, 9th edn. (Ed. M. E. Shils, J. A. Olson, M. Shike & A. C. Ross), pp. 381–9. Lippincott Williams & Wilkins, Philadelphia.

Thornber, E. J., Dunlop, R. H. & Gawthorne, J. M. (1980) Thiamin deficiency in the lamb: changes in thiamin phosphate esters in the brain. *Journal of Neurochemistry*, **35**, 713–17.

Tomasulo, P. A., Kater, R. M. H. & Iber, F. L. (1968) Impairment of thiamine absorption in alcoholism. *American Journal of Clinical Nutrition*, **21**, 1341–4.

Vimokesant, S., Kunjara, S., Rungruangsak, K., Nakornchai, S. & Panijpan, B. (1982) Beriberi caused by antithiamin factors in food and its prevention. *Annals of the New York Academy of Sciences*, **378**, 123–36.

White, H. L., Howard, J. L., Cooper, B. R., Soroko, F. E., McDermed, J. D., Ingold, K. J. & Maxwell, R. A. (1982) A novel inhibitor of gamma-aminobutyrate aminotransferase with anorectic activity. *Journal of Neurochemistry*, **39**, 271–3.

12
Flavins: Riboflavin, FMN and FAD (Vitamin B$_2$)

Key discussion topics

- Specialized membrane transport systems in the intestine and kidney ensure that ingested flavins are efficiently absorbed into the bloodstream and conserved within the body.
- Thyroid hormone regulates the conversion of riboflavin to its functional coenzyme forms, FMN and FAD.
- The production of an oestrogen-dependent riboflavin carrier protein throughout pregnancy ensures delivery of sufficient riboflavin to meet the metabolic demands of the developing fetus.
- Vitamin B$_2$ in its coenzyme forms, FMN and FAD, is involved in key metabolic reactions including carbohydrate, amino acid and lipid metabolism, and in the conversion of folic acid and pyridoxine into their coenzyme forms.

12.1 Historical overview

It became apparent during the 1920s that the polyneuritis preventive factor, which was later designated 'water-soluble B' and subsequently 'vitamin B', could prevent pellagra in humans as well as beriberi. This discovery led to the replacement of the term 'vitamin B' by the terms 'vitamin B$_1$' (the heat-labile, anti-neuritic factor) and 'vitamin B$_2$' (the heat-stable, pellagra-preventive factor). Vitamin B$_2$, present in yeast extracts, was needed to prevent human pellagra and an apparently similar canine disease called 'black tongue'. It was also required by rats to prevent a pellagra-like dermatitis and to promote growth. At that time vitamin B$_2$ was assumed to be a single substance, but it was later found that there are several vitamins present in this heat-stable fraction of yeast.

The presence of water-soluble, fluorescent, yellow pigments in natural materials had been known for some time. These pigments, known generically as flavins, were found in milk, liver, kidney, muscle, yeast and plant materials. They were given specific names according to their sources, e.g. lactoflavin (milk) and hepatoflavin (liver). In 1933, Kuhn, György and Wagner-Jauregg isolated from egg white a fluorescent, yellow, crystalline compound ('ovoflavin') which was a growth-promoting factor for rats. The isolation of other growth-promoting flavins followed. By 1934, Kuhn's group had determined the structures of these various flavins and found them to be chemically identical. Because each molecule contained a ribose-like (ribitol) side chain, the term 'riboflavin' was adopted. Thus riboflavin was the component responsible for the rat growth-promoting activity in the aforementioned vitamin B$_2$ complex. The pellagra-preventive factor and the rat anti-dermatitis factor subsequently became known as niacin and vitamin B$_6$, respectively.

Meanwhile, by 1932, Warburg and Christian had isolated from yeast an enzyme, which dissociated into a protein apoenzyme and a yellow prosthetic group that was chemically similar to a flavin. The yellow pigment isolated from this 'old yellow enzyme' was a vitamin-inactive, photo-derivative of a flavin (lumiflavin). Determination of this compound's structure proved useful to Kuhn for elucidating the structure of riboflavin. The synthesis of riboflavin was accomplished independently by Kuhn's group and Karrer's group in 1935. By 1938, Warburg and Christian had isolated and characterized flavin adenine dinucleotide (FAD) and shown it to be a coenzyme of D-amino acid oxidase. The structure of the simpler coenzyme, riboflavin 5′-phosphate (FMN), was secured in the previous year by Theorell.

12.2   Chemistry

The principal vitamin B$_2$-active flavins found in nature are riboflavin, riboflavin-5′-phosphate (flavin mononucleotide, FMN) and riboflavin-5′-adenosyldiphosphate (flavin adenine dinucleotide, FAD). The structures of these compounds are depicted in Fig. 12.1. The parent riboflavin molecule comprises a substituted isoalloxazine moiety with a ribitol side chain.

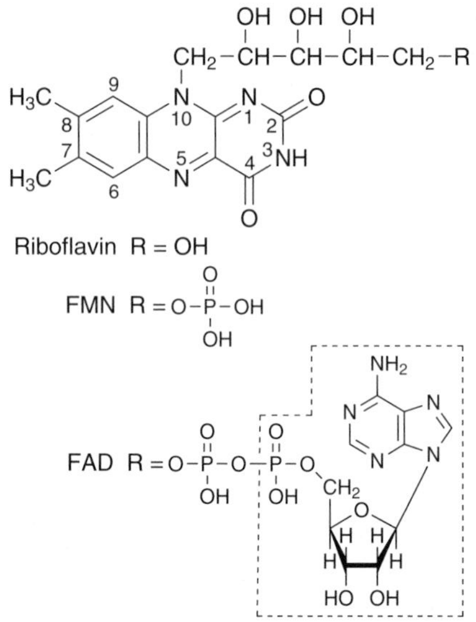

Fig. 12.1 Structures of riboflavin, FMN and FAD.

The 'mononucleotide' and 'dinucleotide' designations for FMN and FAD, respectively, are actually incorrect but are nevertheless still accepted. FMN is not a nucleotide, as the sugar group is not ribose, and the isoalloxazine ring is neither a purine nor a pyrimidine. FAD is composed of a nucleotide (adenosine monophosphate, AMP) and the so-called flavin pseudonucleotide.

In biological tissues, FAD and, to a lesser extent, FMN occur almost entirely as prosthetic groups for a large variety of flavin enzymes (flavoproteins). In most flavoproteins the flavins are bound tightly but noncovalently to the apoenzyme. In mammalian tissues less than 10% of the FAD is covalently attached to specific amino acid residues of four important apoenzymes. These are found within succinate and sarcosine dehydrogenases, monoamine oxidase and gulonolactone oxidase in which FAD is peptide-linked to an N-histidyl or S-cysteinyl residue via the 8-methyl group.

The term 'riboflavin' is confusing as it may be used in two different contexts. It is either synonymous with vitamin B$_2$ (a generic descriptor for all biologically active flavins) or it refers specifically to the parent riboflavin molecule described above. In this text, the names riboflavin, FMN and FAD will be used as specific terms and flavins or vitamin B$_2$ will be used as generic terms. Total riboflavin means the sum of riboflavin, FMN and FAD. There will be no further mention of the 'vitamin B₂' used historically to designate the pellagra-preventive factor.

12.3 Dietary sources and bioavailability

12.3.1 Dietary sources

Living cells require FMN and FAD as the prosthetic groups of a variety of enzymes, and hence the flavins are found, at least in small amounts, in all natural unprocessed foods. In most foods the predominant form of vitamin B₂ is protein-bound FAD. Yeast extract is exceptionally rich in vitamin B₂, and liver and kidney are also rich sources. Wheat bran, eggs, meat, milk and cheese are important sources in diets containing these foods. Cereal grains contain relatively low concentrations of flavins, but are important sources in those parts of the world where cereals constitute the staple diet. The milling of cereals results in considerable loss (up to 60%) of vitamin B₂, so white flour is enriched by addition of the vitamin. The enrichment of bread and breakfast cereals contributes significantly to the dietary supply of vitamin B₂. Polished rice is not usually enriched, since the yellow colour of the vitamin would make the rice visually unacceptable. However, most of the flavin content of the whole brown rice is retained if the rice is steamed prior to milling. This process drives the water-soluble vitamins in the germ and aleurone layers into the endosperm (Cooperman and Lopez, 1991).

12.3.2 Bioavailability

The bioavailability of vitamin B₂ appears to be related to the digestibility of the food, being generally high for meat and dairy products and lower for plant products. Bioavailability is impaired by the excessive consumption of alcohol, which appears to inhibit the intestinal FMN phosphatase and FAD pyrophosphatase necessary to release riboflavin for absorption (Pinto et al., 1984).

12.4 Absorption, transport and metabolism

Humans cannot synthesize vitamin B₂ and thus must obtain the vitamin from exogenous sources via intestinal absorption. The intestine is exposed to flavins from two sources: (1) the diet and (2) the bacterially synthesized flavins in the large intestine. Whether the latter source of vitamin B₂ is available to the host tissues (apart from the colonic epithelial cells) in nutritionally significant amounts is unknown.

12.4.1 Digestion and absorption of dietary vitamin B₂

The FMN and FAD present in the ingested food are released from noncovalent binding to flavoproteins as a consequence of acidification in the stomach and gastric and intestinal proteolysis. Riboflavin is similarly released from its association with binding proteins (Merrill et al., 1981).

The flavin coenzymes are hydrolysed in the upper small intestine to free riboflavin, which is then absorbed. Hydrolysis of both FMN and FAD is effected by alkaline phosphatase (EC 3.1.3.1), which has a broad specificity and is located on the brush-border membrane of the enterocyte (Daniel et al., 1983a). Two additional brush-border enzymes, FMN phosphatase and FAD pyrophosphatase, participate in the degradation of the flavin coenzymes (Akiyama et al., 1982). The considerably smaller amounts of covalently bound flavins are released as 8α-(peptidyl) riboflavins, which are absorbed along with the free riboflavin (Chia et al., 1978).

In vitro studies using rat everted jejunal sacs have shown that absorption of riboflavin takes place by a saturable, energy-dependent process at physiologically relevant concentrations and by simple diffusion at higher concentrations (Daniel et al., 1983b; Said et al., 1985; Middleton, 1990). This dual process of absorption has been confirmed under in vivo conditions (Feder et al., 1991). Casirola et al. (1994) showed that the ribitol side chain and the NH group at position 3 of the isoalloxazine moiety are essential for riboflavin binding to specific sites on the brush-border membrane of rat small intestine.

The absorption of riboflavin is efficient along the length of the small intestine (i.e. jejunum and ileum) in the guinea pig (Hegazy & Schwenk, 1983) and the rabbit (Said et al., 1993a). Absorption is enhanced by the presence of bile salts in the intestinal lumen (Mayersohn et al., 1969). A role of bile salts is also indicated by impaired absorption of riboflavin in cases of biliary obstruction in children (Jusko et al., 1971). Bile salts may increase the absorption of riboflavin in two ways. (1) The detergent action of bile salts enhances the solubility of riboflavin in the intestinal lumen and increases the permeability of the brush-border membrane to the vitamin. (2) Bile salts inhibit gastric emptying and proximal intestinal transit, resulting in an increased residence time of riboflavin at the absorption sites.

Transport of riboflavin across brush-border and basolateral membrane vesicles prepared from rabbit small intestine was found to be independent of sodium and electroneutral in nature (Said et al., 1993a,b). Using human-derived Caco-2 intestinal epithelial cells, Said & Ma (1994) confirmed the involvement of a carrier-mediated process in the initial phase of riboflavin uptake (a 3-min incubation time). Riboflavin uptake was Na^+- and pH-independent and the initial phase occurred without metabolic alteration of the transported riboflavin. Inhibitors of anion transport did not produce inhibition of riboflavin uptake by Caco-2 cells, thus riboflavin does not appear to act as an anion with regard to its intestinal transport.

Some of the absorbed riboflavin is phosphorylated to FMN within the cytosol of the enterocyte by flavokinase (ATP:riboflavin 5′-phosphotransferase, EC 2.7.1.26) and most of the FMN is further converted to FAD by FAD synthetase (ATP:FMN adenylyltransferase, EC 2.7.7.2). Both of these metabolic steps require ATP, i.e. they are energy-dependent. Gastaldi et al. (1999) investigated the energy dependency of the riboflavin uptake process in isolated rat enterocytes by comparing de-energized cells (cells treated with rotenone) with normal cells. Short (3 min) and long (20 min) incubation times were selected as these times represent membrane events and intracellular metabolic events, respectively. The results showed that in the initial (3 min) phase, the saturable uptake of [^{3}H]riboflavin is mainly an energy-independent process with high affinity and low capacity, whereas in the later (20 min) phase the saturable uptake is strictly energy-dependent and has an increased capacity. The presence of a saturable mechanism even when intracellular metabolism is blocked, as in de-energized cells, suggests that the transport across the membrane is due solely to riboflavin binding to carrier proteins on the brush-border membrane. Saturable uptake in the later phase is due to high-affinity binding of riboflavin to the cytosolic enzymes flavokinase and FAD-synthetase. The conversion of riboflavin to FMN

and FAD by these enzymes accounts for the energy dependency of the transport process.

Additional evidence that intracellular phosphorylation is important for the absorption of physiologically relevant concentrations of riboflavin is the observation that riboflavin analogues that are absorbed at low concentrations by the saturable transport process are good substrates for flavokinase, whereas analogues that are absorbed solely through simple diffusion at all concentrations are poor substrates for this enzyme (Kasai et al., 1990). Moreover, both membrane and intracellular events in riboflavin absorption are inhibited by riboflavin analogues that are readily phosphorylated (Gastaldi et al., 1999).

To summarize, the small intestine is well adapted to completely extracting the small amounts of riboflavin that are largely bound within the ingested flavin coenzymes. The coenzymes are dephosphorylated in the lumen and the liberated riboflavin is extracted very efficiently by a high-affinity, carrier-mediated transport system, which is distributed along the entire length of the small intestine. The uptake mechanism is Na^+-independent and electroneutral in nature. After uptake, some of the riboflavin is metabolically trapped within the enterocyte as FMN. The energy used in riboflavin absorption is not required for membrane uptake, but rather for riboflavin metabolism within the enterocyte. Thus, intracellular metabolism is probably the driving force behind the internalization of riboflavin. The vitamin is dephosphorylated to permit exit of riboflavin across the basolateral membrane; this also takes place by a carrier-mediated, Na^+-independent and electroneutral mechanism.

Adaptive regulation of riboflavin absorption

Feeding rats with a vitamin B_2-deficient diet caused a significant and specific up-regulation in riboflavin uptake by rat intestinal brush-border membrane vesicles compared with controls. Conversely, over-supplementing rats with riboflavin caused a down-regulation in the vitamin's uptake. Both up- and down-regulation were mediated through changes in the number of the functional riboflavin uptake carriers and/or their activity (decreased or increased V_{max}) with no effect on the affinity of the transport system (unchanged K_m) (Said & Mohammadkhani, 1993). Similarly, growing Caco-2 monolayers in a riboflavin-deficient medium caused significant enhancement of riboflavin uptake, whereas an over-supplemented medium suppressed riboflavin uptake (Said & Ma, 1994). This adaptive up- or down-regulation of riboflavin uptake was further studied by Said et al. (1994) who established a role for the 'second messenger' cyclic AMP (cAMP) in the regulation mechanism. They found that compounds that increased intracellular cAMP concentration through different mechanisms caused a significant and concentration-dependent inhibition (down-regulation) in riboflavin uptake. This inhibition of riboflavin uptake was in contrast to other findings of stimulation of intestinal uptake of D-glucose by these compounds (Sharp & Debnam, 1994), indicating that the effect of cAMP-stimulating compounds on riboflavin intestinal uptake is not generalized in nature.

12.4.2 Absorption of bacterially synthesized riboflavin in the large intestine

The normal microflora of the large intestine synthesize considerable amounts of vitamin B$_2$, a significant portion of which exists as free riboflavin. The amount of vitamin B$_2$ synthesized depends on the diet, being significantly higher following consumption of a vegetable-based diet compared with a meat-based diet (Iiuma, 1955). In a study with human subjects, Sorrell et al. (1971) showed that riboflavin instilled directly into the lumen of the mid-transverse colon was absorbed, as judged by an increase in plasma riboflavin concentrations. Colonic absorption of FMN sodium has also been demonstrated in the rat (Kasper, 1970).

Said et al. (2000) demonstrated the existence of a high-affinity, carrier-mediated transport system in the large intestine using cultured human colonic epithelial cells (NCM460 cells). Saturable uptake of riboflavin by these cells was energy-dependent and Na$^+$-independent. Transport was regulated by the Ca^{2+}/calmodulin cell signalling pathway but not by the protein kinase C pathway. An adaptive up- and down-regulation of riboflavin uptake took place when NCM460 cells were grown in a riboflavin-deficient or over-supplemented medium, respectively. These findings are similar to those in the small intestine and suggest that the same mechanism may be operating in the large intestine to absorb the bacterially synthesized riboflavin.

12.4.3 Post-absorptive metabolism

Following absorption, B$_2$ vitamers are carried by the portal blood to the liver. About 50% of circulating flavins is riboflavin, with somewhat less FAD and less than 10% FMN. The concentration of riboflavin in human plasma is about 0.03 µM on average (McCormick, 1989). A proportion of the circulating flavins is bound loosely to albumin and tightly to some immunoglobulins. The extent to which flavins are bound to plasma proteins is not believed to be crucial in regulating tissue availability of the vitamin (White & Merrill, 1986). Erythrocytes contain four to five times more flavin than plasma. There is a relatively slow equilibration of free riboflavin between the plasma and erythrocytes, hence flavin levels in erythrocytes are less subject to recent dietary intake. For this reason, the activity of an erythrocyte enzyme, glutathione reductase, is used as an indicator of vitamin B$_2$ status.

Uptake of riboflavin by human-derived cultured liver cells is by means of a carrier-mediated, energy-dependent, Na$^+$-independent system which appears to be regulated by an intracellular Ca^{2+}/calmodulin-mediated transduction pathway and by substrate level in the growth medium (Said et al., 1998). The liver is the major storage site of the vitamin and contains about one-third of the total body flavins, 70–90% of which is in the form of FAD. Free riboflavin constitutes less than 5% of the stored flavins. Other storage sites are the spleen, kidney and cardiac muscle. These depots maintain significant amounts of the vitamin even in severe deficiency states.

Cellular entry of riboflavin in all tissues is followed by metabolic trapping, whereby riboflavin is phosphorylated to FMN (riboflavin phosphate) in an irreversible reaction (reaction 12.1) catalysed by flavokinase.

$$\text{riboflavin} + \text{ATP} \xrightarrow{\text{flavokinase}} \text{FMN} + \text{ADP} \quad (12.1)$$

Some FMN is utilized by certain flavoenzymes; the remainder undergoes a reversible reaction (reaction 12.2) with ATP to give FAD and inorganic pyrophosphate. FAD contributes 70–90% of total flavins in most tissues.

$$\text{FMN} + \text{ATP} \underset{\text{FAD synthetase}}{\rightleftharpoons} \text{FAD} + \text{PPi} \quad (12.2)$$

FAD is inhibitory to the synthetase and thereby confers regulation upon its own synthesis (Yamada et al., 1990).

Free FAD that is not bound to apoenzyme (enzyme protein) is rapidly hydrolysed to FMN and AMP (reaction 12.3) and free FMN is rapidly hydrolysed to riboflavin and inorganic phosphate (reaction 12.4).

Nucleotide pyrophosphatase

$$FAD \xrightarrow{\hspace{3cm}} FMN + AMP \quad (12.3)$$

Non-specific phosphatases

$$FMN \xrightarrow{\hspace{3cm}} riboflavin + Pi \quad (12.4)$$

The activities of enzymes involved in the specific biosynthesis of FMN and FAD are depressed by riboflavin deficiency, while those involved in the non-specific degradation of the flavocoenzymes are not affected by riboflavin status (Lee & McCormick, 1983).

Thyroid hormone regulation of flavocoenzyme biosynthesis

The tight binding of FMN or FAD to their respective apoenzymes confers stability to the holoenzyme and an insufficiency of coenzyme leads to loss of enzyme activity through proteolysis. There is evidence (Rivlin & Langdon, 1966; Rivlin, 1970; Lee & McCormick, 1985) that thyroid hormone regulates the conversion of riboflavin to its functional coenzyme forms. The mechanism of regulation is on biosynthetic rather than degradative steps. Hepatic flavokinase activity was diminished in hypothyroid rats, causing decreased FMN and FAD synthesis and consequent decreases in the activities of a number of FMN- and FAD-dependent enzymes. FAD synthetase activity was also diminished, but to a lesser degree than flavokinase. Furthermore, riboflavin levels were reduced in the livers of hypothyroid rats. Treatment of the hypothyroid rats with thyroid hormone restored coenzyme levels and enzyme activities to normal. In the case of hyperthyroid rats, hepatic levels of FMN and FAD were not increased above normal despite a two-fold increase in the activity of flavokinase. Even when supplemental riboflavin was administered, coenzymes levels were not increased above normal.

Cimino et al. (1987) reported that in hypothyroid adult humans, the activity of the FAD-containing enzyme erythrocyte glutathione reductase was reduced to levels observed during riboflavin deficiency. After 2 weeks of therapy with thyroxine and without supplementation with riboflavin, the enzyme activity reverted to normal.

It is well established that thyroid hormone increases the synthesis of protein at the transcriptional and translational levels. Yet the restoration of flavoprotein enzyme activity produced by thyroid hormone treatment in hypothyroidism was not prevented by inhibiting protein synthesis with actinomycin-D (Rivlin & Langdon, 1966). Apparently, therefore, thyroid hormone does not induce the synthesis of flavokinase apoenzyme; rather it appears to stimulate the conversion of an inactive precursor form of flavokinase to the active form or, alternatively, decrease the proteolytic conversion of active to inactive form (Lee & McCormick (1985). The reduced levels of substrate (riboflavin) could explain the reduced activity of flavokinase in hypothyroidism.

Rivlin & Langdon (1966) offered a plausible explanation for the apparent upper limit in the hepatic concentration of FMN and FAD in hyperthyroidism. The concentration of FMN/FAD remaining in the liver cells is restricted by the quantity of apoenzyme to which it can be stably bound. Excess free coenzyme would not be stored but would be destroyed enzymatically. Thus the elevated flavokinase activity seen in hyperthyroidism is not accompanied by abnormally high levels of coenzyme.

From these data it appears that thyroid hormone regulates FMN and FAD synthesis by altering the activity of flavokinase. Excessive concentrations of FMN/FAD are prevented by the enzymatic destruction of coenzyme that is not stably bound to the limited amounts of apoenzyme.

12.4.4   Brain homeostasis

The concentration of total riboflavin in brain, unlike in liver and kidney, is maintained relatively constant even in the face of severe vitamin B_2 deficiency or after massive doses of intravenous riboflavin. As in other tissues, riboflavin that enters the brain is enzymatically phosphorylated to FMN, which can then be converted to FAD. In rat brain, more than 90% of the total riboflavin is present as FAD and FMN. About 10% of the total riboflavin in the brain of normal rats turns over per hour.

The concentration of total riboflavin in cerebrospinal fluid (CSF) is about 50% of that in plasma. However, because roughly 50% of the total riboflavin in plasma is bound to serum proteins, the concentrations of unbound vitamin in plasma and CSF are approximately equal. Because CSF is constantly leaving the central nervous system, riboflavin must be continually supplied to the newly formed fluid.

Riboflavin, but not FMN or FAD, enters the central nervous system principally through the blood–brain barrier (Spector, 1980a). Uptake of [^{14}C]riboflavin by rabbit brain slices *in vitro* took place by a saturable system that depended on the conversion of accumulated riboflavin to FMN and FAD, i.e. intracellular trapping of riboflavin (Spector, 1980b). These enzymatic conversions require ATP. Energy dependency was shown by the inhibition of uptake by dinitrophenol and low-temperature (1°C) incubation. The system was one-half saturated at the normal plasma concentration of riboflavin (~0.03 µM). This means that the entry of excessive amounts of riboflavin from blood to brain is prohibited.

Spector & Boose (1979) studied the capacity of the isolated choroid plexus, the anatomical locus of the blood–CSF barrier, to transport [^{14}C]riboflavin. With concentrations of [^{14}C]riboflavin of 0.7 µM or greater in the incubation medium, the choroid plexus accumulated [^{14}C]riboflavin against a large concentration gradient, thus demonstrating active transport. Uptake did not depend on intracellular binding or phosphorylation of the vitamin. The half-saturation concentration (K_m) was 78 µM (cf. normal plasma concentration of riboflavin of ~0.03 µM), which means that the system has the potential to transport high concentrations of riboflavin before it becomes saturated. Studies using the isolated choroid plexus do not show direction of transport.

Spector (1980a) injected [^{14}C]riboflavin directly into the ventricular CSF of anaesthetized rabbits. Some of the riboflavin entered the brain by a saturable accumulation system that depended in part on phosphorylation of the riboflavin, but the majority of the labelled vitamin left the CSF extremely rapidly and was not found in the brain. The disappearance of the injected riboflavin means that the choroid plexus must have actively transported the vitamin from the CSF into the bloodstream. Direct pictorial evidence of this property of the choroid plexus was provided by fluorescence microscopy (Spector, 1980c).

In conclusion, the controlled entry and exit of riboflavin from the central nervous system provide the means for maintaining total riboflavin homeostasis in brain cells. The main entry is via the blood–brain barrier followed by high-affinity saturable uptake by brain cells and metabolic trapping. The choroid plexus actively transports riboflavin from blood into the CSF, but perhaps more importantly it has the capacity to transport excess riboflavin in the reverse direction.

12.4.5 Placental transport

A riboflavin carrier protein (RCP) is required to transport riboflavin from the maternal bloodstream across the placental membranes to the developing fetus. The synthesis of RCP in the maternal liver is controlled by the concentration of circulating oestrogen, synthesis being mediated through specific oestrogen receptors in the hepatocytes. An absence of RCP during pregnancy results in resorption of the fetus owing to the lack of riboflavin for fetal FAD/FMN synthesis. Evidence for these statements is based on research carried out by Adiga's group (Adiga, 1994). The following is a summary of this work.

In the adult female monkey, an increase in the concentration of serum oestradiol during the menstrual cycle and early pregnancy could be correlated with enhanced serum RCP. Administration of oestradiol-17β to both immature female and male monkeys specifically elicited elevated levels of serum RCP. Oestrogen appears to be uniquely responsible for the RCP response since administration of progesterone alone to immature male monkeys could not substitute for oestrogen. Ovariectomized female rats also respond to oestrogen administration. Commensurate with two peaks of plasma oestrogen observed during the human menstrual cycle, there were two peaks of RCP.

The fetal liver itself synthesizes RCP in progressively increasing amounts till term. It is conjectured that an RCP–flavokinase complex may facilitate flavin coenzyme biosynthesis in the fetal liver. The endocrine signal for the fetal RCP gene expression *in utero* may also involve oestrogen, since a major portion of oestrogen produced in the placenta is diverted to the fetal circulation. Additionally, the hepatic concentration of oestrogen receptors increases in the fetus as pregnancy progresses.

The importance of adequate circulatory concentrations of RCP for maintenance and progression of pregnancy was revealed in experiments wherein endogenous RCP was immunoneutralized *in vivo* by repeatedly injecting female rats with antiserum to chicken RCP to induce a high titre of anti-RCP antibodies. When such rats were mated they conceived normally. However, serum progesterone concentrations dropped precipitously after day 9 of pregnancy (i.e. soon after the placenta became functional), signifying abrupt pregnancy termination. Autopsy revealed complete fetal resorption. Immunoneutralization of RCP led to drastic curtailment of [^{14}C]riboflavin transport from the maternal circulation to the fetoplacental unit and consequent depletion of FAD to below the critical level required to maintain viability of the fetus. Early termination of pregnancy could be demonstrated repeatedly as long as high antibody titres were maintained by booster injections of the antiserum. Otherwise, the same rats were able to conceive and maintain normal pregnancies. Monkeys also exhibited termination of early pregnancy when immunized with chicken RCP.

A human RCP has been isolated, the concentration of which is higher in umbilical cord serum than in the maternal circulation. There are indications for the existence of a specific membrane receptor for RCP on human first-trimester and term placentae, implying an endocytotic transport mechanism. There is also evidence that the human placenta synthesizes and secretes RCP under the influence of placental oestrogen.

Based on the available data, Adigo (1994) proposed a model (Fig. 12.2) to account for the role of RCP in fetal development. During pregnancy, sustained production of RCP in the maternal liver is dictated by oestrogen produced either directly by the fetoplacental unit or through stimulation of the ovary by follicle-stimulating hormone and luteinizing hormone (luteotropic stimulation). The hepatic RCP secreted into the circulation tightly binds riboflavin and carries it to the placental villous membrane where the carrier–riboflavin complex is endocytosed. The riboflavin is released and then complexed with placental RCP to be transported for fetal utilization. Oestrogen produced by the placenta reaches the fetal circulation and induces RCP in the fetal liver. This RCP conserves the riboflavin in the fetal circulation for efficient utilization by the rapidly growing fetus. Thus, according to this model, an hormonal signal (chorionic gonadotropin) from the fetoplacental unit commands the mother to synthesize hepatic RCP, which facilitates delivery of riboflavin to the fetus.

Role of the riboflavin carrier protein in lactation and spermatogenesis

The rat mammary gland is able to synthesize RCP during pregnancy and lactation, and the carrier

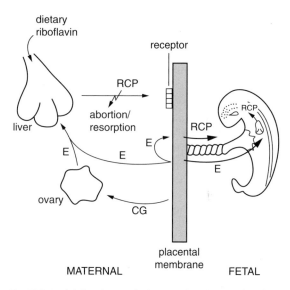

Fig. 12.2 Model of mechanism of induction and involvement of riboflavin carrier protein (RCP) in transplacental transport of riboflavin in pregnant mammals. Explanation given in text. E, (o)estrogen; CG, chorionic gonadotrophin. Reproduced from Adiga (1994), *Vitamin Receptors. Vitamins as Ligands in Cell Communication* (Ed. K. Dakshinamurti), pp. 137–76, by permission of Cambridge University Press.

protein has been detected in the milk of humans and other mammals. The concentration of RCP-bound riboflavin in milk is several-fold higher than in the maternal blood. These observations lend support to the hypothesis that RCP has an additional role as the riboflavin carrier for secretion of the vitamin into milk (Adiga, 1994).

The testicular synthesis of RCP in the rat and its detection in mature spermatozoa of humans and other mammals suggest that RCP may be important in spermatogenesis (Adiga, 1994).

12.4.6   Renal reabsorption and excretion

In the kidney, riboflavin that has been filtered through the glomerulus can undergo either reabsorption or secretion in the proximal tubule before it is finally excreted in the urine. Reabsorption is the process by which riboflavin in the tubular lumen enters the epithelial cell via the brush-border membrane, exits the cell at the basolateral membrane and diffuses into the peritubular capillary. Secretion is the process by which riboflavin in the peritubular capillary is transported across the epithelial cell and into the tubular lumen in the opposite direction to reabsorption. As at least 40% of plasma riboflavin is thought to be unbound in humans (Rose, 1988), renal reabsorption is an important conservation mechanism. Renal secretion removes excess riboflavin from the body at a rate several times higher than the glomerular filtration rate. The kidney, together with the intestine, therefore plays an important role in maintaining riboflavin homeostasis in the body.

Kumar *et al.* (1998) studied riboflavin uptake by cultures of human-derived renal proximal tubule epithelial cells. They demonstrated uptake via an energy-dependent, Na^+-independent, carrier-mediated system that adapted according to the concentration of riboflavin in the growth medium. The adaptive regulatory effect of riboflavin was mediated via changes in the number and/or activity as well as affinity of the riboflavin uptake carriers. Using specific modulators of intracellular signal transduction pathways, it was shown that protein kinase A, protein kinase C and protein tyrosine kinase were not involved in regulating riboflavin uptake. In contrast, inhibition of the Ca^{2+}/calmodulin signal transduction pathway resulted in a significant inhibition of riboflavin uptake, implicating this system in the regulation of riboflavin transport. The effect of one inhibitor, calmidazolium, appeared to be mediated through decreases in both the number/activity and affinity of the riboflavin uptake carriers.

Yanagawa *et al.* (2000) studied riboflavin transport in rabbit renal proximal tubules by using the *in vitro* isolated perfused tubule. This technique is ideal for studying bi-directional tubular transport processes because it allows unidirectional fluxes to be measured separately in a defined tubular segment. Both reabsorption and secretion were found to be influenced by riboflavin concentration. At 0.1 µM riboflavin concentration, secretion was higher than reabsorption so that net riboflavin transport occurred in the direction of secretion. Lowering the riboflavin concentration to 0.01 µM reduced both reabsorption and secretion, but the two fluxes were not significantly different and so no net riboflavin transport occurred. In contrast, both reabsorption and secretion were increased when the riboflavin concentration was raised to 1 µM, leading to a significantly greater net riboflavin secretion. Both fluxes were abolished by the metabolic inhibitor iodoacetate and significantly lowered by lumichrome, indicating dependence on energy and a carrier, respectively. Secretion, but not reabsorption, was inhibited by the anion inhibitor probenecid and *para*-aminohippuric acid (an organic anion), indicating that the organic anion transport system is involved in tubular riboflavin secretion. Changes in luminal pH over the physiological range (7.0–8.0) did not affect reabsorption, but secretion was inhibited when the bath pH was increased to 8.0. Secretion was inhibited by trifluoperazine, indicating that the intracellular Ca^{2+}/calmodulin-dependent pathway may play an important role in mediating the regulation of tubular transport through its effect on riboflavin secretion.

For normal adults eating varied diets, riboflavin accounts for 60–70% of flavin compounds in the urine; the remainder are riboflavin metabolites (McCormick, 1994). Urinary excretion studies carried out in humans have suggested that any riboflavin secreted into the bile is almost fully reabsorbed, i.e. the vitamin is subject to enterohepatic cycling (Jusko & Levy, 1967).

12.5   Biochemical functions

Background information can be found in Section 4.1.

In mammalian tissues, the flavins FAD and FMN function as coenzymes for a wide variety of enzymes known as flavoproteins, which are concerned with oxidoreductive processes. Most of these enzymes require FAD rather than FMN as the coenzyme. The flavins are perhaps better classed as prosthetic groups because they remain tightly bound to the apoenzyme during the catalytic reactions. In most flavoproteins the binding is noncovalent. Less than 10% of the FAD is covalently attached to the protein (apoenzyme) of four important enzymes: succinate and sarcosine dehydrogenases, monoamine oxidase and L-gluconolactone oxidase. The means of attachment is a peptide-link to an *N*-histidyl or *S*-cysteinyl residue via the 8-methyl group of FAD.

Flavins can act as oxidizing agents because of their ability to accept a pair of hydrogen atoms. The isoalloxazine ring is reduced by two successive one-electron transfers with the intermediate formation of a semiquinone free radical (Fig. 12.3).

The flavoproteins play a wide variety of roles in intermediary metabolism. For example, in the oxidative decarboxylation of pyruvate to acetyl-CoA and α-ketoglutarate to succinyl-CoA in the tricarboxylic acid

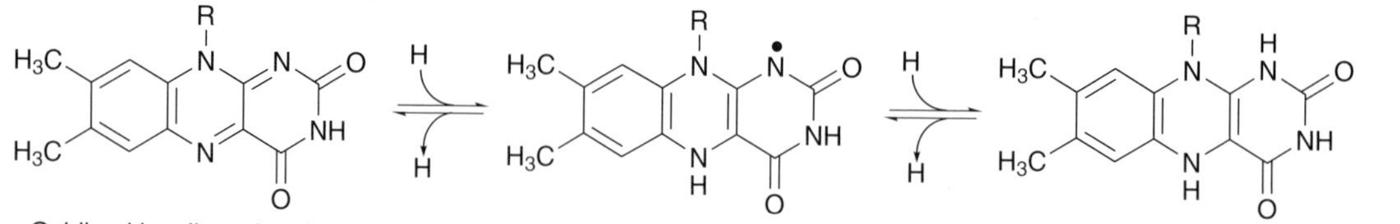

Fig. 12.3 Stages in the reduction of flavins.

cycle, FAD serves as an intermediate electron carrier, passing the electrons to NAD and forming NADH. The NADH is reoxidized by donating its electrons to FMN incorporated within the electron transport chain.

In the following reactions, there is no involvement of NAD, $FADH_2$ being the final reduced product. In the β-oxidation of fatty acids FAD is a coenzyme for the transferase which catalyses the oxidation of saturated fatty acyl-CoA to α,β-unsaturated fatty acyl-CoA (Fig. 12.4). FAD is also a coenzyme for succinate dehydrogenase which catalyses the oxidation of succinate to fumarate in the tricarboxylic acid cycle. The $FADH_2$ produced from these reactions is reoxidized by passing its electrons to coenzyme Q in the electron-transport chain.

As a coenzyme for an oxidase such as xanthine oxidase, FAD transfers electrons directly to oxygen with the formation of hydrogen peroxide. Xanthine oxidase catalyses two steps in the formation of uric acid.

In addition, flavin coenzymes are necessary for reactions involving other vitamins. For example, an FMN-dependent oxidase – pyridoxine phosphate oxidase – catalyses the conversion of pyridoxine phosphate and pyridoxamine phosphate to pyridoxal phosphate, the primary vitamin B_6 coenzyme. An FAD-dependent hydroxylase is involved in the conversion of kynurenine to 3-hydroxykynurenine in the pathway of NAD synthesis from tryptophan. In folate metabolism an FAD-dependent dehydrogenase reduces 5,10-methylenetetrahydrofolate to 5-methyltetrahydrofolate, which interfaces with the vitamin B_{12}-dependent formation of methionine from homocysteine.

12.6   Vitamin B_2 deficiency

No pathologically severe symptoms attributed to vitamin B_2 deficiency have been observed in humans. Deficiency symptoms have been induced experimentally in volunteers whose diets were lacking only in the vitamin or who were fed vitamin B_2 antagonists. Symptoms usually include lesions of the lips (cheilosis) and angles of the mouth (angular stomatitis), a fissured and magenta-coloured tongue (glossitis), seborrhoeic follicular keratosis of the nose and forehead, and dermatitis of the anogenital region. Ophthalmic symptoms are a superficial vascularization of the cornea accompanied by intense photophobia.

12.7   Nutritional aspects

12.7.1   Human requirement

Because of the limited storage capacity for all forms of vitamin B_2, the margin between dietary intake resulting in deficiency (0.55 mg per day) and that resulting in tissue saturation (1.1 mg per day) is very small (Horwitt et al., 1950). In the United States, the vitamin B_2 allowance for healthy people of all ages is based on 0.6 mg per 1000 kcal, even though there is no evidence that the requirement is correlated directly to energy expenditure. This leads to RDAs ranging from 0.4 mg per day for early infants to 1.7 mg per day for young adult males. However, for elderly people and others whose daily caloric intake may be less than 2000 kcal, a minimum of 1.2 mg per day is recommended to ensure tissue saturation.

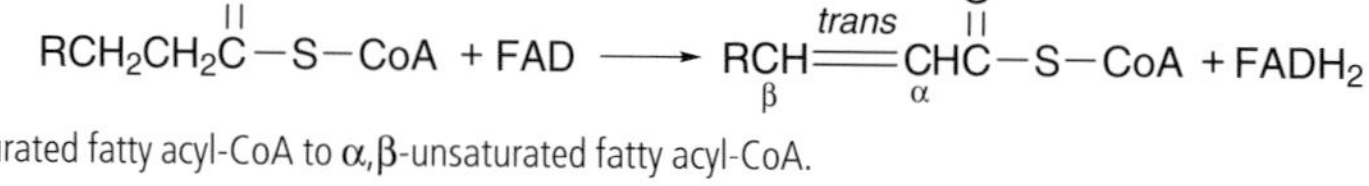

Fig. 12.4 Oxidation of saturated fatty acyl-CoA to α,β-unsaturated fatty acyl-CoA.

12.7.2 Effects of high intake

The low solubility of riboflavin and the limited capacity of intestinal absorption mechanisms probably account for the lack of toxicity following oral doses of up to 20 mg of riboflavin daily (Cumming *et al.*, 1981).

12.7.3 Assessment of nutritional status

The most commonly used current method for assessing vitamin B$_2$ status is based upon the change in activity of the FAD-dependent enzyme erythrocyte glutathione reductase (EGR) as measured by the oxidation of NADPH to NADP. The *in vitro* addition of FAD to freshly lysed erythrocytes, substrate and NADPH provides an activity coefficient, which is inversely proportional to the urinary excretion of riboflavin. Vitamin B$_2$ deficiency is indicated by an activity coefficient >1.2, while tissue saturation results in no additional stimulation and an activity coefficient of 1.0 (Cooperman & Lopez, 1991).

Further reading

Foy, H. & Mbaya, V. (1977) Riboflavin. *Progress in Food & Nutrition Science*, **2**, 357–94.

References

Adiga, P. R. (1994) Riboflavin carrier protein in reproduction. In: *Vitamin Receptors. Vitamins as Ligands in Cell Communication.* (Ed. K. Dakshinamurti), pp. 137–76. Cambridge University Press, Cambridge.

Akiyama, T., Selhub, J. & Rosenberg, I. H. (1982) FMN phosphatase and FAD pyrophosphatase in rat intestinal brush borders: role in intestinal absorption of dietary riboflavin. *Journal of Nutrition*, **112**, 263–8.

Casirola, D., Kasai, S., Gastaldi, G., Ferrari, G. & Matsui, K. (1994) Specificity of riboflavin molecular groups for riboflavin binding to rat small intestinal brush border membrane. *Journal of Nutritional Science and Vitaminology*, **40**, 289–301.

Chia, C. P., Addison, R. & McCormick, D. B. (1978) Absorption, metabolism, and excretion of 8α-(amino acid) riboflavins in the rat. *Journal of Nutrition*, **108**, 373–81.

Cimino, J. A., Jhangiani, S., Schwartz, E. & Cooperman, J. M. (1987) Riboflavin metabolism in the hypothyroid adult. *Proceedings of the Society for Experimental Biology and Medicine*, **184**, 151–3.

Cooperman, J. M. & Lopez, R. (1991) Riboflavin. In: *Handbook of Vitamins*, 2nd edn. (Ed. L. J. Machlin), pp. 283–310. Marcel Dekker, New York.

Cumming, F., Briggs, M. & Briggs, M. (1981) Clinical toxicology of vitamin supplements. In: *Vitamins in Human Biology and Medicine.* (Ed. M. H. Briggs), pp. 187–243. CRC Press, Boca Raton, Florida.

Daniel, H., Binninger, E. & Rehner, G. (1983a) Hydrolysis of FMN and FAD by alkaline phosphatase of the intestinal brush-border membrane. *International Journal of Vitamin and Nutrition Research*, **53**, 109–14.

Daniel, H., Wille, U. & Rehner, G. (1983b) In vitro kinetics of the intestinal transport of riboflavin in rats. *Journal of Nutrition*, **113**, 636–43.

Feder, S., Daniel, H. & Rehner, G. (1991) In vivo kinetics of intestinal absorption of riboflavin in rats. *Journal of Nutrition*, **121**, 72–9.

Gastaldi, G., Laforenza, U., Casirola, D., Ferrari, G., Tosco, M. & Rindi, G. (1999) Energy depletion differently affects membrane transport and intracellular metabolism of riboflavin taken up by isolated rat enterocytes. *Journal of Nutrition*, **129**, 406–9.

Hegazy, E. & Schwenk, M. (1983) Riboflavin uptake by isolated enterocytes of guinea pigs. *Journal of Nutrition*, **113**, 1702–7.

Horwitt, M. K., Harvey, C. C., Hills, O. W. & Liebert, E. (1950) Correlation of urinary excretion of riboflavin with dietary intake and symptoms of ariboflavinosis. *Journal of Nutrition*, **41**, 247–64.

Iinuma, S. (1955) Synthesis of riboflavin by intestinal bacteria. *Journal of Vitaminology*, **1**(2), 6–13.

Jusko, W. J. & Levy, G. (1967) Absorption, metabolism, and excretion of riboflavin-5′-phosphate in man. *Journal of Pharmaceutical Sciences*, **56**, 58–62.

Jusko, W. J., Levy, G., Yaffe, S. J. & Allen, J. E. (1971) Riboflavin absorption in children with biliary obstruction. *American Journal of Diseases of Children*, **121**, 48–52.

Kasai, S., Nakano, H., Maeda, K. & Matsui, K. (1990) Purification, properties, and function of flavokinase from rat intestinal mucosa. *Journal of Biochemistry*, **107**, 298–303.

Kasper, H. (1970) Vitamin absorption in the colon. *American Journal of Proctology*, **21**, 341–5.

Kumar, C. K., Yanagawa, N., Ortiz, A. & Said, H. M. (1998) Mechanism and regulation of riboflavin uptake by human renal proximal tubule epithelial cell line HK-2. *American Journal of Physiology*, **274**, F104–10.

Lee, S.-S. & McCormick, D. B. (1983) Effect of riboflavin status on hepatic activities of flavin-metabolizing enzymes in rats. *Journal of Nutrition*, **113**, 2274–9.

Lee, S.-S. & McCormick, D. B. (1985) Thyroid hormone regulation of flavocoenzyme biosynthesis. *Archives of Biochemistry and Biophysics*, **237**, 197–201.

McCormick, D. B. (1989) Two interconnected B vitamins: riboflavin and pyridoxine. *Physiological Reviews*, **69**, 1170–98.

McCormick, D. B. (1994) Riboflavin. In: *Modern Nutrition in Health and Disease*, 8th edn, Vol. 1. (Ed. M. E. Shils, J. A. Olson & M. Shike), pp. 366–75. Lea & Febiger, Philadelphia.

Mayersohn, M., Feldman, S. & Gibaldi, M. (1969) Bile salt enhancement of riboflavin and flavin mononucleotide absorption in man. *Journal of Nutrition*, **98**, 288–96.

Merrill, A. H. Jr., Lambeth, J. D., Edmondson, D. E. & McCormick, D. B. (1981) Formation and mode of action of flavoproteins. *Annual Review of Nutrition*, **1**, 281–317.

Middleton, H. M. III (1990) Uptake of riboflavin by rat intestinal mucosa in vitro. *Journal of Nutrition*, **120**, 588–93.

Pinto, J., Huang, Y. & Rivlin, R. (1984) Selective effects of ethanol and acetaldehyde upon intestinal enzymes metabolizing riboflavin: mechanism of reduced flavin bioavailability due to ethanol. *American Journal of Clinical Nutrition*, **39**, 685 (abstr).

Rivlin, R. S. (1970) Regulation of flavoprotein enzymes in hypothyroidism and in riboflavin deficiency. *Advances in Enzyme Regulation*, **8**, 239–50.

Rivlin, R. S. & Langdon, R. G. (1966) Regulation of hepatic FAD levels by thyroid hormone. *Advances in Enzyme Regulation*, **4**, 45–58.

Rose, R. C. (1988) Transport of ascorbic acid and other water-soluble vitamins. *Biochimica et Biophysica Acta*, **947**, 335–66.

Said, H. M. & Ma, T. Y. (1994) Mechanism of riboflavine uptake by Caco-2 human intestinal epithelial cells. *American Journal of Physiology*, **266**, G15–21.

Said, H. M. & Mohammadkhani, R. (1993) Uptake of riboflavin across the brush border membrane of rat intestine: regulation by dietary vitamin levels. *Gastroenterology*, **105**, 1294–8.

Said, H. M., Hollander, D. & Duong, Y. (1985) A dual, concentration-dependent transport system for riboflavin in rat intestine *in vitro*. *Nutrition Research*, **5**, 1269–79.

Said, H. M., Mohammadkhani, R. & McCloud, E. (1993a) Mechanism of transport of riboflavin in rabbit intestinal brush border membrane vesicles. *Proceedings of the Society for Experimental Biology and Medicine*, **202**, 428–34.

Said, H. M., Hollander, D. & Mohammadkhani, R. (1993b) Uptake of riboflavin by intestinal basolateral membrane vesicles: a specialized carrier-mediated process. *Biochimica et Biophysica Acta*, **1148**, 263–8.

Said, H. M., Ma, T. Y. & Grant. K. (1994) Regulation of riboflavin intestinal uptake by protein kinase A: studies with Caco-2 cells. *American Journal of Physiology*, **267**, G955–9.

Said, H. M., Ortiz, A., Ma, T. Y. & McCloud, E. (1998) Riboflavin uptake by the human-derived liver cells Hep G2: mechanism and regulation. *Journal of Cellular Physiology*, **176**, 588–94.

Said, H. M., Ortiz, A., Moyer, M. P. & Yanagawa, N. (2000) Riboflavin uptake by human-derived colonic epithelial NCM460 cells. *American Journal of Physiology*, **278**, C270–6.

Sharp, P. A. & Debnam, E. S. (1994) The role of cyclic AMP in the control of sugar transport across the brush border and basolateral membranes of rat jejunal enterocytes. *Experimental Physiology*, **79**, 203–14.

Sorrell, M. F., Frank, O., Thomson, A. D., Aquino, H. & Baker, H. (1971) Absorption of vitamins from the large intestine *in vivo*. *Nutrition Report International*, **3**, 143–8.

Spector, R. (1980a) Riboflavin homeostasis in the central nervous system. *Journal of Neurochemistry*, **35**, 202–9.

Spector, R. (1980b) Riboflavin accumulation by rabbit brain slices *in vitro*. *Journal of Neurochemistry*, **34**, 1768–71.

Spector, R. (1980c) Riboflavin transport in the central nervous system. Characterization and effects of drugs. *Journal of Clinical Investigation*, **66**, 821–31.

Spector, R. & Boose, B. (1979) Active transport of riboflavin by the isolated choroid plexus *in vitro*. *Journal of Biological Chemistry*, **254**(20), 10 286–9.

White, H. B. & Merrill, A. H. Jr. (1986) Riboflavin-binding proteins. *Annual Review of Nutrition*, **8**, 279–99.

Yamada, Y., Merrill, A. H. Jr. & McCormick, D. B. (1990) Probable reaction mechanisms of flavokinase and FAD synthetase from rat liver. *Archives of Biochemistry and Biophysics*, **278**, 125–30.

Yanagawa, N., Shih, R. N G., Jo, O. D. & Said, H. M. (2000) Riboflavin transport by isolated perfused rabbit renal proximal tubules. *American Journal of Physiology*, **279**, C1782–6.

13
Niacin: Nicotinic Acid and Nicotinamide

Key discussion topics

- The major role of reduced NAD is to transfer electrons from metabolic intermediates into the electron-transport chain for the production of ATP. Reduced NADP is mainly employed as a reducing agent in many biosynthetic pathways.
- NAD has a role in DNA repair by donating ADP-ribose for protein modification.
- A deficiency of niacin in the diet gives rise to pellagra.

13.1 Historical overview

The human disease of pellagra was first described in Spain by Casal in 1735 after the introduction of maize into Europe from the Americas. In the 1920s, Goldberger in the USA reported that pellagra and black tongue in dogs responded to treatment with animal protein and also to boiled protein-free extracts of yeast. In 1937, Elvehjem found that the active component in liver extracts used to successfully treat canine black tongue was nicotinamide, and reports that nicotinic acid cured pellagra soon followed.

Nicotinic acid and nicotinamide had been isolated from the coenzymes now known as NAD and NADP by 1934–1935; hence knowledge of their biochemical roles in electron-transfer reactions preceded the discovery of their nutritional significance. By 1946, the metabolism of dietary tryptophan to an active form of the vitamin had been demonstrated.

13.2 Chemistry

Niacin is the generic descriptor for two vitamers,

nicotinic acid and nicotinamide (Fig. 13.1). This no-menclature is not to be confused with American usage of the term niacin to denote specifically nicotinic acid, and niacinamide to denote the amide.

In living tissues nicotinamide is the reactive moiety of the coenzymes NAD and NADP. The structure of NAD can be envisaged as the adenosine diphosphate-ribosyl moiety, hereafter abbreviated as ADP-ribose, attached covalently to nicotinamide through a β-N-glycosidic linkage (Fig. 13.1). This linkage constitutes a high-energy bond, the energy of which supplies the driving force for various ADP-ribosylation reactions (see Section 13.5.2). NAD glycohydrolases hydrolyse the N-glycosidic linkage of NAD, yielding free ADP-ribose, nicotinamide and a proton. Most cellular NAD and NADP is stored in the cytoplasm, bound to protein (Weiner & van Eys, 1983).

In mature cereal grains (those examined included maize, wheat, rice, barley and sorghum) 85–90% of the total niacin content exists in chemically bound

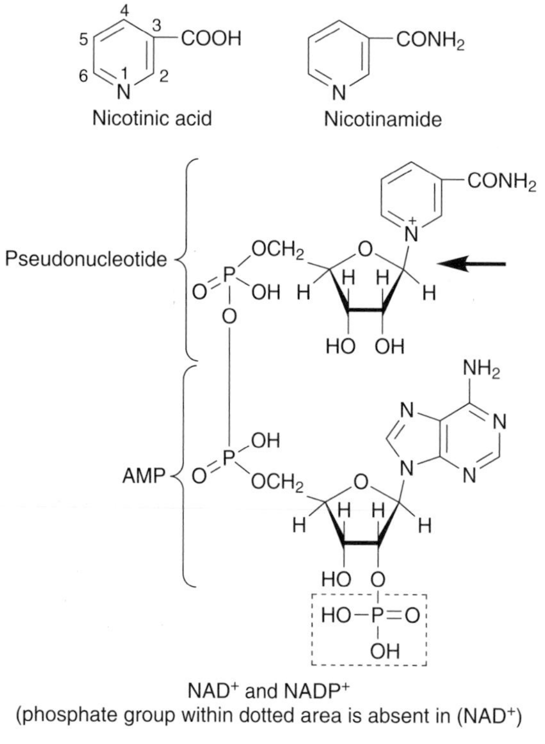

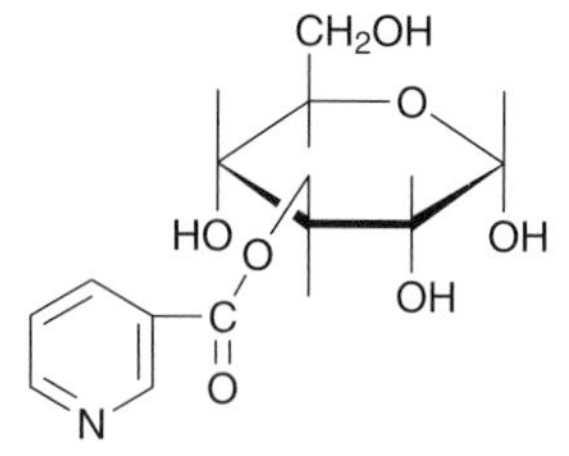

Fig. 13.2 Structure of β-3-O-nicotinoyl-D-glucose.

forms of nicotinic acid, the remainder being present as free nicotinic acid and nicotinamide (Ghosh *et al.*, 1963). Investigations by Mason *et al.* (1973) revealed that the bound nicotinic acid of wheat bran is incorporated in a number of macromolecules that are both polysaccharide and glycopeptide in character. Mason & Kodicek (1973) subjected preparations of bound nicotinic acid of wheat bran to partial acid hydrolysis and identified a subunit as nicotinoyl glucose (Fig. 13.2). The nicotinoyl ester bond linking the nicotinic acid and glucose moieties most probably exists in the polysaccharide and glycopeptide fractions isolated from wheat bran, and is so far the only established linkage in bound nicotinic acid.

13.3   Dietary sources and bioavailability

13.3.1   Dietary sources

Niacin can be synthesized in the human body from the essential amino acid L-tryptophan. Approximately 60 mg of L-tryptophan yield 1 mg of niacin; therefore, to calculate the niacin equivalent of a diet, one adds one-sixtieth of the weight of tryptophan present to the weight of preformed niacin.

Because of the contribution of tryptophan, foods containing balanced protein are important contributors to total niacin equivalent intake. Lean red meat, poultry and liver contain high levels of both niacin and tryptophan and, together with legumes, are important sources of the vitamin. Peanut butter is an excellent source of niacin. Cheese and eggs are relatively poor sources of preformed niacin, but these high-protein foods contain ample amounts of tryptophan and therefore have a high niacin equivalent. Fruits and vegetables provide useful amounts, depending upon the dietary intake. Other useful sources are whole grain cereals, bread, tea and coffee.

Fig. 13.1 Structures of niacin compounds and the nicotinamide nucleotides. The nitrogen in the pyridine ring of nicotinamide is positively charged when it is a component of NAD(P). Arrow shows the β-N-glycosidic linkage separating the ADP-ribose and nicotinamide moieties.

In mature cereal grains most of the niacin is present as bound nicotinic acid and is concentrated in the aleurone and germ layers. Milling to produce white flour removes most of the vitamin with the bran. In the UK it is compulsory by law to add niacin to white flour (mostly 70% extraction rate) at 16 mg kg^{-1}. All flour other than wholemeal (100% extraction) must be enriched (Bender, 1978).

As discussed later, some plant-derived foods contain niacin in chemically bound forms that result in their bioavailabilities being low. Most food composition tables give total niacin, and are compiled from the results of analyses in which nicotinic acid is liberated from unavailable bound forms by hydrolysis with acid or alkali. Therefore, tabulated niacin contents for many plant foods, particularly mature cereals, over-estimate their value in providing biologically available niacin.

13.3.2 Bioavailability

The majority of the bound nicotinic acid in mature cereal grains is biologically unavailable after conventional cooking (Wall & Carpenter, 1988). Nicotinoyl glucose itself is readily utilized, so why should this compound be unavailable when present in plant tissues? Mason & Kodicek (1973) suggested that its incorporation within indigestible celluloses and hemicelluloses prevents access of the gastrointestinal esterases to the nicotinoyl ester bonds. Alternatively, esterase activity may be poor: the methyl ester of nicotinic acid was only 15% as effective as the free acid in supporting the growth of rats (Wall & Carpenter, 1988). About 10% of the total niacin was released as free nicotinic acid after extraction of sorghum meal with 0.1 N HCl (Magboul & Bender, 1982). This suggests that a small proportion of bound nicotinic acid can be hydrolysed by gastric juice and made available.

Pellagra, the disease caused by a deficiency of both niacin and tryptophan, has commonly been found in population groups having maize as their staple food. The generally accepted explanation for this association is the unavailability of niacin in maize, coupled with a very low proportion of tryptophan in zein (the major protein in maize). Mexican and Central American peasants, and also Hopi Indians in Arizona, rely upon maize as a staple food and yet do not experience pellagra. The explanation for this paradox lies in the way in which these people prepare the maize for bread-making. In the traditional preparation of Mexican tortillas (Cravioto et al., 1945), the maize is soaked at alkaline pH in lime-water before baking and this process releases the nicotinic acid from its bound forms. In the making of piki bread the Hopi Indians use wood ash, which is alkaline and also results in the liberation of nicotinic acid. The availability of nicotinic acid in tortillas baked from maize treated with lime-water has been demonstrated in pigs by Kodicek et al. (1959).

13.4 Absorption, transport and metabolism

13.4.1 Digestion and absorption of dietary niacin

Much of the available niacin in the diet will be in the form of the nicotinamide nucleotides (NAD and NADP), with meat and milk containing free nicotinamide. It has been assumed that the digestion process gives rise to nicotinamide after ingestion of these coenzymes, since nicotinamide appears to be the primary circulating vitamer and it is not significantly hydrolysed to nicotinic acid in the intestine of the rat. Studies using various rat tissue preparations (Gross & Henderson, 1983) have led to the following possible pathway of NAD (or NADP) degradation to nicotinamide (Fig. 13.3). The initial step is an attack at the phosphodiester bond of NAD to form nicotinamide mononucleotide and adenosine monophosphate (AMP). The enzyme responsible, NAD pyrophosphatase (EC 3.6.1.22), is present in intestinal secretions and to a much lesser extent in pancreatic juice. Nicotinamide mononucleotide is rapidly hydrolysed to nicotinamide riboside and inorganic phosphate followed by reaction of the riboside with inorganic phosphate to form nicotinamide and ribose-1-phosphate. The latter two reactions require the presence of intestinal cells, indicating that the enzymes are membrane-bound or intracellular.

Schuette & Rose (1983) reported that entry of [^{14}C]nicotinamide into isolated enterocytes was rapid and neither energy-dependent nor saturable at the physiological concentrations employed (11.7 μM). Upon entry into the cells, the nicotinamide was immediately metabolized to NAD. Data obtained from this and other reports (Elbert et al., 1986; Stein et al.,

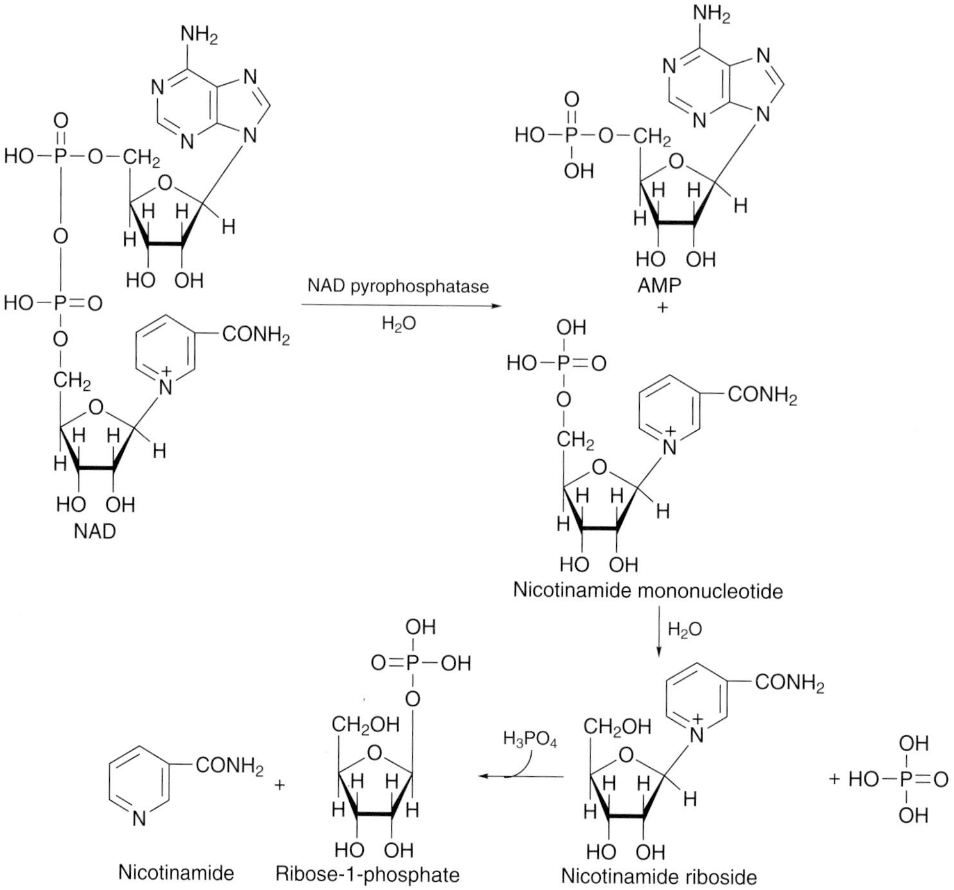

Fig. 13.3 Pathway of NAD degradation to nicotinamide in rat intestine.

1994) have led to the general conclusion that cellular uptake of nicotinamide and nicotinic acid occurs primarily by simple diffusion. This is followed by the rapid conversion of the vitamers to NAD within the cytosol. The NAD and intermediate metabolites are not freely permeable to the cell membrane, resulting in the intracellular trapping of nicotinamide and nicotinic acid. This metabolic trapping creates a concentration gradient across the brush-border membrane, which provides the impetus for passive but rapid uptake of the two vitamers.

13.4.2 Post-absorptive metabolism

In the liver, nicotinic acid and nicotinamide, together with tryptophan, are converted via a common intermediary (nicotinic acid mononucleotide) into NAD,

some of which is utilized by the liver itself. The surplus NAD is hydrolysed in the liver to free nicotinamide, which is then released into the general circulation accompanied by the nicotinic acid that was not metabolized. On reaching the tissues, the niacin vitamers are used for the intracellular synthesis of NAD and NADP. There is a continuous turnover of these nucleotides in the body and very little storage. Excess niacin is converted in the liver to methylated derivatives, which are excreted into the urine (McCormick, 1988).

In the synthesis of nicotinamide nucleotides from tryptophan, the first and rate-limiting enzyme, tryptophan dioxygenase, is sensitive to induction by both glucocorticoid hormones and glucagon. This is true induction of new mRNA and protein synthesis. The mechanisms involved are different and the effects are at least partially additive (Bender, 1992).

13.4.3   Brain homeostasis

Niacin and NAD levels in brain are homeostatically regulated. In niacin-deficient animals, levels of niacin and NAD in the brain are much better maintained than they are in the liver. Conversely, even massive doses (500 mg kg^{-1}) of nicotinamide injected intravenously result in only a 50% increase in brain NAD levels (Spector, 1981).

In plasma and cerebrospinal fluid (CSF), nicotinamide is normally the predominant if not the only form of niacin present. In rabbits, the concentration of nicotinamide in plasma and CSF is 0.5 μM and 0.7 μM, respectively. Phosphorylated forms of nicotinamide or nicotinic acid cannot penetrate brain cells without first being dephosphorylated.

The choroid plexus, the anatomical locus of the blood–CSF barrier, contains separate saturable uptake systems for nicotinic acid and nicotinamide (Spector & Kelley, 1979). The half-saturation concentrations for ^{14}C accumulation by the isolated choroid plexus with [^{14}C]nicotinic acid and [^{14}C]nicotinamide in the medium were 18.1 μM and 0.23 μM, respectively; the respective rate maxima were 439 μmol kg^{-1} per 30 min and 18.6 μmol kg^{-1} per 30 min. Nicotinic acid uptake appeared to depend completely on its immediate intracellular conversion to NAD, whereas nicotinamide uptake was thought to depend partly on its incorporation into intracellular NAD in exchange for the nicotinamide released from NAD by the action of NAD glycohydrolase (EC 3.2.2.5). The intracellular concentration of [^{14}C]nicotinamide was five times the medium concentration, so it seems that nicotinamide is actively transported into choroid plexus before being incorporated into NAD. The isolated choroid plexus released predominantly [^{14}C]nicotinamide whether pre-incubated in [^{14}C]nicotinic acid or [^{14}C]nicotinamide.

Transport studies using rabbit brain slices (Spector & Kelley, 1979) showed that uptake of [^{14}C]nicotinamide by brain cells *in vitro* was saturable and dependent on the production of intracellular energy; the half-saturation concentration of the uptake system was 0.80 μM. Spector (1979) reported that when [^{14}C]nicotinamide was injected into the ventricle of the brain of conscious rabbits, some of the radioactivity was incorporated into intracellular NAD and some left the brain and CSF extremely rapidly by a nonsaturable system. This rapid equilibration of nicotinamide between CSF and plasma suggests that there is no control of the concentration of nicotinamide in the CSF and extracellular space of brain: nicotinamide concentrations in these compartments reflect concentrations in plasma. Once within the extracellular space, nicotinamide enters brain cells by a concentration-dependent, saturable accumulation system. On entry into the brain cells, much of the nicotinamide is incorporated into NAD.

Spector (1987) measured the unidirectional influx of [^{14}C]nicotinamide across cerebral capillaries (the anatomical locus of the blood–brain barrier) using an *in situ* rat brain perfusion technique. Transport of nicotinamide was much faster than could be explained by simple diffusion alone and was not saturable with 10 mM nicotinamide in the perfusate. However, with periods of infusion longer than 30 s, there was substantial backflow of [^{14}C]nicotinamide into the perfusate. At a concentration of 1.7 μM, nicotinamide transport was not inhibited by 3-acetylpyridine. The non-saturability and lack of inhibition in the presence of a structural analogue indicate that nicotinamide transport is not carrier-mediated. The data suggested that most, if not all, of the nicotinamide that enters brain from blood gains access to the extracellular space of brain directly via the blood–brain barrier.

From the above findings the following inferences can be made. The saturability seen in the brain slices and *in vivo* studies is due not to saturation of carrier (probably no carrier exists) but to saturation of the enzymes involved in the intracellular conversion of nicotinamide to NAD. This metabolic conversion requires ATP and so accounts for the observed energy dependency in these experiments. Niacin levels in brain are controlled by the saturable system of nicotinamide uptake by brain cells. Since CSF has a nicotinamide concentration of ~0.7 μM, the uptake system (with half-saturation concentration 0.8 μM) is normally approximately half-saturated. This means that the entry of excessive amounts of nicotinamide into the brain is prohibited. As to the initial uptake mechanism, it can be speculated that nicotinamide that has entered the extracellular space of brain mainly via the blood–brain barrier enters brain cells by diffusion, accelerated by the favourable concentration gradient created by metabolic trapping.

13.4.4 Renal reabsorption

Schuette & Rose (1986) studied brush-border transport and renal metabolism of nicotinic acid in rat kidney brush-border membrane vesicles and renal cortical slices. The data suggested that reabsorption of physiological concentrations of nicotinic acid at the brush border takes place by an active, Na^+-dependent mechanism that is electroneutral in nature. Within the absorptive cell, most of the nicotinic acid is rapidly metabolized to intermediates in the Preiss–Handler pathway for NAD biosynthesis. Cortical tissue concentrated free nicotinic acid only when the involved metabolic pathways were saturated by concentrations of nicotinic acid far in excess of physiological concentrations.

13.5 Biochemical functions

13.5.1 Coenzyme role in oxidation–reduction reactions

Background information can be found in Section 4.1.

The nicotinamide nucleotides, NAD and NADP, serve as coenzymes for hundreds of dehydrogenases that catalyse a wide variety of oxidation–reduction reactions. More precisely, these compounds act as co-substrates as they leave the catalytic site of the enzyme at the end of the reaction. Examples of typical reactions are listed in Table 13.1. The oxidation of a substrate catalysed by an NAD^+- or $NADP^+$-dependent dehydrogenase is shown in Fig. 13.4. Two hydrogen atoms (comprising a total of two protons and two electrons) are removed from the substrate to be oxidized (AH_2). The pyridine ring of the oxidized form of coenzyme accepts a hydride anion (H^-), consisting of the two electrons and one of the protons; the remaining proton is released to the medium. Reduction of the coenzyme is stereospecific with regard to the hydrogen on the carbon-4 of the pyridine ring. Some enzymes have stereospecificity for the A side, others for the B side.

The nicotinamide coenzymes are not tightly bound to their apoenzymes and are not, therefore, prosthetic groups. There is, however, an important exception: glyceraldehyde-3-phosphate dehydrogenase in mammalian muscle contains a binding site for NAD^+ in each of its four subunits and the coenzyme is found in crystalline preparations of the enzyme. This enzyme has the distinction of catalysing the first reaction in the glycolytic pathway in which a high-energy phosphate compound is formed where none previously existed.

Although NAD and NADP undergo similar reversible reduction at the molecular level, their metabolic functions are entirely different. The NADH produced during the tricarboxylic acid cycle is reoxidized by transferring its electrons to the electron transport chain, thereby providing ATP by the coupled process of oxidative phosphorylation. NADH required for gluconeogenesis is generated via the oxidation of

Table 13.1 Reactions catalysed by nicotinamide nucleotide coenzymes within the glycolytic pathway/tricarboxylic acid cycle and pentose phosphate pathway of glucose metabolism.

Enzyme	Substrate	Product	Coenzyme
Glycolysis/TCA cycle			
Glyceraldehyde-3-phosphate dehydrogenase	Glyceraldehyde-3-phosphate	1,3-Diphosphoglycerate	NAD^+
Lactate dehydrogenase	Lactate	Pyruvate	NAD^+
Pyruvate dehydrogenase	Pyruvate	Acetyl-CoA + CO_2	NAD^+
Isocitrate dehydrogenase	Isocitrate	α-Ketoglutarate + CO_2	NAD^+
α-Ketoglutarate dehydrogenase	α-Ketoglutarate	Succinyl-CoA + CO_2	NAD^+
Malate dehydrogenase	Malate	Oxaloacetate	NAD^+
Pentose phosphate pathway			
Glucose-6-phosphate dehydrogenase	Glucose-6-phosphate	6-Phosphogluconic acid[a]	$NADP^+$
6-Phosphogluconic acid dehydrogenase	6-Phosphogluconic acid	Ribulose-5-phosphate + CO_2	$NADP^+$

[a]The δ-lactone of phosphogluconic acid is formed initially.

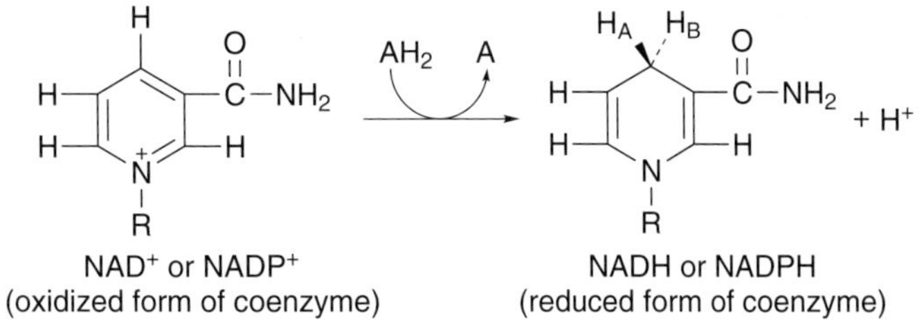

Fig. 13.4 The oxidation of a substrate (AH_2) catalysed by an NAD^+- or $NADP^+$-dependent dehydrogenase. Reduction of the coenzyme is stereospecific with regard to the hydrogen on carbon-4.

NAD$^+$ or NADP$^+$
(oxidized form of coenzyme)

NADH or NADPH
(reduced form of coenzyme)

fatty acids and deamination of amino acids. NADP, on the other hand, participates in the pentose phosphate pathway, which is not primarily a provider of energy. The resulting NADPH is used as a reducing agent to synthesize, among other materials, fatty acids, glutamate, cholesterol (precursor of steroid hormones) and deoxyribonucleotides (precursors of DNA).

13.5.2   Role of NAD in ADP-ribosylation

NAD functions in ADP-ribosylation, a reversible post-translational modification of proteins in which the ADP-ribose moiety of NAD is transferred to acceptor proteins, thereby altering their function. ADP-ribosylation reactions are classified into two major groups: mono-ADP-ribosylation and poly-ADP-ribosylation.

Mono-ADP-ribosylation by bacterial toxins

The transfer of ADP-ribose to the acceptor protein (Fig. 13.5) is catalysed by ADP-ribosyltransferases, which are found in the cytosol, plasma membrane and nuclear envelope of eukaryotic cells. The ADP-ribose reacts with specific amino acid residues on the acceptor protein to form *N*-glycosides. Certain bacterial toxins also possess ADP-ribosyltransferase activity (Ueda & Hayaishi, 1985) and, since more is known about them than eukaryotic ADP-ribosyltransferases, they will be selected as examples.

Two bacterial exotoxins, diphtheria toxin and *Pseudomonas aeruginosa* exotoxin A, prevent protein synthesis in bacterially infected eukaryotic cells by inactivating elongation factor 2, a protein required for polypeptide chain elongation. The uncontrolled action of these exotoxins results in death of the host cells. A mammalian cellular ADP-ribosyltransferase also inactivates elongation factor 2 (Iglewski, 1994), but this is a controlled action required for normal protein synthesis.

Cholera toxin and *Escherichia coli* heat-labile enterotoxin ADP-ribosylate the α subunit of the stimulatory G protein, G_s, which relays the signal from a hormone-activated cell surface receptor to an intracellular effector, in this case adenylyl cyclase (see Section 3.7.5). Cholera toxin-catalysed ADP-ribosylation inhibits the intrinsic GTPase activity of $G_s\alpha$, resulting in stabilization of an active GTP-bound subunit and persistent activation of adenylyl cyclase. ADP-ribosyltransferase activity of cholera toxin is enhanced by ADP-ribosylation factor (ARF), a GTP-dependent eukaryotic protein that functions in intracellular vesicular transport (Moss & Vaughn, 1995).

Pertussis toxin ADP-ribosylates the α subunit of the inhibitory G protein, G_i. The modified G protein uncouples from the receptor, thereby maintaining the protein as its inactive heterotrimer. Because this inhibitory G protein is inactivated, inhibition of adenylyl cyclase is removed and the result is increased cyclase activity.

Role of poly-ADP-ribosylation in DNA repair

The nuclear enzyme, poly(ADP-ribose)polymerase (PARP), has a function in the repair of DNA breaks produced by enzymatic excision of damaged DNA (Shall, 1994). The polymerase binds to and is activated by single and double-strand DNA breaks. It

ADP-ribose-nicotinamide + protein ⟶ ADP-ribose-protein + nicotinamide + H$^+$
     (NAD)

Fig. 13.5 Mono-ADP ribosylation. A single unit of ADP-ribose is transferred to the target protein with the concomitant release of nicotinamide and a proton.

then utilizes NAD for the synthesis of ADP-ribose polymers which are covalently attached to several nuclear proteins, including the enzyme itself (automodification). Automodification results in loss of DNA binding affinity and inactivation of the polymerase. Poly(ADP-ribose)glycohydrolase plays an important role in reversing the automodified state of poly(ADP-ribose)polymerase; this reactivates the polymerase and restores DNA binding.

As discussed in Section 6.1.2, nuclear DNA is condensed into chromatin by winding around histones at intervals along its length. Two molecules each of the core histones form a nucleosome core particle. To allow access of repair proteins to naked DNA, the histones must be temporarily displaced. The automodified poly(ADP-ribose)polymerase displaces histones from DNA by specifically targeting the histone tails responsible for DNA condensation. As a result, the domains surrounding DNA strand breaks become accessible to repair proteins. Poly(ADP-ribose)glycohydrolase attacks ADP-ribose polymers in a specific order and thereby releases histones for re-association with DNA (Althaus et al., 1994).

13.6   Niacin deficiency

A deficiency in niacin results in pellagra, which is a nutritional disease endemic among poor communities who subsist chiefly on maize. The classical features of endemic pellagra are dermatitis, inflammation of the mucous membranes, diarrhoea and psychiatric disturbances. The dermatitis often appears after exposure to sunlight and resembles sunburn. The skin becomes red and blistered and frequently peels off in large areas. In chronic cases the skin becomes rough and thickened with a brown pigmentation. In acute pellagra, the mucous membranes of the gastrointestinal and genitourinary tracts are severely inflamed. The mouth becomes extremely sore and the tongue is swollen and scarlet in colour. Chewing and swallowing are painful and even liquids may be refused. Inflammation of the small and large intestine is manifested by diarrhoea, abdominal pain and soreness of the rectum. Hypermotility of the gastrointestinal tract and the loss of appetite lead to profound loss of weight. Inflammation of the lower urinary tract causes urethritis with increased micturition accompanied by a burning sensation. In the female, severe vaginitis

is observed and amenorrhoea is common. Bender (1984) vividly described neurological and neuropsychiatric signs. Early signs include tremor, irritability, anxiety and depression, with delirium and dementia sometimes occurring in severe and chronic cases. Unless the disease is treated, the inevitable outcome is death. Fortunately, the response to nicotinamide therapy is rapid and dramatic.

The prognosis is complicated by signs of protein-energy malnutrition and by an imbalance of amino acid intake, particularly low levels of tryptophan and high levels of leucine. Because most proteins contain at least 1.0% tryptophan, it is theoretically possible to maintain adequate niacin status on a diet devoid of niacin but containing >100 g of protein. Primary deficiencies are rare (at least in industrialized countries), but secondary deficiencies may arise from gastrointestinal disorders or alcoholism.

13.7   Nutritional aspects

13.7.1   Human requirement

Requirements for niacin are related to energy intake because of the involvement of NAD and NADP as coenzymes in the oxidative release of energy from food. Estimation of niacin requirement is complicated by the conversion of tryptophan to the vitamin. The efficiency of the conversion is affected by a variety of influences, including the amounts of tryptophan and niacin ingested, protein and energy intake, hormonal status, and vitamin B_6 and riboflavin nutriture. A normal intake of protein will probably provide more than enough tryptophan to meet the body's requirement for niacin without the need for any preformed niacin in the diet.

A notable exception to the 60:1 conversion ratio of L-tryptophan to niacin is the state of pregnancy, in which the conversion is about twice as efficient. This increased conversion is presumably due to the stimulation by oestrogen of tryptophan oxygenase, which is a rate-limiting enzyme in the biosynthetic pathway. Conversion is also increased when contraceptive pills are used.

13.7.2   Effects of high intake

Nicotinic acid administered orally at doses as low as 100 mg per day causes peripheral vasodilatation, with the appearance of skin flushing. In high doses, nicotinic acid competes with uric acid for excretion, leading to an increase in the incidence of gouty arthritis. Of greatest concern is possible liver damage, and in one report severe jaundice occurred at doses of 750 mg per day for only 3 months. Nicotinamide does not cause vasodilatation, but is otherwise two to three times as toxic as the acid (Miller & Hayes, 1982; Alhadeff *et al.*, 1984).

13.7.3 Assessment of nutritional status

Biochemical methods for evaluating niacin status are not well established and no reliable blood test has been demonstrated. The most widely used test is measurement of the urinary excretion of N^1-methyl-nicotinamide by fluorimetry or high-performance liquid chromatography (Bender & Bender, 1986).

Further reading

Cervantes-Laurean, D., McElvaney, N. G. & Moss, J. (1999) Niacin. In: *Modern Nutrition in Health and Disease*, 9th edn. (Ed. M. E. Shils, J. A. Olson, M. Shike & A. C. Ross), pp. 401–11. Lippincott Williams & Wilkins, Philadelphia.

Goldsmith, G. A. (1975) Vitamin B complex. Thiamine, riboflavin, niacin, folic acid (folacin), vitamin B_{12}, biotin. *Progress in Food and Nutrition Science*, **1**, 559–609.

Lautier, D., Lagueux, J., Thibodeau, J., Ménard, L. & Poirier, G. G. (1993) Molecular and biochemical features of poly (ADP-ribose) metabolism. *Molecular and Cellular Biochemistry*, **122**, 171–93.

References

Alhadeff, L., Gualtieri, T. & Lipton, M. (1984) Toxic effects of water-soluble vitamins. *Nutrition Reviews*, **42**, 33–40.

Althaus, F. R., Höfferer, L., Kleczkowska, H. E., Malanga, M., Naegeli, H., Panzeter, P. L. & Realini, C. A. (1994) Histone shuttling by poly ADP-ribosylation. *Molecular and Cellular Biochemistry*, **138**, 53–9.

Bender, A. E. (1978) *Food Processing and Nutrition*. Academic Press, London.

Bender, D. A. (1984) B vitamins in the nervous system. *Neurochemistry International*, **6**, 297–321.

Bender, D. A. (1992) *Nutritional Biochemistry of the Vitamins*. Cambridge University Press, Cambridge.

Bender, D. A. & Bender, A. E. (1986) Niacin and tryptophan metabolism: the biochemical basis of niacin requirements and recommendations. *Nutrition Abstracts and Reviews (series A)*, **56**(10), 695–719.

Cravioto, R. O., Anderson, R. K., Lockhart, E. E., Miranda, F. P. & Harris, R. S. (1945) Nutritive value of the Mexican tortilla. *Science*, **102**, 91–3.

Elbert, J., Daniel, H. & Rehner, G. (1986) Intestinal uptake of nicotinic acid as a function of microclimate-pH. *International Journal for Vitamin and Nutrition Research*, **56**, 85–93.

Ghosh, H. P., Sarkar, P. K. & Guha, B. C. (1963) Distribution of the bound form of nicotinic acid in natural materials. *Journal of Nutrition*, **79**, 451–3.

Gross, C. J. & Henderson, L. M. (1983) Digestion and absorption of NAD by the small intestine of the rat. *Journal of Nutrition*, **113**, 412–20.

Iglewski, W. J. (1994) Cellular ADP-ribosylation of elongation factor 2. *Molecular and Cellular Biochemistry*, **138**, 131–3.

Kodicek, E., Braude, R., Kon, S. K. & Mitchell, K. G. (1959) The availability to pigs of nicotinic acid in *tortilla* baked from maize treated with lime-water. *British Journal of Nutrition*, **13**, 363–84.

Magboul, B. I. & Bender, D. A. (1982) The nature of niacin in sorghum. *Proceedings of the Nutrition Society*, **41**, 50A.

Mason, J. B., Gibson, N. & Kodicek, E. (1973) The chemical nature of the bound nicotinic acid of wheat bran: studies of nicotinic acid-containing macromolecules. *British Journal of Nutrition*, **30**, 297–311.

Mason, J. B. & Kodicek, E. (1973) The chemical nature of the bound nicotinic acid of wheat bran: studies of partial hydrolysis products. *Cereal Chemistry*, **50**, 637–46.

McCormick, D. B. (1988) Niacin. In: *Modern Nutrition in Health and Disease*, 7th edn. (Ed. M. E. Shils & V. R. Young), pp. 320–75. Lea & Febiger, Philadelphia.

Miller, D. R. & Hayes, K. C. (1982) Vitamin excess and toxicity. In: *Nutritional Toxicology*, Vol. 1. (Ed. J. N. Hathcock), pp. 81–133. Academic Press, New York.

Moss, J. & Vaughan, M. (1995) Structure and function of ARF proteins: activators of cholera toxin and critical components of intracellular vesicular transport processes. *Journal of Biological Chemistry*, **270**(21), 12 237–30.

Schuette, S. A. & Rose, R. C. (1983) Nicotinamide uptake and metabolism by chick intestine. *American Journal of Physiology*, **245**, G531–8.

Schuette, S. & Rose, R. C. (1986) Renal transport and metabolism of nicotinic acid. *American Journal of Physiology*, **250**, C694–C703.

Shall, S. (1994) The function of poly (ADP-ribosylation) in DNA breakage and rejoining. *Molecular and Cellular Biochemistry*, **138**, 71–5.

Spector, R. (1979) Niacin and niacinamide transport in the central nervous system. *In vivo* studies. *Journal of Neurochemistry*, **33**, 895–904.

Spector, R. (1981) Megavitamin therapy and the central nervous system. In: *Vitamins in Human Biology and Medicine*. (Ed. M. H. Briggs), pp. 137–56. CRC Press, Inc., Boca Raton.

Spector, R. (1987) Niacinamide transport through the blood-brain barrier. *Neurochemical Research*, **12**, 27–31.

Spector, R. & Kelley, P. (1979) Niacin and niacinamide accumulation by rabbit brain slices and choroid plexus *in vitro*. *Journal of Neurochemistry*, **33**, 291–8.

Stein, J., Daniel, H., Whang, E., Wenzel, U., Hahn, A. & Rehner, G. (1994) Rapid postabsorptive metabolism of nicotinic acid in rat small intestine may affect transport by metabolic trapping. *Journal of Nutrition*, **124**, 61–6.

Ueda, K. & Hayaishi, O. (1985) ADP-ribosylation. *Annual Review of Biochemistry*, **54**, 73–100.

Wall, J. S. & Carpenter, K. J. (1988) Variation in availability of niacin in grain products. *Food Technology*, **42**(10), 198–202, 204.

Weiner, M. & van Eys, J. (1983) *Nicotinic Acid. Nutrient – Cofactor – Drug*. Marcel Dekker, Inc., New York.

14
Vitamin B$_6$

Key discussion topics

- A major part of vitamin B$_6$ in plant foods is a glycoside conjugate which has a low bioavailability for humans.
- Vitamin B$_6$ levels in brain are kept relatively constant, even in severe vitamin B$_6$ deficiency, by regulated entry and exit across the blood–cerebrospinal fluid barrier.
- Pyridoxal phosphate is the coenzyme of several enzymes of amino acid metabolism and of glycogen phosphorylase.

- The vitamin B$_6$ incorporated into muscle glycogen phosphorylase is released during starvation to provide coenzyme for amino acid catabolizing reactions that produce precursors for gluconeogenesis.
- Pyridoxal phosphate acts at the level of receptor-mediated transcriptional activation to modulate the biological actions of different steroid hormone receptors.
- Vitamin B$_6$ deficiency impairs the immune system.

14.1 Historical overview

In 1934 Paul György observed the appearance of a scaly dermatitis (acrodynia) in rats fed on diets free from the whole vitamin B complex and supplemented with thiamin and riboflavin. This observation led to the establishment of a 'rat acrodynia-preventative factor' and its designation as vitamin B$_6$. The isolation of the pure crystalline vitamin was first reported by Lepkovsky in 1938, and the synthesis of pyridoxine was accomplished by Harris and Folkers in the following year. Discovery of the existence of pyridoxal and pyridoxamine and the recognition of their phosphorylated forms as coenzymes is largely credited to Esmond E. Snell during 1944–1948.

14.2   Chemistry and biological activity

Vitamin B$_6$ is the generic descriptor for all 3-hydroxy-2-methylpyridine derivatives which exhibit qualitatively in rats the biological activity of pyridoxine. Six B$_6$ vitamers are known, namely pyridoxine or pyridoxol (PN), pyridoxal (PL) and pyridoxamine (PM), which possess, respectively, alcohol, aldehyde and amine group in the 4-position; their respective 5′-phosphate esters are designated as PNP, PLP and PMP (Fig. 14.1).

In its role as a coenzyme, PLP is attached to the apoenzyme by a Schiff base (aldimine) linkage (−N=CH−) formed through condensation of the 4-carbonyl group with the ε-amino group of specific lysine residues (Fig. 14.2).

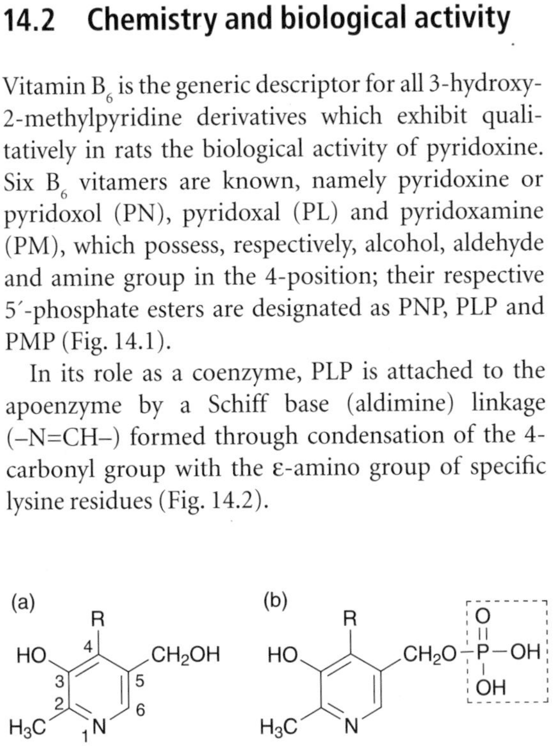

Fig. 14.1 Structures of vitamin B$_6$ compounds showing (a) nonphosphorylated and (b) phosphorylated forms.

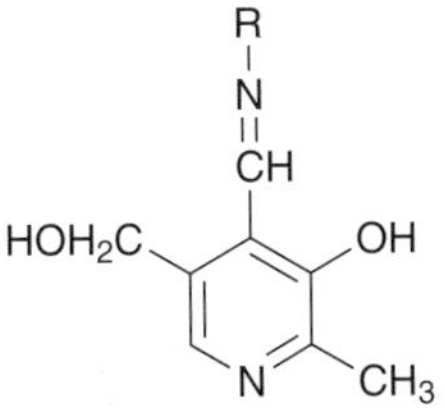

Fig. 14.2 Attachment of PLP to the apoenzyme by a Schiff base (aldimine) linkage.

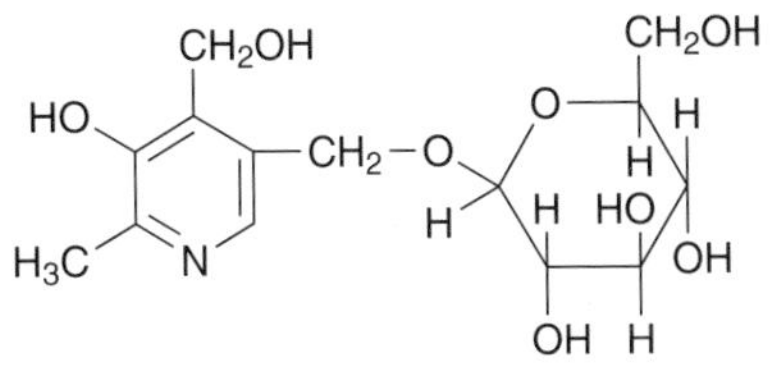

Fig. 14.3 Structure of 5′-*O*-(β-D-glucopyranosyl) pyridoxine.

A ubiquitous bound form of PN that occurs in plant tissues is a glucoside conjugate, 5′-*O*-(β-D-glucopyranosyl)pyridoxine (Fig. 14.3), designated in this text as PN-glucoside. A more complex derivative of PN-glucoside containing cellobiose and 5-hydroxydioxindole-3-acetic acid moieties has been identified as a major form of vitamin B$_6$ in rice bran and a minor form in wheat bran and legumes (Tadera & Orite, 1991).

All of the six B$_6$ vitamers are considered to have approximately equivalent biological activity in humans as a result of their ultimate conversion to coenzymes.

14.3   Dietary sources and bioavailability

14.3.1   Dietary sources

Vitamin B$_6$ is present in all natural unprocessed foods, with yeast extract, wheat bran and liver containing particularly high concentrations. Other important sources include whole-grain cereals, nuts, pulses, lean meat, fish, kidney, potatoes and other vegetables. In cereal grains over 90% of the vitamin B$_6$ is found in the bran and germ (Polansky & Toepfer, 1969), and 75–90% of the B$_6$ content of the whole grain is lost in the milling of wheat to low-extraction flour (Sauberlich, 1985). Thus, white bread is considerably lower in vitamin B$_6$ content than is whole wheat bread. Milk, eggs and fruits contain relatively low concentrations of the vitamin.

In raw animal and fish tissue the major form of vitamin B$_6$ is PLP. Apart from very low concentrations in liver, PN and PNP are virtually absent in animal tissues.

Plant tissue contains mostly PN, a proportion of which may be present as PN-glucoside and/or other conjugates. PN-glucoside has not been found in animal products. No generalizations can be made as to one group of foods consistently having a high

PN-glucoside content. Typical sources of PN-glucoside (expressed as a percentage of the total vitamin B_6 present) are bananas (5%), raw broccoli (35%), raw green beans (58%), raw carrots (70%) and orange juice (69%) (Gregory & Ink, 1987). PN-glucoside accounted for 10–15% of the total vitamin B_6 in the typical mixed diets used in an American human study (Gregory *et al.*, 1991), but would be proportionally higher in vegetarian diets.

14.3.2   Bioavailability

Losses of vitamin B_6 content caused by thermal instability occur during food processing, but the remaining vitamin B_6 does not necessarily exhibit incomplete bioavailability.

The bioavailability of vitamin B_6 in foods is highly variable, owing largely to the presence of poorly utilized PN-glucoside in plant tissues. As expected, vitamin B_6 generally has a lower availability from plant-derived foods than from animal tissues (Nguyen & Gregory, 1983). Based on plasma PLP levels in male human subjects, the bioavailability of the vitamin in an average American diet ranged from 61% to 81%, with a mean of 71% (Tarr *et al.*, 1981).

Gregory *et al.* (1991) determined the bioavailability of PN-glucoside in humans through the use of a stable-isotope method. The utilization of orally administered deuterated PN-glucoside was 58 ± 13% (mean ± SEM) relative to that of deuterated PN. Intravenously administered PN-glucoside underwent approximately half the metabolic utilization of oral PN-glucoside, which suggested a role of β-glucosidase(s) of the intestinal mucosa, microflora, or both, in the release of free PN from dietary PN-glucoside. Stable isotope methodology provided evidence that PN-glucoside weakly retards the metabolic utilization of non-glycosylated forms of vitamin B_6 in humans (Gilbert *et al.*, 1991). Despite the relatively high consumption of glycosylated vitamin B_6, vegetarian women did not demonstrate any significant difference in vitamin B_6 status compared with non-vegetarian women (Shultz & Leklem, 1987; Löwik *et al.*, 1990). In addition, the intake of glycosylated vitamin B_6 had little, if any, effect upon maternal plasma PLP concentration and maternal urinary excretion of total vitamin B_6 and 4-pyridoxic acid in lactating women (Andon *et al.*, 1989). These observations suggest that

there may be little practical significance to the human consumption of glycosylated vitamin B_6.

14.4   Absorption, transport and metabolism

Humans cannot synthesize vitamin B_6 and thus must obtain the vitamin from exogenous sources via intestinal absorption. The intestine is exposed to vitamin B_6 from two sources: (1) the diet and (2) the bacterially synthesized vitamin B_6 in the large intestine. Whether the latter source of vitamin B_6 is available to the host tissues (apart from the colonic epithelial cells) in nutritionally significant amounts is unknown.

14.4.1   Digestion and absorption of dietary vitamin B_6

Vitamin B_6 is present in foods mainly as the PN, PLP and PMP vitamers. In many fruits and vegetables, 30% or more of the total vitamin B_6 is present as PN-glucoside. The binding of PLP to protein through aldimine (Schiff base) and substituted aldamine linkages is reversibly dependent on pH, the vitamin–protein complexes being readily dissociated under normal gastric acid (low pH) conditions. The release of PLP from its association with protein is an important step in the subsequent absorption of vitamin B_6, as binding to protein inhibits the next step, hydrolysis of PLP by alkaline phosphatase (Middleton, 1986). It would appear, therefore, that the widespread practice of raising the post-prandial gastric and upper small intestinal pH by the use of pharmaceutical antacids may impair vitamin B_6 absorption.

Physiological amounts of PLP and PMP are largely hydrolysed by alkaline phosphatase in the intestinal lumen before absorption of free PL and PM (Hamm *et al.*, 1979; Mehanso *et al.*, 1979). When present in the lumen at non-physiological levels which saturate the hydrolytic enzymes, substantial amounts of PLP and PMP are absorbed intact, but at a slower rate than their non-phosphorylated forms.

The absorption of PN, PL and PM takes place mainly in the jejunum and is a dynamic process involving several interrelated events. The vitamers cross the brush-border membrane by simple diffusion as shown, for example, in everted intestinal sacs (Tsuji *et* al., 1973), brush-border membrane vesicles (Yoshida et al., 1981) and isolated intestinal loops (Middleton, 1979). In humans, PM is absorbed more slowly or metabolized differently, or both, than either PL or PN (Wozenski et al., 1980). Middleton (1983) noted a significant positive correlation between PLP luminal disappearance and both alkaline phosphatase activity and net water absorption in perfused segments of rat jejunum. It is conjectural that increased water absorption results in a greater concentration of PL within the lumen, allowing absorption to proceed more rapidly. Within the enterocyte PN, PL and PM are converted to their corresponding phosphates by the catalytic action of cytoplasmic pyridoxal kinase, and transaminases interconvert PLP and PMP. The conversion of a particular vitamer to other forms by intracellular metabolism creates a concentration gradient across the brush border for that vitamer, thus enhancing its uptake by diffusion (Middleton, 1985). The phosphorylated vitamers formed in the cell are largely dephosphorylated by non-specific phosphatases, thus permitting easy diffusion of vitamin B$_6$ compounds across the basolateral membrane. The major form of vitamin B$_6$ released to the portal circulation is the non-phosphorylated form of the vitamer predominant in the intestinal lumen.

Absorption capacity in rats was not affected directly by dietary vitamin B$_6$ supply (Roth-Maier et al., 1982) and so it is supposed that homeostatic regulation of vitamin B$_6$ is not due to a variation of absorption.

14.4.2 Absorption of bacterially synthesized vitamin B$_6$ in the large intestine

The normal microflora of the large intestine synthesizes vitamin B$_6$, but it is not known how much, if any, of this endogenous vitamin is available to the host. In human subjects, absorption of vitamin B$_6$ takes place equally well whether the vitamin is given orally or instilled directly into the lumen of the mid-transverse colon (Sorrell et al., 1971).

14.4.3 Post-absorptive metabolism

Newly absorbed vitamin B$_6$ is conveyed to the liver in the portal blood in the form of free non-phosphorylated vitamers. The liver, being the primary site of vitamin B$_6$ metabolism, supplies the active form of vitamin B$_6$, PLP, to the circulation for delivery to other tissues (Lumeng et al., 1974). Uptake and accumulation of the vitamers by the liver takes place by diffusion and conversion to phosphorylated forms (metabolic trapping). A single enzyme, pyridoxal kinase (EC 2.7.1.35), catalyses the phosphorylation of PN, PL and PM. The PNP and PMP are oxidized to PLP by pyridoxine (pyridoxamine) 5′-phosphate oxidase (EC 1.4.3.5). The newly formed PLP is contained in small, rapidly mobilized pools that have a rapid rate of turnover and are not freely exchangeable with the endogenous coenzyme pools. A proportion of the newly formed PLP is released into the bloodstream in regulated amounts bound to plasma albumin. PLP is the principal circulatory B$_6$ vitamer in normal adults on regular diets (McCormick, 1989). The remaining unbound PLP is rapidly dephosphorylated and oxidized irreversibly to 4-pyridoxic acid by aldehyde oxidase and/or aldehyde dehydrogenase (Merrill et al., 1984). The pyridoxic acid is released into the plasma and excreted in the urine. As the major end-product of vitamin B$_6$ metabolism, urinary 4-pyridoxic acid reflects the in vivo metabolic utilization of the vitamin.

Prior to uptake by extracellular tissues, PLP is dissociated from the plasma albumin and dephosphorylated by alkaline phosphatase. Cellular uptake of PL is by diffusion and metabolic trapping by phosphorylation. Interconversion between PLP and PMP occurs within the tissues. Some 80% of the total body pool of about 250 mg of the vitamin is in skeletal muscle, mostly in the form of PLP bound to glycogen phosphorylase. The liver contains a further 10% of the body pool. The cellular content of hepatic PLP is kept constant by the joint action of protein-binding, which protects the coenzyme against degradation by phosphatase, and enzymatic hydrolysis of PLP synthesized in excess (Li et al., 1974).

Effects of alcohol

The excessive consumption of alcohol meets most of the human energy needs and decreases food intake by as much as 50%. Alcoholic beverages that replace food are practically devoid of vitamin B$_6$ and the alcoholic is therefore likely to be consuming a diet that is deficient in the vitamin.

Chronic excessive alcohol ingestion can interfere with the normal processes of vitamin B$_6$ metabolism, thus leading to an increased requirement for the vitamin (Li, 1978). The conversion of intravenously administered pyridoxine to PLP in the plasma is impaired in alcoholic patients, suggesting that alcohol or its oxidation products may interfere directly with the metabolism of vitamin B_6. There is *in vitro* evidence that acetaldehyde facilitates the dissociation of PLP from its binding with protein, thereby making the PLP available for hydrolysis by membrane-bound alkaline phosphatase (Hoyumpa, 1986). Thus the generation of acetaldehyde associated with alcoholism accelerates the degradation of PLP, lowering plasma concentrations and also body stores. Ethanol may also stimulate the urinary excretion of non-phosphorylated B_6 vitamers (Hoyumpa, 1986).

14.4.4   *Brain homeostasis*

Vitamin B_6 levels in brain are homeostatically regulated. Although it is relatively easy to produce symptomatic vitamin B_6 deficiency in animals, levels of the vitamin in brain (and heart) are somewhat better maintained in deficiency states than they are in liver and kidney. Conversely, massive parenteral doses (daily intravenous injections of 200 mg kg^{-1} of PN for 3 days to rabbits) elevated the brain levels of PLP by an average of only 39% (Spector & Shikuma, 1978).

In brain, vitamin B_6 exists predominantly in the enzymatically active forms PLP and PMP at concentrations much higher than in plasma and cerebrospinal fluid (CSF). In rabbits, the concentrations of vitamin B_6 in plasma, CSF, brain and choroid plexus were, respectively, 0.30, 0.39, 8.90 and 15.10 µmol L^{-1} or kg^{-1} (Spector, 1978a).

Spector studied the *in vitro* uptake and release of tritium-labelled vitamin B_6 in rabbit brain slices and isolated choroid plexuses (Spector, 1978b; Spector & Greenwald, 1978). Uptake of [³H]PN by both tissues was inhibited by (1) low temperature (2°C) and dinitrophenol, demonstrating energy dependence; (2) pyridoxal azine, demonstrating dependence on the activity of intracellular pyridoxal kinase; and (3) unlabelled non-phosphorylated B_6 vitamers and, to lesser extent, phosphorylated B_6 vitamers, demonstrating saturability of the uptake system. There was no detectable metabolism of [³H]PN to [³H]pyridoxic acid in brain slices or choroid plexus. From 70 to 80% of the labelled vitamin B_6 in both tissues was phosphorylated after a 30-minute incubation in [³H]PN. Phosphorylated B_6 vitamers were taken up much less readily than non-phosphorylated vitamers. These

studies are not conclusive in separating active transport from metabolic trapping because both pyridoxal kinase and active transport require ATP, and therefore depletion of ATP could affect either process. Furthermore, dinitrophenol is known to inhibit mammalian pyridoxal kinase as well as preventing ATP synthesis by uncoupling oxidative phosphorylation from electron flow through the electron-transport chain.

The activity of pyridoxal kinase in brain is unimpaired by moderate and severe vitamin B_6 deficiency (McCormick *et al.*, 1961). Spector & Shikuma (1978) showed that pyridoxal kinase activity and vitamin B_6 accumulation by brain slices and choroid plexus are not affected by various drugs that alter the concentrations of PLP or biogenic amines in brain.

Spector (1978a) showed that, during one pass through the cerebral circulation, [³H]PN was cleared from the circulation no more rapidly than mannitol. Mannitol, a molecule of similar size and shape to PN, is known to be transported by diffusion. Spector (1978a) also confirmed *in vivo*, by injection directly into the ventricular CSF of rabbits, that non-phosphorylated B_6 vitamers enter brain cells by a saturable accumulation process. Kinetic studies conducted by Spector & Greenwald (1978) revealed marked differences in the uptake of vitamin B_6 by choroid plexus and brain. The half-saturation concentrations and rate maxima for accumulation were ~0.2 µM and 1.0–2.0 µmol kg^{-1} per 30 min for brain slices and 7.0 µM and 40 µmol kg^{-1} per 30 min for isolated choroid plexus. Assuming the absence of a membrane carrier for vitamin B_6 uptake, the kinetic constants refer to the binding of substrate to pyridoxal kinase and are therefore values of K_m and V_{max}. The differences in the constants for vitamin B_6 uptake by brain cells and choroid plexus are presumably due to factors (e.g. intracellular pH) that cause variations in enzyme activity.

The addition of carrier (unlabelled) PN to the incubation medium not only inhibited uptake of [³H]PN by brain slices and choroid plexus, but accelerated dephosphorylation and release of previously accumulated labelled vitamin B_6 (Spector, 1978b). These two mechanisms, acting together, would tend to keep the total intracellular vitamin B_6 concentrations constant. One striking difference in the release mechanism was that choroid plexus released predominantly phosphorylated B_6 vitamers, whereas brain slices released only non-phosphorylated B_6 vitamers (Spector, 1978b).

This makes the choroid plexus, rather than brain cells, the likely source of the phosphorylated B₆ vitamers in CSF.

Vitamin B₆ is transported in the reverse direction (i.e. from brain and/or CSF into blood) more rapidly than mannitol (Spector, 1978a). This suggests that the transport mechanism for vitamin B₆ in this direction involves a mechanism other than simple diffusion.

In conclusion, Spector's data show that circulating vitamin B₆ can enter the brain via the blood–CSF barrier (choroid plexus). The finding that PN was extracted no more rapidly than mannitol during one pass through the cerebral circulation argues against significant entry of PN via the blood–brain barrier. There is a saturable transport system ($K_m = 0.7\ \mu M$) within the choroid plexus that regulates the entry of free (unbound) non-phosphorylated B₆ vitamers from plasma into the CSF. The vitamers finds their way into the extracellular space of brain and enter brain cells by a high-affinity ($K_m = \sim 0.2\ \mu M$) saturable accumulation system. The transport system in both choroid plexus and brain cells appears to be simple (or possibly facilitated) diffusion accelerated by the concentration gradient created by phosphorylation of the transported B₆ vitamers (metabolic trapping). PN, PL and PM have comparable affinity for the vitamin B₆ transport systems, as they also do for pyridoxal kinase. Excessive concentrations of phosphorylated B₆ vitamers within brain cells are dephosphorylated intracellularly and transported out of the cells.

14.4.5   Renal reabsorption

Bowman & McCormick (1989) studied the uptake of [³H]PN by freshly isolated rat renal proximal tubular cells. Uptake was temperature-dependent and exhibited saturation kinetics with a half-saturation concentration of 1.3 μM. Inhibition of uptake by 4′-deoxypyridoxine, an inhibitor of pyridoxal kinase, indicated dependence upon this enzyme. Amiloride, a competitive inhibitor of sodium–hydrogen exchange, inhibited PN uptake in a concentration-related fashion. Partial substitution of RbCl for NaCl also caused a significant inhibition. These data are consistent with a saturable uptake process that may be uniquely mediated by the plasma membrane sodium–hydrogen exchanger. Cellular uptake is followed by intracellular metabolic trapping catalysed by pyridoxal kinase.

14.5   Biochemical functions

As illustrated in the examples given below, vitamin B₆ is involved in a wide variety of biochemical functions.

14.5.1   Role in amino acid metabolism

Vitamin B₆, in the form of PLP, functions as a coenzyme for over 100 enzymes involved in amino acid metabolism. Reactions catalysed by PLP include deamination, transamination, decarboxylation, transulphuration and desulphuration. In certain aminotransferases the coenzyme is PMP.

Metabolism of tryptophan
PLP is a coenzyme for kynureninase, the enzyme which catalyses the conversion of 3-hydroxykynurenine to 3-hydroxyanthranilic acid in the oxidative metabolism of tryptophan (Fig. 14.4). In vitamin B₆ deficiency the production of NAD from tryptophan is impaired at the 3-hydroxykynurenine stage because the activity of PLP-dependent kynureninase is lower than that of the normally rate-limiting tryptophan dioxygenase. The resultant accumulation of both 3-hydroxykynurenine and kynurenine leads to increased metabolic flux through kynurenine aminotransferase and the appearance of kynurenic acid and xanthurenic acid in the urine. Kynurenine aminotransferase is also PLP-dependent but for some reason it is little affected in vitamin B₆ deficiency. Measurement of urinary kynurenic and xanthurenic acids after a test dose of tryptophan provides an early indication of vitamin B₆ deficiency and is known as the tryptophan load test. Abnormal results of this test are subject to misinterpretation because hormonal factors unrelated to vitamin B₆ deficiency can affect the enzymes involved. For example, during stress or illness the secretion of glucocorticoid hormones induces tryptophan dioxygenase, resulting in an increased formation of the metabolites being measured (Bender, 1992).

Metabolism of methionine
The metabolism of methionine includes two PLP-dependent steps (Fig. 14.5). Activity of cystathionine γ-lyase falls in vitamin B₆ deficiency and this results in an increased urinary excretion of cystathionine. Activity of cystathionine β-synthetase is little affected by vitamin B₆ deficiency. Measurement of urinary

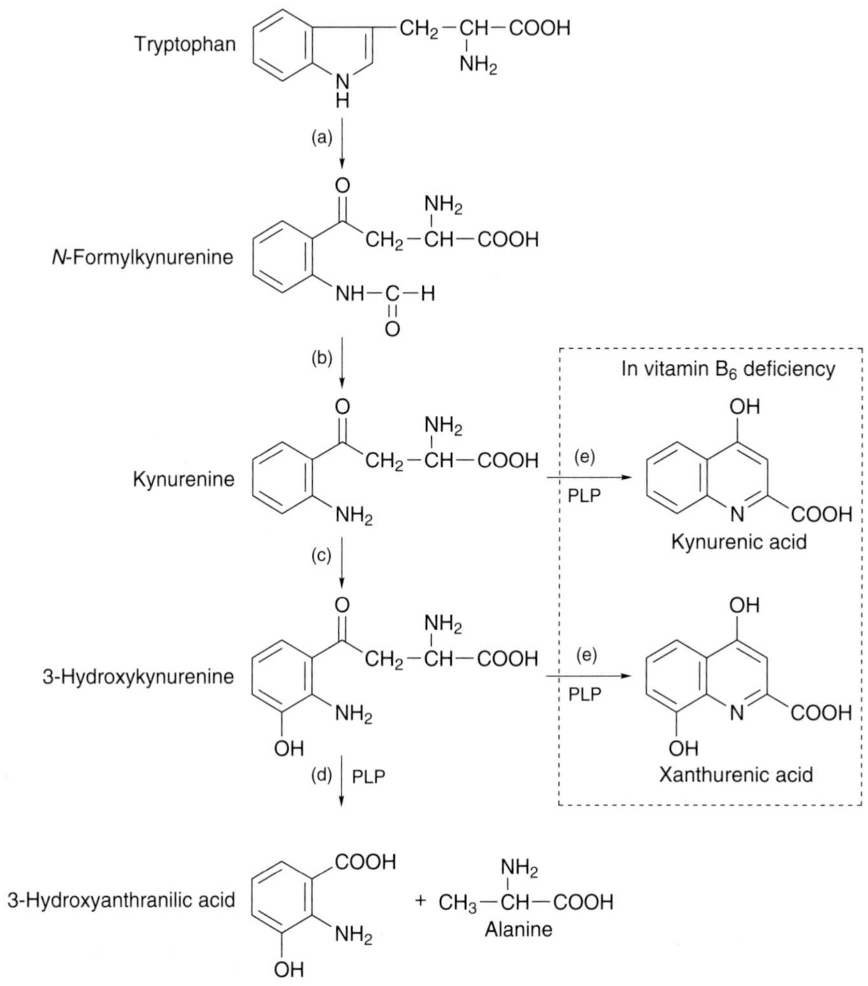

Fig. 14.4 Effect of vitamin B_6 deficiency on the biochemical conversion of tryptophan to NAD in the liver. In vitamin B_6 deficiency the tryptophan metabolites kynurenic acid and xanthurenic acid appear in the urine. Enzymes: (a) tryptophan dioxygenase; (b) formylkynurenine formamidase; (c) kynurenine hydroxylase; (d) kynureninase; (e) kynurenine aminotransferase.

cystathionine after a test dose of methionine provides another means of assessing vitamin B_6 nutritional status, which is less subject to misinterpretation than the tryptophan load test.

Biosynthesis of porphyrin

The haem proteins (e.g. cytochromes, haemoglobin and myoglobin) have in common a cyclic tetrapyrrole structure called a porphyrin. In the biosynthesis of porphyrin (Fig. 14.6) PLP is a coenzyme for δ-aminolevulinic acid synthase, which catalyses the formation of δ-aminolevulinic acid from succinyl-CoA and glycine. In the presence of the appropriate enzyme,

two molecules of δ-aminolevulinic acid condense by dehydration and porphobilinogen is formed. Several additional enzymes acting sequentially combine four molecules of porphobilinogen into protoporphyrin IX. Finally, to form haem, a specific ferrochetalase inserts the ferrous iron into the tetrapyrrole ring.

Biosynthesis of biogenic amines

Several physiologically important amines, collectively referred to as biogenic amines (Table 14.1 and Fig. 14.7), are formed by the non-oxidative decarboxylation of amino acids (reaction 14.1). The enzymes, amino acid decarboxylases, all require PLP as coenzyme.

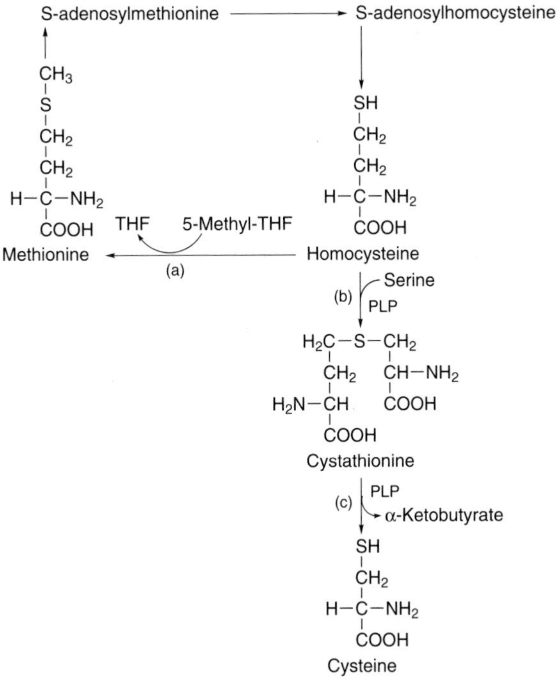

Fig. 14.5 Effect of vitamin B$_6$ deficiency on the biosynthesis of cysteine from methionine. In vitamin B$_6$ deficiency there is an increase in the urinary excretion of cystathionine. Enzymes: (a) methionine synthetase; (b) cystathionine β-synthetase; (c) cystathionine γ-lyase.

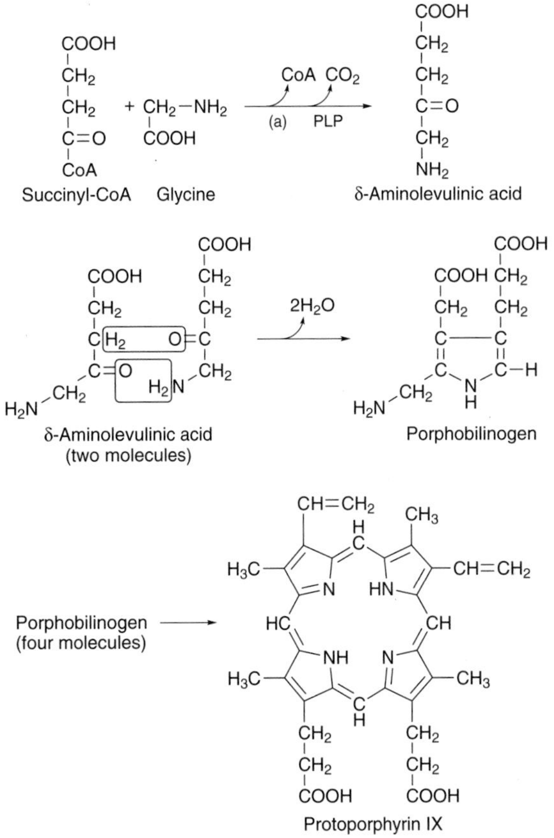

Fig. 14.6 PLP as a coenzyme in the biosynthesis of porphyrin. Enzyme: (a) δ-aminolevulinic acid synthase.

$$H\!-\!\overset{\displaystyle R}{\underset{\displaystyle COO^-}{C}}\!-\!NH_3^+ \rightarrow H\!-\!\overset{\displaystyle R}{\underset{\displaystyle H}{C}}\!-\!NH_2 + CO_2 \qquad [14.1]$$

Biosynthesis of nucleic acids

The β-carbon of serine is the major source of one-carbon units which are utilized in the biosynthesis of the purines (adenine and guanine) and thymine, the base constituents of DNA. PLP is a coenzyme for serine hydroxymethyltransferase, which catalyses the transfer of the one-carbon β-hydroxymethyl group of serine to tetrahydrofolate. The role of tetrahydrofolate

Table 14.1   Biogenic amines derived from amino acids or amino acid derivatives by PLP-dependent nonoxidative decarboxylation.

Amino acid	Amine	Function of amine
Glutamic acid	γ-Aminobutyric acid (GABA)	Inhibitory neurotransmitter in the brain and spinal cord.
Histidine	Histamine	Amplifies the immunoresponse by increasing capillary permeability and smooth muscle contraction. Stimulates gastric acid secretion.
Dihydroxyphenylalanine (DOPA)	Dihydroxyphenylethylamine (dopamine)	Intermediary in the biosynthesis of noradrenaline and adrenaline (neurohormonal agents). Is active itself as an inhibitory transmitter in certain parts of the brain.
5-Hydroxytryptophan	5-Hydroxytryptamine (serotonin)	Inhibition of pain signals in the spinal cord. Associated with promotion of sleep.

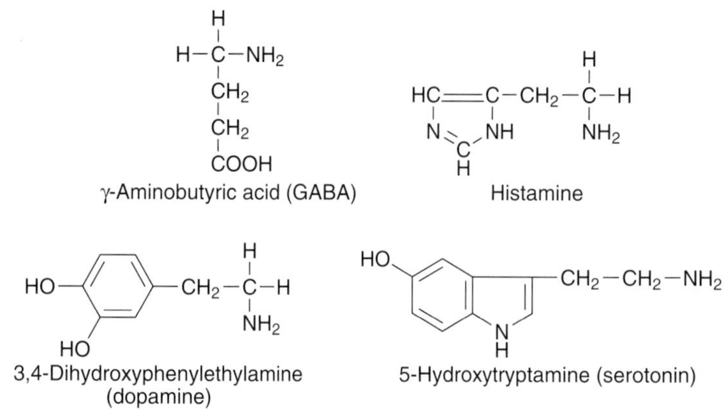

Fig. 14.7 Structures of some biogenic amines.

in one-carbon metabolism is discussed in Section 17.5.2.

14.5.2   Role in glycogenolysis

After entry into a cell, glucose that is not used immediately for energy production can be stored in the form of glycogen. The glycogen molecule is a branched-chain polymer with a molecular weight of around 5 million. The glucose units are linked as shown in Fig. 14.8. All cells of the body are capable of storing at least some glycogen, but most is produced and stored in liver and muscle. The glycogen precipitates in the form of solid granules, making it possible to store large quantities of polymerized glucose without significantly altering the osmotic pressure of the intracellular fluids.

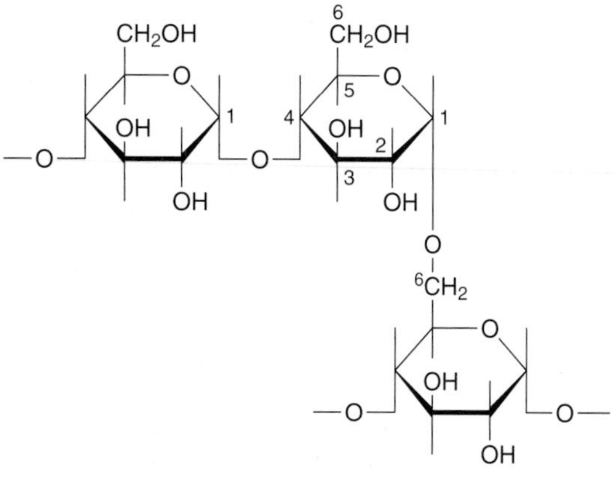

Fig. 14.8 The branched-chain structure of glycogen. Glucose units are joined by α-1,4 linkages and branch points are provided by α-1,6 linkages. For the sake of clarity, lone hydrogen atoms have been omitted.

Glycogenolysis refers to the breakdown of the cell's stored glycogen to glucose-1-phosphate. This compound is converted to glucose-6-phosphate, which then enters either the glycolytic or pentose phosphate pathway. Glycogenolysis does not occur by reversal of reactions involved in the synthesis of glycogen. Rather, each terminal glucose unit on each branch of the polymer is split from its neighbour by the introduction of inorganic phosphate. In this way a branch of the polymer chain is progressively shortened by one glucose unit at a time. This process, phosphorolysis, is catalysed by glycogen phosphorylase which requires PLP as a coenzyme. Unlike the role of PLP in amino acid metabolism, the initial Schiff base between PLP and lysine in the phosphorylase is not involved in the enzyme action. Phosphorylase attacks only the α-1,4-glucosidic linkages of the polymer chain; a debranching enzyme is required to split the α-1,6 linkages and achieve complete breakdown of the glycogen molecule.

Behaviour of muscle glycogen phosphorylase as a reservoir for vitamin B$_6$

The PLP bound in stoichiometric amounts to glycogen phosphorylase in skeletal muscle constitutes a reservoir for vitamin B$_6$ in the animal. The enzyme accumulates in muscle during abundance of vitamin B$_6$ in the diet (Black et al., 1977). There have been reports that vitamin B$_6$ deficiency causes depletion of muscle glycogen phosphorylase, but this in fact is not so. The reported fall in enzyme concentration per gram of tissue was caused by tissue growth, which diluted the enzyme present; it did not result from net depletion of enzyme during vitamin deficiency. Black *et al.* (1978) presented evidence that vitamin B₆ deficiency is ineffective in reducing total phosphorylase in gastrocnemius muscle of young rats over a period of at least 8 weeks. Prolonged deficiency did ultimately lead to enzyme depletion, but this was after anorexia had developed and weight loss had occurred. When rats were partially starved for 1 to 4 days (fed 10% of normal energy intake) they lost muscle phosphorylase but retained alanine aminotransferase and aspartate aminotransferase. When totally starved, the rats lost more phosphorylase than during partial starvation, but completely retained alanine aminotransferase, and lost some aspartate aminotransferase. Several other investigators cited by Black *et al.* (1978) have reported increased levels of PLP-containing enzymes during starvation.

From a variety of data, Black *et al.* (1978) and other groups have postulated that the reservoir of muscle glycogen phosphorylase provides an endogenous source of PLP to meet the urgent need for glucose synthesis during starvation. The PLP released from the muscle combines with appropriate apoenzymes to boost the amounts of amino acid catabolizing enzymes. The relevant enzymes act upon glucogenic amino acids (e.g. glutamate) to produce precursors (e.g. α-ketoglutarate) for glucose synthesis by gluconeogenesis (see Section 4.2.4).

14.5.3   Role in lipid metabolism

PLP is a coenzyme for the decarboxylation of phosphatidylserine to phosphatidylethanolamine, a precursor of phosphatidylcholine. Hydrolysis of phosphatidylcholine releases free choline which can be used to form the neurotransmitter, acetylcholine. PLP is also a coenzyme in one of the steps leading to the synthesis of sphingosine. A deficiency of vitamin B₆ leads to impaired development of brain lipids and incomplete myelination of nerve fibres (Dakshinamurti, 1982). Hence vitamin B₆ plays a critical role in the structural and functional integrity of the central and peripheral nervous systems.

14.6   Regulation of steroid hormone action

Steroid hormones (androgens, oestrogens, progestins and the corticosteroids) are able to enter cells, bind

to receptors and directly regulate gene transcription. The synthesized proteins carry out the ultimate effect of the hormone. Evidence accrued in the following studies suggest a physiological role for vitamin B₆ in modulating steroid hormone action.

The influence of B₆ vitamers and analogues on the physical properties of the glucocorticoid receptor has been studied using *in vitro* receptor preparations (Allgood *et al.*, 1990a). The combined data showed that, among these compounds, only PLP can directly associate with the glucocorticoid receptor and alter several of its properties, including molecular conformation, surface charge, susceptibility to exogenous proteolysis, DNA binding capacity and subcellular localization. The last two properties are requisites for regulation of target gene expression.

In a number of rat studies, Bender's group produced *in vivo* evidence that vitamin B₆ may be involved in the normal physiological action of steroid hormones. In male rats, Symes *et al.* (1984) showed that the uptake and accumulation of tracer [1,2,6,7-³H]testosterone in the nucleus of the prostate gland were significantly increased in vitamin B₆-deficient animals compared with vitamin B₆-adequate controls. In a corresponding study of female rats (Bowden *et al.*, 1986), the animals were segregated according to the phase of the oestrous cycle to avoid the inherent variations of both plasma concentration of oestrogen and the concentration of oestrogen receptor in the uterus during the course of the oestrous cycle. As for testosterone in the male, uptake and accumulation of tracer [2,4,6,7-³H]17β-oestradiol in uterine nuclei were significantly increased in vitamin B₆-deficient animals throughout the oestrous cycle; there were no significant differences at anoestrus.

Bender's group also found evidence of enhanced sensitivity to steroid hormone action in vitamin B₆-deficient rats of both sexes. In the male, testosterone is secreted by the interstitial cells of Leydig in the testes, but only when these cells are stimulated by luteinizing hormone (LH) released by the anterior pituitary gland in response to hypothalamic gonadotropin-releasing hormone (Gn-RH). Circulating testosterone exerts negative feedback control at the level of the hypothalamus, switching off the supply of pituitary LH and thereby stopping testicular secretion of testosterone (Fig. 14.9). Symes *et al.* (1984) found that the plasma concentration of testosterone in vitamin B₆-deficient male rats was only 25% of that in vitamin

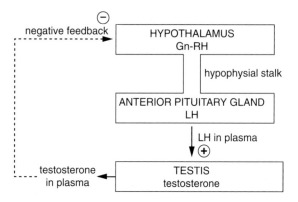

Fig. 14.9 Negative feedback of luteinizing hormone (LH) secretion by testosterone. −, inhibition; +, stimulation. Gn-RH, gonadotrophin-releasing hormone.

B_6-adequate controls. This unexplainable reduction in plasma testosterone was not accompanied by a reduction in the relative weight of the prostate gland as might have been expected; neither was it accompanied by a rise in plasma LH. These two observations suggest that there may be enhanced sensitivity of the hypothalamus to negative feedback by testosterone in vitamin B_6 deficiency, leading to normal (or reduced) plasma concentrations of LH and normal growth of the prostate despite considerably reduced circulating concentrations of testosterone.

In the female rat, ovarian secretion of oestrogen is stimulated by LH and follicle-stimulating hormone (FSH) released from the anterior pituitary gland in response to hypothalamic Gn-RH. During most of the oestrous cycle, circulating oestrogen exerts negative feedback control at the level of the hypothalamus, suppressing the release of LH and FSH. The major event of ovulation is preceded by a massive outflow of LH from the pituitary (the pre-ovulatory surge) caused by positive feedback of oestrogen upon the hypothalamus. Bowden *et al.* (1986) reported that in ovariectomized rats, doses of ethynyl-oestradiol that had no effect on circulating LH in control animals (i.e. submaximal doses) lowered plasma LH levels in vitamin B_6-deficient animals. As in the male rat, this suggests that vitamin B_6 deficiency leads to enhanced sensitivity of the hypothalamus to negative feedback by steroid hormone.

Allgood *et al.* (1990b) investigated the influence of PLP on glucocorticoid receptor-dependent gene expression by introducing a reporter gene with a defined promoter into a cell culture line. The results showed that, under conditions of moderate vitamin B_6 deficiency, the glucocorticoid receptor becomes a more efficient activator of gene transcription. Conversely, high concentrations of vitamin B_6 suppress activation of transcription. The modulatory effects of PLP concentration occurred through a novel mechanism that did not involve changes in glucocorticoid receptor mRNA or protein levels, or the receptor's ligand binding capacity. Analogous effects of PLP were found with the oestrogen, androgen and progesterone receptors (Allgood & Cidlowski, 1992). Vitamin B_6 appears to modulate steroid hormone-mediated gene expression through its influence on a functional or co-operative interaction between steroid hormone receptors and the transcription factor NF1 (Allgood *et al.*, 1993).

14.7   Immune function

Background information can be found in Chapter 5.

Vitamin B_6 deficiency is accompanied by impairment of both humoral and cell-mediated immunity (Chandra & Sudhakaran, 1990; Rall & Meydani, 1993).

14.7.1   Animal studies

Kumar & Axelrod (1968) reported a lowered level of circulating antibodies and a dramatic reduction in the number of antibody-forming cells in the spleens of vitamin B_6-deficient rats immunized with sheep erythrocytes. This decreased cellular immune response was independent of the inanition associated with the deficiency and was restored to normal by the administration of PN shortly before immunization.

Robson & Schwarz (1975) reported a dramatic 85–95% reduction in the number of thoracic duct lymphocytes and a significant reduction in cellular immunocompetence in vitamin B_6-deficient rats. These conclusions were based on the results of two tests: (1) the *in vitro* mixed lymphocyte reaction (MLR) and (2) the *in vivo* normal lymphocyte transfer reaction (NLT). In the MLR, lymphocytes from test Lewis strain rats (in this case, vitamin B_6-deficient and control rats) are cultured with genetically dissimilar lymphocytes taken from normally nourished F1 hybrid rats. If the lymphocytes are immunocompetent, they will become activated and then they will proliferate and transform into the larger lymphoblasts. The extent of blastogenesis is quantitated by exposing the cultures to [^{3}H]thymidine and then measuring the incorporation of the radioactivity into DNA. In the NLT, lymphocytes from donor Lewis rats (the test rats) are injected into the ventral abdominal wall of F1 hybrid rats. Immunologically competent donor cells produce a graft-versus-host reaction in the skin of the F1 rat. The impaired proliferation of lymphocytes and loss of cellular immunocompetence may perhaps be attributed to a cessation of T-lymphocyte development within the thymus of the vitamin B$_6$-deficient animal.

The development of functional T lymphocytes depends on humoral factors secreted by thymic epithelial (TE) cells. To investigate the effects of dietary vitamin B$_6$ deficiency on TE cell function, Willis-Carr & St. Pierre (1978) used three groups of Lewis strain rats as cell donors: (1) normal (control) rats, (2) rats maintained for 2 weeks on a vitamin B$_6$-deficient diet and (3) rats whose thymus glands had been surgically removed 24 hours after birth (neonatally thymectomized rats). Spleen, bone marrow and mesenteric lymph nodes were removed from each donor and washed cells from these lymphoid tissues were exposed to monolayers of TE cells. The TE monolayers were made from (1) normal, (2) vitamin B$_6$-deficient and (3) 'post B$_6$' rats, i.e. rats placed back on a regular diet for 3 weeks after the original 2-week B$_6$-deficient diet. Exposure of T-lymphocyte precursors from B$_6$-deficient or neonatally thymectomized donors to normal TE monolayers resulted in their conversion to functional T lymphocytes, as measured by their response in MLR and to mitogens. However, TE monolayers from B$_6$-deficient rats were unable to effect such a maturation of T lymphocytes. When the deficient rats were returned to a normal diet, TE cell function was restored. The authors suggested that the cause of defective cellular immunocompetence following vitamin B$_6$ deprivation is the inability of TE cells to effect the differentiation of T-lymphocyte precursors to functional T lymphocytes. Vitamin B$_6$ deficiency did not impair T-lymphocyte precursors, which could be stimulated to differentiate by exposure to normal TE cell monolayers. Presumably, the observed effect of vitamin B$_6$ deficiency is due to a blocking of the biosynthesis and/or release of a humoral factor that is produced by TE cells. Chandra & Puri (1985) found

significantly reduced serum thymic factor activity in rats fed diets restricted in vitamin B$_6$ and given 4-deoxypyridoxine hydrochloride in their drinking water.

Vitamin B$_6$-deficient mice exhibited impaired production and reduced activity of cytotoxic T lymphocytes (Sergeev et al., 1978; Ha et al., 1984). Antibody-mediated cytotoxicity, macrophage phagocytosis and natural killer cell activity were not affected by the level of vitamin B$_6$ intake (Ha et al., 1984).

14.7.2 Human studies

Talbott et al. (1987) investigated the effect of pyridoxine supplementation on lymphocyte responsiveness to mitogens in elderly persons who are likely to have a depressed vitamin B$_6$ status (Rose et al., 1976) and reduced immunocompetence. In vitro lymphocyte proliferation from both T- and B-cell mitogens increased as a result of vitamin B$_6$ supplementation, particularly in individuals with initially low plasma PLP concentrations. After 2 months of supplementation there was an increase in the percentages of CD3$^+$ and CD4$^+$ T helper cells and no change in the percentage of CD8$^+$ cytotoxic T cells. The increased production of helper T cells suggests that vitamin B$_6$ supplementation may have influenced the differentiation of immature T lymphocytes to mature T cells.

Meydani et al. (1991) reported that vitamin B$_6$ depletion in healthy elderly adults significantly decreased lymphocyte proliferation, mitogenic responses of lymphocytes to T- and B-cell mitogens, and interleukin 2 production. These parameters returned to baseline levels after three 21-day stages of vitamin B$_6$ repletion, when the total vitamin B$_6$ intakes were 1.90 mg per day for women and 2.88 mg per day for men. It would appear that for maintenance of normal immune function, elderly people may require amounts of vitamin B$_6$ higher than those currently recommended (see Section 14.9.1).

It can be inferred from the above observations that a deficiency of vitamin B$_6$ impairs the production of T helper lymphocytes that in turn are responsible for producing cytokines such as interleukin 2. The reduced immunocompetence seen in vitamin B$_6$ deficiency could be attributed ultimately to the role of PLP in the formation from serine of one-carbon units required for the synthesis of nucleic acids. Axelrod & Trakatellis (1964) showed that both DNA and RNA synthesis are decreased in vitamin B$_6$-deficient rats. Impairment of DNA and RNA production would cause a decrease in protein synthesis and this could adversely affect lymphocyte proliferation and biosynthesis of cytokines. Whatever the mechanism, the results suggest that elderly persons would benefit from vitamin B_6 supplements in terms of improved immunocompetence.

14.8   Vitamin B_6 deficiency

Vitamin B_6 is widely distributed in foods, and any diet so poor as to be insufficient in this vitamin would most likely lack adequate amounts of other B-group vitamins. For this reason, a primary clinical deficiency of B_6 in the adult human is rarely encountered under normal circumstances.

In a well-controlled study conducted by Hodges *et al.* (1962), six healthy male volunteers were divided into pairs and given a basic formulated diet administered by nasogastric tube twice daily. The first pair of men received a complete formula including pyridoxine; the second pair received the same diet without pyridoxine; and the third pair were given the anti-vitamin deoxypyridoxine in addition to the pyridoxine-free diet. The men receiving pyridoxine-free diets, but not those receiving complete diets, developed adverse symptoms and signs of illness, which were more severe in the men given the anti-vitamin. The most obvious symptoms were gastrointestinal disturbances and epithelial changes. Both men in the anti-vitamin group had scaling of the skin, foul breath, severe gingivitis, soreness and discoloration of the tongue and dry cracked lips. No objective neurological changes could be demonstrated. After vitamin B_6 was restored to their diet and the anti-vitamin discontinued, one man recovered promptly and the other recovered gradually.

Vitamin B_6 deprivation imposed at certain stages of brain development interferes with the orderly process of neuronal development (Kirksey *et al.*, 1990). In the 1950s, an occurrence of convulsions in infants was traced to an unfortified liquid milk-based canned formula that had undergone autoclaving in manufacture (Coursin, 1954). There is some circumstantial evidence that convulsions resulting from vitamin B_6 deficiency may be caused by an insufficient production of γ-aminobutyric acid, the major neurotransmitter in the brain (Ebadi, 1978). However, a meaningful correlation among vitamin B_6 deficiency, concentration of γ-aminobutyric acid and convulsion has not been established.

14.9   Nutritional aspects

14.9.1   Human requirement

It is well established that the human requirement for vitamin B_6 increases as the intake of protein increases (Miller *et al.*, 1985; Hansen *et al.*, 1996). This relationship is readily explained by the coenzyme role of the vitamin in amino acid metabolism. There appears to be an age-dependent difference in the protein intake-related needs for vitamin B_6 in humans, whereby elderly subjects need less of the vitamin at a higher protein intake as compared with young adults (Pannemans *et al.*, 1994). A dietary vitamin B_6 ratio of 16 µg per g protein appears to ensure acceptable nutritional status in adults of both sexes.

The current RDA for vitamin B_6 in the United States is 1.3 mg per day for men and women in the age range 19–50 years. For men and women aged 51 upwards the RDAs are 1.7 and 1.5 mg per day, respectively. RDAs for pregnant and lactating women are 1.9 and 2.0 mg per day, respectively (Food and Nutrition Board, 1998).

14.9.2   Effects of high intake

Symptoms of neuropathy due to vitamin B_6 overdose have been observed in women receiving upwards of 50 mg of the vitamin per day for 6 months or more (Dalton & Dalton, 1987). These observations suggest that chronic dosing with vitamin B_6 above 50 mg per day is potentially dangerous. Acute toxicity of the vitamin is, however, low (McCormick, 1988).

14.9.3   Assessment of nutritional status

Various biochemical methods, such as plasma PLP concentrations, urinary excretion of 4-pyridoxic acid, measurement of aminotransferase activity and metabolic load tests, have been used to assess vitamin B_6 status in humans (Bender, 1993; Leklem, 1994).

Metabolic load tests are based on an individual's ability to metabolize a test dose of a substrate whose catabolism is dependent on vitamin B_6. In the tryptophan load test, a 2-g oral load of L-tryptophan is administered and the urinary excretion of the metabolites xanthurenic acid and kynurenic acid is determined. The sensitivity of the test to intakes of vitamin B$_6$ between 1.0 and 2.5 mg (common intakes in adults) is not known, so the test may only apply to situations in which the intake of the vitamin is low (<0.8 mg per day). In certain cases the test may give results suggesting a vitamin B$_6$ deficiency where no such deficiency exists. For example, during stress or illness the secretion of glucocorticoid hormones induces tryptophan dioxygenase, resulting in an increased formation of the metabolites being measured. The ability to metabolize a test dose of methionine is an alternative test, which does not seem to be as prone to misinterpretation as the tryptophan load test (Bender, 1993; Leklem, 1994).

Because the catabolism of homocysteine through cystathionine synthesis requires PLP (Section 17.6.1 and Fig. 17.10), one might expect fasting plasma homocysteine to be a good indicator of vitamin B$_6$ status. However, fasting plasma homocysteine concentrations are not elevated in vitamin B$_6$ deficiency (Miller *et al.*, 1992), probably because of the ability of S-adenosylmethionine to activate the homocysteine catabolic enzyme cystathionine β-synthase, despite a decrease in availability of this enzyme's cofactor, PLP.

Further reading

Allgood, V. E. & Cidlowski, J. A. (1991) Novel role for vitamin B$_6$ in steroid hormone action: a link between nutrition and the endocrine system. *Journal of Nutritional Biochemistry*, **2**, 523–34.

Merrill, A. H. Jr. & Henderson, J. M. (1987) Diseases associated with defects in vitamin B$_6$ metabolism or utilization. *Annual Review of Nutrition*, **7**, 137–56.

References

Allgood, V. E. & Cidlowski, J. A. (1992) Vitamin B$_6$ modulates transcriptional activation by multiple members of the steroid hormone receptor superfamily. *Journal of Biological Chemistry*, **267**(6), 3819–24.

Allgood, V. E., Powell-Oliver, F. E. & Cidlowski, J. A. (1990a) The influence of vitamin B$_6$ on the structure and function of the glucocorticoid receptor. *Annals of the New York Academy of Sciences*, **585**, 452–65.

Allgood, V. E., Powell-Oliver, F. E. & Cidlowski, J. A. (1990b) Vitamin B$_6$ influences glucocorticoid receptor-dependent gene expression. *Journal of Biological Chemistry*, **265**(21), 12 424–33.

Allgood, V. E., Oakley, R. H. & Cidlowski, J. A. (1993) Modulation by vitamin B$_6$ of glucocorticoid receptor-mediated gene expression requires transcription factors in addition to the glucocorticoid receptor. *Journal of Biological Chemistry*, **268**(28), 20 870–6.

Andon, M. B., Reynolds, R. D., Moser-Veillon, P. B. & Howard, M. P. (1989) Dietary intake of total and glycosylated vitamin B-6 and the vitamin B-6 nutritional status of unsupplemented lactating women and their infants. *American Journal of Clinical Nutrition*, **50**, 1050–8.

Axelrod, A. E. & Trakatellis, A. C. (1964) Relationships of pyridoxine to immunological phenomena. *Vitamins and Hormones*, **2**, 591–607.

Bender, D. A. (1992) *Nutritional Biochemistry of the Vitamins*. Cambridge University Press, Cambridge.

Bender, D. A. (1993) Vitamin B$_6$. Physiology. In: *Encyclopedia of Food Science, Food Technology and Nutrition*, Vol. 7. (Ed. R. Macrae, R. K. Robinson & M. J. Sadler), pp. 4795–804. Academic Press, London.

Black, A. L., Guirard, B. M. & Snell, E. E. (1977) Increased muscle phosphorylase in rats fed high levels of vitamin B$_6$. *Journal of Nutrition*, **107**, 1962–8.

Black, A. L., Guirard, B. M. & Snell, E. E. (1978) The behavior of muscle phosphorylase as a reservoir for vitamin B$_6$ in the rat. *Journal of Nutrition*, **108**, 670–7.

Bowden, J.-F., Bender, D. A., Coulson, W. F. & Symes, E. K. (1986) Increased uterine uptake and nuclear retention of [^{3}H]oestradiol through the oestrous cycle and enhanced end-organ sensitivity to oestrogen stimulation in vitamin B$_6$ deficient rats. *Journal of Steroid Biochemistry*, **25**, 359–65.

Bowman, B. B. & McCormick, D. B. (1989) Pyridoxine uptake by rat renal proximal tubular cells. *Journal of Nutrition*, **119**, 745–9.

Chandra, R. K. & Puri, S. (1985) Vitamin B-6 modulation of immune responses and infection. In: *Vitamin B-6: Its Role in Health and Disease*. (Ed. R. D Reynolds & J. E. Leklem), pp. 163–75. Alan R. Liss, Inc., New York.

Chandra, R. K. & Sudhakaran, L. (1990) Regulation of immune responses by vitamin B$_6$. *Annals of the New York Academy of Sciences*, **585**, 404–23.

Coursin, D. B. (1954) Convulsive seizures in infants with pyridoxine-deficient diet. *Journal of the American Medical Association*, **154**, 406–8.

Dakshinamurti, K. (1982) Neurobiology of pyridoxine. In: *Advances in Nutritional Research*, Vol. 4. (Ed. H.H. Draper), pp. 143–79. Plenum Press, New York.

Dalton, K. & Dalton, M. J. T. (1987) Characteristics of pyridoxine overdose neuropathy syndrome. *Acta Neurologica Scandinavica*, **76**, 8–11.

Ebadi, M. (1978) Vitamin B$_6$ and biogenic amines in brain metabolism. In: *Human Vitamin B$_6$ Requirements*. Committee on Dietary Allowances, Food and Nutrition Board, National Research Council, pp. 129–61. National Academy of Sciences, Washington, DC.

Food and Nutrition Board (1998) Vitamin B$_6$. In: *Dietary Reference Intakes for Thiamin, Riboflavin, Niacin, Vitamin B$_6$, Folate, Vitamin B$_{12}$, Pantothenic Acid, Biotin, and Choline*, pp. 150–95. National Academy Press, Washington, DC.

Gilbert, J. A., Gregory, J. F. III, Bailey, L. B., Toth, J. P. & Cerda, J. J. (1991) Effects of pyridoxine-β-glucoside on the utilization of deuterium-labeled pyridoxine in the human. *FASEB Journal*, **5**, A586 (abstr.).

Gregory, J. F. III & Ink, S. L. (1987) Identification and quantification of pyridoxine-β-glucoside as a major form of vitamin B6 in plant-derived foods. *Journal of Agricultural and Food Chemistry*, **35**, 76–82.

Gregory, J. F. III, Trumbo, P. R., Bailey, L. B., Toth, J. P., Baumgartner, T. G. & Cerda, J. J. (1991) Bioavailability of pyridoxine-5′-β-D-glucoside determined in humans by stable-isotopic methods. *Journal of Nutrition*, **121**, 177–86.

Ha, C., Miller, L. T. & Kerkvliet, N. I. (1984) The effect of vitamin B_6 deficiency on cytotoxic immune responses of T cells, antibodies, and natural killer cells, and phagocytosis by macrophages. *Cellular Immunology*, **85**, 318–29.

Hamm, M. W., Mehanso, H. & Henderson, L. M. (1979) Transport and metabolism of pyridoxamine and pyridoxamine phosphate in the small intestine of the rat. *Journal of Nutrition*, **109**, 1552–9.

Hansen, C. M., Leklem, J. E. & Miller, L. T. (1996) Vitamin B-6 status of women with a constant intake of vitamin B-6 changes with three levels of dietary protein. *Journal of Nutrition*, **126**, 1891–901.

Hodges, R. E., Bean, W. B., Ohlson, M. A. & Bleiler, R. E. (1962) Factors affecting human antibody response. IV. Pyridoxine deficiency. *American Journal of Clinical Nutrition*, **11**, 180–6.

Hoyumpa, A. M. (1986) Mechanisms of vitamin deficiencies in alcoholism. *Alcoholism: Clinical and Experimental Research*, **10**, 573–81.

Kirksey, A., Morré, D. M. & Wasynczuk, A. Z. (1990) Neuronal development in vitamin B_6 deficiency. *Annals of the New York Academy of Sciences*, **585**, 202–18.

Kumar, M. & Axelrod, A. E. (1968) Cellular antibody synthesis in vitamin B_6-deficient rats. *Journal of Nutrition*, **96**, 53–9.

Leklem, J. E. (1994) Vitamin B_6. In: *Modern Nutrition in Health and Disease*, 8th edn, Vol. 1. (Ed. M. E. Shils, J. A. Olson & M. Shike), pp. 383–94. Lea & Febiger, Philadelphia.

Li, T.-K. (1978) Factors influencing vitamin B_6 requirement in alcoholism. In: *Human Vitamin B_6 Requirements*. Committee on Dietary Allowances, Food and Nutrition Board, National Research Council, pp. 210–25. National Academy of Sciences, Washington, DC.

Li, T.-K., Lumeng, L. & Veitch, R. L. (1974) Regulation of pyridoxal 5′-phosphate metabolism in liver. *Biochemical and Biophysical Research Communications*, **61**, 677–84.

Löwik, M. R. H., Schrijver, J., van den Berg, H., Hulshof, K. F. A. M., Wedel, M. & Ockhuizen, T. (1990) Effect of dietary fiber on the vitamin B_6 status among vegetarian and nonvegetarian elderly (Dutch Nutrition Surveillance System). *Journal of the American College of Nutrition*, **9**, 241–9.

Lumeng, L., Brashear, R. E. & Li, T.-K. (1974) Pyridoxal 5′-phosphate in plasma: source, protein-binding, and cellular transport. *Journal of Laboratory and Clinical Medicine*, **84**, 334–43.

McCormick, D. B. (1988) Vitamin B_6. In: *Modern Nutrition in Health and Disease*, 7th edn. (Ed. M. E. Shils & V. R. Young), pp. 376–82. Lea & Febiger, Philadelphia.

McCormick, D. B. (1989) Two interconnected B vitamins: riboflavin and pyridoxine. *Physiological Reviews*, **69**, 1170–98.

McCormick, D. B., Gregory, M. E. & Snell, E. E. (1961) Pyridoxal phosphokinases. I. Assay, distribution, purification, and properties. *Journal of Biological Chemistry*, **236**(7), 2076–84.

Mehanso, H., Hamm, M. W. & Henderson, L. M. (1979) Transport and metabolism of pyridoxal and pyridoxal phosphate in the small intestine of the rat. *Journal of Nutrition*, **109**, 1542–51.

Merrill, A. H. Jr., Henderson, J. M., Wang, E., McDonald, B. W. & Millikan, W. J. (1984) Metabolism of vitamin B-6 by human liver. *Journal of Nutrition*, **114**, 1664–74.

Meydani, S. N., Ribaya-Mercado, J. D., Russell, R. M., Sahyoun, N., Morrow, F. D. & Gershoff, S. N. (1991) Vitamin B-6 deficiency impairs interleukin 2 production and lymphocyte proliferation in elderly adults. *American Journal of Clinical Nutrition*, **53**, 1275–80.

Middleton, H. M. III (1979) In vivo absorption and phosphoryla-

tion of pyridoxine·HCl in rat jejunum. *Gastroenterology*, **76**, 43–9.

Middleton, H. M. III (1983) Pyridoxal 5′-phosphate disappearance from perfused rat jejunal segments: Correlation with perfusate alkaline phosphatase and water absorption. *Proceedings of the Society for Experimental Biology and Medicine*, **174**, 249–57.

Middleton, H. M. III (1985) Uptake of pyridoxine by in vivo perfused segments of rat small intestine: a possible role for intracellular vitamin metabolism. *Journal of Nutrition*, **115**, 1079–88.

Middleton, H. M. III (1986) Intestinal hydrolysis of pyridoxal 5′-phosphate in vitro and in vivo in the rat. Effect of protein binding and pH. *Gastroenterology*, **91**, 343–50.

Miller, L. T., Leklem, J. E. & Shultz, T. D. (1985) The effect of dietary protein on the metabolism of vitamin B-6 in humans. *Journal of Nutrition*, **115**, 1663–72.

Miller, J. W., Ribaya-Mercado, J. D., Russell, R. M., Shepard, D. C., Morrow, F. D., Cochary, E. F., Sadowski, J. A., Gershoff, S. N. & Selhub, J. (1992) Effect of vitamin B-6 deficiency on fasting plasma homocysteine concentrations. *American Journal of Clinical Nutrition*, **55**, 1154–60.

Nguyen, L. B. & Gregory, J. F. III (1983) Effects of food composition on the bioavailability of vitamin B-6 in the rat. *Journal of Nutrition*, **113**, 1550–60.

Pannemans, D. L. E., van den Berg, H. & Westerterp, K. R. (1994) The influence of protein intake on vitamin B-6 metabolism differs in young and elderly humans. *Journal of Nutrition*, **124**, 1207–14.

Polansky, M. M. & Toepfer, E. W. (1969) Nutrient composition of selected wheats and wheat products. IV. Vitamin B-6 compounds. *Cereal Chemistry*, **46**, 664–74.

Rall, L. C. & Meydani, S. N. (1993) Vitamin B_6 and immune competence. *Nutrition Reviews*, **51**, 217–25.

Robson, L. C. & Schwarz, M. R. (1975) Vitamin B_6 deficiency and the lymphoid system. 1. Effects on cellular immunity and *in vitro* incorporation of ^{3}H-uridine by small lymphocytes. *Cellular Immunology*, **16**, 135–44.

Rose, C. S., György, P., Butler, M., Andres, R., Norris, A. H., Shock, N. W., Tobin, J., Brin, M. & Spiegel, H. (1976) Age differences in vitamin B_6 status of 617 men. *American Journal of Clinical Nutrition*, **29**, 847–53.

Roth-Maier, D. A., Zinner, P. M. & Kirchgessner, M. (1982) Effect of varying dietary vitamin B_6 supply on intestinal absorption of vitamin B_6. *International Journal for Vitamin and Nutrition Research*, **52**, 272–9.

Sauberlich, H. E. (1985) Bioavailability of vitamins. *Progress in Food and Nutrition Science*, **9**, 1–33.

Sergeev, A. V., Bykovskaja, S. N., Luchanskaja, L. M. & Rauschenbach, M. O. (1978) Pyridoxine deficiency and cytotoxicity of T lymphocytes *in vitro*. *Cellular Immunology*, **38**, 187–92.

Shultz, T. D. & Leklem, J. E. (1987) Vitamin B-6 status and bioavailability in vegetarian women. *American Journal of Clinical Nutrition*, **46**, 647–51.

Sorrell, M. F., Frank, O., Thomson, A. D., Aquino, H. & Baker, H. (1971) Absorption of vitamins from the large intestine *in vivo*. *Nutrition Report International*, **3**, 143–8.

Spector, R. (1978a) Vitamin B_6 transport in the central nervous system: *in vivo* studies. *Journal of Neurochemistry*, **30**, 881–7.

Spector, R. (1978b) Vitamin B_6 transport in the central nervous system: *in vitro* studies. *Journal of Neurochemistry*, **30**, 889–97.

Spector, R. & Greenwald, L. L. (1978) Transport and metabolism of vitamin B_6 in rabbit brain and choroid plexus. *Journal of Biological Chemistry*, **253**(7), 2373–9.

Spector, R. & Shikuma, S. N. (1978) The stability of vitamin B_6 accumulation and pyridoxal kinase activity in rabbit brain and choroid plexus. *Journal of Neurochemistry*, **31**, 1403–10.

Symes, E. K., Bender, D. A., Bowden, J.-F. & Coulson, W. F. (1984) Increased target tissue uptake of, and sensitivity to, testosterone in the vitamin B$_6$ deficient rat. *Journal of Steroid Biochemistry*, **20**, 1089–93.

Tadera, K. & Orite, K. (1991) Isolation and structure of a new vitamin B$_6$ conjugate in rice bran. *Journal of Food Science*, **56**, 268–9.

Talbott, M. C., Miller, L. T. & Kerkvliet, N. I. (1987) Pyridoxine supplementation: effect on lymphocyte responses in elderly persons. *American Journal of Clinical Nutrition*, **46**, 659–64.

Tarr, J. B., Tamura, T. & Stokstad, E. L. R. (1981) Availability of vitamin B-6 and pantothenate in an average American diet in man. *American Journal of Clinical Nutrition*, **34**, 1328–37.

Tsuji, T., Yamada, R. & Nose, Y. (1973) Intestinal absorption of vitamin B$_6$. I. Pyridoxol uptake by rat intestinal tissue. *Journal of Nutritional Science and Vitaminology*, **19**, 401–17.

Willis-Carr, J. I. & St. Pierre, R. L. (1978) Effects of vitamin B6 deficiency on thymic epithelial cells and T lymphocyte differentiation. *Journal of Immunology*, **120**, 1153–9.

Wozenski, J. R., Leklem, J. E. & Miller, L. T. (1980) The metabolism of small doses of vitamin B-6 in men. *Journal of Nutrition*, **110**, 275–85.

Yoshida, S., Hayashi, K. & Kawasaki, T. (1981) Pyridoxine transport in brush border membrane vesicles of guinea pig jejunum. *Journal of Nutritional Science and Vitaminology*, **27**, 311–17.

15
Pantothenic Acid and Coenzyme A

Key discussion topics

- The biological activity of pantothenic acid is attributable to its incorporation into the molecular structures of coenzyme A and acyl carrier protein.
- A multivitamin transporter mediates the uptake of pantothenate, biotin and lipoate by apparently all cell types.

- Many diverse cellular proteins are modified by the covalent attachment of lipids donated by CoA or requiring CoA for their synthesis.

15.1   Historical overview

In 1933 R. J. Williams and his research team isolated from a variety of biological materials an acidic substance that acted as a growth factor for yeast. Williams' team elucidated the chemical structure of the purified substance and named it pantothenic acid because of its apparently widespread occurrence (Greek *pantos*, everywhere). Pantothenic acid was established as a vitamin in 1939, when it was shown to be identical to a 'filtrate factor' required by rats for normal growth, and to a chick anti-dermatitis factor. The chemical synthesis of pantothenic acid was reported by Williams and Major in 1940 and its biochemical role as a constituent of coenzyme A was identified by Fritz Lipmann in 1947.

15.2   Chemistry

Structures of pantothenic acid and compounds containing a pantothenate moiety are shown in Fig. 15.1. Pantothenic acid comprises a derivative of butyric acid (pantoic acid) joined by a peptide linkage to the amino acid β-alanine. In nature, pantothenic acid occurs only rarely in the free state, but it is very widely distributed as an integral part of the structures of coenzyme A (CoA) and 4-phosphopantetheine. The latter serves as a covalently attached prosthetic group of acyl carrier protein. The steric configuration of the pantothenic acid moiety is important for enzymatic recognition in biochemical reactions involving CoA and acyl carrier protein.

15.3   Dietary sources and bioavailability

15.3.1   Dietary sources

Coenzyme A is the major pantothenic acid-containing compound present in foods of both animal and plant origin, accompanied by small amounts of other bound forms (phosphopantothenic acid, pantetheine and phosphopantetheine). Notable exceptions are human and bovine milk in which free (unbound) pantothenic acid constitutes around 90% of the total pantothenate content.

Pantothenic acid is widely distributed in foods. It is particularly abundant in animal organs (liver, kidney, heart, brain) and also in egg yolk, peanuts

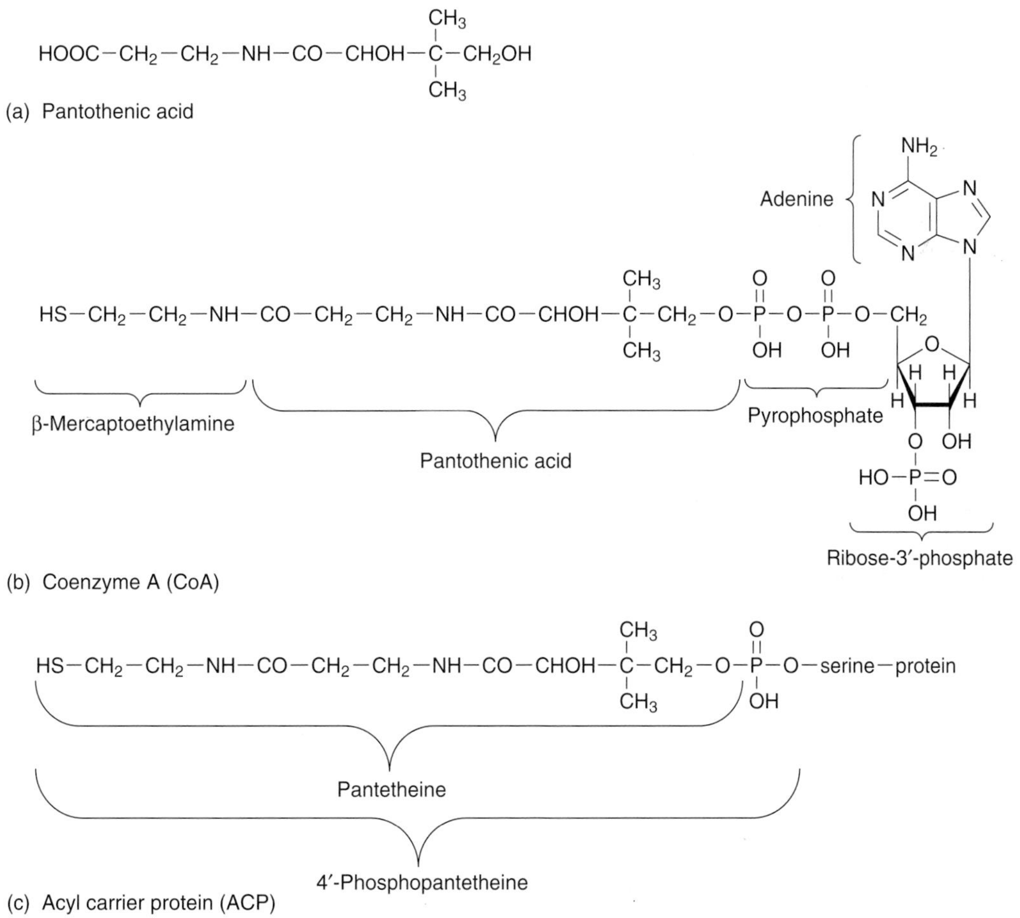

Fig. 15.1 Structures of (a) pantothenic acid, (b) coenzyme A and (c) acyl carrier protein.

and broad beans. Lean meat, milk, potatoes and green leafy vegetables contain lesser amounts, but these will be important food sources if consumed in sufficient quantity. Highly refined foods such as sugar, fats and oils, and cornstarch are totally devoid of the vitamin.

15.3.2 Bioavailability

Little information is at hand regarding the nutritional availability to the human of pantothenic acid in food commodities. Based on the urinary excretion of pantothenic acid, the availability for male human subjects ingesting the 'average American diet' ranged from 40% to 61% with a mean of 50% (Tarr et al., 1981).

15.4 Absorption, transport and metabolism

Humans and other mammals cannot synthesize pantothenic acid and therefore they rely on dietary sources of the vitamin. Pantothenic acid is synthesized by the normal microflora in the large intestine but the quantitative contribution of this endogenous vitamin to the host tissues is unknown.

15.4.1 Digestion and absorption of dietary pantothenic acid

Ingested CoA, the major dietary form of pantothenic acid, is hydrolysed in the intestinal lumen to pantetheine by the non-specific action of pyrophosphatases and phosphatase. Pantetheine is then split into pantothenic acid and β-mercaptoethylamine by the action of pantetheinase secreted from the intestinal mucosa into the lumen (Shibata et al., 1983). Absorption of the liberated pantothenic acid takes place mainly in the jejunum, although there is no significant difference in the rate of uptake in the upper, middle or lower intestine. Within the alkaline medium of the intestinal chyme, the vitamin exists primarily as the pantothenate anion.

Fenstermacher & Rose (1986) evaluated the properties of pantothenic acid absorption in the intestine of rat and chicken using several experimental approaches. Sodium dependency and saturation kinetics were demonstrated for the unidirectional influx of [^{3}H]pantothenic acid across the brush-border membrane of rat jejunum. Potassium gradients were employed in isolated ATP-depleted chicken enterocytes

to evaluate the effects of cell membrane potential on pantothenic acid uptake. Uptake was not influenced by the artificially induced electrical gradients and so it appeared that the coupling ratio of Na$^+$:pantothenate$^-$ is 1:1, making the process electroneutral. The process by which pantothenic acid exits the enterocyte at the basolateral membrane has not been established.

The sodium-dependent multivitamin transporter

A so-called sodium-dependent multivitamin transporter (SMVT) which mediates placental and intestinal uptake of pantothenate, biotin, certain biotin analogues and the essential metabolite lipoate has been cloned from rat (Prasad et al., 1998) and human (Wang et al., 1999) placenta and from rabbit intestine (Prasad et al., 1999). Transfection of the cloned intestinal cDNA into COS-7 cells has confirmed that the functional characteristics of the cloned transporter are similar to those observed in native intestinal membranes regarding substrate specificity, kinetics and inhibitor profiles (Chatterjee et al., 1999). The transporter appears to interact primarily, though not exclusively, with the long side-chain of the substrate containing the carboxylate group, which is present in pantothenate, biotin and lipoate. mRNA transcripts of SMVT were shown to be present in all of the tissues that were tested (intestine, liver, kidney, heart, lung, skeletal muscle, brain and placenta), suggesting that this carrier protein may be involved in the uptake of pantothenate, biotin and lipoate by all cell types (Prasad et al., 1998). Chatterjee et al. (1999) identified four distinct variants (I–IV) of the SMVT and determined their tissue distribution. Variants II, III and IV were present in the small intestine, with II predominating; variant I was present in the placenta, but not in the small intestine.

The number of Na$^+$ ions interacting with SMVT was calculated to be 1.6 for the uptake of pantothenate and 2.0 for the uptake of biotin (Prasad et al., 1999). This indicates that, for every pantothenate or biotin molecule transported, two Na$^+$ ions are co-transported, i.e. a Na$^+$:vitamin stoichiometry of 2:1. Since both pantothenic acid and biotin are monovalent anions at physiological pH, the transport process involving this carrier is electrogenic. Thus, both the Na$^+$ gradient and the potential difference across the brush-border membrane drive the transport process.

Whether the SMVT is actually responsible for pantothenate uptake by the enterocyte in vivo is not known for certain. If it does fulfil this function, the reason that previous studies failed to show the electrogenicity of the transport process may be that the experimental concentrations of Na^+ were not low enough to observe the sigmoidicity of the plot of the Na^+ concentration/uptake rate (Prasad et al., 1999).

Absence of adaptive regulation of pantothenic acid absorption

Unlike the other water-soluble vitamins which are absorbed by specific carrier-mediated systems (ascorbic acid, biotin and thiamin), the absorption of pantothenic acid is not adaptively regulated by its level of dietary intake (Stein & Diamond, 1989). The absence of clear-cut deficiency symptoms in humans and the lack of toxicity at high doses could explain why an adaptively regulated absorption mechanism has not evolved for pantothenic acid.

15.4.2   Absorption of bacterially synthesized pantothenic acid in the large intestine

The normal microflora of the large intestine synthesizes pantothenic acid, but it is not known how much, if any, of this endogenous vitamin is available to the host tissues. In human subjects, absorption of pantothenic acid takes place equally well whether the vitamin is given orally or instilled directly into the lumen of the mid-transverse colon (Sorrell et al., 1971). Said et al. (1998) showed that human colonic epithelial NCM460 cells took up pantothenic acid by a Na^+-dependent, carrier-mediated process that was shared by biotin. The existence of this uptake system was corroborated by the identification of mRNA transcripts complementary to the cloned intestinal cDNA in rat colon (Chatterjee et al., 1999).

15.4.3   Post-absorptive metabolism

After absorption, free pantothenic acid is conveyed in the portal circulation to the liver where the majority is taken up by sodium-coupled, secondary active transport (Smith & Milner, 1985). The heart takes up pantothenic acid by a similar mechanism (Lopaschuk et al., 1987). Beinlich et al. (1990) observed that pantothenic acid inhibited biotin accumulation in the perfused rat heart, suggesting that these two vitamins share a common uptake mechanism in the heart.

Uptake of pantothenic acid by red blood cells, unlike other tissues and cell types, takes place by simple diffusion (Annous & Song, 1995).

In mammalian tissues (but not in red blood cells) CoA is synthesized from pantothenic acid in five enzymatic steps. Three substrates are needed to synthesize CoA: pantothenic acid, ATP and cysteine. The rate-controlling step in the synthesis is the conversion of pantothenic acid to 4′-phosphopantothenic acid by pantothenate kinase. Tissue levels of CoA are kept in check by feedback inhibition of pantothenate kinase by CoA, acetyl-CoA or a related metabolite (Robishaw & Neely, 1985).

In the event of a drastically reduced intake of pantothenic acid, such as would occur during food deprivation, the liver, and possibly other tissues, is able to maintain nearly constant CoA levels for some considerable time. In fasting rats, pantothenic acid uptake by the liver is stimulated by the natural rise in glucagon, and incorporation of pantothenic acid into CoA is stimulated by glucagon and cortisol (Smith & Savage, 1980). In contrast to the liver, uptake of pantothenic acid by heart and skeletal muscle of fasting rats is reduced, and yet the rate of pantothenic acid conversion to CoA is increased (Reibel et al., 1981). Evidently, myocardial and muscle CoA synthesis is not governed by the availability of pantothenic acid to these tissues, but rather is controlled intracellularly by regulation of enzymes involved in the CoA synthetic and/or degradative pathways. Reibel et al. (1981) postulated that the large amounts of pantothenic acid stored in muscle can be shifted to the liver where endogenous concentrations of the vitamin are normally low.

15.4.4   Brain homeostasis

Spector et al. (1986) measured the unidirectional influx of [³H]pantothenic acid across cerebral capillaries (the anatomical locus of the blood–brain barrier) using an in situ rat brain perfusion technique. Transport took place by a low-capacity, saturable system that was inhibited by biotin and medium-chain fatty acids. The data suggested that most, if not all, of the pantothenic acid in brain gains entry through the blood–brain barrier. The half-saturation concentration for the transport process was 19 μM, which is an order of magnitude greater than the plasma concentration of 2 μM. Normally, the concentration of plasma pantothenic acid is regulated by the kidneys, but if one were to increase plasma levels by parenteral means, unnaturally high concentrations would gain access to the extracelluar space of brain. Thus transport across the blood–brain barrier plays no role in the regulation of brain CoA levels; rather, subsequent enzymatic steps in the brain cells regulate the conversion of pantothenic acid to CoA. This conversion is very slow, unlike that in other tissues such as the liver and heart, and could at least partly explain why the brain is the organ most difficult to deplete of pantothenic acid and CoA. The inhibition of pantothenic acid transport by biotin provided further evidence that these two vitamins share the SMVT characterized by Prasad et al. (1998). The inhibitory effect of medium-chain fatty acids has clinical significance, as in several disease states (e.g. liver failure) there are enormous increases in plasma concentrations of medium-chain and long-chain fatty acids.

The entry of pantothenic acid from blood into cerebrospinal fluid via the choroid plexus and from the extracellular space of brain into brain cells themselves are both saturable transport processes (Spector, 1986).

15.4.5 Placental transport

Evidence of an electrogenic Na^+-pantothenate (2: 1) co-transport mechanism was reported in human placental microvillous membrane vesicles (Grassl, 1992) and two human placental cell lines (Prasad et al., 1997). The system was inhibited by biotin and lipoate. Prasad et al. (1999) deduced from amino acid sequencing that the SMVT involved in Na^+-coupled transport of pantothenate and biotin in the intestine is also shared by these vitamins in placental transport.

15.4.6 Renal reabsorption and excretion

Reabsorption of pantothenic acid in the brush-border membrane of the proximal convoluted tubule takes place by a carrier-mediated, Na^+-dependent transport system that is electrogenic and has a 2:1 Na^+:pantothenate$^-$ stoichiometry (Barbarat & Podevin, 1986).

Pantothenic acid derived from the degradation of CoA is excreted intact in urine. The amount excreted varies proportionally with dietary intake over a wide range of intake values (Tahiliani & Beinlich, 1991). Both fasting and diabetes result in decreased excre-

tion (Reibel et al., 1981), thus conserving whole-body pantothenic acid under these conditions.

15.5 Biochemical functions of coenzyme A and acyl carrier protein in cellular metabolism

15.5.1 Coenzyme A

Background information can be found in Section 4.1.

CoA (HS–CoA in biochemical reactions) forms energy-rich thioesters with weakly reactive carboxylic acids, so that the acyl (R–CO–) groups can participate in numerous biochemical reactions. Some of these reactions are involved in the release of energy from carbohydrates, fats and amino acids.

- In carbohydrate metabolism, the pyruvate produced by glycolysis must undergo an oxidative decarboxylation reaction with CoA to form acetyl-CoA (CH_3–CO–S–CoA in biochemical reactions) before the acetyl moiety can react with oxaloacetate to produce citrate in the tricarboxylic acid cycle.
- Another tricarboxylic acid cycle intermediate, α-ketoglutarate, undergoes an oxidative decarboxylation with CoA to form succinyl-CoA. Succinyl-CoA reacts with glycine to form (via an intermediate) δ-aminolevulinic acid, which is a precursor of the porphyrin ring system of haemoglobin and cytochromes.
- CoA is required at two steps in each cycle of the β-oxidation of fatty acids, in which two carbon units are removed per cycle to yield ultimately acetyl-CoA.
- In amino acid metabolism, leucine is deaminated to form the keto acid isovalerylformic acid, which reacts with CoA to yield a series of intermediates, ultimately giving rise to acetoacetic acid and acetyl-CoA.
- Acetyl-CoA is required for the acetylation of choline to form the neurotransmitter acetylcholine.
- The amino sugars D-glucosamine and D-galactosamine react with acetyl-CoA to form acetylated products, which are structural components of various mucopolysaccharides. For example, hyaluronic acid, which is found in connective tissue, the vitreous humour of the eye, and Wharton's jelly in the

umbilical cord, consists of alternating residues of N-acetyl-D-glucosamine and D-glucuronic acid.

- Chondroitin sulphate, found in the matrix of cartilage and bone, heart valves, tendons, and the cornea, is built up from sulphated esters of N-acetyl-D-galactosamine and D-glucuronic acid.
- The biosynthesis of cholesterol begins with the condensation of two molecules of acetyl-CoA to form acetoacetyl-CoA. The latter reacts with a third molecule of acetyl-CoA to form β-hydroxy-β-methylglutaryl-CoA (HMG-CoA), which in turn is reduced to mevalonic acid.

Mevalonic acid is an important intermediate because it gives rise to isoprenoids that are involved in the modification of functional proteins (Section 15.6). As well as being synthesized within the cell, cholesterol enters the cell from receptor-mediated uptake of plasma low-density lipoprotein (LDL). The cell must balance the endogenous and exogenous sources of cholesterol to avoid over-accumulation of the sterol, while sustaining adequate mevalonic acid synthesis. This balance is achieved through feedback regulation of at least two sequential enzymes in mevalonic acid synthesis, HMG-CoA synthase and HMG-CoA reductase, and also of LDL receptors (Fig. 15.2). In the absence of LDL, animal cells maintain high activities of the two enzymes, thereby synthesizing mevalonic acid for production of cholesterol as well as the essential isoprenoids. When LDL is present, the synthase and reductase activities decline by more than 90%, and the cells produce only the small amounts of mevalonic acid needed for the non-sterol end-products. When cellular sterol levels rise or when cell growth ceases and cholesterol demand declines, the LDL receptor gene is repressed, further averting cholesterol accumulation.

15.5.2 Acyl carrier protein

Acyl carrier protein, as an integral part of fatty acid synthase, is involved in the biosynthesis of fatty acids. Apart from dietary fat, the major source of fatty acids in the animal body is carbohydrate, which is broken down to pyruvate by the glycolytic pathway in the cytoplasm of all cells. Pyruvate moves by passive diffusion from the cytosol into the matrix of the mitochondrion where it is (1) oxidized to acetyl-CoA and (2) carboxylated to oxaloacetate. Acetyl-CoA is the

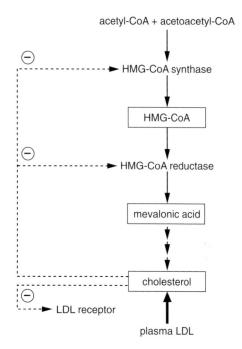

Fig. 15.2 Regulation of the mevalonic acid pathway showing cholesterol-mediated feedback repression of the genes for HMG-CoA synthase, HMG-CoA reductase and the LDL receptors.

starting material for the synthesis of fatty acids. The formation of acetyl-CoA in the mitochondrion poses a problem because the enzyme complex required for fatty acid synthesis (fatty acid synthase) is located in the cytosol. The cell circumvents this problem in the following way. The acetyl-CoA and oxaloacetate react together to form CoA and citrate, and the latter is transported out of the mitochondrion to the cytosol. In the cytosol citrate reacts with CoA to form oxaloacetate and acetyl-Co. Acetyl-CoA, with the required amounts of ATP and NADPH, is now ready to serve as substrate to form palmitate.

The fatty acid synthase enzyme complex in vertebrates consists of two identical subunits, each with a molecular weight of 240 000 and each containing the full complement of enzymes required for fatty acid synthesis. Each subunit is totally inactive in synthesizing a fatty acid: only when the two subunits combine in an antiparallel orientation to form a homodimer is activity expressed. In addition to ACP, the fatty acid synthase complex contains condensing enzyme, which also possesses a free sulphydryl (–SH) group.

The involvement of ACP in fatty acid biosynthesis is depicted in Fig. 15.3. Malonyl-CoA is formed by the

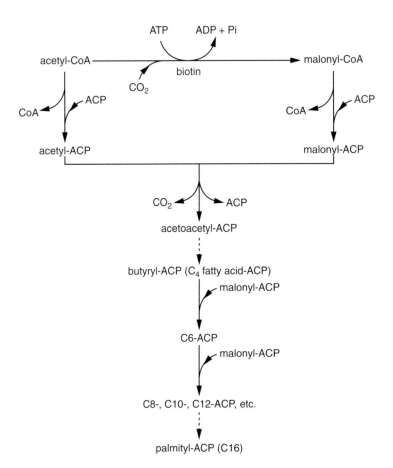

Fig. 15.3 The role of acyl carrier protein (ACP) in the biosynthesis of fatty acids. For simplicity, the contribution of condensing enzyme is not shown.

biotin-dependent carboxylation of acetyl-CoA and the acyl groups of acetyl-CoA and malonyl-CoA are transferred to the –SH group of acyl carrier protein (ACP). The resultant acetyl-ACP and malonyl-ACP molecules react together with the release of CO_2 to form acetoacetyl-ACP, which undergoes further reduction and dehydration reactions to yield butyryl-ACP. This, in turn, reacts with malonyl-ACP, with a repetition of the same sequence of events, to yield a six-carbon fatty acyl ACP derivative. The process is repeated, adding two carbon atoms at a time to the growing chain, until the palmityl derivative with 16 carbon atoms is formed. The ACP moiety then splits off and the palmitic acid is released. The palmitic acid can be lengthened by fatty acid elongation systems to stearic acid and even longer saturated fatty acids. Furthermore, by desaturation reactions, palmitate and stearate can be converted to their corresponding Δ^9 mono-unsaturated fatty acids – palmitoleic and oleic acids, respectively.

15.6 Physiological roles of coenzyme A in the modification of proteins

15.6.1 Protein modification

Many diverse cellular proteins are modified by the covalent attachment of lipids donated by CoA or requiring CoA for their synthesis. The modifications fall into three main categories: acetylation, acylation and isoprenylation (Magee, 1990; Casey, 1994). The alterations in protein structure may be relevant to the association of proteins with the plasma membrane or with subcellular membranes, protein–protein binding, or the targeting of proteins to specific intracellular locations. In some cases the modifications are co-translational, i.e. they take place on the growing polypeptide chain associated with the ribosome during protein synthesis; in other cases they are post-translational.

Most soluble proteins are acetylated at their amino termini as a means of altering their binding affinity for receptors or other proteins. Internal acetylation of nuclear histones weakens their association with DNA. The two long-chain fatty acids most commonly attached to proteins are myristic acid (14:0) and palmitic acid (16:0). The enzyme linking myristate to amino-terminal glycine residues by an amide bond is *N*-myristoyl transferase, which has strict sequence requirements in the protein substrate. Palmitoyl transferases link palmitate to the side chains of cysteine residues by a thioester bond. The cysteine residues can reside at any point in the primary structure of the protein; there is little evidence for any specific sequence requirements. Unlike the highly stable amide linkages to myristate, modifications of proteins by palmitate occur in thioester or oxyester linkages that are subject to hydrolysis by esterases. Cycles of palmitoylation and depalmitoylation allow the modified protein to have a regulating function. Addition of an isoprenoid chain to the cysteine residue of the primary motif CAAX (C, cysteine; AA, an aliphatic amino acid; X, the carboxy terminal amino acid) is the first step in the modification of proteins bearing this C-terminal motif. Either the 15-carbon farnesyl or the 20-carbon geranylgeranyl chain is added, depending on the sequence of the CAAX motif.

Myristoylated proteins include G protein α subunits (signal transduction), ADP-ribosylation factors (vesicular transport), myristoylated alanine-rich C kinase substrate protein (cytoskeletal rearrangements), recoverin (vision), proteins of the immune system, and several enzymes. Palmitoylated proteins include G protein α subunits, many plasma membrane-anchored receptors, cytoskeletal proteins, gap junction proteins, neuronal proteins, and the enzymes acetylcholinesterase and glutamic acid decarboxylase. Palmitate modification is also a prerequisite for the budding of transport vesicles from Golgi cisternae. Isoprenylated proteins include Ras proteins (signal transduction), Rab proteins (vesicular transport), nuclear lamins A and B (assembly and stabilization of the nuclear envelope), G protein γ subunits, and the enzymes phosphorylase kinase and rhodopsin kinase.

15.6.2 Physiological implications of protein modification

The physiological implications of protein modifications involving coenzyme A are illustrated in the following examples.

Acetylation of β-endorphin

Amino-terminal acetylation plays an important role in regulating the biological activity of the brain neurotransmitter β-endorphin. This peptide has morphine-like analgesic activity and also affects sexual behaviour and learning. Acetylation deactivates β-endorphin by rendering it unable to bind to specific receptors. The modification is post-translational and occurs before or during the packaging of the peptide into the secretory granules of neurotransmitter neurons in the pituitary gland (Glembotski, 1982; Chappell *et al.*, 1986).

Histone acetylation

Background information can be found in Section 6.6.4.

The DNA in cell nuclei does not exist in the 'naked' state – rather it is compacted into chromatin by winding around specific DNA-binding proteins called histones. The fundamental repeating unit of chromatin is the nucleosome. The organization of chromatin into nucleosomes is an essential feature in the regulation of gene transcription – the step in protein synthesis in which messenger RNA is synthesized from DNA.

It is necessary to control gene transcription so that only those proteins needed by a particular cell for a specific purpose are synthesized. When a protein is not needed, nucleosomes prevent transcription by impeding the access of factors required to initiate and regulate this process. When protein synthesis is required, changes in cell physiology cause a partial and localized alteration of chromatin structure (chromatin remodelling) in a manner that permits the binding of initiating and regulatory factors. One important chromatin remodelling system involves the enzyme-catalysed acetylation/deacetylation of core histones. Histone acetylation, which results in activation of transcription, requires acetyl-CoA as the acetyl donor (see Fig. 6.14).

α-Tubulin acetylation

Microtubules are constituents of the cytoskeleton and are composed of polymerized α- and β-tubulin dimers (Section 3.1.1). A subset of the α-tubulin is modified, like the histones, by post-translational acetylation of the ε-amino group of specific lysine residues. In contrast to histone acetylation, the acetylation of α-tubulin stabilizes the polymeric structure of the microtubule; deacetylation is coupled to depolymerization (Plesofsky-Vig & Brambl, 1988).

Acylation of G proteins

Background information can be found in Section 3.7.5.

The biological activity of peptide hormones is mediated by second messengers such as cyclic AMP whose formation is triggered by the action of a G protein upon an effector enzyme. The reversible translocation of the G protein α-subunit between the plasma membrane and the cytoplasm is facilitated by the detachment and re-attachment of a palmitate group. Coenzyme A is required as the palmitate donor when Gα is palmitoylated by palmitoyl transferase (see Fig. 3.29).

The α-subunit of the G_i family of G proteins is further modified by the covalent attachment of myristic acid, which takes place during or immediately after translation. This modification is usually irreversible and therefore an unlikely target for regulation. Myristoylation promotes membrane attachment of the α subunit by increasing its affinity for membrane-bound βγ subunits; it also facilitates productive interaction with adenylate cyclase (Wilson & Bourne, 1995).

Farnesylation of rhodopsin kinase

Rhodopsin kinase, the enzyme which phosphorylates the photon-stimulated receptor rhodopsin and desensitizes the visual signal, is translocated from the cytosol to the rod outer segment membrane upon light exposure. This light-induced translocation is facilitated by farnesylation of the enzyme's CAAX motif (Inglese et al., 1992). The synthesis of farnesol (an isoprenyl compound) requires CoA.

15.7 Deficiency in animals and humans

15.7.1 Animals

Pantothenic acid deficiency has been induced experimentally in many species of animals and birds by feeding diets containing low levels of the vitamin. The wide range of deficiency signs, histopathological abnormalities and metabolic changes indicate disorders of the nervous system, reproductive system, gastrointestinal tract and immune system. Immune defects in deficient animals have been attributed primarily to a block in the secretion of newly synthesized proteins out of the cell, resulting in their accumulation in the smooth endoplasmic reticulum (Axelrod, 1971). Rodents are particularly prone to necrosis and haemorrhage of the adrenal glands with consequent impairment of adrenal endocrine function. In young animals, the earliest sign of deficiency is a decline in the rate of growth. Distinctive visible signs are depigmentation of fur in rats and mice, and rough plumage and exudative lesions around the beak and eyelids of chickens. 'Goose-stepping' of the hind legs in pigs and ataxia in chicks are associated with demyelination of the motor neurons.

15.7.2 Humans

Human pantothenic acid deficiency has been carefully studied in healthy male volunteers given an emulsified artificial diet by stomach tube. In one study (Hodges et al., 1958), two subjects received the basic diet devoid of pantothenic acid, a second pair received the same diet with added antagonist (omega-methyl pantothenic acid), and a third pair (the controls) received the diet supplemented with pantothenic acid. After about 4 weeks, subjects receiving the antagonist and those in the deficient group began to show similar symptoms of illness. Clinical observations were irritability, restlessness, drowsiness, insomnia, impaired motor co-ordination, and neurological manifestations such as numbness and 'burning feet' syndrome. The most persistent and troublesome symptoms were fatigue, headache and the sensation of weakness. Among the laboratory tests, the loss of eosinopenic response to adrenocorticotropic hormone indicated adrenocortical insufficiency.

15.8 Dietary intake

A Recommended Dietary Allowance (RDA) for a nutrient is derived from an Estimated Average Requirement (EAR), which is an estimate of the intake at which the risk of inadequacy to an individual is 50%. In the case of pantothenic acid, no data have been found on which to base an EAR, and an Adequate Intake (AI) is used instead of an RDA in the USA. The AI for infants up to 12 months old (1.7–1.8 mg per day) reflects the observed mean intake of breast-fed infants. The AI for children aged 1 to 3 years (2 mg per day) is extrapolated from adult values. The AIs for children aged 4 to 13 years (3–4 mg per day), and adolescents and adults of both sexes (5 mg per day) are based on pantothenic acid intake sufficient to replace urinary excretion. AIs for women during pregnancy and lactation are 6 mg per day and 7 mg per day, respectively (Institute of Medicine, 1998).

There are no known toxic effects of oral pantothenic acid in humans or animals.

Further reading

Plesofsky-Vig, N. (1999) Pantothenic acid. In: *Modern Nutrition in Health and Disease*, 9th edn. (Ed. M. E. Shils, J. A. Olson, M. Shike & A. C. Ross), pp. 423–32. Lippincott Williams & Wilkins, Philadelphia.

Smith, C. M. & Song, W. O. (1996) Comparative nutrition of pantothenic acid. *Journal of Nutritional Biochemistry*, 7, 312–21.

References

Annous, K. F. & Song, W. O. (1995) Pantothenic acid uptake and metabolism by red blood cells of rats. *Journal of Nutrition*, 125, 2586–93.

Axelrod, A. E. (1971) Immune processes in vitamin deficiency states. *American Journal of Clinical Nutrition*, 24, 265–71.

Barbarat, B. & Podevin, R.-A. (1986) Pantothenate-sodium cotransport in renal brush-border membranes. *Journal of Biological Chemistry*, 261(31), 14 455–60.

Beinlich, C. J., Naumovitz, R. D., Song, W. O. & Neely, J. R. (1990) Myocardial metabolism of pantothenic acid in chronically diabetic rats. *Journal of Molecular and Cellular Cardiology*, 22, 323–32.

Casey, P. J. (1994) Lipid modifications of G proteins. *Current Opinion in Cell Biology*, 6, 219–25.

Chappell, M. C., O'Donohue, T. L., Millington, W. M. & Kempner, E. S. (1986) The size of enzymes acetylating α-melanocyte-stimulating hormone and β-endorphin. *Journal of Biological Chemistry*, 261(3), 1088–90.

Chatterjee, N. S., Kumar, C. K., Ortiz, A., Rubin, S. A. & Said, H. M. (1999) Molecular mechanism of the intestinal biotin transport process. *American Journal of Physiology*, 277, C605–13.

Fenstermacher, D. K. & Rose, R. C. (1986) Absorption of pantothenic acid in rat and chick intestine. *American Journal of Physiology*, 250, G155–60.

Glembotski, C. C. (1982) Characterization of the peptide acetyltransferase activity in bovine and rat intermediate pituitaries responsible for the acetylation of β-endorphin and α-melanotropin. *Journal of Biological Chemistry*, 257(17), 10 501–9.

Grassl, S. M. (1992) Human placental brush-border membrane Na^+-pantothenate cotransport. *Journal of Biological Chemistry*, 267(32), 22 902–6.

Hodges, R. E., Ohlson, M. A. & Bean, W. B. (1958) Pantothenic acid deficiency in man. *Journal of Clinical Investigation*, 37, 1642–57.

Inglese, J., Glickman, J. F., Lorenz, W., Caron, M. G. & Lefkowitz, R. J. (1992) Isoprenylation of a protein kinase. Requirement of farnesylation/α-carboxyl methylation for full enzymatic activity of rhodopsin kinase. *Journal of Biological Chemistry*, 267(3), 1422–5.

Institute of Medicine (1998) *Dietary Reference Intakes for Thiamin, Riboflavin, Niacin, Vitamin B_6, Folate, Vitamin B_{12}, Pantothenic Acid, Biotin, and Choline*. National Academy Press, Washington, DC.

Lopaschuk, G. D., Michalak, M. & Tsang, H. (1987) Regulation of pantothenic acid transport in the heart. Involvement of a Na^+-cotransport system. *Journal of Biological Chemistry*, 262(8), 3615–19.

Magee. A. I. (1990) Lipid modification of proteins and its relevance to protein targeting. *Journal of Cell Science*, 97, 581–4.

Plesofsky-Vig, N. & Brambl, R. (1988) Pantothenic acid and coenzyme A in cellular modification of proteins. *Annual Review of Nutrition*, 8, 461–82.

Prasad, P. D., Ramamoorthy, S., Leibach, F. H. & Ganapathy, V. (1997) Characterization of a sodium-dependent vitamin transporter mediating the uptake of pantothenate, biotin and lipoate in human placental choriocarcinoma cells. *Placenta*, 18, 527–33.

Prasad, P. D., Wang, H., Kekuda, R., Fujita, T., Fei, Y.-J., Devoe, L. D., Leibach, F. H. & Ganapathy, V. (1998) Cloning and functional expression of a cDNA encoding a mammalian sodium-dependent vitamin transporter mediating the uptake of pantothenate, biotin, and lipoate. *Journal of Biological Chemistry*, 273(13), 7501–6.

Prasad, P. D., Wang, H., Huang, W., Fei, Y.-J., Leibach, F. H., Devoe, L. D. & Ganapathy, V. (1999) Molecular and functional characterization of the intestinal Na^+-dependent multivitamin transporter. *Archives of Biochemistry and Biophysics*, 366, 95–106.

Reibel, D. K., Wyse, B. W., Berkich, D. A. & Palko, W. M. (1981) Effects of diabetes and fasting on pantothenic acid metabolism in rats. *American Journal of Physiology*, 240, E597–E601.

Robishaw, J. D. & Neely, J. R. (1985) Coenzyme A metabolism. *American Journal of Physiology*, 248, E1–E9.

Said, H. M., Ortiz, A., McCloud, E., Dyer, D., Moyer, M. P. & Rubin, S. (1998) Biotin uptake by human colonic epithelial NCM460 cells: a carrier-mediated process shared with pantothenic acid. *American Journal of Physiology*, 275, C1365–71.

Shibata, K., Gross, C. J. & Henderson, L. M. (1983) Hydrolysis and absorption of pantothenate and its coenzymes in the rat small intestine. *Journal of Nutrition*, 113, 2107–15.

Smith, C. M. & Milner, R. E. (1985) The mechanism of pantothenate transport by rat liver parenchymal cells in primary culture. *Journal of Biological Chemistry*, 260(8), 4823–31.

Smith, C. M. & Savage, C. R. Jr. (1980) Regulation of Coenzyme A biosynthesis by glucagon and glucocorticoid in adult rat liver parenchymal cells. *Biochemical Journal*, 188, 175–84.

Sorrell, M. F., Frank, O., Thomson, A. D., Aquino, H. & Baker, H. (1971) Absorption of vitamins from the large intestine in vivo. *Nutrition Reports International*, 3, 143–8.

Spector, R. (1986) Pantothenic acid transport and metabolism in the central nervous system. *American Journal of Physiology*, 250, R292–7.

Spector, R., Sivesind, C. & Kinzenbaw, D. (1986) Pantothenic acid transport through the blood–brain barrier. *Journal of Neurochemistry*, 47, 966–71.

Stein, E. D. & Diamond, J. M. (1989) Do dietary levels of pantothenic acid regulate its intestinal uptake in mice? *Journal of Nutrition*, 119, 1973–83.

Tahiliani, A. G. & Beinlich, C. J. (1991) Pantothenic acid in health and disease. *Vitamins and Hormones*, 46, 165–228.

Tarr, J. B., Tamura, T. & Stokstad, E. L. R. (1981) Availability of vitamin B-6 and pantothenate in an average American diet in man.

American Journal of Clinical Nutrition, **34**, 1328–37.

Wang, H., Huang, W., Fei, Y.-J., Xia, H., Yang-Feng, T. L., Leibach, F. H., Devoe, L. D., Ganapathy, V. & Prasad, P. D. (1999) Human placental Na⁺-dependent multivitamin transporter. Cloning, functional expression, gene structure, and chromosomal locali-zation. *Journal of Biological Chemistry*, **274**(21), 14875–83.

Wilson, P. T. & Bourne, H. R. (1995) Fatty acylation of α$_z$. Effects of palmitoylation and myristoylation on α$_z$ signaling. *Journal of Biological Chemistry*, **270**(16), 9667–75.

16
Biotin

Key discussion topics

- Biotin is a coenzyme for four carboxylases that play key roles in gluconeogenesis, fatty acid biosynthesis, amino acid metabolism and odd-chain fatty acid catabolism.
- Metabolic recycling of biotin is essential for maintaining an adequate biotin supply.
- Biotin deficiency leads to serious clinical complications including growth retardation, neurological disorders and skin abnormalities.

16.1 Historical overview

The discovery and recognition of biotin as a member of the water-soluble vitamin B complex resulted from several independent lines of investigation. In 1933, Franklin E. Allison and his colleagues at the US Department of Agriculture reported that the growth and respiration of *Rhizobium trifolii*, a nitrogen-fixing bacterium found in the root nodules of legumes, were stimulated by a factor, 'coenzyme R', extractable from various organic sources. By the early 1920s, several investigators had isolated from various organic sources crude fractions that contained a novel growth factor for yeast. Eventually, in 1936, Fritz Kögl and B. Tönnis, organic chemists at the University of Utrecht in Germany, isolated from dried egg yolk a crystalline substance that strongly stimulated the growth of yeast. This growth factor, which Kögl and Tönnis named 'biotin', was later shown to have exactly the same stimulatory effect on *Rhizobium* as coenzyme R. In this respect, at least, the two factors were identical.

Further progress came from the field of animal nutrition. In 1927, Margaret A. Boas at the Lister Institute of Preventive Medicine in London observed toxicity in rats when raw egg white was used as a source of protein in the animals' diet. After a few weeks the rats developed dermatitis and haemorrhages of the skin, their hair fell out, their limbs became paralysed, they lost considerable weight, and eventually they died. Only raw or cold-dried egg white produced the toxicity; cooking made the egg white harmless. This toxicity, which Boas called egg white injury, was prevented by a 'protective factor X' present in liver and other sources. Paul György showed that biotin had the same protective action against egg white injury as did protective factor X, which he renamed 'vitamin H' (German *Haut*, skin). György also showed that vitamin H concentrates supported the growth of biotin-requiring bacteria. In 1940 György and Vincent du Vigneaud independently isolated crystalline vitamin H from liver concentrates. It was soon proven that biotin and vitamin H were one and the same compound.

The chemical structure of biotin was established by du Vigneaud's group in 1942 and in the following year the vitamin was synthesized at the Merck Company, USA.

16.2 Chemistry

The biotin molecule (Fig. 16.1) is a fusion of an imidazolidone ring with a tetrahydrothiophene ring bearing a pentanoic acid side chain. The molecule contains three asymmetric carbon atoms, and hence eight stereoisomers are possible. Of these, only the dextrorotatory *d*-(+)-biotin occurs in nature and possesses vitamin activity. Biotin synthesized industrially by the Hoffmann–La-Roche process is also in the *d*-form (Achuta Murthy & Mistry, 1977).

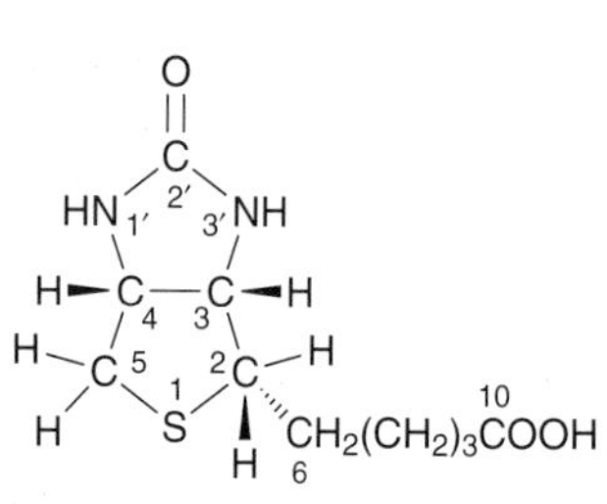

Fig. 16.1 Structure of *d*-biotin.

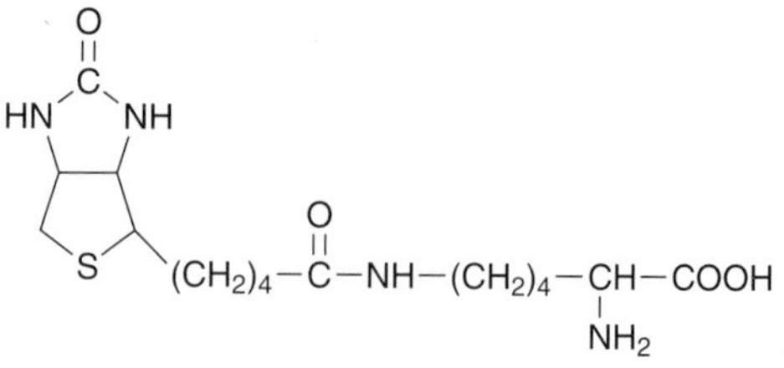

Fig. 16.2 Structure of biocytin.

In animal and plant tissues only a small proportion of the biotin present occurs in the free state. The majority is covalently bound to the protein structure (apoenzyme) of biotin-dependent enzymes via an amide bond between the carboxyl group of biotin and the ε-amino group of a lysine residue. Proteolysis of such enzymes liberates a natural water-soluble fragment called biocytin (ε-*N*-biotinyl-L-lysine) (Fig. 16.2), which is biologically active.

16.3 Dietary sources and bioavailability

16.3.1 Dietary sources

Biotin is present in all natural foodstuffs, but the content of even the richest sources is very low when compared with the content of most other water-soluble vitamins. Biotin is not commonly used in fortified foods, apart from infant formulas. Typical values of some rich natural sources of biotin include ox liver (33 μg per 100 g), whole eggs (20 μg per 100 g), dried soya beans (65 μg per 100 g) and peanuts (72 μg per 100 g) (Holland *et al.*, 1991). Other good sources include yeast, wheat bran, oatmeal and some vegetables. Muscle meats, fish, dairy products and cereals contain smaller amounts, but are important contributors to the dietary intake. Most of the biotin content of animal products, nuts, cereals and yeast is in a protein-bound form. A higher percentage of free, water-extractable biotin occurs in vegetables, green plants, fruit, milk and rice bran (Lampen *et al.*, 1942).

16.3.2 Bioavailability

The bioavailability of biotin in various foods and the effect of protein binding on bioavailability have not been studied directly in human subjects. Studies of animal feed ingredients using growth assays have shown that biotin in various cereals (but not in maize) is largely unavailable to the chicken (Frigg, 1984), turkey (Misir & Blair, 1988a) and weanling pig (Misir & Blair, 1988b). Most, if not all, of the biotin content of human milk is in the free form and thus is likely to be completely bioavailable to the infant (Heard *et al.*, 1987).

16.4   Absorption, transport and metabolism

Humans and other mammals cannot synthesize biotin and thus must obtain the vitamin from exogenous sources via intestinal absorption. The liver extracts the majority of the newly absorbed biotin from the portal blood and is the major site of biotin utilization and metabolism. Biotin is synthesized by the microflora that normally inhabit the large intestine. Presumably, this endogenous vitamin is not available to the host tissues in nutritionally significant amounts because an inherited impairment of biotin recycling results in symptoms of biotin deficiency.

16.4.1   *Digestion and absorption of dietary biotin*

Biotin in foods exists as the free vitamin and as protein-bound forms in variable proportions. Because the amide bond linking biotin and lysine residues is not hydrolysed by gastrointestinal proteases, proteolytic digestion of protein-bound biotin releases not biotin, but biocytin and biotin-containing short peptides (biotinyl peptides). Biotinidase, which is present in pancreatic juice and in intestinal mucosa, is capable of hydrolysing biocytin to yield free biotin. The release of biotin might occur during the luminal phase of proteolysis by the action of pancreatic biotinidase or in the intestinal mucosa by the action of mucosal biotinidase. Biocytin may also be absorbed intact and be acted upon by biotinidase present in plasma. Biotinyl peptides can also be absorbed directly.

Avidin, the glycoprotein in egg white, uniquely binds biotin, both in the free form and as the prosthetic group of enzymes. The complex is stable over a wide pH range and is not dissociated in the gastrointestinal tract. When eggs are cooked, the avidin is denatured and the biotin is liberated.

Intestinal absorption of biotin in the rat proceeds largely by a saturable (carrier-mediated) process at concentrations less than 5 µM, whereas at concentrations above 25 µM, non-saturable uptake (simple diffusion) predominates (Bowman *et al.*, 1986). The rate of biotin transport in human intestine was shown to increase with a decrease in pH of the incubation medium from 8 to 5.5 (Said *et al.*, 1988a). This effect presumably occurs through an increase in the transport of biotin by simple diffusion and is due to an increase in the percentage of the easily diffusible un-ionized form of the vitamin under acidic conditions. In adult humans, biotin absorption is significantly greater in the duodenum and jejunum than in the ileum, owing to a decrease in V_{max} (the number of biotin transport carriers) distally with no changes in the apparent K_m (affinity of the carrier towards its substrate) (Said *et al.*, 1988a). The sodium-dependent multivitamin transporter, which handles pantothenate, biotin and lipoate (Section 15.4.1), mediates an electrogenic process with an assumed Na$^+$:biotin$^-$ stoichiometry of 2:1 (Prasad *et al.*, 1999).

Experiments using specific activators and inhibitors have shown that biotin absorption in human-derived Caco-2 cells is regulated by the protein kinase C and Ca^{2+}/calmodulin cell signalling pathways, but not by the protein kinase A pathway (Said, 1999). Activation of protein kinase C by a phorbol ester (phorbol 12-myristate 13-acetate) inhibited biotin uptake; conversely, inhibition of protein kinase C with staurosporine and chelerythrin stimulated biotin uptake. The inhibition was due to a decrease in the number of functional biotin uptake carriers (decreased V_{max}) with no effect upon their affinity (apparent K_m unchanged). In contrast, inhibition of the Ca^{2+}/calmodulin pathway by calmidazolium and trifluoperazine inhibited biotin uptake, also through a decrease in the number of functional carriers. Simultaneous addition of phorbol ester and calmidazolium to the cultured cells produced a greater degree of inhibition than addition of either compound alone, which suggested that these compounds use different mechanisms to exert their effects.

The exit of biotin from the human enterocyte, i.e. transport across the basolateral membrane, is a carrier-mediated process which has a higher affinity for the substrate than the transport system at the brush-border membrane. The basolateral transport process is independent of sodium, electrogenic in nature, and not capable of accumulating biotin against a concentration gradient (Said *et al.*, 1988b).

There are conflicting data from rat studies regarding the intestinal transport of biocytin. Dakshinamurti *et al.* (1987) concluded that the transport is carrier-mediated and more efficient than the uptake of free biotin. Said *et al.* (1993), on the other hand, found that the transport of biocytin occurs by a non-mediated process that is independent of sodium, pH, energy and temperature, and is significantly less efficient than that of free biotin. The mechanism for the transport of biotinyl peptides is unknown; it might involve a non-specific pathway for peptide absorption or possibly a specific biotin transporter (Mock, 1990).

Adaptive regulation of biotin absorption

Transport in both the jejunum and the ileum of the rat is appropriately increased and suppressed by biotin deficiency and biotin excess, respectively, due to changes in the number of functional carriers (Said *et al.*, 1989).

16.4.2 Absorption of bacterially synthesized biotin in the large intestine

The normal microflora of the large intestine (mainly in the caecum) can synthesize large amounts of biotin, much of which exists as the unbound molecule. This is inferred by the faecal content of biotin exceeding dietary intake three- to six-fold. Balance studies in humans have shown that urinary content often exceeds dietary intake, suggesting that enterically synthesized biotin can be absorbed and utilized to some extent by the host. In a study with human subjects (Sorrell *et al.*, 1971), when biotin was instilled directly into the lumen of the mid-transverse colon, the concentration of plasma biotin increased, although not as much as when the same dose of vitamin was given orally. Bowman & Rosenberg (1987) examined biotin absorption using the rat intestinal loop, an *in vivo* preparation in which the intestinal blood supply and lymphatics remain intact. Their data showed that the large intestine of the rat is capable of absorbing nutritionally significant amounts of biotin.

Said *et al.* (1998) studied the mechanism and regulation of biotin transport in the large intestine using the human colonic epithelial cell line NCM460 as an *in vitro* model system. Uptake of biotin by these cells involved a Na$^+$-dependent, carrier-mediated transport

system that was competitively inhibited by pantothenic acid and appeared to be under the regulation of an intracellular protein kinase C-mediated pathway. These findings are similar to those in the small intestine and suggest that a common mechanism mediated by the sodium-dependent multivitamin transporter may be involved in the transport of biotin and pantothenic acid in the small and large intestinal epithelia.

16.4.3 Biotinidase as a biotin carrier in plasma

Approximately 81% of the total biotin in plasma is free (unbound), 7% is reversibly bound to plasma proteins, and 12% is covalently bound (Mock & Malik, 1992). In plasma, at pH 7.4, biotinidase (biotin-amidohydrolase, EC 3.5.1.12) cleaves biocytin (the only enzyme known to do so), but instead of releasing the biotin, a complex, biotinyl-biotinidase (Fig. 16.3), is formed through the sulphydryl group of a cysteine moiety in the protein (Hymes *et al.*, 1995). The stability of the thioester bond at >pH 7 allows biotinidase to act as a carrier protein for biotin in plasma.

16.4.4 Brain homeostasis

Spector & Mock (1987) measured the unidirectional influx of [³H]biotin across cerebral capillaries (the anatomical locus of the blood–brain barrier) using an *in situ* rat brain perfusion technique. Transport took place by a low-capacity, saturable system that was inhibited by pantothenic acid. This inhibition suggests that the sodium-dependent multivitamin transporter characterized by Prasad *et al.* (1998) is responsible for the shared transport of biotin and pantothenic acid into the brain. The concentration of plasma biotin necessary to one-half saturate the entry of tracer [³H]biotin into brain, 100 μM, is several orders of magnitude higher than the normal plasma

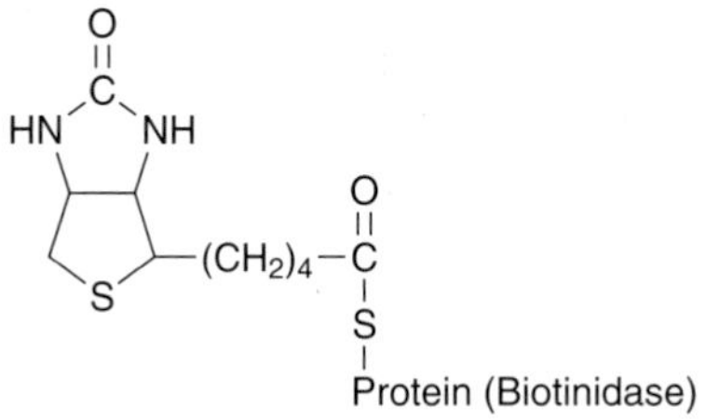

Fig. 16.3 Structure of biotinyl-biotinidase.

concentration of biotin (0.02 μM). This means that blood–brain transport plays no part in brain homeostasis of total biotin. If one were to increase plasma biotin levels by parenteral means, unnaturally high concentrations would enter the extracellular space of brain. Normally, the brain relies on the kidneys to maintain constant plasma levels of biotin. Biotin is similar to pantothenic acid in this respect, but differs from thiamin, folate and vitamin C whose blood–brain transport systems play an important homeostatic role.

The isolated rabbit choroid plexus was unable to accumulate [³H]biotin from a medium concentration of 1 nM (Spector & Mock, 1987). This implies that there is no active transport process for transferring biotin between blood and cerebrospinal fluid: the route of biotin entry into the brain is mainly, if not exclusively, via the blood–brain barrier.

Spector & Mock (1988) investigated the observed resistance of brain to depletion of total biotin in deficiency states. They concluded that the resistance is due to the minimal incorporation of biotin into the appropriate apoenzymes and hence slow turnover of the holoenzymes in brain; it is not due to the extremely slow turnover of biotin in the cerebrospinal fluid and brain.

16.4.5   Placental transport

Evidence of an electrogenic Na⁺–biotin (2:1) cotransport system was reported in human placental microvillous membrane vesicles (Grassl, 1992) and two human placental cell lines (Prasad et al., 1997). The transport system was inhibited by pantothenic acid and lipoate. Prasad et al. (1999) proved that the same transporter, the sodium-dependent multivitamin transporter, is responsible for the uptake of biotin and pantothenate in placenta and intestine.

16.4.6   Renal reabsorption and excretion

The renal reabsorption of biotin plays an essential role in biotin homeostasis and conservation. Concentrative uptake of free biotin into brush-border membrane vesicles isolated from human kidney cortex was shown to be carrier-mediated and Na⁺-dependent (Baur & Baumgartner, 1993). Intracellular biotin is thought to diffuse passively across the basolateral membrane into the peritubular fluid to complete the

process of renal reabsorption (Podevin & Barbarat, 1986).

Biotin is excreted in the urine primarily unchanged, with only a small amount as metabolites (Dakshinamurti, 1994). The biliary excretion of biotin and metabolites is only a minor route in the overall elimination of biotin from the body (Zemplini et al., 1997).

16.5   Biochemical and physiological functions

16.5.1   Biotin as coenzyme for carboxylases

In mammals, biotin functions as a covalently bound prosthetic group in four carboxylase enzymes, which are capable of taking up bicarbonate ions as the carboxyl donor and transferring them to specific substrates. A single enzyme, holocarboxylase synthetase (EC 6.3.4.10), acts on the apoenzymes of all four carboxylases to form the active holoenzymes. An overall scheme of biotin-dependent carboxylase reactions is shown in Fig. 16.4; detailed reactions are presented in Figs 16.5–16.8.

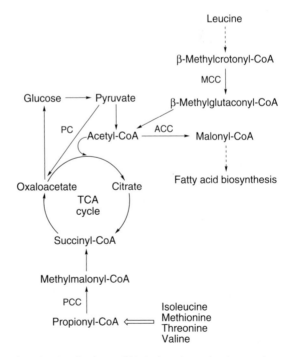

Fig. 16.4 Overall scheme of biotin-dependent carboxylase reactions. MCC, β-methylcrotonyl-CoA carboxylase; PC, pyruvate carboxylase; ACC, acetyl-CoA carboxylase; PCC, propionyl-CoA carboxylase.

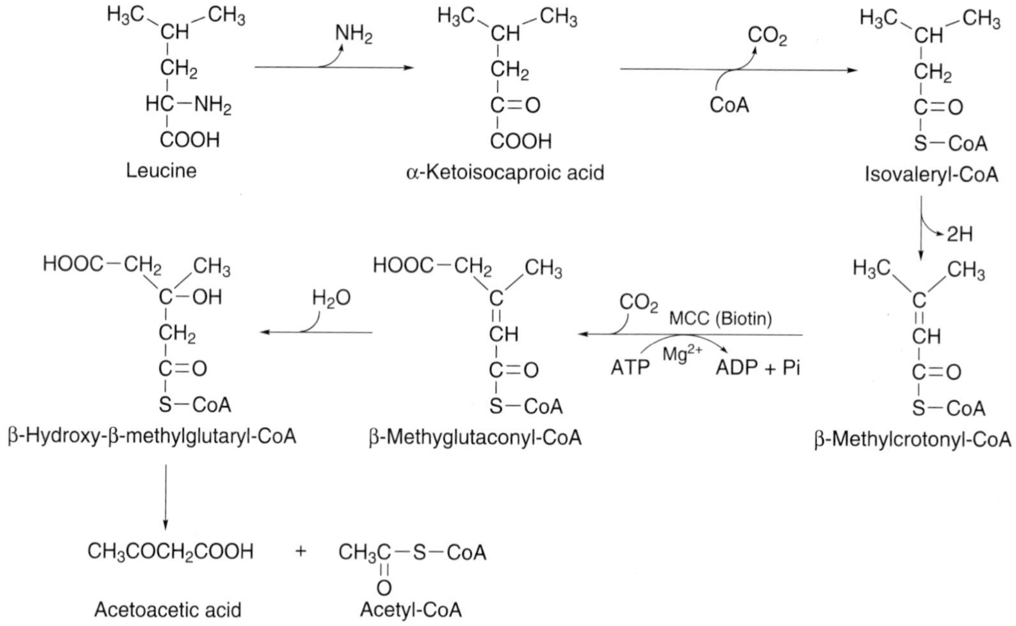

Fig. 16.5 Pathway for the catabolism of leucine. MCC, β-methylcrotonyl-CoA carboxylase.

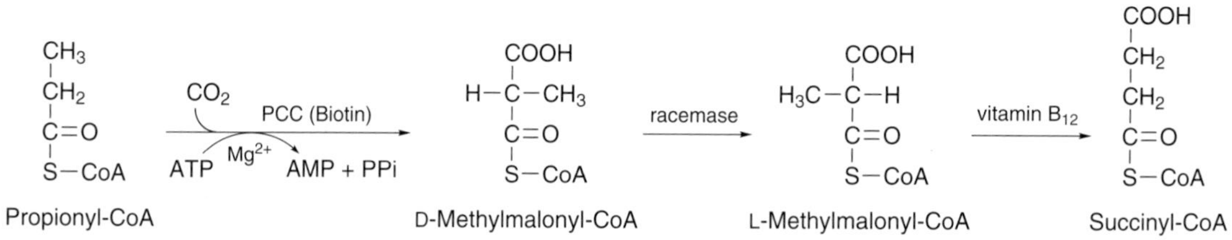

Fig. 16.6 Oxidation of propionyl-CoA. PCC, propionyl-CoA carboxylase.

In the liver, the regeneration of glucose (gluco-neogenesis) from lactate produced during exercise requires means of bypassing several energy barriers in the glycolytic pathway. The bypassing of the phosphoenolpyruvate to pyruvate step is achieved by the actions of two enzymes that are unique to gluconeogenesis. The biotin-dependent pyruvate carboxylase (EC 6.4.1.1) catalyses the conversion of pyruvate to oxaloacetate, which is then converted by the second (biotin-independent) enzyme to phosphoenolpyruvate (Fig. 16.7). Pyruvate carboxylase is allosterically activated by acetyl-CoA, which will be abundant when energy intake exceeds demand. The glucose thus produced in the liver is returned to the muscle for energy storage in the form of glycogen. The

formation of oxaloacetate is also important in lipid biosynthesis through its role in transporting acetyl-CoA from within the mitochondrion to the cytosol. This involves the continuous removal of oxaloacetate from the mitochondrion, and its replacement by the action of pyruvate carboxylase is necessary to maintain normal tricarboxylic acid cycle activity (Achuta Murthy & Mistry, 1977).

In fatty acid biosynthesis the first and rate-limiting step is the conversion of acetyl-CoA to malonyl-CoA catalysed by biotin-dependent acetyl-CoA carboxylase (EC 6.4.1.2) (Fig. 16.8).

The amino acids valine, isoleucine and methionine are metabolized to propionyl-CoA, which is converted by biotin-dependent propionyl-CoA carboxylase

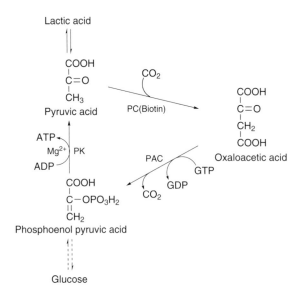

Fig. 16.7 The role of biotin in gluconeogenesis. PK, pyruvate kinase; PC, pyruvate carboxylase; PAC, phosphoenolpyruvate carboxylase.

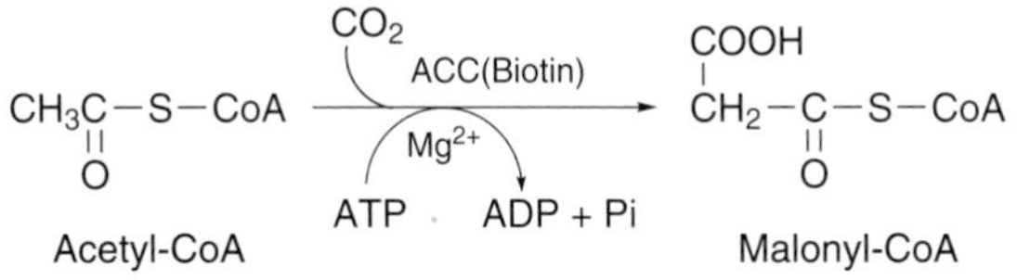

$$CH_3C-S-CoA \xrightarrow[\substack{Mg^{2+} \\ ATP \quad ADP + Pi}]{\substack{CO_2 \\ ACC(Biotin)}} CH_2-C-S-CoA$$

Acetyl-CoA   Malonyl-CoA

Fig. 16.8 Carboxylation of acetyl-CoA. ACC, acetyl-CoA carboxylase.

(EC 6.4.1.3) to methylmalonyl-CoA. This compound is isomerized to succinyl-CoA, which enters the tricarboxylic acid cycle.

The fourth biotin-dependent enzyme, β-methylcrotonyl-CoA carboxylase (6.4.1.4), catalyses the conversion of β-methylcrotonyl-CoA, arising from the catabolism of leucine, to β-methylglutaconyl-CoA. This reaction product is hydroxylated to a compound which is cleaved to form acetyl-CoA and acetoacetate.

16.5.2   Activation of guanylyl cyclase

Biotin increases the activity of guanylyl cyclase in tissues, causing an increased generation of cyclic guanosine monophosphate (cyclic GMP) (Vesely, 1982). Spence & Koudelka (1984) reported that the addition of biotin to cultured rat hepatocytes increased the intracellular levels of cyclic GMP and also the activity of glucokinase. Glucokinase, an enzyme found almost exclusively in the liver, catalyses the conversion of glucose to glucose-6-phosphate. The enzyme plays an important role in removing excess glucose from the bloodstream and storing it as liver glycogen. It appears that the activity of glucokinase can be substituted by the action of biotin, through its ability to activate guanylyl cyclase. These *in vitro* effects were elicited at a micromolar concentration of biotin, which is about two orders of magnitude higher than the normal concentration of biotin. Physiological concentrations of biotin enhance glucokinase activity in biotin-deficient rats (Dakshinamurti & Chauhan, 1994).

16.5.3   Role of biotin in the nucleus

The protein histone is a specific acceptor for biotin from biotinyl-biotinidase and histones are biotinylated when incubated with biotinidase and biocytin at pH > 7 (Hymes & Wolf, 1999). Histones are essential components of chromatin in the nucleus. It can be speculated that biotin is involved in the packaging of DNA into chromatin because histones have been shown to dissociate from the DNA in biotin-deficient rats (Petrelli *et al.*, 1976). Biotin deficiency was also associated with decreased phosphorylation and methylation, and increased acetylation of histones (Petrelli *et al.*, 1978). The ability of biotin to up-regulate the synthesis of glucokinase at the transcriptional stage in the starved rat (Chauhan & Dakshinamurti, 1991) is further evidence for a role of the vitamin in the nucleus.

16.6   Biotin deficiency

16.6.1   Dietary deficiency

Biotin is so widely distributed in foods that it is doubtful whether a true dietary deficiency of the vitamin has ever occurred in human adults capable of utilizing it. Artificial biotin deficiency states have been induced in healthy volunteers by feeding low-biotin diets containing a high proportion of raw egg white. An initial dry scaly dermatitis was followed by non-specific symptoms that included anorexia and extreme lassitude. All of the symptoms responded to injections of 150–300 μg of biotin per day.

A unique opportunity to study dietary biotin deficiency was presented to Baugh et al. (1968) by a 62-year-old female patient who had consumed six raw eggs and 4 pints of skimmed milk daily for 18 months. This diet had been recommended by a physician (ill-advisedly, as we now know) as a dietary supplement to provide a high intake of essential amino acids to aid liver regeneration following a diagnosis of liver cirrhosis. During this dietary period, the patient took vitamin supplements, which included biotin, and she also received 100 µg of vitamin B_{12} by injection monthly. Thus the stage was set, unintentionally, for the development of biotin deficiency due to the avidin content of raw egg whites, uncomplicated by deficiencies of other vitamins or common nutrients. Clinical manifestations included anorexia, nausea, vomiting, glossitis, pallor, depression, lassitude, substernal pain, scaly dermatitis and desquamation of the lips. All symptoms cleared or improved markedly after 2 to 5 days of parenteral (by injection) vitamin therapy providing 200 µg of biotin daily, while the patient continued her pre-treatment diet. In contrast to other case reports, the patient did not exhibit anaemia, muscle pains, hypercholesterolaemia or electrocardiographic abnormalities.

Seborrhoeic dermatitis of the scalp and a more generalized dermatitis known as Leiner's disease have been reported in breast-fed infants when the mother is malnourished. These symptoms are relieved when biotin is administered to the mother.

16.6.2   Inherited defects of biotin metabolism

There are two known congenital disorders of biotin metabolism: (1) holocarboxylase synthetase (HCS) deficiency and (2) biotinidase deficiency. Both disorders are inherited as an autosomal recessive trait and both lead to deficiency of the four biotin-dependent carboxylases, a condition known as multiple carboxylase deficiency (MCD). Because of the vital role of these enzymes in protein, carbohydrate and lipid metabolism, their deficiency leads to severe life-threatening disease.

The two forms of MCD usually become symptomatic in early infancy or childhood. The incidence of biotinidase deficiency is about one in 60 000 and that of HCS deficiency seems to be even lower. The underlying cause of HCS deficiency is decreased affinity of HCS for biotin resulting in reduced formation of holocarboxylases with physiological concentrations of biotin. In biotinidase deficiency, MCD results from progressive development of biotin deficiency due to inability to liberate biotin from the biocytin or short biotinyl peptides that remain after metabolic degradation of biotin-containing carboxylases. The recycling of biotin salvaged from degraded enzymes is essential to maintain an adequate supply of the vitamin. A lack of biotinidase results in excessive urinary excretion of biocytin and this raises the requirement for biotin to above normal intakes.

The two forms of MCD differ biochemically in that the HCS-deficient patients have normal plasma biotin concentrations but decreased carboxylase activities, whereas patients with biotinidase deficiency have subnormal plasma biotin concentrations and normal carboxylase activities. MCD arising from either inherited defect causes a block in the biotin-dependent metabolic pathways with characteristic accumulation and urinary excretion of organic acids such as lactate, 3-hydroxyisovalerate, 3-methylcrotonylglycine and methylcitrate.

The clinical presentation and age of onset of MCD are extremely variable. HCS deficiency may present in the first days of life, while biotinidase deficiency usually becomes manifest between the second and fifth months of age, depending on the amount of free biotin in the diet. However, onset of HCS deficiency is delayed (2–21 months) in some cases and therefore classifying the two disorders as neonatal- or early-onset and infantile- or late-onset MCD should be discouraged. Clinical symptoms common to both disorders include neurological abnormalities (hypotonia, seizures, ataxia) and cutaneous changes (skin rash, alopecia). In healthy persons receiving an adequate diet, biotinidase activity in the brain is relatively very low (Suchy et al., 1985) and so the brain relies largely on biotin that is transferred across the blood–brain barrier. This feature of the brain could explain the rapid onset of neurological symptoms observed in biotinidase deficiency.

MCD attributable to either cause is treatable by oral daily doses of 10 mg of biotin continued through life.

Further reading

Baumgartner, E. R. & Suormala, T. (1997) Multiple carboxylase deficiency; inherited and acquired disorders of biotin metabolism. *International Journal for Vitamin and Nutrition Research*, **67**, 377–84.

Dakshinamurti, K. & Chauhan, J. (1989) Biotin. *Vitamins and Hormones*, **45**, 337–84.

Mock, D. M. (1999) Biotin. In: *Modern Nutrition in Health and Disease*, 9th edn. (Ed. M. E. Shils, J. A. Olson, M. Shike & A. C. Ross), pp. 459–66. Lippincott Williams & Wilkins, Philadelphia.

References

Achuta Murthy, P. N. & Mistry, S. P. (1977) Biotin. *Progress in Food and Nutrition Science*, **2**, 405–55.

Baugh, C. M., Malone, J. H. & Butterworth, C. E. Jr. (1968) Human biotin deficiency. A case history of biotin deficiency induced by raw egg consumption in a cirrhotic patient. *American Journal of Clinical Nutrition*, **21**, 173–82.

Baur, B. & Baumgartner, E. R. (1993) Na$^+$-dependent biotin transport into brush-border membrane vesicles from human kidney cortex. *European Journal of Physiology*, **422**, 499–505.

Bowman, B. B. & Rosenberg, I. H. (1987) Biotin absorption by distal rat intestine. *Journal of Nutrition*, **117**, 2121–6.

Bowman, B. B., Selhub, J. & Rosenberg, I. H. (1986) Intestinal absorption of biotin in the rat. *Journal of Nutrition*, **116**, 1266–71.

Chauhan, J. & Dakshinamurti, K. (1991) Transcriptional regulation of the glucokinase gene by biotin in starved rats. *Journal of Biological Chemistry*, **266**(16), 10 035–8.

Dakshinamurti, K. (1994) Biotin. In: *Modern Nutrition in Health and Disease*, 8th edn, Vol. 1. (Ed. M. E. Shils, J. A. Olson & M. Shike), pp. 426–31. Lea & Febiger, Philadelphia.

Dakshinamurti, K. & Chauhan, J. (1994) Biotin-binding proteins. In: *Vitamin Receptors. Vitamins as Ligands in Cell Communication*. (Ed. K. Dakshinamurti), pp. 200–49. Cambridge University Press, Cambridge.

Dakshinamurti, K., Chauhan, J. & Ebrahim, H. (1987) Intestinal absorption of biotin and biocytin in the rat. *Bioscience Reports*, **7**, 667–73.

Frigg, M. (1984) Available biotin content of various feed ingredients. *Poultry Science*, **63**, 750–3.

Grassl, S. M. (1992) Human placental brush-border membrane Na$^+$-biotin cotransport. *Journal of Biological Chemistry*, **267**(25), 17 760–5.

Heard, G. S., Redmond, J. B. & Wolf, B. (1987) Distribution and bioavailability of biotin in human milk. *Federation Proceedings*, **46**, 897 (abstr).

Holland, B., Welch, A. A., Unwin, I. D., Buss, D. H., Paul, A. A. & Southgate, D. A. T. (1991) *McCance and Widdowson's The Composition of Foods*, 5th edn, Royal Society of Chemistry and Ministry of Agriculture, Fisheries and Food.

Hymes, J. & Wolf, B. (1999) Human biotinidase isn't just for recycling biotin. *Journal of Nutrition*, **129**, 485S–9S.

Hymes, J., Fleischhauer, K. & Wolf, B. (1995) Biotinylation of biotinidase following incubation with biocytin. *Clinica Chimica Acta*, **233**, 39–45.

Lampen, J. O., Bahler, G. P. & Peterson, W. H. (1942) The occurrence of free and bound biotin. *Journal of Nutrition*, **23**, 11–21.

Misir, R. & Blair, R. (1988a) Biotin bioavailability of protein supplements and cereal grains for starting turkey poults. *Poultry Science*, **67**, 1274–80.

Misir, R. & Blair, R. (1988b) Biotin bioavailability from protein supplements and cereal grains for weanling pigs. *Canadian Journal of Animal Science*, **68**, 523–32.

Mock, D. M. (1990) Biotin. In: *Present Knowledge in Nutrition*, 6th edn. (Ed. M. L. Brown), pp. 189–207. International Life Sciences Institute, Nutrition Foundation, Washington, D.C.

Mock, D. M. & Malik, M. I. (1992) Distribution of biotin in human plasma: most of the biotin is not bound to protein. *American Journal of Clinical Nutrition*, **56**, 427–32.

Petrelli, F., Marsili, G. & Moretti, P. (1976) RNA, DNA, histones and interactions between histone proteins and DNA in the liver of biotin deficient rats. *Biochemistry and Experimental Biology*, **12**, 461–5.

Petrelli, F., Coderoni, S., Moretti, P. & Paparelli, M. (1978) Effect of biotin on phosphorylation, acetylation, methylation of rat liver histones. *Molecular Biology Reports*, **4**, 87–92.

Podevin, R.-A. & Barbarat, B. (1986) Biotin uptake mechanisms in brush-border and basolateral membrane vesicles isolated from rabbit kidney cortex. *Biochimica et Biophysica Acta*, **856**, 471–81.

Prasad, P. D., Ramamoorthy, S., Leibach, F. H. & Ganapathy, V. (1997) Characterization of a sodium-dependent vitamin transporter mediating the uptake of pantothenate, biotin and lipoate in human choriocarcinoma cells. *Placenta*, **18**, 527–33,

Prasad, P. D., Wang, H., Kekuda, R., Fujita, T., Fei, Y.-J., Devoe, L. D., Leibach, F. H. & Ganapathy, V. (1998) Cloning and functional expression of a cDNA encoding a mammalian sodium-dependent vitamin transporter mediating the uptake of pantothenate, biotin, and lipoate. *Journal of Biological Chemistry*, **273**(13), 7501–6.

Prasad, P. D., Wang, H., Huang, W., Fei, Y.-J., Leibach, F. H., Devoe, L. D. & Ganapathy, V. (1999) Molecular and functional characterization of the intestinal Na$^+$-dependent multivitamin transporter. *Archives of Biochemistry and Biophysics*, **366**, 95–106.

Said, H. M. (1999) Cellular uptake of biotin: mechanisms and regulation. *Journal of Nutrition*, **129**, 490S–3S.

Said, H. M., Redha, R. & Nylander, W. (1988a) Biotin transport in the human intestine: site of maximum transport and effect of pH. *Gastroenterology*, **95**, 1312–17.

Said, H. M., Redha, R. & Nylander, W. (1988b) Biotin transport in basolateral membrane vesicles of human intestine. *Gastroenterology*, **94**, 1157–63.

Said, H. M., Mock, D. M. & Collins, J. C. (1989) Regulation of intestinal biotin transport in the rat: effect of biotin deficiency and supplementation. *American Journal of Physiology*, **256**, G306–11.

Said, H. M., Thuy, L. P., Sweetman, L. & Schatzman, B. (1993) Transport of the biotin dietary derivative (*N*-biotinyl-L-lysine) in rat small intestine. *Gastroenterology*, **104**, 75–80.

Said, H. M., Ortiz, A., McCloud, E., Dyer, D., Moyer, M. P. & Rubin, S. (1998) Biotin uptake by human colonic epithelial NCM460 cells: a carrier-mediated process shared with pantothenic acid. *American Journal of Physiology*, **275**, C1365–71.

Sorrell, M. F., Frank, O., Thomson, A. D., Aquino, H. & Baker, H. (1971) Absorption of vitamins from the large intestine in vivo. *Nutrition Report International*, **3**, 143–8.

Spector, R. & Mock, D. (1987) Biotin transport through the blood–brain barrier. *Journal of Neurochemistry*, **48**, 400–4.

Spector, R. & Mock, D. M. (1988) Biotin transport and metabolism in the central nervous system. *Neurochemical Research*, **13**, 213–19.

Spence, J. T. & Koudelka, A. P. (1984) Effects of biotin upon the intracellular level of cGMP and the activity of glucokinase in cultured rat hepatocytes. *Journal of Biological Chemistry*,

259(10), 6393–6.

Suchy, S. F., McVoy, J. S. & Wolf, B. (1985) Neurologic symptoms of biotinidase deficiency: possible explanation. *Neurology*, **35**, 1510–11.

Vesely, D. L. (1982) Biotin enhances guanylate cyclase activity. *Science*, **216**, 1329–30.

Zemplini, J., Green, G. M., Spannagel, A. W. & Mock, D. M. (1997) Biliary excretion of biotin and biotin metabolites is quantitatively minor in rats and pigs. *Journal of Nutrition*, **127**, 1496–500.

17
Folate

Key discussion topics

- Cellular uptake of folate involves two functionally different membrane transport systems: the reduced folate carrier and the membrane folate receptor.
- The folate vitamers act as enzyme co-substrates by accepting or donating single-carbon units in many metabolic reactions of amino acids and nucleotides.
- Folate is an essential factor for the *de novo* biosynthesis of purines and one pyrimidine nucleotide required for DNA synthesis.
- Folate is critical for the synthesis of *S*-adenosylmethionine, a methyl donor for a variety of biologically important acceptors.

- A dietary deficiency of folate leads to an elevation of plasma homocysteine concentrations, which is an early risk factor for atherosclerosis.
- A poor maternal folate status in early pregnancy is related to the occurrence of neural tube defects in the fetus.
- Polymorphisms in genes encoding key enzymes in folate and homocysteine metabolism play a role in occlusive vascular disease and neural tube defects.
- Folate deficiency has the potential to cause DNA strand breaks and DNA hypomethylation, both of which may lead to mutations and cancer.

17.1   Historical overview

In 1931, a research group led by Lucy Wills showed that an autolysed yeast preparation (Marmite™), which was therapeutically ineffective against the pernicious anaemia caused by vitamin B_{12} deficiency, was effective against nutritional megaloblastic anaemia in pregnant women. These researchers induced a similar anaemia in monkeys which then responded to crude liver extracts. Other substances that cured specific deficiency anaemias in monkeys and chicks were isolated from yeast by different research groups and assigned the names 'vitamin M' and 'vitamin B_c'. Another substance isolated from liver was shown to be essential to the growth of *Lactobacillus casei* and therefore called the '*L. casei* factor'. In 1941, Mitchell and co-workers processed four tons of spinach leaves to obtain a purified substance with acidic properties which was an active growth factor for rats and *L. casei*. They named the factor 'folic acid' (from *folium*, the Latin word for leaf). Eventually, all of the above substances proved to be the same when Angier's group in 1946 accomplished the synthesis and chemical structure of folic acid.

17.2   Chemistry

The term 'folate' is used as the generic descriptor for all derivatives of pteroic acid that demonstrate vitamin activity in humans. The structure of the parent folate compound, folic acid, comprises a bicyclic pterin moiety joined by a methylene bridge to *p*-aminobenzoic acid, which in turn is coupled via an α-peptide bond to a single molecule of L-glutamic acid (Fig. 17.1, top).

(Note: In the present context, the term 'folic acid' refers specifically to pteroylmonoglutamic acid which, with reference to the pteroic acid and glutamate moieties, can be abbreviated to PteGlu. 'Folate' is a non-specific term referring to any folate compound with vitamin activity. 'Folacin' is a non-approved term synonymous with 'folate'.)

Folic acid is not a common natural physiological form of the vitamin. In most natural foods, the pteridine ring is reduced to give either the 7,8-dihydrofolate (DHF) or 5,6,7,8-tetrahydrofolate (THF) (see Fig. 17.1). These reduced forms can be substituted with a covalently bonded one-carbon adduct attached to nitrogen positions 5 or 10 or bridged across both positions. The following substituted forms of THF are important intermediates in folate metabolism: 10-formyl-THF, 5-methyl-THF, 5-formimino-THF, 5,10-methylene-THF and 5,10-methenyl-THF (see Fig. 17.1).

An important structural aspect of the 5,6,7,8-tetrahydrofolates is the stereochemical orientation at the C-6 asymmetric carbon of the pteridine ring. Of the two stereoisomers, 6*S* and 6*R* (formerly called 6*l* and 6*d*), only the 6*S* is biologically active and occurs in nature. Methods of chemical synthesis of tetrahydrofolates, whether by catalytic hydrogenation or chemical reduction, yield a racemic product (i.e. a mixture of both stereoisomers).

All folate compounds exist predominantly as polyglutamates, containing typically from five to seven glutamate residues in γ-peptide linkage. The γ-peptide bond is unique in mammalian biochemistry. Folate conjugates are abbreviated to PteGlu$_n$ derivatives, where *n* is the number of glutamate residues; for example, 5-CH$_3$-H$_4$PteGlu$_3$ refers to triglutamyl-5-methyltetrahydrofolic acid.

Methotrexate (4-amino-10-methylfolic acid; Fig. 17.2) is a folate antagonist which is used as an anticancer drug.

17.3   Dietary sources and bioavailability

17.3.1   Dietary sources

Polyglutamyl folate is an essential biochemical constituent of living cells, and most foods contribute some folate. The folates generally exist in nature bound to proteins (Baugh & Krumdieck, 1971) and they are also bound to storage polysaccharides (various types of starch and glycogen) in foods (Černá & Káš, 1983). In the United States, dried beans, eggs, greens, orange juice, sweet corn, peas and peanut products are good sources of folate that are inexpensive and available all the year round.

Although liver, all types of fortified breakfast cereals, cooked dried beans, asparagus, spinach, broccoli and avocado provide the highest amount of folate per average serving, several of these foods do not rank highly in terms of actual dietary folate intake in the United States because of their low rate of consumption. In fact, orange juice ranks the highest, contributing 9.70% to dietary folate intake (Subar *et al.*,

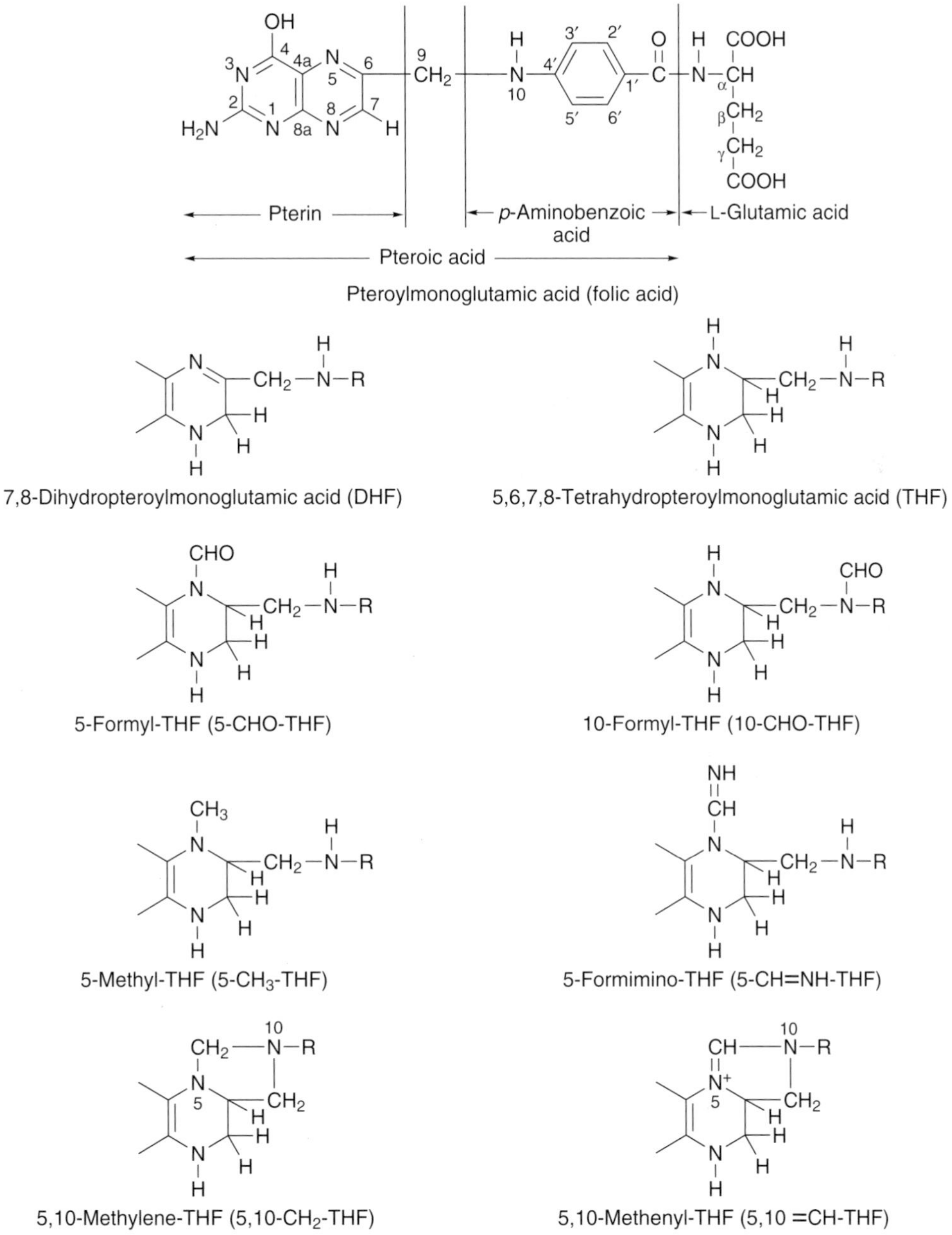

Fig. 17.1 Structures of folate compounds.

1989). The distribution of the various folate forms in selected foods is shown in Table 17.1.

17.3.2 Bioavailability

The bioavailability of folate depends, among other factors, on whether the folate is in the polyglutamyl form (i.e. food folate in natural sources) or in the monoglutamyl form (i.e. synthetic folic acid in supplements and fortified foods). Polyglutamyl folates, unlike folic acid, must undergo enzymatic deconjugation in the small intestine before they can be absorbed.

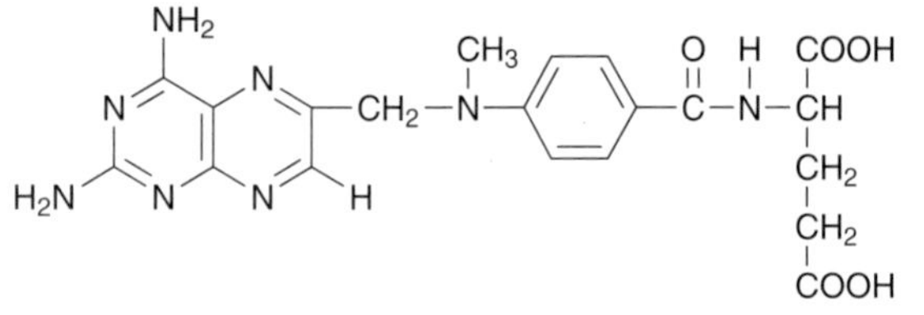

Fig. 17.2 Structure of methotrexate.

Organic acids present in many foods can inhibit conjugase activity (Wei & Gregory, 1998) and this may partly explain why the polyglutamyl folate present in natural food sources is less bioavailable than the folic acid present in fortified foods and supplements (Cuskelly et al., 1996). Physical entrapment of folates in the cellular structure of plant materials can adversely affect the rate of folate absorption (van het Hof et al., 1999; Castenmiller et al., 2000). Gregory et al. (1991) reported a bioavailability of around 50% for

PteGlu₆ relative to PteGlu as judged by urinary excretion when stable isotopes of these compounds were administered orally to human subjects. In a 92-day metabolic study in women, dietary folate appeared to be no more than 50% bioavailable when compared with folic acid in a formulated diet (Sauberlich et al., 1987). Brouwer et al. (1999a) calculated the bioavailability of folate from vegetables and citrus fruits to be 60–98% relative to folic acid in tablet form. Pfeiffer et al. (1997) reported that folic acid added to cereal is highly bioavailable and the matrix of cereal-grain foods has little inhibitory effect on intestinal absorption of the added folate.

There is little information regarding the effects of food on the bioavailability of folic acid in supplements. Absorption of a dose of $[^{13}C_5]$folic acid was reduced by an insignificant 15% when taken immediately after a light meal (Pfeiffer et al., 1997), providing an estimated 85% for the bioavailability of folic acid supplement consumed with food.

Table 17.1 Distribution of folates in various foods (from Seyoum & Selhub, 1998).

Form[a]	Percent of total folate[b]						
	Egg yolk	Cow's liver	Cabbage	Lettuce	Orange juice	Lima beans	Baker's yeast
DHF₁ and THF₁		63.4					
Folic acid₁				2.6	4.0		
5-methyl-THF₁	100	36.6	15.0	36.0	20.2		
5-methyl-THF₂			3.9	7.1	19.3		
5-methyl-THF₃			40.2	2.2	10.5		
5-methyl-THF₄			3.0	10.1	8.4		
THF₅						8.3	
5- and 10-formyl-THF₅						61.4	
5-methyl-THF₅			3.9	37.8	32.4	30.3	
THF₆							3.2
5- and 10-formyl-THF₆							0.1
5-methyl-THF₆			11.0	4.3	5.3		13.6
THF₇							14.7
5- and 10-formyl-THF₇							0.2
5-methyl-THF₇			17.0				53.7
THF₈							1.9
5- and 10-formyl-THF₈							2.5
5-methyl-THF₈			6.1				10.1
Total folate (nmol g⁻¹)	3.8	9.7	0.8	3.0	0.3	1.8	55.5

[a]Subscripts denote total number of glutamate residues.
[b]Mean of 5 values.

17.4   Absorption, transport and metabolism

Background information can be found in Section 3.1.5.

Humans and other mammals cannot synthesize folate in their tissues and thus they must obtain the vitamin from exogenous sources via intestinal absorption. The intestine is exposed to two sources of folate: (1) dietary folate and (2) folate synthesized by bacteria in the large intestine. The latter source is available to the host tissues through direct absorption in the colon.

It is fundamental in folate metabolism that folate monoglutamates are the circulatory and membrane-transportable forms of the vitamin, whereas polyglutamates are the intracellular biochemical and storage forms.

17.4.1   Folate transport proteins

Cellular uptake of folate involves two functionally different membrane transport proteins: (1) the reduced folate carrier, which is an organic anion exchange protein present in the plasma membrane of a wide variety of cells, and (2) the less ubiquitous folate receptor, which internalizes folate by a receptor-mediated process. The affinities of these proteins for folates and antifolates differ significantly (Table 17.2). After internalization, folates are retained in the cytoplasm by polyglutamylation.

In certain specific cell types, such as human placental trophoblast cells, a functional coordination between the two transport proteins has been proposed. Enterocytes and hepatocytes lack the folate receptor and so folate transport in the human intestine and liver is mediated solely by the reduced folate carrier.

The folate receptor
Since the initial report of a soluble folate binding protein in milk (Ford *et al.*, 1969), membrane-bound folate-binding proteins have been discovered in various tissues. The recognition that these binding proteins were involved in the accumulative uptake of folate by certain cells led to their designation as folate receptors (FRs).

The FRs are proteins of molecular weight 38–44 kDA that initiate cellular accumulation of 5-methyl-THF, the predominant folate vitamer in blood, in a number of epithelial cell types *in vitro*. Rothberg *et al.* (1990), using immunocytochemistry on cultured MA104 cells (a monkey kidney epithelial cell line), showed a clustering of the FR on the cell surface, preferentially associated with uncoated membrane invaginations rather than clathrin-coated pits; the FR was not located in endosomes or lysosomes. This suggests that the FR mediates folate uptake by potocytosis, the process by which the FR–folate complex is enclosed within a caveola that remains associated with the plasma membrane and does not merge with other endocytotic compartments. The caveola closes transiently, during which the acidic milieu causes the FR–folate complex to dissociate. An organic anion carrier (the reduced folate carrier) transports folate from the caveola across the membrane into the cytoplasm (Kamen *et al.*, 1991), using the energy generated by an H^+ gradient (Section 17.4.8). The FR is maximally expressed on the surface of folate-depleted tissue culture cells and so data from such cells may not extrapolate to normal cells which are not so rich in these folate-binding sites.

The three known isoforms of the human folate receptor, FR-α, FR-β and FR-γ, are differentially expressed in different tissues. The α and β isoforms are concentrated in caveolae and are anchored to the plasma membrane by a covalently attached glycosylphosphatidylinositol linkage; the γ isoform is not anchored but secreted due to lack of an efficient signal for glycosylphosphatidylinositol modification (Antony, 1996). FR-γ is also generally expressed at levels

Table 17.2   Affinities of the reduced folate carrier and folate receptor for folates and antifolate.[a]

Folate	Reduced folate carrier (RFC)	Folate receptor (FR)
Folic acid	Low affinity (K_m 200–400 μM)	High affinity (K_m 0.1–1 nM)
Reduced folates (e.g. 5-methyl-THF, 5-formyl-THF)	Relatively high affinity (K_m 1–10 μM)	High affinity (K_m 1–10 nM)
Methotrexate (antifolate)	Relatively high affinity (K_m 1–10 μM)	Relatively low affinity (K_m >100 nM)

[a]Values from Rijnboutt *et al.* (1996)

Table 17.3 Folate receptor expression in human tissues[a] (from Weitman et al., 1992).

Site	Cellular localization
Choroid plexus	Epithelial cells
Epididymis	Epithelial cells
Vas deferens	Basal cells of the epithelium
Fallopian tube	Epithelial cells
Uterus	Epithelial cells of the endometrium
Placenta	Syncytiotrophoblastic cells
Mammary gland	Acinar cells
Salivary gland	Serous acinar cells of the submandibular gland
Lung	Bronchial and bronchiolar epithelium; alveolar lining cells; acinar cells of bronchial glands
Kidney	Epithelial cells of the proximal convoluted tubule

[a]The tissues listed have strong immunoreactivity. Limited but focal reactivity was noted in the ovary, thyroid and pancreas. The liver and small intestine failed to show any specific immunohistochemical reactivity for the folate receptor.

much lower than FR-α and FR-β. Human tissues expressing the folate receptor are listed in Table 17.3. The best studied transport system is the maternal-to-fetal transfer of 5-methyl-THF across the placenta, which is mediated by FR-α (Prasad et al., 1994a). FR-α and FR-β display relatively similar affinities for folic acid. However, they differ in their stereospecificity for reduced folate coenzymes, with FR-α having a 50-fold higher affinity than FR-β for the physiological (6S) diastereoisomer of 5-methyl-THF (Wang et al., 1992).

The cellular expression of folate receptor is regulated inversely by the extracellular folate concentration. Up-regulation of the receptor in response to low extracellular folate can result from increased rates of gene transcription and/or increased stability of receptor mRNA. In addition, translational or post-translational changes may be involved (Antony, 1996).

The folate antagonist methotrexate has a chemotherapeutic potential in the treatment of malignant disease. Methotrexate binds to and inhibits the cytosolic enzyme dihydrofolate reductase, thereby interfering with the synthesis of reduced folate coenzymes that are necessary for the synthesis of purines and a pyrimidine. Unbound intracellular methotrexate concentrations in excess of the maximum binding by dihydrofolate reductase is necessary to completely inhibit the enzyme activity. Methotrexate is transported by the folate receptor, but its affinity for the receptor is relatively low (see Table 17.2). However, malignant cells express very high levels of folate receptor com-

pared to the corresponding normal tissue (Ross et al., 1994), and this over-expression allows methotrexate to enter the cells and inhibit their proliferation (Kane et al., 1986).

17.4.2 Digestion and absorption of dietary folate and milk folate

Deconjugation of polyglutamyl folate

The folates naturally present in foods exist largely in protein-bound form, the predominant vitamers being polyglutamyl forms of THF, 5-methyl-THF and 10-formyl-THF (Gregory, 1984). Folylpolyglutamates, being large and strongly electronegative molecules, are not transportable into cells and, before they can be absorbed, they must be hydrolysed to monoglutamate forms. None of the known proteases in saliva, gastric juice or pancreatic secretions are capable of splitting the γ-peptide bonds in the polyglutamyl side chain. Polyglutamyl folate can, however, be hydrolysed by folate conjugase, which is a trivial name for pteroylpolyglutamate hydrolase, EC 3.4.12.10 (also known as folylpoly-γ-glutamyl carboxypeptidase). As much as 50–75% of dietary polyglutamyl folate can be absorbed after deconjugation to monoglutamyl folate (Butterworth et al., 1969). The presence of conjugase activity in many raw foods of both plant and animal origin results in a high proportion of the dietary folate being already monoglutamyl when presented to the intestinal mucosa (Gregory, 1989).

Two folate conjugases have been found in human jejunal tissue fractions. One, a brush-border exopeptidase, has a pH optimum of 6.7–7.0 and is activated by Zn^{2+}. The other, an intracellular endopeptidase of mainly lysosomal origin, has a pH optimum of 4.5 and no defined metal requirement. The brush-border conjugase splits off terminal glutamate residues one at a time and is thought to be the principal enzyme in the hydrolysis of polyglutamyl folate. Brush-border conjugases from the jejunum of the human and pig possess similar enzymatic properties (Gregory et al., 1987) and thus the porcine enzyme can be used to study folate bioavailability in humans. Interestingly, the human and the pig are the only species in which intestinal brush-border conjugase activity has been demonstrated. Bhandari & Gregory (1990) showed that extracts from certain foods (e.g. legumes, tomatoes and orange juice) can inhibit brush-border conjugase activity from human and porcine intestine *in vitro*. Organic acids may be responsible for this inhibition (Wei & Gregory, 1998). Such inhibition may be a factor affecting the bioavailability of polyglutamyl folates in diets containing these foods. The intracellular conjugase may play no role in the digestion of dietary folate, being, instead, concerned with folate metabolism within the enterocyte (Halsted, 1990).

Significant conjugase activity has also been reported in the pancreatic juice of pigs and humans (Gregory, 1995). Bhandari *et al.* (1990) found the porcine pancreatic enzyme to be Zn^{2+}-dependent with maximum activity at pH 4.0–4.5. Feeding stimulated secretion of pancreatic juice, including conjugase activity. Chandler *et al.* (1991) calculated that conjugase activity in porcine pancreatic juice was minor relative to the activity of the jejunal brush-border conjugase.

Absorption of dietary folate

In the human, the entire small intestine is capable of absorbing monoglutamyl folate. Absorption is somewhat greater in the proximal than in the distal jejunum which, in turn, is much greater than in the ileum. Folate transport across the brush-border membrane of the enterocyte proceeds by two parallel processes (Selhub & Rosenberg, 1981). At physiological concentrations ($<5\ \mu M$) of luminal folate, transport occurs primarily by a saturable process, whereas at higher concentrations, transport occurs by a non-saturable process with characteristics of simple diffusion. Zimmerman *et al.* (1986) produced data which suggest that the latter process occurs in part through a conductance pathway that involves anionic folate and a cation (perhaps Na^+) whose membrane permeation properties affect the rate of folate transport. The saturable component is discussed in the following with no further mention of unsaturable transport.

Transport of folate is mediated by the reduced folate carrier and is markedly influenced by changes in pH (Schron, 1991). Folate exists primarily as an anion at the pH of the lumenal contents. *In vitro* studies using everted rat jejunal rings showed that absorption was maximal at pH 6.3 and fell off sharply between pH 6.3 and 7.6 (Russell *et al.*, 1979). In studies using brush-border membrane vesicles (Said *et al.*, 1987), folate uptake increased as the pH of the incubation buffer was decreased from 7.4 to 5.5. This increase in folate uptake appeared to be partly mediated through $folate^-/OH^-$ exchange and/or $folate^-/H^+$ co-transport mechanisms driven by the proton gradient across the membrane and partly through a direct effect of acidic pH on the carrier. Inhibition of folate transport by the anion transport inhibitor DIDS suggested the involvement of the $folate^-/OH^-$ exchange mechanism. Data reported by Mason *et al.* (1990) suggest that the effect of pH on the carrier is attributable to an increased affinity of the carrier for its folate substrate. The physiological relevance of the pH dependency may be related to the existence of the acidic microclimate at the luminal surface of the jejunum. This so-called 'unstirred layer' has a pH that is approximately 2 units lower than the bulk luminal pH and therefore provides the necessary extracellular acidic conditions for folate uptake.

Said *et al.* (1987) also found that folate transport across the brush-border membrane was saturable, competitively inhibited by structural analogues of folic acid, unaffected by transmembrane electrical potential, and Na^+-independent. The human intestinal reduced folate carrier has been cloned and characterized at the molecular level (Nguyen *et al.*, 1997).

Said *et al.* (1997) studied the intracellular regulation of intestinal folate uptake using monolayers of cultured mature IEC-6 epithelial cells. These cells are derived from the proximal small intestine of a normal rat and possess all of the cellular structures of native enterocytes. Uptake of folic acid by IEC-6 cells was similar to that of the native small intestine. Intracellular cyclic AMP was found to affect the uptake of folic acid independently of protein kinase A. Protein tyrosine kinase also affected uptake, but protein kinase C and Ca^{2+}/calmodulin mediated pathways had no significant effect.

During intestinal transport some of the folate is converted within the enterocyte to 5-methyl-THF in a pH-dependent manner (Strum, 1979). This conversion is extensive at pH 6.0 and negligible at pH 7.5 presumably because dihydrofolate reductase, the rate-limiting enzyme in the reduction and methylation process, has an acidic pH optimum. The percent conversion is reduced by increasing the concentration of folate in the mucosal medium, thus indicating saturation of the process. Since at higher concentrations most transported folate remains unmodified, intestinal conversion of absorbed folic acid is not obligatory for transport into the circulation.

The mechanism of folate exit from the enterocyte into the lamina propria of the villus is also carrier-mediated and sensitive to the effect of anion exchange inhibition. In addition, the exit mechanism is electroneutral and Na^+-independent and has a higher affinity for the substrate than has the system at the brush-border membrane (Said & Redha, 1987).

Absorption of milk folate by the suckling infant

Milk from humans and several species of other mammals contains a folate-binding protein (FBP) which may be important for folate absorption by the suckling infant. In neonates, the uptake of folate bound to milk FBP occurs preferentially in the ileum as opposed to the jejunum. The incomplete development of pancreatic and intestinal absorptive functions could allow the FBP to reach the ileum without being digested. This situation was demonstrated by Salter & Mowlem (1983) who showed that a proportion of goat's milk FBP administered orally to neonatal goats survived along the length of the small intestine. Protease inhibitors inherent to colostrum may assist the passage of bound folate along the small intestine (Laskowski & Laskowski, 1951). *In vitro*, the addition of goat's milk FBP to the medium enhanced the transport of 5-methyl-THF in brush-border membrane vesicles isolated from the small intestine of neonatal goats (Salter & Blakeborough, 1988). Mason & Selhub (1988) observed that the characteristics of FBP-bound folate absorption in the suckling rat resemble in some respects the characteristics of endocytotic absorption of macromolecules – a well-documented feature of the suckling mammal's intestinal physiology.

Adaptive regulation of folate absorption

Said *et al.* (2000) induced folate deficiency in rats by feeding a folate-deficient diet that contained an antibiotic to decrease the bacterial synthesis of folate in the intestine. Using everted intestinal sacs and brush-border membrane vesicles, they showed that folate deprivation causes a specific up-regulation in the transport of physiological concentrations of folic acid across the brush-border membrane of both the small and large intestines. The effect in the small intestine took place not only in the jejunum, but also in the ileum, a region that does not usually absorb folate. The up-regulation was mediated through an increase in the number and/or activity of functional reduced folate carriers (increased V_{max}) with no significant effect on the affinity of the transport system (unchanged K_m). The up-regulation was associated with a marked increase in the levels of carrier mRNA and protein,

suggesting a possible involvement of transcriptional regulatory mechanisms. In addition to the up-regulation of transepithelial folate transport, folate deficiency was associated with a 10-fold increase in the activity of brush-border membrane conjugase. The intestine is therefore able to maximize its ability to extract the limited amount of folate ingested during periods of deprivation.

Effects of alcohol

Both hydrolysis of polyglutamyl folate by brush-border jejunal conjugase and jejunal uptake of folate are affected by chronic alcoholism. Naughton *et al.* (1989) demonstrated a significant (50%) decrease in conjugase activity in jejunal brush-border vesicles obtained from miniature pigs that had been fed ethanol as 50% of dietary energy for 1 year. Conjugase activity was also decreased by the addition of a physiological concentration of ethanol (445 mmol L^{-1}) to brush-border vesicles from control-fed pigs. These data suggest that polyglutamyl folate hydrolysis is inhibited by chronic and acute exposure to alcohol.

In a clinical study conducted by Halsted *et al.* (1973), jejunal uptake of orally administered radioactive folic acid was decreased in two hospitalized patients who developed megaloblastic bone marrow while consuming a folate-deficient diet supplemented with ethanol. Uptake was unchanged in a third patient who received the folate-deficient diet without added ethanol, and in a fourth patient who received an adequate diet with added ethanol. These findings suggest that folate malabsorption in alcoholics is the result of a dietary inadequacy and chronic alcohol ingestion acting synergistically.

17.4.3 Absorption of bacterially synthesized folate in the large intestine

A significant proportion of the bacterially synthesized folate in the large intestine exists in the form of monoglutamyl folate. Rong *et al.* (1991) have shown that a portion of this folate is absorbed by the rat and is incorporated into the various tissues. In studies using a human-derived colonic epithelial cell line NCM460 (Kumar *et al.*, 1997) and purified apical membrane vesicles isolated from the colon of human organ donors (Dudeja *et al.*, 1997), clear evidence was presented to show the existence of a specific, pH-dependent, carrier-mediated system for folate uptake.

The uptake system was found to be similar in most respects to that of the small intestine, including intracellular regulation by protein tyrosine kinase and cyclic AMP. Energy dependency was also demonstrated using different metabolic inhibitors. The K_m for the brush-border transport system of the human colon was ~8 μM compared with 1.9 μM for the small intestinal system, indicating a relatively low affinity of the colonic carrier for the folate substrate. On the other hand, the maximal velocity (V_{max}) of the colonic system was three to four times higher compared with the small intestinal system, indicating a greater capacity. The mechanism for folate exit across the basolateral membrane of the human colon was similar to that for uptake (Kode *et al.*, 1997).

A role for the colonic transport system in human folate nutrition was suggested by a report of a significant association between serum folate levels and consumption of dietary fibre (Houghton *et al.*, 1997). These authors suggested that an increase in fibre intake may promote increased folate biosynthesis by the large intestinal microflora and subsequent absorption of some of this folate.

17.4.4 Plasma transport and intracellular metabolism

Following the ingestion of foods containing natural amounts of folate, the vitamin circulates in the plasma as reduced monoglutamates, primarily 5-methyl-THF, in concentrations ranging from 10 nM to 35 nM. High oral doses of folic acid bypass the normal folate absorption mechanism, resulting in both folic acid and 5-methyl-THF appearing in the bloodstream (Kelly *et al.*, 1997). Folate in plasma seems to be distributed in three fractions: free folate and that loosely bound to plasma proteins such as albumin exist in similar proportions; less than 5% is bound to high-affinity binders (Herbert, 1999). Folate is not taken up by circulating erythrocytes during their 120-day life span; it is only taken by the developing erythrocytes in the bone marrow.

Approximately 10–20% of the reduced monoglutamyl folate in the portal blood is taken up by the liver during the first pass through this organ. The remainder is taken up by the extrahepatic tissues and demethylated by the action of vitamin B_{12}-dependent methionine synthetase (Steinberg, 1984). The resultant THF can now have glutamate residues (usually five to eight) added to it. The resultant polyglutamated THF is the functional coenzyme, accepting and transferring one-carbon units in intermediary metabolism.

The glutamate moieties of polyglutamyl folates are linked covalently by γ-peptide bonds forming an oligo-γ-glutamyl chain. The chain length changes in response to folate, methionine and vitamin B_{12} status and to changes in growth rates. The enzyme responsible for the stepwise addition of glutamate residues to intracellular folates is folylpolyglutamyl synthetase (FPGS). This enzyme is located mainly in the cytosol, although some activity is found in the mitochondrial fraction. The enzyme requires ATP as a source of energy and has optimal activity at pH 8.5–9.0.

$$H_4PteGlu_n + ATP + glutamate$$
$$(THF)$$
$$\rightarrow H_4PteGlu_{n+1} + ADP + Pi \qquad (17.1)$$

FPGS activity is particular high in the liver. The folylglutamates in rat liver are mainly pentaglutamates with smaller amounts of hexaglutamates and trace amounts of heptaglutamates. When rats are dosed with radioactive folate, pentaglutamates account for most of the label in the liver after about 6 hours. Labelled hexaglutamates appear in the liver after 2 to 3 days and heptaglutamates after about 4 weeks (Shane, 1989).

The preferred substrate for FPGS is THF; DHF and 10-formyl-THF are also effective substrates, but 5-methyl-THF, 5,10-methylene-THF and folic acid are very poor substrates. When THF is incubated with purified FPGS, the hexaglutamate and smaller amounts of the heptaglutamate accumulate. The substrate specificity determines which folylpolyglutamates are predominant in a particular tissue.

Polyglutamylation fulfils three important roles in folate metabolism. Firstly, the addition of at least three glutamate residues to monoglutamyl folate is necessary in order for folates to be retained by cells after uptake. Secondly, folylpolyglutamates have greater affinities for enzymes than their monoglutamyl counterparts; for most (but not all) folate-dependent enzymes, hexaglutamates are the most effective substrates. Thirdly, polyglutamylation facilitates the channelling of substrates between different enzymes that are organized into clusters. Channelling is the process whereby the reaction product of one enzyme is transferred directly to the next enzyme without achieving equilibrium with the cell medium.

17.4.5   Folate homeostasis

The majority of 5-methyl-THF arriving at the liver from the intestine and taken up is not demethylated and converted to polyglutamate; instead it is quickly released for distribution to extrahepatic tissues. The initial route for this distribution is the enterohepatic circulation, whereby the folate is discharged into the bile and subsequently reabsorbed by the small intestine before re-entering the systemic circulation. Accompanying 5-methyl-THF in the bile are larger amounts of non-methylated tetrahydrofolates which represent folates salvaged from dying cells such as senescent erythrocytes and hepatocytes (Shin *et al.*, 1995). Any folic acid that might have been absorbed and released into the portal circulation without modification is exclusively taken up by the liver and either converted into one-carbon derivatives of THF prior to rapid release into bile or polyglutamated and incorporated into the hepatic folate pool (Steinberg, 1984). Hepatic reduction and derivatization of folic acid provides another source of non-methylated tetrahydrofolates present in bile (Shin *et al.*, 1995).

The recycling of folate via the enterohepatic pathway may account for as much as 50% of the folate that ultimately reaches the extrahepatic tissues. Disruption of the enterohepatic cycle by bile drainage results in a fall of the serum folate level to 30–40% of normal within 6 hours – a much more dramatic drop than that seen with a folate-deficient diet. Eventually, the serum folate level stabilizes, despite continuing losses in the bile. This suggests a net flux of folate into the plasma compartment from tissue pools. Release of stored folate from cells of any tissue requires hydrolysis of the polyglutamates to monoglutamates by intracellular conjugase.

The maintenance of a normal level of plasma folate depends on regular increments of exogenous folate from the diet. The enterohepatic circulation of folate evens out the intermittent intake of dietary folate. The liver plays a major role in maintaining folate homeostasis because of its capacity to store about 50% of the total body folate, its relatively rapid folate turnover, and the large folate flux through the enterohepatic circulation (Steinberg, 1984). In situations of dietary

folate deficiency, the liver does not respond by releasing its folate stores. Rather, the non-proliferating, less metabolically active tissues mobilize their folate stores and return monoglutamyl folate to the liver. This folate is released by the liver via the enterohepatic cycle and distributed to the tissues that most require it – in particular, those with actively proliferating cells. Preferential uptake of folate by certain tissues (e.g. placenta and choroid plexus) is made possible by the presence of the folate receptor on their cellular surfaces. The kidney plays its part in conserving body folate by actively reabsorbing folate from the glomerular filtrate. In addition, a pathway exists that is capable of salvaging folate released from senescent erythrocytes.

17.4.6   Hepatic uptake of 5-methyltetrahydrofolate

Uptake of 5-methyl-THF by sinusoidal membrane vesicles isolated from human liver is an electroneutral active transport process, which is pH-dependent, sodium-independent and appears to involve co-transport with hydrogen ions mediated by the reduced folate carrier (Horne *et al.*, 1993). This would require a mechanism for maintaining a gradient of H^+ across the basolateral membrane, but how this is accomplished is not known for certain. Sinusoidal membrane vesicles isolated from rat hepatocytes contain a Na^+–H^+ exchange system (Arias & Forgac, 1984) and it can be speculated that the H^+ could be conducted along the membrane and interact with the carrier, thereby generating a 'localized' proton gradient that could energize active transport of 5-methyl-THF.

17.4.7   Transport of 5-methyltetrahydrofolate across the blood–cerebrospinal fluid barrier

One important physiological role of folate in mammalian brain is the recycling of methionine from homocysteine (Spector *et al.*, 1980). Conversely, it is essential to prevent excessive amounts of folate from entering the brain. Toxicity can be demonstrated by the seizures induced by injecting folate directly into the brain. Folate homeostasis in brain is implied by the fact that it is much more difficult to cause folate depletion in brain than in other organs, such as the liver and bone marrow. On the other hand, it is difficult to raise the concentration of 5-methyl-THF in brain by raising the plasma levels of this metabolite.

In brain, the folates exist mainly as derivatives of polyglutamyl DHF and THF, 5-methyl-THF being predominant. The concentration of folate in cerebrospinal fluid (CSF) is usually 3 to 5 times higher than in plasma (Spector, 1981). The brain cannot convert folic acid to reduced folate coenzymes as it lacks the enzyme (dihydrofolate reductase) that catalyses the reduction of folic acid to THF (Makulu et al., 1973). The high concentrations of reduced folate in CSF and brain are due to active transport of reduced folate (mainly 5-methyl-THF) from blood across the blood–CSF barrier via the choroid plexus. Once within the CSF, folate is taken up by the brain cells, but the mechanism of uptake is not known. The transport mechanism across the choroid plexus is specific for reduced folate, saturable and energy-dependent (Spector & Lorenzo, 1975a, b). A high-affinity binding protein for folate has been characterized in human choroid plexus (Holm et al., 1991) and its cross-reactivity with rabbit antibodies against the 25-kDa human milk folate-binding protein showed it to be the folate receptor. The affinity of the receptor for folate changes with pH. At the extracellular pH of 7.4 in the body, the binding of folate would be very tight; however, the binding would be appreciably less tight at the intracellular pH of the choroid plexus, pH 6.3.

The entry of 5-methyl-THF from blood into CSF is approximately one-half saturated at the normal plasma concentration of ~0.02 μM. Thus if plasma folate levels are increased to much above normal levels by intravenous injection of folate, the uptake mechanism becomes fully saturated and the brain is protected from excessive amounts of folate. Diffusion of folate across the choroid plexus is prevented by the tight junctions of adjacent choroid epithelial cells. The saturable entry of 5-methyl-THF into the central nervous system complements the regulation of plasma 5-methyl-THF levels by the intestine, liver and kidney.

Folic acid, which the brain cannot utilize, is not transported in the manner of 5-methyl-THF. If injected into the CSF, folic acid is rapidly transported via the choroid plexus to blood by a saturable system (Spector & Lorenzo, 1975b).

17.4.8 Placental transport of 5-methyltetrahydrofolate

Total folate concentrations in fetal plasma or whole blood are generally five- to six-fold higher than those in the mother, with the placental concentration being several-fold higher. This implies that active transport processes across the placenta from mother to fetus are responsible for maintaining the higher fetal concentrations.

Prasad et al. (1994a, b) investigated the mechanism of transport of 5-methyl-THF in cultured human placental trophoblast cells and JAR human placental choriocarcinoma cells. The presence of the folate receptor-α isoform (FR-α) was demonstrated in the trophoblast cells. The transport of 5-methyl-THF into the cytoplasm of the JAR cells was mediated by an anion transporter and was dependent on a transmembrane H^+ gradient generated by a V-type H^+-ATPase (proton pump). Inhibitors of receptor-mediated endocytosis had no effect on the cytosolic transport nor on the accumulation. There was also evidence of a V-type proton pump in brush-border membrane vesicles isolated from human placentas (Simon et al., 1992). Proton pumps require an accompanying movement of Cl^- in the same direction. Illsley et al. (1988) demonstrated the presence of a saturable chloride conductance and an electroneutral chloride–bicarbonate exchanger in placental brush-border membrane vesicles. Prasad et al. (1995) accomplished the molecular cloning of the human placental reduced folate carrier. All in all, these results strongly suggest that the transport of 5-methyl-THF from mother to fetus across the placental syncytiotrophoblast occurs by potocytosis involving a functional coupling between the folate receptor, the reduced folate carrier and the proton pump.

17.4.9 Renal reabsorption and secretion

Circulating free folate, but not the protein-bound fraction, is filterable at the glomerulus. Failure to reabsorb filtered folate would result in urinary losses of approximately 1 mg per day and the subsequent rapid depletion of body stores. Folic acid undergoes net tubular reabsorption in the luminal-to-serosal direction against a concentration gradient during free urinary flow, indicative of active transport. The reabsorption system becomes saturated at plasma concentrations above 0.2 mM. When the urinary flow is experimentally stopped, there is net tubular secretion of folic acid in the serosal-to-luminal direction, i.e. basolateral to apical transport (Williams & Huang, 1982).

There is strong evidence that the folate receptor (FR) plays an important role in the renal reabsorption of folate. The FR is abundant on the luminal (brush-border) surface of the proximal tubule epithelial cell (Selhub & Franklin, 1984) where its function is to capture folate molecules in the glomerular filtrate. Treatment of cultured proximal tubule cells with colchicine, which disrupts the vesicular trafficking that takes place during endocytosis, inhibits folate transport across the apical membrane, but not across the basolateral membrane (Morshed *et al.*, 1997). This suggests that folate uptake by the apical membrane of the tubular epithelial cell involves internalization of the FR–folate complex by some form of endocytosis.

Experimental evidence points to receptor-mediated endocytosis (not potocytosis) as a major transport mechanism for 5-methyl-THF transport across the tubular apical membrane. Let us look at some of the evidence. (1) Autoradiography and electron microscopy of rat kidney 10 min after intravenous infusion of [³H]folic acid revealed that the label was significantly concentrated only in the brush border, endocytic vesicles and lysosomes (Hjelle *et al.*, 1991). (2) Application of immunocytochemistry and electron microscopy after microinjection of a polyclonal anti-FR into rat proximal tubules *in situ* and fixation of the tubules at various times showed that anti-FR is conveyed sequentially from endocytic invaginations into vacuoles and thence into dense apical tubules within 15 s. There was no obvious clustering of anti-FR on brush-border membranes (Birn *et al.*, 1993). (3) Microinjection of folate-coupled colloidal gold particles into rat proximal tubules *in situ* and examination in the electron microscope revealed the location of the internalized gold particles exclusively to brush border, endocytic invaginations, vesicles, vacuoles, lysosomes and dense apical tubules. The coupling to folate increased internalization of the gold particles six-fold compared with non-coupled controls. A large fraction of the invaginations or vesicles containing gold particles were coated (Birn *et al.*, 1997). On the basis of these and other findings, it can be postulated that folate in the glomerular filtrate binds to the FR in the apical membrane of the proximal convoluted

tubule and the FR–folate complex is subsequently internalized by receptor-mediated endocytosis. After dissociation in the endosomes, folate is transported across the basolateral membrane for release into the renal vascular circulation, while the receptor migrates back into the apical membrane through dense apical tubules.

Although the above electron microscope studies point to FR-mediated endocytosis as a major player in the apical transport of 5-methyl-THF in proximal tubule epithelial cells, Morshed *et al.* (1997) reported evidence for an additional pathway or pathways. For example, although folic acid completely blocked the binding of 5-methyl-THF to the FR, it inhibited apical transport by only 50%. Involvement of the reduced folate carrier is implied by the observation that probenecid (an inhibitor of anion transport) decreased the apical transport of 5-methyl-THF by about 50%, without altering binding to the FR.

The reduced folate carrier seems to be primarily responsible for the transport of 5-methyl-THF across the basolateral membrane of the proximal tubule cell. Transport was not inhibited by colchicine and FR is not abundant in the basolateral membrane, which rules out an endocytotic pathway. Furthermore, transport was 80% inhibited by probenecid (Morshed *et al.*, 1997).

Morshed & McMartin (1997) demonstrated that secretory transport of 5-methyl-THF in human proximal tubule cells occurred as readily as reabsorptive transport. Hence urinary excretion of excess folate could result from either a decreased tubular reabsorption or an increased serosal-to-luminal secretion.

17.4.10   Excretion

Except in cases of malabsorption, the body is very adept at conserving folate of dietary origin. Folate secreted into the bile is reabsorbed in the small intestine; much of the circulating folate binds to plasma proteins and so cannot be filtered in the kidney; and the free circulating folate that is filtered is captured by the folate receptors in the renal tubules and reabsorbed into the bloodstream. The result is very little folate loss by faecal or urinary excretion.

The initial step in folate catabolism is cleavage of intracellular folylpolyglutamates at the C-9–N-10 bond, catalysed by carboxypeptidase G (EC 3.4.17.11). The resulting *p*-aminobenzoylglutamates are hydrolysed to the monoglutamates, which are *N*-acetylated before excretion; the pterin is excreted either unchanged or as biologically inactive derivatives.

Effects of alcohol

The feeding of acute doses of ethanol to fasting rats produced a marked increase in urinary folate levels, in amounts that accounted for a subsequent decrease in plasma folate levels (McMartin, 1984). Eisenga *et al.* (1989) presented evidence that acute ethanol treatment decreases proximal tubular reabsorption of 5-methyl-THF in the rat, thus enhancing the urinary excretion of this compound. McMartin *et al.* (1986) showed that repeated daily doses of ethanol produced a cumulative increase in urinary folate excretion in fed and fasted rats, although the effect in fed rats was less marked. There was no adaptation to the loss of folate during the subacute treatment. Chronic ethanol treatment (McMartin *et al.*, 1989) also led to increased urinary folate excretion in rats fed folate-containing diets, but the rats did not become folate deficient. In contrast, when ethanol-treated rats were fed folate-deficient diets for 2 weeks, only very small amounts of folate were excreted in the urine. Thus, in the absence of a dietary supply of folate, the rat adapts its renal processing of folate to conserve the vitamin. The adaptive mechanism evidently opposes and overcomes the normal effect of ethanol on the renal processing of folate.

Russell *et al.* (1983) reported that urinary folate excretion was moderately increased in human volunteers given folic acid supplements and alcohol for 2 weeks.

17.5   Biochemical functions

Folate plays an essential role in the mobilization of one-carbon units in intermediary metabolism. Such reactions are essential for the synthesis of the purines (adenine and guanine) and one of the pyrimidine nucleotides (deoxythymidine monophosphate), which are required for DNA synthesis. Folate is also directly involved in the metabolism of certain amino acids. The role of folate in the metabolism of homocysteine is discussed in Section 17.6.1.

Folic acid, the parent compound, is not biochemically active, but becomes so after reduction to THF and substitution of one-carbon units on the N-5

and/or the N-10 positions. THF accepts one-carbon groups from various degradative reactions in amino acid metabolism. The THF derivatives thus formed are coenzymes that serve as donors of one-carbon units in a variety of synthetic reactions. The folate coenzymes are interconvertible by virtue of reversible reactions. There is, however, one important exception: 5-methyl-THF cannot be converted back to 5,10-methylene-THF under physiological conditions.

17.5.1   Reduction of folic acid to THF

Folic acid and subsequently DHF are both reduced by dihydrofolate reductase (EC 1.5.1.3) to generate THF.

$$PteGlu + NADPH + H^+ \rightarrow H_2PteGlu + NADP^+$$
$$\text{(folic acid)} \qquad \text{(DHF)} \qquad (17.2)$$

$$H_2PteGlu + NADPH + H^+ \rightarrow H_4PteGlu + NADP^+$$
$$\text{(DHF)} \qquad \text{(THF)} \qquad (17.3)$$

Reaction 17.2 is essential for utilizing the synthetic form of the vitamin, folic acid. The enzyme is the target of the anticancer drug methotrexate, which binds extremely tightly to the active site. By inhibiting the enzyme, methotrexate produces a partial depletion of intracellular reduced folates, thereby impeding folate-dependent one-carbon reactions and conferring cytotoxicity. Methotrexate treatment also results in the accumulation of DHF and 10-formyl-DHF. The latter compound, which is not found in normal tissues, may be responsible for the drug-related cytotoxicity, since it inhibits both glycinamide ribotide transformylase and thymidylate synthase (Baram *et al.*, 1988). Chemotherapy consists of alternating periods of administration of methotrexate and 5-formyl-THF (leucovorin) in order to replete the normal tissues.

17.5.2   Folate coenzymes in one-carbon transfer reactions

Interconversion of serine and glycine

Reaction 17.4 (Fig. 17.3) is the major pathway for serine catabolism under normal conditions and the β-carbon of serine is the major source of one-carbon units for folate metabolism. The reversible reaction between serine and glycine is catalysed by serine hydroxymethyltransferase (EC 2.1.2.1) which

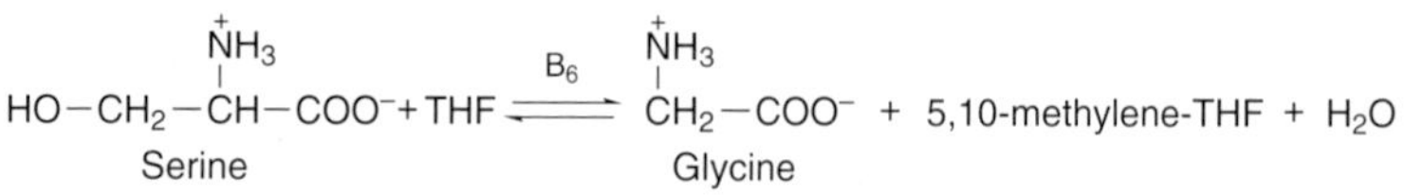

Fig. 17.3 Interconversion of serine to glycine.

requires pyridoxal phosphate (vitamin B_6) as cofactor. Mammalian cells contain two isozymes of the hydroxymethyltransferase, one cytosolic and one mitochondrial, encoded by separate genes. The cytosolic isozyme appears to be the predominant one in liver. The formation of 5,10-methylene-THF plays a central role in one-carbon metabolism as its one-carbon moiety can be directed into pathways for the synthesis of methionine, purine and pyrimidine nucleotide.

$$\text{serine} + \text{THF} \xrightleftharpoons{B_6} \text{glycine} + 5,10\text{-methylene-THF} + H_2O \quad (17.4)$$

5-Methyl-THF is a potent inhibitor of serine hydroxymethyltransferase, so when there is an adequate concentration of substituted folates from other sources, serine can be spared for energy-yielding metabolism or gluconeogenesis.

Synthesis of 5,10-methenyl-THF from a product of histidine catabolism

Formiminoglutamate, a product of histidine catabolism, provides an alternative source of one-carbon units to the principal source, serine. Transfer of the formimino group of formiminoglutamate to THF (reaction 17.5) (Fig. 17.4) and removal of the =NH group by the bifunctional enzyme 5-formimino-THF cyclodeaminase/transferase yields 5,10-methenyl-THF (reaction 17.6).

$$N\text{-formiminoglutamate} + \text{THF} \rightarrow \text{glutamate} + 5\text{-formimino-THF} \quad (17.5)$$

$$5\text{-formimino-THF} + 2H^+ \rightarrow 5,10\text{-methenyl-THF} + NH_4^+ \quad (17.6)$$

Synthesis of deoxythymidine monophosphate

Deoxythymidine monophosphate (dTMP) is the nucleotide of the pyrimidine thymine and is one of the four nucleotide constituents of DNA. (Note: deoxythymidine monophosphate is frequently and confusingly referred to as thymidine monophosphate and also as thymidylate.) The transfer of a one-carbon unit from deoxyuridine monophosphate (dUMP) to

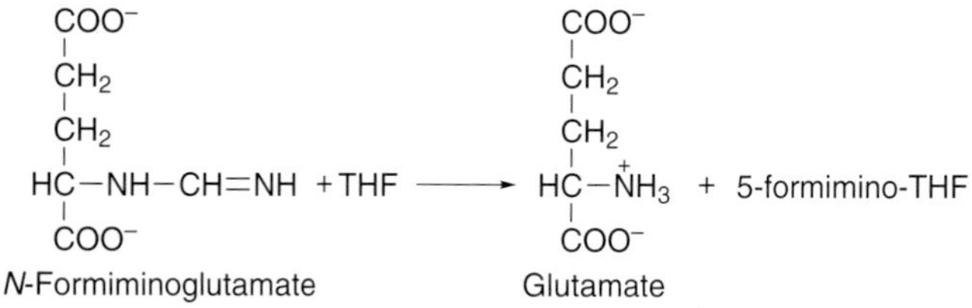

Fig. 17.4 Formimination of THF.

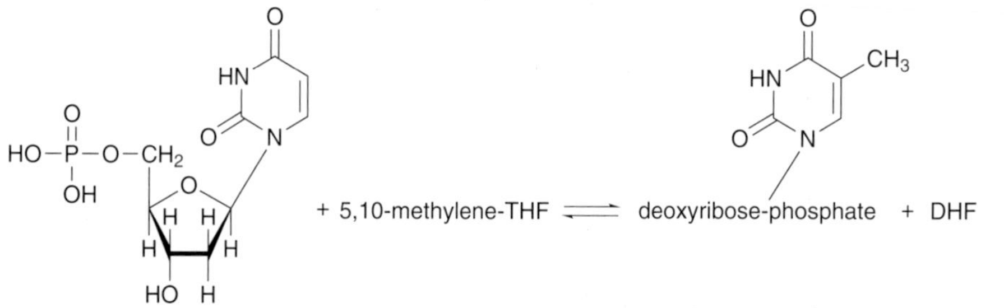

Deoxyuridine monophosphate (dUMP)

Deoxythymidine monophosphate (dTMP)

Fig. 17.5 Methylation of deoxyuridine monophosphate (dUMP) to deoxythymidine monophosphate (dTMP).

dTMP (reaction 17.7) (Fig. 17.5) is required for DNA synthesis. The enzyme responsible for the methylation, thymidylate synthase (EC 2.1.1.45), is rate limiting in the synthesis of DNA by the action of DNA polymerase. The transferred methylene group (CH_2) is reduced to a methyl group (CH_3), the reducing component being supplied by the reduced pteridine ring of 5,10-methylene-THF, which is converted to DHF. The DHF is then rapidly reduced to THF by dihydrofolate reductase, after which 5,10-methylene-THF can be regenerated through reaction 17.4.

$$dUMP + 5,10\text{-methylene-THF} \rightarrow dTMP + DHF \quad (17.7)$$

dTMP is not an immediate precursor for DNA synthesis. The nucleotide must first be converted to deoxythymidine triphosphate (dTTP) by two consecutive reactions with ATP. The high-energy bonds of the β and γ terminal phosphates of dTTP and other nucleotide triphosphates provide the energy required to form each phosphodiester bond of the growing strand of complementary DNA. The loss of the pyrophosphate results in the nucleotide monophosphates being incorporated into the new polynucleotide chain.

Purine biosynthesis

Adenine and guanine are the two common purine base constituents of DNA and RNA. In the second step of purine biosynthesis, glycine reacts with 5-phosphoribosyl-1-amine to produce glycinamide ribonucleotide (GAR). GAR then reacts with 10-formyl-THF to produce formylglycinamide ribonucleotide (FGAR). The transfer of the formyl group from the folate coenzyme to GAR is catalysed by GAR transformylase (EC 2.1.2.2). This reaction (reaction 17.8) (Fig. 17.6) gives rise to the C-8 position of the eventual purine ring.

glycinamide ribonucleotide + 10-formyl-THF →
(GAR)
    formylglycinamide ribonucleotide + THF
    (FGAR)   (17.8)

A similar folate-dependent reaction (reaction 17.9) (Fig. 17.7) is involved in the penultimate (ninth) step of purine biosynthesis, giving rise to the C-2 position of the nearly formed purine ring. In this reaction, the transference of formate to 5-amino-4-imidazole carboxamide ribonucleotide (AICAR) to produce FAICAR is catalysed by AICAR transformylase (EC 2.1.2.3).

5-amino-4-imidazole carboxamide ribonucleotide (AICAR)
+ 10-formyl-THF →
    formyl-5-amino-4-imidazole carboxamide
    ribonucleotide + THF   (17.9)
    (FAICAR)

The 10-formyl-THF used in the biosynthesis of purines can be produced by reactions catalysed by a trifunctional enzyme known as C_1-THF synthase

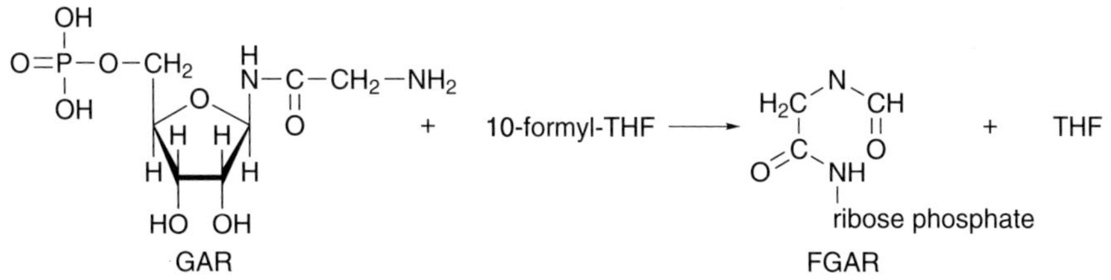

Fig. 17.6 Conversion of glycinamide ribonucleotide (GAR) to formylglycinamide ribonucleotride (FGAR).

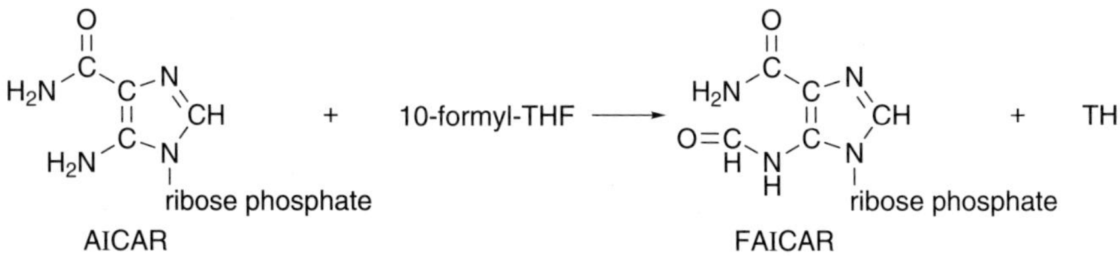

Fig. 17.7 Conversion of AICAR to FAICAR.

(Shane, 1989). This enzyme has two domains in its protein structure, each containing a folate-binding site. One domain contains two enzyme activities: (1) 5,10-methylene-THF dehydrogenase (EC 1.5.1.5), which converts 5,10-methylene-THF to 5,10-methenyl-THF (reaction 17.10) and (2) 5,10-methenyl-THF cyclohydrolase (EC 3.5.4.9), which converts 5,10-methenyl-THF to 10-formyl-THF (reaction 17.11). The second domain contains the third enzyme activity, namely 10-formyl-THF synthetase (EC 6.3.4.3) which catalyses the conversion of formate to 10-formyl-THF (reaction 17.12).

$$5,10\text{-methylene-THF} + NADP^+ \rightarrow$$
$$5,10\text{-methenyl-THF} + NADPH \quad (17.10)$$

$$5,10\text{-methenyl-THF} + H_2O \rightarrow$$
$$10\text{-formyl-THF} + H^+ \quad (17.11)$$

$$THF + HCOOH + ATP \rightarrow 10\text{-formyl-THF}$$
$$(\text{formate}) \qquad + ADP + Pi \quad (17.12)$$

Formate is derived metabolically from the indole ring of tryptophan. Under normal physiological conditions, formate constitutes only a minor source of 1-carbon units for folate metabolism in mammalian tissues.

Disposal of excess one-carbon units

Excess one-carbon units formed during the catabolism of histidine, tryptophan, glycine, serine or formate can be eliminated by reaction 17.13, which is catalysed by 10-formyl-THF dehydrogenase (EC 1.5.1.6). This enzyme is inhibited by the product THF and regulated by the ratio of 10-formyl-THF to free THF in the tissue.

$$10\text{-formyl-THF} + NADP^+ + H_2O \rightarrow$$
$$THF + NADPH + H^+ + CO_2 \quad (17.13)$$

Choline catabolism

Choline catabolism takes place exclusively in liver mitochondria (Wagner, 1996). Choline first undergoes a two-step oxidation to betaine (trimethylglycine), followed by the transfer of one of the methyl groups of betaine to homocysteine to generate methionine and dimethylglycine. The dimethylglycine undergoes an oxidative demethylation to sarcosine (N-methylglycine) which in turn is similarly converted to glycine. Reactions 17.14 and 17.15 (Fig. 17.8) are catalysed respectively by the flavoproteins dimethylglycine dehydrogenase (EC 1.5.99.2) and sarcosine dehydrogenase (EC 1.5.99.1). These enzymes can function at a maximal rate in the absence of folate. However, THF effectively traps the formaldehyde produced and thus minimizes the accumulation of this potentially toxic compound in the cell (Brody, 1991).

$$N,N\text{-dimethylglycine} + THF + FAD \rightarrow$$
$$\text{sarcosine} + 5,10\text{-methylene-THF} + FADH_2 \quad (17.14)$$

$$\text{sarcosine} + THF + FAD \rightarrow$$
$$\text{glycine} + 5,10\text{-methylene-THF} + FADH_2 \quad (17.15)$$

Cytoplasmic sarcosine, if transported into the mitochondria, is an additional potential source of one-carbon units for mitochondrial metabolism. Cytoplasmic sarcosine is formed by methylation of glycine by S-adenosylmethionine in a reaction catalysed by glycine N-methyltransferase (Shane, 1989).

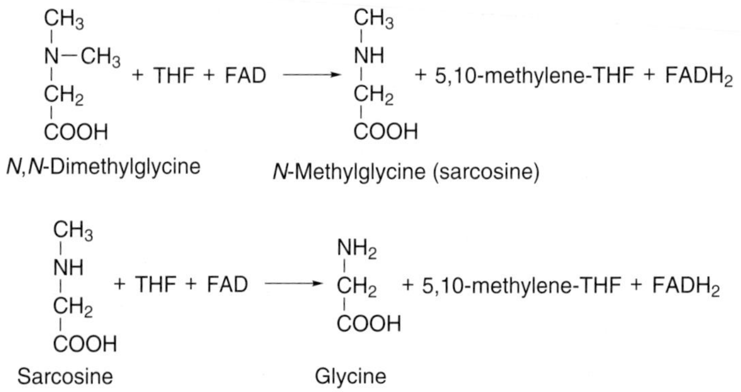

Fig. 17.8 Two-step conversion of dimethylglycine to glycine.

Serine and glycine metabolism

Mitochondria contain a serine hydroxymethyltrans-ferase isozyme for the reversible interconversion of serine and glycine (see reaction 17.4). The major pathway of glycine metabolism is via the oxidative decarboxylation of glycine catalysed by a multisub-unit enzyme complex known as the glycine cleavage system (Okamura-Ikeda *et al.*, 1987). The result of glycine catabolism is that the α-carbon of glycine is converted to a one-carbon compound which enters the intracellular folate pool.

The glycine cleavage system comprises three en-zymes, designated P-, T- and L-proteins, and a car-rier protein, known as the H-protein. The H-protein contains covalently bound lipoic acid, which exists in either the oxidized or reduced form (Fig. 17.9). The four proteins participate in reactions 17.16 to 17.18 in the following manner. In reaction 17.16, glycine forms a Schiff base with pyridoxal phosphate (vitamin B_6), the coenzyme of P-protein. The disulphide (oxidized) form of lipoate on the H-protein then combines with the Schiff base, liberating CO_2 from the glycine car-boxyl group. In reaction 17.17, the H-protein–inter-mediate complex serves as a substrate for T-protein which, in the presence of THF, catalyses the decompo-sition of the complex to H-protein, ammonia and for-maldehyde. The formaldehyde is transferred to THF forming 5,10-methylene-THF. In reaction 17.18, the disulphydryl lipoate on H-protein is reoxidized by the NAD^+-dependent L-protein.

$$CH_2(NH_2)COOH + \text{H-protein-lipoylS}_2 \xrightarrow{\text{P-protein (}B_6\text{)}}$$
$$\text{H-protein-lipoyl(SH)S–CH}_2NH_2 + CO_2 \quad (17.16)$$

$$\text{H-protein-lipoyl(SH)S–CH}_2NH_2 + THF \xrightarrow{\text{T-protein}}$$
$$\text{5,10-methenyl-THF} + \text{H-protein-lipoyl(SH)}_2 + NH_3 \quad (17.17)$$

$$\text{H-protein-lipoyl(SH)}_2 + NAD^+ \xrightarrow{\text{L-protein}}$$
$$\text{H-protein-lipoylS}_2 + NADH + H^+ \quad (17.18)$$

The overall reaction is:

$$\text{glycine} + THF + NAD^+ \rightarrow$$
$$\text{5,10-methenyl-THF} + NH_3 + CO_2 + NADH + H^+ \quad (17.19)$$

The glycine cleavage system, although reversible *in vitro*, is not utilized for glycine synthesis *in vivo*. However, coupling of the mitochondrial serine hy-droxymethyltransferase and glycine cleavage system provides a mechanism for the synthesis of serine from glycine. One molecule of serine can arise by reversal of the transferase-catalysed reaction. The 5,10-meth-ylene-THF required for the reversed reaction arises from oxidative decarboxylation of an additional molecule of glycine via the cleavage system (Shane, 1989).

17.6 Homocysteine-related occlusive arterial and thrombotic diseases

17.6.1 Cellular metabolism of homocysteine

Homocysteine is a sulphur-containing amino acid formed as an intermediate during the conversion of methionine to cysteine. It is not a constituent of pro-tein and hence is not present in the diet. If the balance between synthesis and turnover of homocysteine is interrupted, homocysteine and its derivatives begin to accumulate in cells. The cell is able to export poten-tially toxic homocysteine, leading to the appearance of excess homocysteine in the blood (hyperhomo-cysteinaemia).

In humans, the metabolism of homocysteine in-volves two pathways in which homocysteine under-goes (1) remethylation and (2) trans-sulphuration (Selhub & Miller, 1992). The overall metabolism of homocysteine is shown in Fig. 17.10. Individual reac-tions are shown in Fig. 17.11.

In remethylation, homocysteine acquires a methyl group from 5-methyl-THF or from betaine to form methionine. Remethylation by either route is essential

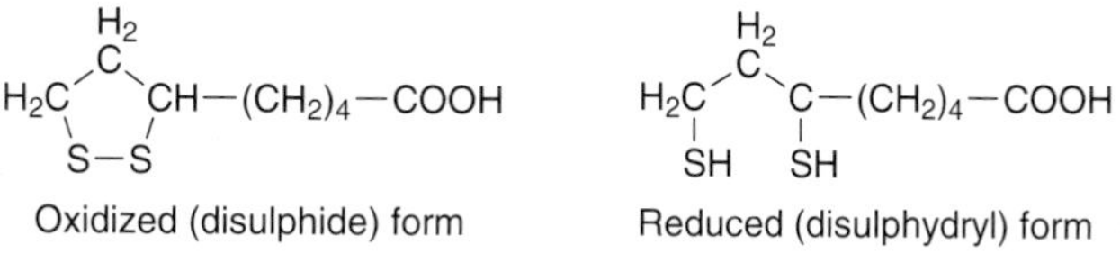

Fig. 17.9 Structures of oxidized and reduced lipoic acid.

Oxidized (disulphide) form   Reduced (disulphydryl) form

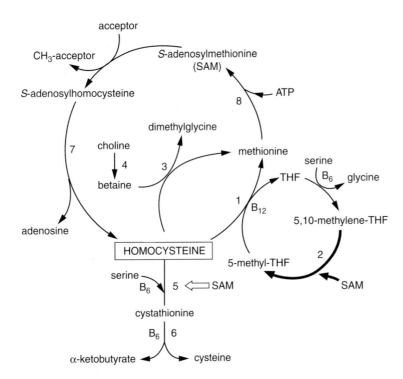

Fig. 17.10 Pathways of homocysteine metabolism showing involvement of vitamins B_6 and B_{12} as coenzymes. Enzyme reactions that are regulated by S-adenosylmethionine (SAM) are indicated by large arrows; closed arrow indicates inhibition, open arrow indicates activation. Enzymes: (1) methionine synthase, (2) 5,10-methylene-THF reductase, (3) betaine: homocysteine methyltransferase, (4) choline dehydrogenase, (5) cystathionine β-synthase, (6) γ-cystathionase, (7) S-adenosylhomocysteine hydrolase, (8) methionine-adenosyl transferase. THF, tetrahydrofolate. The reduction of 5,10-methylene-THF is irreversible under physiological conditions. (From Selhub & Miller, 1992). Reproduced with permission by the *Americal Journal of Clinical Nutrition.* © Am J Clin Nutr. American Society for Clinical Nutrition.

for maintaining adequate intracellular pools of methionine as well as for maintaining concentrations of homocysteine at non-toxic concentrations.

A considerable proportion of methionine is activated by ATP to form S-adenosylmethionine (SAM). SAM serves primarily as a methyl donor to a variety of acceptors, including DNA, neurotransmitters, phospholipids and hormones. S-Adenosylhomocysteine, the by-product of these methyl transfer reactions, is hydrolysed, thus regenerating homocysteine, which can be utilized to start a new cycle of methyl-group transfer.

The remethylation of homocysteine to methionine is catalysed by methionine synthase (EC 2.1.1.13) which has an enzyme-bound methylcobalamin (vitamin B_{12}) cofactor. The cofactor acts as an intermediate methyl-group carrier between 5-methyl-THF and homocysteine. Over time, the essential methylcob(I)alamin cofactor becomes oxidized to methylcob(II)alamin, rendering methyl synthase inactive. An auxiliary enzyme, methionine synthase reductase, catalyses the regeneration of functional cobalamin cofactor by reductive methylation via a reaction in which SAM is employed as a methyl donor.

The methyl group of 5-methyl-THF is synthesized *de novo* when a carbon unit is transferred from a carbon source, such as serine, to THF. The product, 5,10-methylene-THF, is subsequently reduced to 5-methyl-THF, which is a poor substrate for polyglutamylation. Since methionine synthase is unique in converting 5-methyl-THF to THF, which *is* readily polyglutamated, the enzyme is rate-limiting for the cellular accumulation of polyglutamyl folates.

The reaction with betaine uses preformed methyl groups because betaine is derived from choline, which in part is obtained from the diet and in part is synthesized through successive methylations of phosphatidylethanolamine.

The reduction of 5,10-methylene-THF to 5-methyl-THF (reaction 17.20) is catalysed by 5,10-methylenetetrahydrofolate reductase (MTHFR) (EC 1.1.1.68) and is irreversible under physiological conditions. A non-covalently bound flavin adenine nucleotide (FAD) coenzyme accepts reducing equivalents from NADPH and transfers them to 5,10-methylene-THF.

$$\text{5,10-methylene-THF} + \text{FADH}_2 + \text{NADPH} + \text{H}^+ \rightarrow$$
$$\text{5-methyl-THF} + \text{FAD} + \text{NADP}^+ \quad (17.20)$$

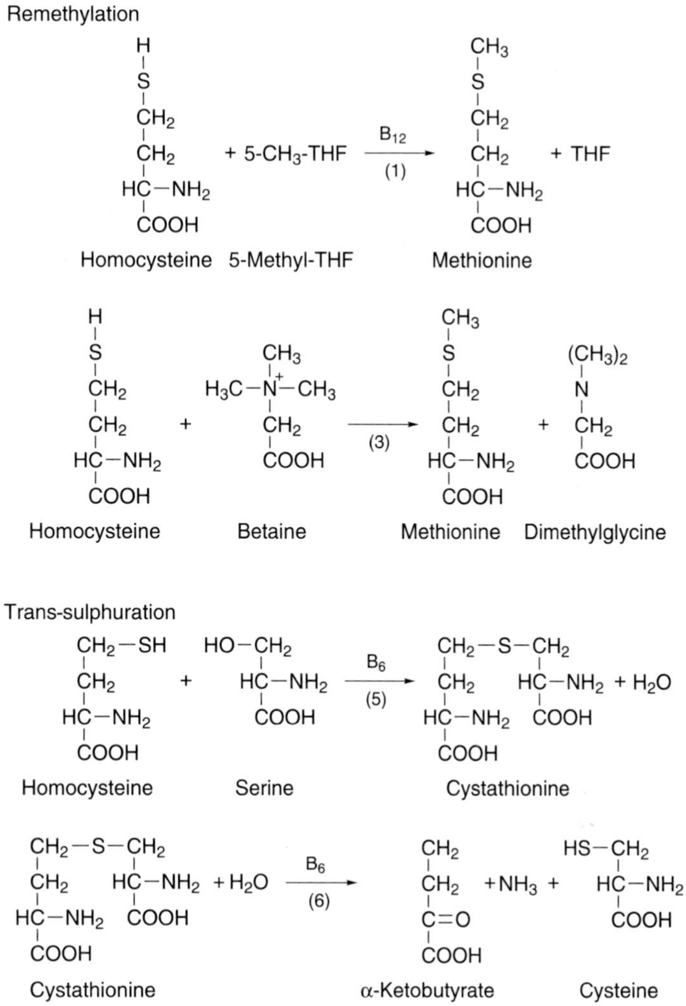

Remethylation

```
H                                          CH3
|                                          |
S                                          S
|                                          |
CH2                            B12         CH2
|                                          |
CH2        + 5-CH3-THF       ———>          CH2        + THF
|                            (1)           |
HC—NH2                                     HC—NH2
|                                          |
COOH                                       COOH

Homocysteine  5-Methyl-THF              Methionine
```

```
H                                          CH3
|                                          |
S                  CH3                      S              (CH3)2
|                  |+                       |              |
CH2          H3C—N—CH3                      CH2            N
|       +          |          ———>          |         +    |
CH2                CH2        (3)            CH2            CH2
|                  |                         |             |
HC—NH2             COOH                      HC—NH2        COOH
|                                            |
COOH                                         COOH

Homocysteine      Betaine              Methionine   Dimethylglycine
```

Trans-sulphuration

```
CH2—SH       HO—CH2                    CH2—S—CH2
|            |              B6         |
CH2     +    HC—NH2       ———>         CH2     HC—NH2 + H2O
|            |             (5)         |       |
HC—NH2       COOH                      HC—NH2  COOH
|                                      |
COOH                                   COOH

Homocysteine    Serine                    Cystathionine
```

```
CH2—S—CH2                              CH2              HS—CH2
|        |            B6               |                |
CH2      HC—NH2 +H2O ———>              CH2    +NH3 +     HC—NH2
|        |            (6)              |                |
HC—NH2   COOH                          C=O              COOH
|                                      |
COOH                                   COOH

Cystathionine                       α-Ketobutyrate      Cysteine
```

Fig. 17.11 Individual reactions involved in homocysteine metabolism. Numbers in parentheses correspond to the enzymes numbered in Fig. 17.10.

Reaction 17.20 is the only reaction capable of producing 5-methyl-THF in the body. The 5-methyl-THF is used exclusively for the regeneration of methionine from homocysteine.

In the trans-sulphuration pathway, homocysteine condenses with serine to form cystathionine in a vitamin B_6-dependent irreversible reaction. Cystathionine is then hydrolysed by a second vitamin B_6-dependent enzyme to form cysteine and α-ketobutyrate. Excess cysteine is oxidized to taurine and eventually to inorganic sulphates. Thus, in addition to the synthesis of cysteine, this trans-sulphuration pathway effectively catabolizes potentially toxic homocysteine, which is not required for methyl group transfer.

SAM is both an allosteric inhibitor of MTHFR and an activator of cystathionine β-synthase. The ability of SAM to act as an enzyme effector provides a means by which remethylation and trans-sulphuration can be coordinated. When cellular SAM concentration is low, the synthesis of 5-methyl-THF will proceed uninhibited, whereas cystathionine synthesis will be suppressed. This will result in the conservation of homocysteine for methionine synthesis. Conversely, when SAM concentration is high, inhibition of 5-methyl-THF synthesis is accompanied by the diversion of homocysteine through the trans-sulphuration pathway because of stimulated cystathionine synthesis.

Increased synthesis of deoxythymidine monophosphate (dTMP) in actively proliferating cells elevates DHF levels (see reaction 17.7). Inhibition of the allosteric MTHFR by DHF provides a regulatory mechanism for ensuring that priority is given to DNA synthesis over methionine formation in proliferating tissues (Matthews & Baugh, 1980).

17.6.2   Hyperhomocysteinaemia

In plasma, 70–80% of homocysteine is bound to plasma proteins, chiefly albumin; only about 1% circulates as free homocysteine. The remaining 20–30% circulates as homocysteine disulphide (homocystine) or as the mixed disulphide, homocysteine–cysteine. Plasma homocysteine assays measure total homocysteine, which is the sum of the homocysteine moieties present in all of the above forms. Because variable changes in plasma homocysteine concentration have been observed post-prandially, it is customary to obtain measurements in the fasting state. Normal levels of fasting plasma homocysteine are considered to be between 5 and 15 µmol L^{-1}. Higher fasting values are classified arbitrarily as moderate (16–30), intermediate (31–100) and severe (>100 µmol L^{-1}) hyperhomocysteinaemia. The methionine loading test has been used to accentuate abnormalities of the homocysteine metabolic pathways. The test measures fasting plasma homocysteine before and 2 hours after an oral dose of methionine (100 mg per kg body weight). An elevated post-loading homocysteine level indicates an abnormality.

Hyperhomocysteinaemia can result from inherited defects in enzymes necessary for either trans-sulphuration or remethylation and from acquired deficiencies in vitamin coenzymes. Renal insufficiency can also lead to hyperhomocysteinaemia. Subclinical folate deficiency is commonly associated with hyperhomocysteinaemia, presumably because of decreased remethylation of homocysteine. Kang et al. (1987) found elevated total homocysteine levels in 84% of subjects with subnormal folate levels. The mean homocysteine level in the low-folate subjects was about four-fold greater than the mean level in the control subjects.

An association between mild hyperhomocysteinaemia and increased risk of occlusive vascular disease in the coronary, cerebral and peripheral arteries has been demonstrated in case-control (Selhub et al., 1995; European Concerted Action Project, 1997) and prospective (Stampfer et al., 1992; Arneson et al., 1995; Perry et al., 1995) studies. Plasma homocysteine concentration is a strong predictor of mortality in patients with angiographically confirmed coronary artery disease

(Nygard et al., 1997). Whether hyperhomocysteinaemia is a causal risk factor for the disease or simply a marker of another prothrombotic risk factor(s) is debatable (Kuller & Evans, 1998).

Up to 30% of patients with coronary artery disease had homocysteine elevations that were 10–50% greater than the level observed among normal subjects (Clarke et al., 1991). Subjects with hyperhomocysteinaemia have a two-fold to three-fold increase in risk of developing cardiovascular disease or venous thrombosis (den Heijer et al., 1998). In vitro studies have shown that high concentrations of homocysteine can promote a prothrombotic state at the luminal surface of the blood vessel (Lentz, 1998). An association between impaired endothelium-dependent vasodilation and hyperhomocysteinaemia was demonstrated in children with homozygous homocystinuria (Celermajer et al., 1993), in monkeys fed a methionine-enriched diet (Lentz et al., 1996), in methionine-loaded healthy humans (Bellamy et al., 1998; Chambers et al., 1998) and in non-induced hyperhomocysteinaemic healthy middle-aged (Woo et al., 1997) and elderly (Tawakol et al., 1997) humans. In healthy human subjects, even physiological increments in plasma homocysteine following oral administration of methionine or an animal protein meal impaired endothelium-dependent vasodilatation (Chambers et al., 1999a). Plasma homocysteine concentration can be decreased by dietary supplementation with folic acid, which suggests that hyperhomocysteinaemia may be a treatable risk factor for vascular disease.

17.6.3   Effects of homocysteine on vascular function

The following in vivo observations provide insight into potential mechanisms of vascular dysfunction in moderate hyperhomocysteinaemia. Infusion of homocystine caused patchy desquamation of arterial endothelial cells, proliferation of arterial smooth muscle cells and intimal thickening in baboons (Harker et al., 1976). The endothelial injury, by exposing the subcellular matrix, could lead to platelet aggregation. In rats, acute methionine-induced hyperhomocysteinaemia enhanced platelet aggregation in response to thrombin and ADP as well as the thrombin-induced platelet synthesis of thromboxane. It also stimulated the basal and lipopolysaccharide-induced tissue factor activity of macrophages (Durand et al., 1997). In healthy humans, coagulation and circulating adhesion molecules significantly increased after methionine loading, but not after placebo or methionine ingestion with antioxidant vitamins C and E (Nappo *et al.*, 1999). Hyperhomocysteinaemia in minipigs caused deterioration of elastic material of the arterial wall (Charpiot *et al.*, 1998).

Homocysteine can be viewed as an early risk factor for atherosclerosis. When added to plasma it undergoes auto-oxidation, forming homocystine, homocysteine-mixed disulphides and homocysteine thiolactone. During oxidation of the sulphydryl group, superoxide and hydrogen peroxide are generated. Both of these oxygen-derived molecules give rise to the harmful hydroxyl radical, the former by reacting with nitric oxide. The hydroxyl radical initiates lipid peroxidation at the endothelial cell surface, thus accounting for the cytotoxic effects of superoxide and hydrogen peroxide. Upchurch *et al.* (1997) showed that, compared with control cells, cultured aortic endothelial cells treated with homocysteine showed a significant reduction in glutathione peroxidase activity. Thus, in addition to increasing the generation of hydrogen peroxide, homocysteine may selectively impair the endothelial cell's ability to detoxify hydrogen peroxide.

Acute methionine-induced hyperhomocysteinaemia impaired vascular responses to L-arginine, the natural precursor of nitric oxide, in healthy humans (Nappo *et al.*, 1999). The impairment of endothelial function was prevented by a 1 g (Chambers *et al.*, 1999b) or 2 g (Kanani *et al.*, 1999) daily supplement of ascorbic acid, suggesting that the effects of hyperhomocysteinaemia are produced through an increase in oxidative stress. By scavenging reactive oxygen species, ascorbic acid may prevent the formation of the cytotoxic hydroxyl radical. *In vivo* evidence for oxidative stress during hyperhomocysteinaemia was the demonstrations of increased lipid peroxidation after methionine loading in humans (Domagala *et al.*, 1997) and rats (Durand *et al.*, 1997).

17.6.4 Genetic effects

Polymorphisms involved in folate and homocysteine metabolism

In 1988, a thermolabile variant of MTHFR was discovered which had reduced (~50%) specific enzyme activity (Kang *et al.*, 1988). This variant was associated with intermediate hyperhomocysteinaemia, which could be corrected by oral folic acid supplementation. It was found to be present in 17% of 212 patients with proven coronary artery disease and in 5% of 202 control subjects without evidence of atherosclerotic vascular disease (Kang *et al.*, 1991). The enzyme variant was shown to be the result of a common polymorphism in the gene encoding this important rate-limiting enzyme (Frosst *et al.*, 1995). In the mutant gene a cytosine base constituent is substituted at nucleotide 677 by a thymine (C677T MTHFR). This changes the code triplet of bases from one specifying alanine to one specifying valine, and results in an alanine to valine substitution at amino acid position 222 within the catalytic domain of the protein. Individuals homozygous (TT) and heterozygous (CT) for this polymorphism exhibited mean MTHFR activities of 30% and 65%, respectively, relative to the mean activity of normal homozygotes (CC). This tiered reduction in MTHFR activity between genotypes indicates incomplete dominance at the biochemical level. Approximately 12% of individuals in the general North American population have the TT genotype, while 40–45% have the CT genotype (Rozen, 1997).

A second polymorphism in the MTHFR gene leading to an A→C base substitution at nucleotide 1298 (A1298C MTHFR) results in the coding of a glutamic acid residue instead of an alanine within the regulatory domain of the protein (van der Put *et al.*, 1998). The A1298C mutation reduces MTHFR activity, albeit to a lesser extent than C677T, but neither homozygous recessive nor heterozygous individuals have significantly higher plasma homocysteine levels compared to controls (Weisberg *et al.*, 1998). However, individuals who carry C677T and A1298C mutations on different alleles (compound heterozygotes) have slightly elevated plasma homocysteine levels. The two polymorphisms have never been observed to occur on the same allele (compound homozygosity) and any such cases would be exceedingly rare.

A common mutation of the gene encoding methionine synthase is A2756G, in which the adenine (A) to guanine (G) transition at base pair 2756 results in the replacement of aspartic acid by glycine at position 919 in the protein (van der Put *et al.*, 1997). This mutation breaks a long helix that extends from the cobalamin domain to the SAM-binding domain in the protein and is associated with an increased plasma homocysteine level. Methionine synthase reductase is the auxiliary enzyme that reductively activates me-thionine synthase. A mutant gene that encodes this enzyme, A66G, has an adenine (A) to guanine (G) substitution at nucleotide 66, changing an isoleucine to a methionine residue at amino acid position 22 within the protein (Wilson *et al.*, 1999).

Effects of the C677T 5,10-methylene-tetrahydrofolate reductase polymorphism

Under conditions of inadequate folate status, indi-viduals who are homozygous for C677T MTHFR (TT homozygotes) invariably have higher total plasma homocysteine levels than CT heterozygotes, which in turn have higher levels than normal CC homozygotes. Frosst *et al.* (1995) reported plasma homocysteine levels (μmol L^{-1}, mean $\pm$ standard error) of 22.4 ± 2.9 for TT, 13.8 ± 1.0 for CT and 12.6 ± 1.1 for CC. When folate status is adequate, plasma homocysteine levels are normal and independent of genotype. Jacques *et al.* (1996) reported that TT homozygotes with folate plasma concentrations <15.4 nmol L^{-1} had total fast-ing homocysteine levels that were 24% greater than normal CC homozygotes. Homocysteine levels were not increased in TT homozygotes whose folate plasma levels were $\geq$15.4 nmol L^{-1}. Folate protects the ther-molabile variant of MTHFR against loss of its FAD cofactor, thereby stabilizing the enzyme (Guenther *et al.*, 1999).

Although the thermolabile C677T MTHFR variant is associated with moderate or intermediate hyper-homocysteinaemia, and elevated total homocysteine is associated with increased risk of vascular disease, there is controversy concerning the influence of the C677T MTHFR polymorphism in vascular disease.

In a study of 339 American subjects (Kang *et al.*, 1993), the prevalence of thermolabile MTHFR was 18.1% and 13.4% in groups of patients with severe and mild-to-moderate coronary artery stenosis, respectively; in patients with non-stenotic coronary arteries, the prevalence was 7.9%. This positive asso-ciation between the severity of coronary artery steno-sis and the presence of thermolabile MTHFR was in-dependent of the major coronary risk factors, namely diabetes, hypertension, hyperlipidaemia and cigarette smoking. In a study of 216 Irish subjects (Gallagher *et al.*, 1996), 17% of patients with premature coronary artery disease and 7% of non-matched control sub-jects had the homozygous genotype for the C677T polymorphism (the TT genotype), giving an odds

ratio of 2.9 (95% confidence interval 1.2 to 7.2). Klui-jtmans *et al.* (1996) studied 60 Dutch patients with documented premature vascular disease (myocardial infarction, cerebral and peripheral arterial occlusive disease) who did not have any of the known risk fac-tors for vascular disease, and 111 control subjects. The TT genotype was found in 15% of the patients and 5% of the controls, giving an odds ratio of 3.1 (95% con-fidence interval 1.0 to 9.2). Kluijtmans *et al.* (1997) performed a meta-analysis of eight case-control stud-ies reporting data on the MTHFR genotype distribu-tion to estimate the relative risk of the TT genotype for coronary artery disease. The TT genotype was present in 12% of 2496 patients and in 10.4% of 2481 control subjects, resulting in a modest but significant odds ratio of 1.22 (95% confidence interval 1.01 to 1.47) relative to the normal CC genotype. Homocysteine concentrations were significantly elevated in both homozygotes (TT) and heterozygotes (CT) relative to CC individuals. In a total study sample of 2453 par-ticipants, Gardemann *et al.* (1999) could not detect an association of the C677T MTHFR polymorphism with the risk of coronary artery disease and myocar-dial infarction. However, an association was found between the TT genotypes for this polymorphism and the extent of coronary atherosclerosis in patients defined by means of coronary angiography as being at high risk for coronary artery disease. The frequency of the TT genotype was also correlated with the sever-ity of coronary artery stenosis in a study of Japanese patients (Morita *et al.*, 1997).

Other studies have shown a lack of correlation between the C677T MTHFR polymorphism and increased cardiovascular risk. In a largely white, mid-dle-class American sample of 190 cases with myocar-dial infarction and 188 healthy age- and sex-matched controls, Schmitz *et al.* (1996) found no evidence for association between the TT genotype and increased risk of myocardial infarction. The same lack of as-sociation was also reported by Ma *et al.* (1996) in American physicians, although a non-significantly increased risk was found among individuals with low folate status. In this study, the frequency of the three genotypes of C677T MTHFR were CC, 47%; CT, 40%; and TT, 13%, with a similar distribution among both patients and control subjects. In another American study of 247 older subjects with vascular disease and 594 non-age-matched healthy subjects (in three control groups), Delougherty *et al.* (1996) also found no evidence for association between the TT genotype and late-onset vascular disease. In a study of 565 white Australian men and women with established coronary artery disease and 225 healthy control subjects, Wilcken *et al.* (1996) could not identify any relationship between the mutation and the occurrence or severity of the disease. In a meta-analysis of 23 studies (Brattström *et al.*, 1998), the TT genotype was present in 11.9% of 5869 patients with cardiovascular disease and in 11.7% of 6644 control subjects, a non-significant difference.

Any association between frequency of the TT genotype and onset of vascular disease likely depends on the individual's folate status. Presumably, those studies in which a positive correlation between frequency of the TT genotype and onset of vascular disease was demonstrated included many subjects whose folate status was suboptimal. Conversely, those studies which showed no such correlation may have included many well-nourished subjects. Pursuing this line of thought, well-nourished TT homozygotes, who have no other defects of homocysteine-metabolizing enzymes, seem to be able to tolerate the reduced C677T MTHFR activity without adverse biochemical or clinical consequences. In individuals with insufficient intake of folate, the homozygous MTHFR polymorphism may contribute to hyperhomocysteinaemia and possibly heightened cardiovascular risk. The results of the various studies raise the possibility that TT homozygotes may be able to compensate for the disturbed homocysteine metabolism through increasing their intake of folate.

Effects of the A2756G methionine synthase and A66G methionine synthase reductase polymorphisms

In their prospective study of American male physicians, Chen *et al.* (2001) reported descending plasma homocysteine and ascending plasma folate across AA, AG and GG genotypes for the A2756G methionine synthase polymorphism. This suggests that the polymorphism may increase the activity of methionine synthase, leading to a lower level of homocysteine and conferring a protective effect against vascular disease. The frequencies of AA, AG and GG genotypes among control subjects were 67%, 29% and 4%, respectively. A non-significant 49% reduction in myocardial infarction risk was found among the GG subjects. Hyndman *et al.* (2000) reported that AG genotypes

are 3.4 times less likely to have recurrent myocardial infarction, heart failure, or bypass surgery (95% confidence interval 1.09 to 10.9) than AA genotypes. Yates & Lucock (2002) found that the prevalence of the mutant G allele was lower in subjects who had experienced a thromboembolic event (i.e. deep vein thrombosis) than in controls. Salomon *et al.* (2001) found that homozygosity for A2756G methionine synthase does not constitute a risk factor for idiopathic venous thromboembolism. In contrast to the apparent protective effect of the methionine synthase polymorphism, homozygosity for A66G methionine synthase reductase was found to increase the risk of premature coronary artery disease by a mechanism independent of the detrimental vascular effects of hyperhomocysteinaemia (Brown *et al.*, 2000).

17.6.5 Response to vitamin supplementation

In a meta-analysis (Homocysteine Lowering Trialists' Collaboration, 1998) individual data on 1114 people included in 12 randomized controlled trials were analysed to assess the effects of folic acid-based supplements on plasma homocysteine concentrations. The proportional and absolute reductions in blood homocysteine produced by the supplements were greater at higher pre-treatment homocysteine concentrations and at lower pre-treatment blood folate concentrations. After standardization to pre-treatment blood concentrations of homocysteine and folate, folic acid at doses ranging between 0.5 and 5 mg per day reduced blood homocysteine concentrations by 25%. Vitamin B_{12} (mean 0.5 mg daily) produced an additional 7% (3% to 10%) reduction in blood homocysteine. Vitamin B_6 (mean 16.5 mg daily) did not have a significant effect.

In a study of women with a history of unexplained recurrent miscarriages, Nelen *et al.* (1998) showed that the C677T MTHFR polymorphism affects the change in blood homocysteine and folate concentrations resulting from folic acid supplementation. Before supplementation, subjects with the TT genotype had the highest fasting plasma homocysteine concentrations and the lowest serum folate concentrations compared with the CT or CC genotypes. After 2 months of daily supplementation of 500 μg folic acid, the homocysteine-lowering effect was more pronounced in subjects with the TT genotype (41%

reduction) than in those with the CT or CC genotypes (26% reduction). The TT homozygotes exhibited the lowest absolute increase in serum folate concentration after supplementation, presumably due to impaired production of 5-methyl-THF, the primary folate form in the circulation.

Brouwer *et al.* (1999b) studied the effect of low-dose folic acid administration on plasma homocysteine concentrations in healthy women. After 4 weeks of supplementation with an average daily dose of 250 or 500 µg, plasma total homocysteine concentrations decreased significantly by 11% and 22%, respectively. Eight weeks after the treatment (week 12) plasma homocysteine levels in the supplemented group had not returned to baseline. The effectiveness of these low doses of folic acid suggests that increased intake of dietary folate from vegetables and citrus fruits would improve the folate status and decrease homocysteine concentrations. This suggestion was confirmed in a dietary controlled trial (Brouwer *et al.*, 1999a). Ward *et al.* (1997) showed that a folic acid dose as low as 200 µg per day is effective in lowering plasma homocysteine concentrations in apparently healthy adult males. The subjects were non-consumers of folic acid-fortified foods and were not taking any form of B-vitamin supplement. Thus optimal homocysteine lowering was obtained with 200 µg of supplemental folic acid over and above the subjects' mean dietary folate intake of 281 µg per day (range 191 to 421 µg per day). A supplemental folic acid dose of 100 µg per day was suboptimal.

In a review of therapeutic studies in patients with vascular disease, Mayer *et al.* (1996) concluded that folic acid at a dose of at least 400 µg per day would produce a maximal homocysteine-lowering effect. Schorah *et al.* (1998) studied the plasma responsiveness of healthy subjects to the consumption of breakfast cereals fortified with folic acid at the UK reference nutrient intake of 200 µg per day. The resultant increase in serum folate (66%) and subsequent red cell folate (24%) was associated with a small (10%) but significant decrease in plasma homocysteine. The homocysteine decrease persisted until the end of the 24-week study. The addition of vitamins B_6 and B_{12}, which have the potential for lowering plasma homocysteine levels, did not add to the folate effect. Lobo *et al.* (1999) reported that a daily 400 µg folic acid supplement containing 500 µg of vitamin B_{12} and 12.5 mg of vitamin B_6 lowered homocysteine concentrations by approximately 30% in patients with documented coronary artery disease. The reduction was similar to that obtained with 1 and 5 mg supplements of folic acid. Malinow *et al.* (1998) assessed the effects of breakfast cereals fortified with three levels of folic acid, and also containing the recommended dietary allowances of vitamins B_6 and B_{12}, in reducing plasma homocysteine levels in patients with coronary heart disease. Cereals providing 127 µg of folic acid daily, approximating the predicted increase (80–100 µg per day) that may result from the FDA's 1998 enrichment policy (Section 17.7.3), increased plasma folic acid by 31% but decreased plasma homocysteine by only 3.7%. However, cereals providing 499 and 665 µg of folic acid daily increased plasma folic acid by 65% and 106%, respectively, and decreased plasma homocysteine by 11.0% and 14.0%, respectively.

Bostom *et al.* (2002) investigated the effect of vitamin supplementation on homocysteine lowering in coronary artery disease patients chronically exposed to cereal grain flour products fortified with folic acid at 140 µg per 100 g flour. A daily supplement containing folic acid (2.5 mg), riboflavin (5 mg) and vitamin B_{12} (0.4 mg), with or without vitamin B_6 (50 mg), taken for 12 weeks provided only a very modest (1.0 µmol L^{-1}), albeit statistically significant, reduction in mean fasting total homocysteine levels relative to placebo treatment. The supplement did not significantly reduce the 2-hour post-methionine load increase in total plasma homocysteine. This modest homocysteine-lowering effect is presumably attributable to adequate folate status and highlights the impact of flour fortification with folic acid in the USA.

Observational studies (Rimm *et al.*, 1998) suggest that folate may reduce the risk of coronary heart disease. However, we await more solid evidence based on large-scale intervention trials. There is, however, plenty of evidence that folic acid improves vascular endothelial function. The improvement in endothelial function seen after folic acid supplementation is likely mediated through multiple mechanisms. In addition to its homocysteine-lowering effect, folic acid can increase nitric oxide formation by stimulating the recycling of tetrahydrobiopterin, an essential cofactor of nitric oxide synthase (Kaufman, 1991). Folate can also prevent the oxidative degradation of nitric oxide by reducing superoxide generated from nitric oxide synthase or xanthine oxidase (Verhaar *et al.*, 1998).

Constans *et al.* (1999) reported that 3 months supplementation with a combination of folic acid (5 mg) and vitamin B$_6$ (250 mg) improves biological markers of endothelial dysfunction in hyperhomocysteinaemic patients. Undas *et al.* (1999) investigated the effect of homocysteine-lowering treatment on thrombin generation in adults with hyperhomocysteinaemia, some of whom had symptomatic atherosclerotic vascular disease. The treatment consisted of daily doses of a combination of folic acid (5 mg), vitamin B$_6$ (300 mg) and vitamin B$_{12}$ (1 mg). Following the 8-week treatment, the median plasma homocysteine concentrations became significantly reduced from 20 to 10 μmol L^{-1}. The treatment also attenuated thrombin generation, both in peripheral blood and at sites of haemostatic plug formation. Using venous occlusion plethysmography to assess forearm vascular function, Verhaar *et al.* (1999) showed that 4 weeks of oral folic acid treatment (5 mg per day) restored impaired endothelial function in patients with increased risk of atherosclerosis due to familial hypercholesterolaemia. This beneficial effect occurred without changes in plasma lipid levels. Oral folate therapy would seem to be particularly appropriate for hypercholesterolaemic patients in whom lipid-lowering medication is not recommended.

Brachial artery endothelial-dependent dilatation can be measured by vascular ultrasound, a non-invasive test that relates mainly to endothelial nitric oxide release in response to shear stress. Endothelial function in the brachial artery correlates significantly with that in the coronary vasculature (Anderson *et al.*, 1995) as well as with the extent of coronary artery disease assessed angiographically (Neunteufl *et al.*, 1997). Vascular ultrasound was used to demonstrate that 5 mg (Bellamy *et al.*, 1999) and 10 mg (Woo *et al.*, 1999) daily supplements of folic acid improve endothelial function in healthy adults with mild hyperhomocysteinaemia. Chambers *et al.* (2000) showed that supplementation with a combination of folic acid (5 mg) and vitamin B$_{12}$ (1 mg), daily for 8 weeks, improved endothelial dysfunction in patients with established coronary heart disease. An independent relationship was found between flow-mediated dilatation and concentration of free, but not protein-bound, homocysteine. Thus free plasma homocysteine may be a more accurate index of the *in vivo* biological activity of homocysteine than total homocysteine.

It must be pointed out that the 5 mg daily dose of folic acid used to demonstrate improvements in vascular endothelial function exceeds the Tolerable Upper Intake Level for adults of 1 mg per day of folate from fortified foods or supplements set by the Institute of Medicine (1998). Any folic acid treatment to lower plasma homocysteine must include vitamin B$_{12}$ to avoid the possible development of neurological damage in persons with a chronic B$_{12}$ deficiency (see Section 17.9.2).

17.7 Folate and neural tube defects

17.7.1 Introduction

Neural tube defects (NTDs) comprise a range of congenital malformations resulting from a failure of the neural tube to close during embryonic development, late in the fourth week after conception. NTDs include spina bifida, in which the developing neural tube fails to close posteriorly, causing the herniation of meninges (meningocele), neural tissue (myelocele) or both (myelomeningocele). Spina bifida causes varying degrees of motor paralysis as well as impaired bowel, bladder and sexual function. Failure of the anterior cranial portion of the neural tube to close leads to anencephaly, a fatal condition in which the brain is exposed and incompletely developed, and encephalocele, in which meninges and neural tissue herniate through a defect in the skull.

NTDs are among the most common of severe birth defects, affecting about 4000 pregnancies in the United States each year. Of these pregnancies, approximately 2500 result in babies born with spina bifida and anencephaly; the remaining NTD-affected pregnancies are electively terminated (Mulinare, 1995). In many countries the prevalence of NTD is approximately 1 in 1000 births. Over 95% of NTD-affected pregnancies occur in women who have not previously had an affected pregnancy. Women who have had a previous NTD-affected pregnancy are 10–20 times more likely to have a subsequent affected pregnancy than those who have not. Some rare cases of NTD (e.g. Meckel–Gruber syndrome) have a purely genetic basis. However, the majority of cases have an underlying genetic basis that can be influenced by a variety of environmental (nutritional, geographical and socioeconomic) factors (Scott *et al.*, 1990).

17.7.2   Genetic determinants

Because of the association between low maternal folate status, hyperhomocysteinaemia and increased incidence of NTDs (Eskes, 1998), the search for the genetic determinants of NTD risk has focused on polymorphisms involved in folate and homocysteine metabolism.

Homozygosity for the C677T MTHFR polymorphism in infants is associated with a moderately increased risk for spina bifida (Botto & Yang, 2000). In a study of 271 NTD cases in the Irish population (Shields et al., 1999), the level of risk conferred by the embryonic TT genotype was expressed as an odds ratio of 2.57 (95% confidence interval 1.48 to 4.45). A significant bias in the transmission of the T allele from heterozygous parents to NTD offspring in 218 families confirmed the pathogenic involvement of the MTHFR polymorphism. The data were consistent with a biological model of NTD pathogenesis in which suboptimal maternal folate status imposes biochemical stress on the developing embryo, a stress the embryo is ill-equipped to overcome if it is a TT homozygote expressing the thermolabile form of MTHFR.

Christensen et al. (1999) found that the risk for NTD was higher (odds ratio 6.0; 95% confidence interval 1.26 to 28.53) if both mother and child were homozygous for C667T MTHFR than if one of them was homozygous (odds ratio 2.0; 95% confidence interval 0.47 to 11.54). In contrast, Shields et al. (1999) found that the maternal TT genotype was not a significant independent contributor to NTD risk. Compound heterozygosity for the C677T and A1298A mutations of MTHFR was found in 28% of NTD patients compared with 20% among controls, giving an odds ratio of 2.04 (95% confidence interval 0.9 to 4.7) (van der Put et al., 1998).

The effect of the C677T MTHFR polymorphism on NTDs depends on folate status. The NTD risk for infant TT homozygotes is lower if the mothers periconceptionally use vitamin supplements containing folic acid than if the mothers do not use supplements (Shaw et al., 1998). Christensen et al. (1999) found that the combination of TT homozygosity and low folate status in mother or offspring may be a greater risk factor than either variable alone, suggesting a genetic–nutrient interactive effect. Mothers with this combination had higher plasma homocysteine levels compared to mothers with only the mutant genotype. Molloy et al. (1998) showed that homozygosity for C677T MTHFR cannot account for reduced blood folate levels in many NTD-affected mothers and Lucock et al. (2000) found little difference between NTD and control groups with respect to the frequency of MTHFR polymorphism. It seems that either low maternal folate status is itself the major determinant of NTD risk or other folate-dependent genetic variants confer risk through the reduction of folate levels.

The A2756G polymorphism in methionine synthase does not seem to be a risk factor for NTDs (van der Put et al., 1997; Lucock et al., 2000). However, the A66G polymorphism in the auxiliary enzyme, methionine synthase reductase, when combined with low vitamin B_{12} status or in the presence of the C677T MTHFR polymorphism, greatly increases the risk of an NTD (Wilson et al., 1999).

17.7.3   Nutritional studies

A possible link between folate deficiency and NTDs in humans was first reported in 1965 (Hibbard & Smithells, 1965). Because closure of the embryonic neural tube takes place very early in pregnancy, at a time when many women will be unaware that they are pregnant, any intervention to prevent NTDs must be initiated around the periconceptional period – an 8-week period 4 weeks before and after conception (Mulinare et al., 1988). Beginning in the 1980s, numerous studies have investigated the effect of periconceptional folic acid supplementation on recurrence or occurrence risk for NTDs (Institute of Medicine, 1998). Two representative studies are those reported by the Vitamin Study Research Group of the Medical Research Council in the United Kingdom (MRC, 1991) and the National Institute of Hygiene, a World Health Organization Collaborating Centre for the Community Control of Hereditary Diseases in Hungary (Czeizel & Dudás, 1992).

The MRC (1991) study was a randomized double-blind prevention trial conducted at 33 centres in 7 countries. The study was designed to determine whether folic acid prevented recurring NTDs using high-risk women who had previously had an affected pregnancy. The 1817 volunteers, who were all planning a pregnancy, were randomly allocated to one of four groups to receive capsules containing folic acid (4 mg), folic acid plus a mixture of other vitamins, other vitamins without folic acid, and placebo. The capsules were to be taken daily from the date of randomization until 12 weeks of pregnancy, estimated from the first day of the last menstrual period. Among the 1195 completed pregnancies, 6 of the 593 women who received folic acid had pregnancies with NTDs, giving a recurrence rate of 1%. In contrast, 21 of the 602 women who did not receive folic acid had affected pregnancies, a recurrence rate of 3.5%. The overall result was a significant (72%) reduction in NTD recurrence by periconceptional supplementation with folic acid (4 mg daily), but not with other vitamins.

The Hungarian study (Czeizel & Dudás, 1992) was a randomized double-blind prevention trial comparing a multivitamin preparation containing 800 µg of folic acid with a trace element preparation. In contrast to the MRC (1991) study, none of the 4156 volunteers had previously experienced an NTD-affected pregnancy. The objective was to test the efficacy of periconceptional multivitamin supplementation in reducing the incidence of a first occurrence of an NTD. The outcome was no NTD-affected pregnancies in the 2104 women receiving daily folic acid supplements and 6 affected pregnancies in the 2052 women receiving the trace element preparation. Overall, periconceptional folic acid supplementation reduced the incidence of NTDs over 90%.

The above studies confirmed that folic acid reduces both the occurrence and recurrence of NTDs. This important finding led to a number of recommendations regarding folic acid supplementation and the prevention of NTDs (summarized by Picciano et al., 1994). The 1998 US recommended dietary allowance (RDA) for folate during pregnancy is 600 µg per day, with an upper limit of 1000 µg per day (Institute of Medicine, 1998). In order to achieve this recommended intake, women are advised to take a 400 µg folic acid supplement daily in addition to consuming food folate from a varied diet. To boost the contribution of food folate to total folate intake, the Food and Drug Administration (FDA) in the United States decreed in March 1996 that folic acid must be added to all enriched cereal grains (e.g. enriched bread, pasta, flour, breakfast cereals and rice) at 1.4 mg kg^{-1} of grain, with compliance mandatory from January 1 1998. Cereal products were chosen for folate fortification because they are widely consumed in the United States and because they are suitable vehicles for this purpose. It was estimated that this public health measure would

increase the folate intake of most US women by about 80 to 100 µg per day. This estimate was based on the assumption that the fortified products would actually contain the amount of folic acid required by the FDA's regulation. However, it is standard manufacturing practice to add more than the stipulated amount of vitamin to allow for potential vitamin loss during processing and throughout the shelf-life. In practice, the increased intake of folate resulting from fortification is approximately twice as high as projected (Choumenkovitch et al., 2002). Honein et al. (2001) reported a 19% decrease in the birth prevalence of NTDs following folic acid fortification of the US food supply.

Analysis of data from a case-control study involving 56 049 pregnant women showed that a woman's risk of having a child with an NTD is inversely correlated with early pregnancy erythrocyte folate levels, an indicator of folate body status (Daly et al., 1995). At erythrocyte folate levels below 150 µg L^{-1}, the risk of an NTD was 6.6 per 1000 births, whereas at levels greater than 400 µg L^{-1} the risk was only 0.8 per 1000 births. The average risk among all the women in the study was 1.9 per 1000 births. It was calculated that if all the women had erythrocyte folate levels above 400 µg L^{-1}, the risk of an NTD would be reduced by around 60%. A study by Brown et al. (1997) indicated that an erythrocyte folate concentration of 400 µg L^{-1} could be achieved by taking a daily 400 µg folic acid supplement in addition to the usual diet. Daly et al. (1997) reported that women receiving 100, 200 or 400 µg daily of additional folic acid for 6 months had median post-treatment erythrocyte folate concentrations of 375 µg L^{-1} (354–444), 475 µg L^{-1} (432–503) and 571 µg L^{-1} (481–654) respectively. The authors estimated that delivery of these amounts of folic acid via fortification would yield reductions in NTD incidence of 22%, 41% and 47%, respectively.

In the UK there is no current policy for mandatory folate fortification. Recommendations by the Department of Health (1992) suggest that the daily intake of an extra 400 µg of folate can be achieved through the ample consumption of naturally folate-rich foods. However, Cuskelly et al. (1996) reported that, compared with supplements and fortified food, consumption of extra folate as natural food folate is ineffective at increasing folate status. This is because the polyglutamyl folate present in natural food sources is less bioavailable than the monoglutamyl folic acid present in supplements and fortified foods. Even though protection can be achieved through the use of supplements, there is no guarantee that women will actually take the supplements. An audit of compliance with the UK Department of Health recommendation for routine folate prophylaxis indicated that, at least 6 months after its issue, very few women had complied (Clark & Fisk, 1994).

Despite the beneficial effects of supplemental folate in reducing the incidence of NTDs, no direct link has been found to connect maternal folate deficiency with NTDs. A study of non-pregnant women who had had two NTD-affected pregnancies did not exhibit folate deficiency (erythrocyte folate levels were not depressed). However, unlike control women, there was no correlation between dietary intake of folate and both serum and erythrocyte folate levels (Wild *et al.*, 1994). It appeared that women at increased risk for NTD may have defective folate metabolism and an increased requirement for folate.

Exactly how folate therapy reduces NTD risk is not known. The teratogenic effect of folate deficiency could result from an insufficient supply of nucleic acid precursors to the rapidly dividing embryonic cells. However, the highly specific and predictable nature of the congenital defects caused by folate deficiency argues against a general limitation of nucleic acid availability. Rosenquist *et al.* (1996) showed that treatment of avian embryos with physiological concentrations of exogenous homocysteine induces NTDs that are typical of folate deficiency. This implies that the congenital defects that arise from maternal folate deficiency are a result of hyperhomocysteinaemia and, conversely, that folate supplementation protects against dysmorphogenesis by lowering maternal plasma homocysteine levels. Bearing in mind that homocysteine promotes proliferation of cultured vascular smooth muscle cells (Tsai *et al.*, 1994), Rosenquist and colleagues postulated that the teratogenic effect of homocysteine is based on a growth factor-like effect, altering with this effect the expression of genes critical to the process of neural tube closure/neural crest migration.

17.8 Folate deficiency

Folate deficiency is associated with increased risk of occlusive vascular disease and neural tube defects, as previously discussed. The classic deficiency disease is megaloblastic anaemia.

17.8.1 Megaloblastic anaemia

A deficiency of folate gives rise to a type of anaemia known as megaloblastic anaemia. A clinically indistinguishable anaemia is also produced by vitamin B_{12} deficiency but, because it is accompanied by neurological damage, it is referred to as pernicious anaemia. Both types of anaemia are the result of abnormal nuclear maturation caused by impaired DNA synthesis. The impaired DNA synthesis is presumed to be attributable to reduced intracellular levels of polyglutamyl 5,10-methylene-THF. As shown in reaction 17.7, this important folate is involved in the formation of deoxythymidine monophosphate, one of the two pyrimidine nucleotide constituents of DNA. The defect in DNA synthesis leads to a variety of secondary disturbances which result in the premature death of many haemopoietic cells in the bone marrow, possibly without ever completing the S phase of cell replication.

Megaloblastic anaemia caused by folate deficiency manifests as megaloblastosis of the bone marrow and macrocytosis of the circulating erythrocytes. Examination of the bone marrow is of great diagnostic importance. The erythrocyte precursor cells (erythroblasts) in the bone marrow fail to proliferate rapidly and exist as gigantic cells called megaloblasts at all stages of maturation. It is the existence of such cells that gives rise to the term megaloblastic anaemia. The increased size of megaloblasts is apparent both in the cytoplasm and in the nucleus. The nuclei contain smaller quantities of condensed chromatin than the nuclei of normoblasts of similar maturity and thus have an open, sieve-like appearance.

The circulating erythrocytes which are derived from mature megaloblasts are also abnormally large and are referred to as macrocytes. The mean corpuscular volume of macrocytes ranges from 100 to 160 μm^3 compared with 90 to 95 μm^3 for normal erythrocytes. The macrocytes are generally oval in shape (erythrocytes are biconcave discs) but some fragmented and irregularly shaped cells are also present. There is a reduction in red cell count and sometimes incredibly low values are found. The haemoglobin content of individual macrocytes is increased owing to their larger size, but there is little change in the haemoglobin concentration of whole blood.

White cells and platelets are also produced in the bone marrow. In the differentiating granulocyte series of white blood cells (neutrophils, eosinophils and basophils) giant, abnormally shaped metamyelocytes are found. Megakaryocytes (precursors of platelets) may also be larger than usual. In advanced folate/B_{12} deficiency, the total white cell count and platelet count may be low. Circulating neutrophils are characterized by an increased number of nuclear segments. The presence of hypersegmented neutrophils is a valuable clue in diagnosing folate/B_{12} deficiency when red cell changes are masked by a coexistent iron deficiency or the anaemia of chronic disease.

As in all cases of anaemia, the body adjusts its cardiopulmonary system to compensate for the diminished oxygen-carrying capacity of the blood, so in mild anaemia the subject may not be aware of any problems. Eventually, however, the progressing anaemia leads to symptoms of weakness, fatigue, shortness of breath and palpitations. The sufferer may also experience headache, irritability and an inability to concentrate. Visible signs of megaloblastic anaemia in white-skinned people are a marked pallor and a slight jaundice, giving the skin a distinctive lemon-yellow tinge.

Megaloblastosis is not confined to developing cells in the bone marrow – all other rapidly dividing cell types will be affected, including epithelial cells lining the gastrointestinal, respiratory, and urinogenital tracts. A notable feature is glossitis where the tongue is sore at the edges, bright red in colour and smooth in texture. Gastrointestinal disturbances caused by defective gut epithelia have adverse consequences upon overall nutritional status. Male infertility results from impaired spermatogenesis.

Folate deficiency can result, in the absence of disease, from reduced ingestion or absorption, or from increased utilization. Dietary folate deficiency is common among people who, for various reasons, eat little fruit or fresh vegetables. Absorption is impaired in alcoholics. There is an increased utilization of folate during pregnancy owing to the need to transfer an extra 100–300 µg of folate per day to the fetus (Beatty & Wickramasinghe, 1993). Experimental folate deficiency is difficult to produce under normal circumstances, but the study of patients suffering from malabsorption problems such as tropical sprue or the use of folate antagonists has yielded much clinical information.

17.8.2 Chromosome damage: implications for cancer

Division of cells with unrepaired or misrepaired DNA damage leads to mutations. If these relate to critical genes, such as proto-oncogenes or tumour suppressor genes, cancer may result. Folate is essential for DNA synthesis and repair through its role in purine and pyrimidine synthesis. Its role in the synthesis of S-adenosylmethionine (SAM) is also relevant to cancer. SAM donates its methyl group to DNA, among other acceptors, and a deficiency of folate can lead to hypomethylation of DNA. As DNA methylation is a mechanism for silencing transcription (Ng & Bird, 1999), hypomethylation of DNA has the potential to alter the normal control of gene expression. Hypomethylation also alters chromatin conformation, thereby allowing access of DNA-damaging agents and endonucleases, which destabilize the DNA and make it more susceptible to strand breaks (Kim et al., 1997). Imbalanced DNA methylation is a common occurrence in carcinogenesis (Laird & Jaenisch, 1994).

Low cytosolic levels of 5,10-methylene-THF associated with folate deficiency result in decreased synthesis of deoxythymidine monophosphate (dTMP) and the accumulation of deoxyuridine monophosphate (dUMP). This leads to DNA polymerase-mediated incorporation of dUMP into the DNA molecule in place of dTMP. Normal DNA repair processes remove the misincorporated dUMP, forming transient single-strand breaks (nicks) that could result in a double-strand break if two opposing nicks are formed. Kim et al. (1997) showed that, in rats, dietary folate depletion is capable of producing DNA strand breaks and hypomethylation within a highly conserved region of the p53 tumour suppressor gene. The p53 gene was chosen for study because alterations in it have been implicated in >50% of human cancers. On a genome-wide basis such alterations either did not occur or were delayed, indicating some selectivity for the exons examined within the p53 gene.

In epidemiological studies, dietary folate deficiency is associated with an increased risk of several specific malignancies, notably cancer of the cervix, lung, colorectum and brain (Glynn & Albanes, 1994). The presence of micronucleated erythrocytes in marginal folate deficiency is indicative of chromosomal damage (Everson *et al.*, 1988). Both high DNA dUMP levels and elevated erythrocyte/reticulocyte micronucleus frequency are reversed by folate administration (Blount *et al.*, 1997). Duthie & Hawdon (1998) showed that a dietary intake of folate adequate for the prevention of clinical deficiency may not be sufficient to maintain DNA stability.

In a study of American male physicians, Ma *et al.* (1997) showed that the C677T polymorphism in the MTHFR gene reduces the risk of colorectal cancer. Subjects with the homozygous mutation (15% in controls) had half the risk of colorectal cancer (odds ratio 0.49; 95% confidence interval 0.27 to 0.87) compared with the homozygous normal or heterozygous genotypes. The protection due to the polymorphism was absent in subjects with folate deficiency and reduced in those with high alcohol consumption. It can be reasoned that, provided folate status is adequate, the reduced activity of the thermolabile MTHFR enzyme variant would lead to an increased level of intracellular 5,10-methylene-THF and this would reduce the likelihood of dUMP misincorporation into DNA.

17.8.3 Cognitive function

Folate is important for cognitive function and some studies have found an association between folate deficiency, psychogeriatric disease, depression and the enhanced activity of neurotoxins (see Blount *et al.*, 1997 for references).

17.9 Dietary intake

17.9.1 Human requirement

The results of many studies have led to the universal conclusion that an intake of folate adequate for the prevention of clinical deficiency (megaloblastic anaemia) may be suboptimal for long-term health. Epidemiological studies have shown that dietary folate deficiency is associated with an increased risk of certain types of cancer. It will be interesting to see what impact the US 1998 cereal-food fortification

policy (also adopted in Canada) has on the health and life expectancy of American and Canadian people.

17.9.2 Effects of high intake

Folate is generally considered to have a low acute and chronic toxicity for humans. No adverse effects have been associated with the consumption of folate normally found in fortified foods (Butterworth & Tamura, 1989). Safety is concerned primarily with ingestion of folate supplements and is related to the occasional presence of metabolically unaltered folic acid in the circulation (Kelly *et al.*, 1997).

People with undiagnosed vitamin B_{12} deficiency are particularly at risk if they take folic acid supplements without concomitant vitamin B_{12} supplementation because the obvious symptoms of megaloblastic anaemia will be cured by folic acid, leaving the hidden neurological symptoms of B_{12} deficiency to progress. This applies particularly to the elderly because of their propensity to vitamin B_{12} malabsorption. It is important to make sure that folic acid or multivitamin supplements contain sufficient vitamin B_{12} to provide adequate absorption even in the total absence of intrinsic factor. The RDA for vitamin B_{12} is 2.4 µg per day. Assuming that 1% of ingested vitamin B_{12} is absorbed passively, a supplemental level of 500 µg would provide twice the RDA in the event of pernicious anaemia.

It is possible that anticonvulsant drugs become less effective if the patient is taking high doses of folic acid, giving rise to increased fit frequency in epileptics (Butterworth & Tamura, 1989). Folic acid supplements should therefore be used with caution in patients with epilepsy. Reports of an association between supplemental folate intake and impaired intestinal zinc absorption have not been substantiated in the more recent literature (Institute of Medicine, 1998).

Further reading

Bailey. L. B. & Gregory, J. F. III (1999) Polymorphisms of methylenetetrahydrofolate reductase and other enzymes: metabolic significance, risks and impact on folate requirement. *Journal of Nutrition*, **129**, 919–22.

Lucock, M. (2000) Folic acid: nutritional biochemistry, molecular biology, and role in disease processes. *Molecular Genetics and Metabolism*, **71**, 121–38.

Stehouwer, C. D. A. & Jacobs, C. (1998) Abnormalities of vascular function in hyperhomocysteinaemia: relationship to athero-thrombotic disease. *European Journal of Pediatrics*, 157 (Suppl. 2) S107–S111.

Steinberg, S. E. (1984) Mechanisms of folate homeostasis. *American Journal of Physiology*, 246, G319–24.

Welch, G. N. & Loscalzo, J. (1998) Homocysteine and atherothrombosis. *New England Journal of Medicine*, 338, 1042–50.

References

Anderson, T. J., Uehata, A., Gerhard, M. D., Meredith, I. T., Knab, S., Delagrange, D., Lieberman, E. H., Ganz, P., Creager, M. A., Yeung, A. C. & Selwyn, A. P. (1995) Close relation of endothelial function in the human coronary and peripheral circulations. *Journal of the American College of Cardiology*, 26, 1235–41.

Antony, A. C. (1996) Folate receptors. *Annual Review of Nutrition*, 16, 501–21.

Arias, I. M. & Forgac, M. (1984) The sinusoidal domain of the plasma membrane of rat hepatocytes contains an amiloride-sensitive Na^+/H^+ antiport. *Journal of Biological Chemistry*, 259(9), 5406–8.

Arnesen, E., Refsum, H., Bønaa, K. H., Ueland, P. M., Førde, O. H. & Nordrehaug, J. E. (1995) Serum total homocysteine and coronary heart disease. *International Journal of Epidemiology*, 24, 704–9.

Baram, J., Chabner, B. A., Drake, J. C., Fitzhugh, A. L., Sholar, P. W. & Allegra, C. J. (1988) Identification and biochemical properties of 10-formyldihydrofolate, a novel folate found in methotrexate-treated cells. *Journal of Biological Chemistry*, 263(15), 7105–7111.

Baugh, C. M. & Krumdieck, C. L. (1971) Naturally occurring folates. *Annals of the New York Academy of Sciences*, 186, 7–28.

Beatty, C. & Wickramasinghe, S. N. (1993) Megaloblastic anaemias. In: *Encyclopaedia of Food Science, Food Technology and Nutrition*, Vol. 1. (Ed. R. Macrea, R. K. Robinson & M. J. Sadler), pp. 171–7. Academic Press, London.

Bellamy, M. F., McDowell, I. W. F., Ramsey, M. W., Brownlee, M., Bones, C., Newcombe, R. G. & Lewis, M. J. (1998) Hyperhomocysteinemia after an oral methionine load acutely impairs endothelial function in healthy adults. *Circulation*, 98, 1848–52.

Bellamy, M. F., McDowell, I. F. W., Ramsey, M. W., Brownlee, M., Newcombe, R. G. & Lewis, M. J. (1999) Oral folate enhances endothelial function in hyperhomocysteinaemic subjects. *European Journal of Clinical Investigation*, 29, 659–62.

Bhandari, S. D. & Gregory, J. F. III (1990) Inhibition by selected food components of human and porcine intestinal pteroylpolyglutamate hydrolase activity. *American Journal of Clinical Nutrition*, 51, 87–94.

Bhandari, S. D., Gregory, J. F. III, Renuart, D. R. & Merritt, A. M. (1990) Properties of pteroylpolyglutamate hydrolase in pancreatic juice of the pig. *Journal of Nutrition*, 120, 467–75.

Birn, H., Selhub, J. & Christensen, E. I. (1993) Internalization and intracellular transport of folate-binding protein in rat kidney proximal tubule. *American Journal of Physiology*, 264, C302–10.

Birn, H., Nielsen, S. & Christensen, E. I. (1997) Internalization and apical-to-basolateral transport of folate in rat kidney proximal tubule. *American Journal of Physiology*, 272, F70–8.

Blount, B. C., Mack, M. M., Wehr, C. M., MacGregor, J. T., Hiatt, R. A., Wang, G., Wickramasinghe, S. N., Everson, R. B. & Ames, B. N. (1997) Folate deficiency causes uracil misincorporation into human DNA and chromosome breakage: implications for cancer and neuronal damage. *Proceedings of the National Academy of Sciences of the U.S.A.*, 94, 3290–5.

Bostom, A. G., Jacques, P. F., Liaugaudas, G., Rogers, G., Rosenberg, I. R. & Selhub, J. (2002) Total homocysteine lowering treatment among coronary artery disease patients in the era of folic acid-fortified cereal grain flour. *Arteriosclerosis, Thrombosis, and Vascular Biology*, 22, 488–91.

Botto, L. D. & Yang, Q. (2000) 5,10-Methylenetetrahydrofolate reductase gene variants and congenital anomalies: a HuGE review. *American Journal of Epidemiology*, 151, 862–77.

Brattström, L., Wilcken, D. E. L., Öhrvik, J. & Brudin, L. (1998) Common methylenetetrahydrofolate reductase gene mutation leads to hyperhomocysteinemia but not to vascular disease. The result of a meta-analysis. *Circulation*, 98, 2520–6.

Brody, T. (1991) Folic acid. In: *Handbook of Vitamins*, 2nd edn. (Ed. L. J. Machlin), pp. 453–89. Marcel Dekker, Inc., New York.

Brouwer, I. A., van Dusseldorp, M., West, C. E., Meyboom, S., Thomas, C. M. G., Duran, M., van het Hof, K. H., Eskes, T. K. A. B., Hautvast, J. G. A. J. & Steegers-Theunissen, R. P. M. (1999a) Dietary folate from vegetables and citrus fruit decreases plasma homocysteine concentrations in humans in a dietary controlled trial. *Journal of Nutrition*, 129, 1135–9.

Brouwer, I. A., van Dusseldorp, M., Thomas, C. M. G., Duran, M., Hautvast, J. G. A. J., Eskes, T. K. A. B. & Steegers-Theunissen, R. P. M. (1999b) Low-dose folic acid supplementation decreases plasma homocysteine concentrations: a randomized trial. *American Journal of Clinical Nutrition*, 69, 99–104.

Brown, C. A., McKinney, K. Q., Kaufman, J. S., Gravel, R. A. & Rozen, R. (2000) A common polymorphism in methionine synthase reductase increases risk of premature coronary artery disease. *Journal of Cardiovascular Risk*, 7, 197–200.

Brown, J. E., Jacobs, D. R. Jr., Hartman, T. J., Barosso, G. M., Stang, J. S., Gross, M. D. & Zeuske, M. A. (1997) Predictors of red cell folate level in women attempting pregnancy. *Journal of the American Medical Association*, 277, 548–52.

Butterworth, C. E. Jr. & Tamura, T. (1989) Folic acid safety and toxicity: a brief review. *American Journal of Clinical Nutrition*, 50, 353–8.

Butterworth, C. E. Jr., Baugh, C. M. & Krumdieck, C. (1969) A study of folate absorption and metabolism in man utilizing carbon-14-labeled polyglutamates synthesized by the solid phase method. *Journal of Clinical Investigation*, 48, 1131–42.

Castenmiller, J. J. M., van den Poll, C. J., West, C. E., Brouwer, I. A., Thomas, C. M. G. & van Dusseldorp, M. (2000) Bioavailability of folate from processed spinach in humans. *Annals of Nutrition and Metabolism*, 44, 163–9.

Celermajer, D. S., Sorensen, K., Ryalls, M., Robinson, J., Thomas, O., Leonard, J. V. & Deanfield, J. E. (1993) Impaired endothelial function occurs in the systemic arteries of children with homozygous homocystinuria but not in their heterozygous parents. *Journal of the American College of Cardiology*, 22, 854–8.

Černá, J. & Káš, J. (1983) New conception of folacin assay in starch or glycogen containing food samples. *Nahrung*, 27, 957–64.

Chambers, J. C., McGregor, A., Jean-Marie, J. & Kooner, J. S. (1998) Acute hyperhomocysteinaemia and endothelial dysfunction. *Lancet*, 351, 36–7.

Chambers, J. C., Obeid, O. A. & Kooner, J. S. (1999a) Physiological increments in plasma homocysteine induce vascular endothelial dysfunction in normal human subjects. *Arteriosclerosis and Thrombosis*, 19, 2922–7.

Chambers, J. C., McGregor, A., Jean-Marie, J., Obeid, O. A. & Kooner, J. S. (1999b) Demonstration of rapid onset vascular endothelial dysfunction after hyperhomocysteinemia. An effect reversible with vitamin C therapy. *Circulation*, 99, 1156–60.

Chambers, J. C., Ueland, P. M., Obeid, O. A., Wrigley, J., Refsum, H. & Kooner, J. S. (2000) Improved vascular endothelial function after oral B vitamins. An effect mediated through reduced concentrations of free plasma homocysteine. *Circulation*, **102**, 2479–83.

Chandler, C. J., Harrison, D. A., Buffington, C. A., Santiago, N. A. & Halsted, C. H. (1991) Functional specificity of jejunal brush-border pteroylpolyglutamate hydrolase in pig. *American Journal of Physiology*, **260**, G865–72.

Charpiot, P., Bescond, A., Augier, T., Chareyre, C., Fraterno, M., Rolland, P.-H. & Garcon, D. (1998) Hyperhomocysteinemia induces elastolysis in minipig arteries: structural consequences, arterial site specificity and effect of captopril-hydrochlorothiazide. *Matrix Biology*, **17**, 559–74.

Chen, J., Stampfer, M. J., Ma, J., Selhub, J., Malinow, M. R., Hennekens, C. H. & Hunter, D. J. (2001) Influence of a methionine synthase (D919G) polymorphism on plasma homocysteine and folate levels and relation to risk of myocardial infarction. *Atherosclerosis*, **154**, 667–72.

Choumenkovitch, S. F., Selhub, J., Wilson, P. W. F., Rader, J. I., Rosenberg, I. H. & Jacques, P. F. (2002) Folic acid intake from fortification in United States exceeds predictions. *Journal of Nutrition*, **132**, 2792–8.

Christensen, B., Arbour, L., Tran, P., Leclerc, D., Sabbaghian, N., Platt, R., Gilfix, B. M., Rosenblatt, D. S., Gravel, R. A., Forbes, P. & Rozen, R. (1999) Genetic polymorphisms in methylenetetrahydrofolate reductase and methionine synthase, folate levels in red blood cells, and risk of neural tube defects. *American Journal of Medical Genetics*, **84**, 151–7.

Clark, N. A. C. & Fisk, N. M. (1994) Minimal compliance with the Department of Health recommendation for routine folate prophylaxis to prevent fetal neural tube defects. *British Journal of Obstetrics and Gynaecology*, **101**, 709–10.

Clarke, R., Daly, L., Robinson, K., Naughten, E., Cahalane, S., Fowler, B. & Graham, I. (1991) Hyperhomocysteinemia: an independent risk factor for vascular disease. *New England Journal of Medicine*, **324**, 1149–55.

Constans, J., Blann, A. D., Resplandy, F., Parrot, F., Renard, M., Seigneur, M., Guérin, V., Boisseau, M. & Conri, C. (1999) Three months supplementation of hyperhomocysteinaemic patients with folic acid and vitamin B$_6$ improves biological markers of endothelial dysfunction. *British Journal of Haematology*, **107**, 776–8.

Cuskelly, G. J., McNulty, H. & Scott, J. M. (1996) Effect of increasing dietary folate on red-cell folate: implications for prevention of neural tube defects. *Lancet*, **347**, 657–9.

Czeizel, A. E. & Dudás, I. (1992) Prevention of the first occurrence of neural-tube defects by periconceptional vitamin supplementation. *New England Journal of Medicine*, **327**, 1832–5.

Daly, L. E., Kirke, P. N., Molloy, A., Weir, D. G. & Scott, J. M. (1995) Folate levels and neural tube defects. Implications for prevention. *Journal of the American Medical Association*, **274**, 1698–702.

Daly, S., Mills, J. L., Molloy, A. M., Conley, M., Lee, Y. J., Kirke, P. N., Weir, D. G. & Scott, J. M. (1997) Minimum effective dose of folic acid for food fortification to prevent neural-tube defects. *Lancet*, **350**, 1666–9.

Deloughery, T. G., Evans, A., Sadeghi, A., McWilliams, J., Henner, W. D., Taylor, L. M. Jr. & Press, R. D. (1996) Common mutation in methylenetetrahydrofolate reductase. Correlation with homocysteine metabolism and late-onset vascular disease. *Circulation*, **94**, 3074–8.

den Heijer, M., Brouwer, I. A., Bos, G. M. J., Blom, H. J., van der Put, N. M. J., Spaans, A. P., Rosendaal, F. R., Thomas, C. M. G., Haak, H. L., Wijermans, P. W. & Gerrits, W. B. J. (1998) Vitamin supplementation reduces blood homocysteine levels. A controlled trial in patients with venous thrombosis and healthy volunteers.

Arteriosclerosis, Thrombosis, and Vascular Biology, **18**, 356–61.

Department of Health (1992) *Folic acid and the prevention of neural tube defects.* Report from an expert advisory group. Department of Health, London.

Domagala, T. B., Libura, M. & Szczeklik, A. (1997) Hyperhomocysteinemia following oral methionine load is associated with increased lipid peroxidation. *Thrombosis Research*, **87**, 411–16.

Dudeja, P. K., Torania, S. A. & Said, H. M. (1997) Evidence for the existence of a carrier-mediated folate uptake mechanism in human colonic luminal membranes. *American Journal of Physiology*, **272**, G1408–15.

Durand, P., Lussier-Cacan, S. & Blache, D. (1997) Acute methionine load-induced hyperhomocysteinemia enhances platelet aggregation, thromboxane biosynthesis, and macrophage-derived tissue factor activity in rats. *FASEB Journal*, **11**, 1157–68.

Duthie, S. J. & Hawdon, A. (1998) DNA instability (strand breakage, uracil misincorporation, and defective repair) is increased by folic acid depletion in human lymphocytes *in vitro*. *FASEB Journal*, **12**, 1491–7.

Eisenga, B. H., Collins, T. D. & McMartin, K. E. (1989) Effects of acute ethanol on urinary excretion of 5-methyltetrahydrofolic acid and folate derivatives in the rat. *Journal of Nutrition*, **119**, 1498–505.

Eskes, T. K. A. B. (1998) Neural tube defects, vitamins and homocysteine. *European Journal of Pediatrics*, **157** (Suppl. 2), S139–41.

European Concerted Action Project (1997) Plasma homocysteine as a risk factor for vascular disease. *Journal of the American Medical Association*, **277**, 1775–81.

Everson, R. B., Wehr, C. M., Erexson, G. L. & MacGregor, J. T. (1988) Association of marginal folate depletion with increased human chromosomal damage in vivo: demonstration by analysis of micronucleated erythrocytes. *Journal of the National Cancer Institute*, **80**, 525–9.

Ford, J. E., Salter, D. N. & Scott, K. J. (1969) The folate-binding protein in milk. *Journal of Dairy Research*, **36**, 435–46.

Frosst, P., Blom, H. J., Milos, R., Goyette, P., Sheppard, C. A., Matthews, R. G., Boers, G. J. H., den Heijer, M., Kluijtmans, L. A. J., van den Heuvel, L. P. & Rozen, R. (1995) A candidate genetic risk factor for vascular disease: a common mutation in methylenetetrahydrofolate reductase. *Nature Genetics*, **10**, 111–13.

Gallagher, P. M., Meleady, R., Shields, D. C., Tan, K. S., McMaster, D., Rozen, R., Evans, A., Graham, I. M. & Whitehead, A. S. (1996) Homocysteine and risk of premature coronary heart disease. Evidence for a common gene mutation. *Circulation*, **94**, 2154–8.

Gardemann, A., Weidemann, H., Philipp, M., Katz, N., Tillmanns, H., Hehrlein, F. W. & Haberbosch, W. (1999) The TT genotype of the methylenetetrahydrofolate reductase C$_{677}$T gene polymorphism is associated with the extent of coronary atherosclerosis in patients at high risk for coronary artery disease. *European Heart Journal*, **20**, 584–92.

Glynn, S. A. & Albanes, D. (1994) Folate and cancer: a review of the literature. *Nutrition and Cancer*, **22**, 101–119.

Gregory, J. F. III (1984) Determination of folacin in foods and other biological materials. *Journal of the Association of Official Analytical Chemists*, **67**, 1015–19.

Gregory, J. F. III (1989) Chemical and nutritional aspects of folate research: analytical procedures, methods of folate synthesis, stability, and bioavailability of dietary folates. *Advances in Food and Nutrition Research*, **33**, 1–101.

Gregory, J. F. III (1995) The bioavailability of folate. In: *Folate in Health and Disease*. (Ed. L. B. Bailey), pp. 195–235. Marcel Dekker, Inc., New York.

Gregory, J. F. III, Ink, S. L. & Cerda, J. J. (1987) Comparison of pteroylpolyglutamate hydrolase (folate conjugase) from porcine and human intestinal brush border membrane. *Comparative Biochemistry and Physiology*, **88B**, 1135–41.

Gregory, J. F. III, Bhandari, S. D., Bailey, L. B., Toth, J. P., Baumgartner, T. G. & Cerda, J. J. (1991) Relative bioavailability of deuterium-labeled monoglutamyl and hexaglutamyl folates in human subjects. *American Journal of Clinical Nutrition*, **53**, 736–40.

Guenther, B. D., Sheppard, C. A., Tran, P., Rozen, R., Matthews, R. G. & Ludwig, M. L. (1999) The structure and properties of methylenetetrahydrofolate reductase from *Escherichia coli* suggest how folate ameliorates human hyperhomocysteinemia. *Nature Structural Biology*, **6**, 359–65.

Halsted, C. H. (1990) Intestinal absorption of dietary folates. In: *Folic Acid Metabolism in Health and Disease*. (Ed. M. F. Picciano, E. L. R. Stokstad & J. F. Gregory III), pp. 23–45. Wiley-Liss, Inc., New York.

Halsted, C. H., Robles, E. A. & Mezey, E. (1973) Intestinal malabsorption in folate-deficient alcoholics. *Gastroenterology*, **64**, 526–32.

Harker, L. A., Ross, R., Slichter, S. J. & Scott, C. R. (1976) Homocystine-induced arteriosclerosis. The role of endothelial cell injury and platelet response in its genesis. *Journal of Clinical Investigation*, **58**, 731–41.

Herbert, V. (1999) Folic acid. In: *Modern Nutrition in Health and Disease*, 9th edn. (Ed. M. E. Shils, J. A. Olson, M. Shike & A. C. Ross), pp. 433–46. Lippincott Williams & Wilkins, Philadelphia.

Hibbard, E. D. & Smithells, R. W. (1965) Folic acid metabolism and embryopathy. *Lancet*, **I**(7398), 1254.

Hjelle, J. T., Christensen, E. I., Carone, F. A. & Selhub, J. (1991) Cell fractionation and electron microscope studies of kidney folate-binding protein. *American Journal of Physiology*, **260**, C338–46.

Holm, J. S., Hansen, S. I., Hoier-Madsen, M. & Bostad, L. (1991) High-affinity folate binding in human choroid plexus. Characterization of radioligand binding, immunoreactivity, molecular heterogeneity and hydrophobic domain of the binding protein. *Biochemical Journal*, **280**, 267–71.

Homocysteine Lowering Trialists' Collaboration (1998) Lowering blood homocysteine with folic acid based supplements: meta-analysis of randomized trials. *British Medical Journal*, **316**, 894–8.

Honein, M. A., Paulozzi, L. J., Mathews, T. J., Erickson, J. D. & Wong, L.-Y. C. (2001) Impact of folic acid fortification of the US food supply on the occurrence of neural tube defects. *Journal of the American Medical Association*, **285**, 2981–6.

Horne, D. W., Reed, K. A., Hoefs, J. & Said, H. M. (1993) 5-Methyltetrahydrofolate transport in basolateral membrane vesicles from human liver. *American Journal of Clinical Nutrition*, **58**, 80–4.

Houghton, L. A., Green, T. J., Donovan, U. M., Gibson, R. S., Stephen, A. M. & O'Connor, D. L. (1997) Association between dietary fiber intake and the folate status of a group of female adolescents. *American Journal of Clinical Nutrition*, **66**, 1414–21.

Hyndman, M. E., Bridge, P. J., Warnica, J. W., Fick, G. & Parsons, H. G. (2000) Effect of heterozygosity for the methionine synthase 2756A→G mutation on the risk for recurrent cardiovascular events. *American Journal of Cardiology*, **86**, 1144–6.

Illsley, N. P., Glaubensklee, C., Davis, B. & Verkman, A. S. (1988) Chloride transport across placental microvillous membranes measured by fluorescence. *American Journal of Physiology*, **255**, C789–97.

Institute of Medicine (1998) *Dietary Reference Intakes for Thiamin, Riboflavin, Niacin, Vitamin B_6, Folate, Vitamin B_{12}, Pantothenic Acid, Biotin, and Choline*. National Academy Press, Washington, D.C.

Jacques, P. F., Bostom, A. G., Williams, R. R., Ellison, R. C., Eckfeldt, J. H., Rosenberg, I. H., Selhub, J. & Rozen, R. (1996) Relation between folate status, a common mutation in methylenetetrahydrofolate reductase, and plasma homocysteine concentrations. *Circulation*, **93**, 7–9.

Kamen, B. A., Smith, A. K. & Anderson, R. G. W. (1991) The folate receptor works in tandem with a probenecid-sensitive carrier in MA104 cells in vitro. *Journal of Clinical Investigation*, **87**, 1442–9.

Kanani, P. M., Sinkey, C. A., Browning, R. L., Allaman, M., Knapp, H. R. & Haynes, W. G. (1999) Role of oxidant stress in endothelial dysfunction produced by experimental hyperhomocyst(e)inemia in humans. *Circulation*, **100**, 1161–8.

Kane, M. A., Portillo, R. M., Elwood, P. C., Antony, A. C. & Kolhouse, J. F. (1986) The influence of extracellular folate concentration on methotrexate uptake by human KB cells. Partial characterization of a membrane-associated methotrexate binding protein. *Journal of Biological Chemistry*, **261**(1), 44–9.

Kang, S.-S., Wong, P. W. K. & Norusis, M. (1987) Homocysteinemia due to folate deficiency. *Metabolism*, **36**, 458–62.

Kang, S.-S., Zhou, J., Wong, P. W. K., Kowalisyn, J. & Strokosch, G. (1988) Intermediate homocysteinemia: a thermolabile variant of methylenetetrahydrofolate reductase. *American Journal of Human Genetics*, **43**, 414–21.

Kang, S.-S., Wong, P. W. K., Susmano, A., Sora, J., Norusis, M. & Ruggie, N. (1991) Thermolabile methylenetetrahydrofolate reductase; an inherited risk factor for coronary artery disease. *American Journal of Human Genetics*, **48**, 536–45.

Kang, S.-S., Passen, E. L., Ruggie, N., Wong, P. W. K. & Sora, H. (1993) Thermolabile defect of methylenetetrahydrofolate reductase in coronary artery disease. *Circulation*, **88**, 1463–9.

Kaufman, S. (1991) Some metabolic relationships between biopterin and folate: implications for the 'methyl trap hypothesis'. *Neurochemical Research*, **16**, 1031–6.

Kelly, P., McPartlin, J., Goggins, M., Weir, D. G. & Scott, J. M. (1997) Unmetabolized folic acid in serum: acute studies in subjects consuming fortified food and supplements. *American Journal of Clinical Nutrition*, **65**, 1790–5.

Kim, Y.-I., Pogribny, I. P., Basnakian, A. G., Miller, J. W., Selhub, J., James, S. J. & Mason, J. B. (1997) Folate deficiency in rats induces DNA strand breaks and hypomethylation within the p53 tumor suppressor gene. *American Journal of Clinical Nutrition*, **72**, 46–52.

Kluijtmans, L. A. J., van den Heuvel, L. P. W. J., Boers, G. H. J., Frosst, P., Stevens, E. M. B., van Oost, B. A., den Heijer, M., Trijbels, F. J. M., Rozen, R. & Blom, H. J. (1996) Molecular genetic analysis in mild hyperhomocysteinemia: a common mutation in the methylenetetrahydrofolate reductase gene is a genetic risk factor for cardiovascular disease. *American Journal of Human Genetics*, **58**, 35–41.

Kluijtmans, L. A. J., Kastelein, J. J. P., Lindemans, J., Boers, G. H. J., Heil, S. G., Bruschke, A. V. G., Jukema, J. W., van den Heuvel, L. P. W. J., Trijbels, F. J. M., Boerma, G. J. M., Verheugt, F. W. A., Willems, F. & Blom, H. J. (1997) Thermolabile methylenetetrahydrofolate reductase in coronary artery disease. *Circulation*, **96**, 2573–7.

Kode, A., Alnounou, M., Tyagi, S., Torania, S., Said, H. M. & Dudeja, P. K. (1997) Mechanism of folate transport across the human colonic basolateral membrane. *FASEB Journal*, **11**, A35.

Kuller, L. H. & Evans, R. W. (1998) Homocysteine, vitamins, and cardiovascular disease. *Circulation*, **98**, 196–9.

Kumar, C. K., Moyer, M. P., Dudeja, P. K. & Said, H. M. (1997) A protein-tyrosine kinase-regulated, pH-dependent, carrier-mediated uptake system for folate in human normal colonic epithelial cell line NCM460. *Journal of Biological Chemistry*,

272(10), 6226–31.

Laird, P. W. & Jaenisch, R. (1994) DNA methylation and cancer. *Human Molecular Genetics*, **3**, 1487–95.

Laskowski, M. & Laskowski, M. (1951) Crystalline trypsin inhibitor from colostrum. *Journal of Biological Chemistry*, **190**, 563–73.

Lentz, S. R. (1998) Mechanisms of thrombosis in hyperhomocysteinemia. *Current Opinion in Hematology*, **5**, 343–9.

Lentz, S. R., Sobey, C. G., Piegors, D. J., Bhopatkar, M. Y., Faraci, F. M., Malinow, M. R. & Heistad, D. D. (1996) Vascular dysfunction in monkeys with diet-induced hyperhomocyst(e)inemia. *Journal of Clinical Investigation*, **98**, 24–9.

Lobo, A., Naso, A., Arheart, K., Kruger, W. D., Abou-Ghazala, T., Alsous, F., Nahlawi, M., Gupta, A., Moustapha, A., van Lente, F., Jacobsen, D. W. & Robinson, K. (1999) Reduction of homocysteine levels in coronary artery disease by low-dose folic acid combined with vitamins B$_6$ and B$_{12}$. *American Journal of Cardiology*, **83**, 821–5.

Lucock, M., Daskalakis, I., Briggs, D., Yates, Z. & Levene, M. (2000) Altered folate metabolism and disposition in mothers affected by a spina bifida pregnancy: influence of 677c→t methylenetetrahydrofolate reductase and 2756a→g methionine synthase genotypes. *Molecular Genetics and Metabolism*, **70**, 27–44.

Ma, J., Stampfer, M. J., Hennekens, C. H., Frosst, P., Selhub, J., Horsford, J., Malinow, M. R., Willett, W. C. & Rozen, R. (1996) Methylenetetrahydrofolate reductase polymorphism, plasma folate, homocysteine, and risk of myocardial infarction in US physicians. *Circulation*, **94**, 2410–16.

Ma, J., Stampfer, M. J., Giovannucci, E., Artigas, C., Hunter, D. J., Fuchs, C., Willett, W. C., Selhub, J., Hennekens, C. H. & Rozen, R. (1997) Methylenetetrahydrofolate reductase polymorphism, dietary interactions, and risk of colorectal cancer. *Cancer Research*, **57**, 1098–102.

Makulu, D. R., Smith, E. F. & Bertino, J. R. (1973) Lack of dihydrofolate reductase activity in brain tissue of mammalian species: possible implications. *Journal of Neurochemistry*, **21**, 241–5.

Malinow, M. R., Duell, P. B., Hess, D. L., Anderson, P. H., Kruger, W. D., Phillipson, B. E., Gluckman, R. A., Block, P. C. & Upson, B. M. (1998) Reduction of plasma homocyst(e)ine levels by breakfast cereal fortified with folic acid in patients with coronary heart disease. *New England Journal of Medicine*, **338**, 1009–15.

Mason, J. B. & Selhub, J. (1988) Folate-binding protein and the absorption of folic acid in the small intestine of the suckling rat. *American Journal of Clinical Nutrition*, **48**, 620–5.

Mason, J. B., Shoda, R., Haskell, M., Selhub, J. & Rosenberg, I. H. (1990) Carrier affinity as a mechanism for the pH-dependence of folate transport in the small intestine. *Biochimica et Biophysica Acta*, **1024**, 331–5.

Matthews, R. G. & Baugh, C. M. (1980) Interactions of pig liver methylenetetrahydrofolate reductase with methylenetetrahydropteroylpolyglutamate substrates and with dihydropteroylpolyglutamate inhibitors. *Biochemistry*, **19**, 2040–5.

Mayer, E. L., Jacobsen, D. W. & Robinson, K. (1996) Homocysteine and coronary atherosclerosis. *Journal of the American College of Cardiology*, **27**, 517–27.

McMartin, K. E. (1984) Increased urinary folate excretion and decreased plasma folate levels in the rat after acute ethanol treatment. *Alcoholism: Clinical and Experimental Research*, **8**, 172–8.

McMartin, K. E., Collins, T. D. & Bairnsfather, L. (1986) Cumulative excess urinary excretion of folate in rats after repeated ethanol treatment. *Journal of Nutrition*, **116**, 1316–25.

McMartin, K. E., Collins, T. D., Eisenga, B. H., Fortney, T., Bates, W. R. & Bairnsfather, L. (1989) Effects of chronic ethanol and diet treatment on urinary folate excretion and development of folate deficiency in the rat. *Journal of Nutrition*, **119**, 1490–7.

Molloy, A. M., Mills, J. L., Kirke, P. N., Ramsbottom, D., McPartlin, J.

M., Burke, H., Conley, M., Whitehead, A. S., Weir, D. G. & Scott, J. M. (1998) Low blood folates in NTD pregnancies are only partly explained by thermolabile 5,10-methylenetetrahydrofolate reductase: low folate status alone may be the critical factor. *American Journal of Medical Genetics*, **78**, 155–9.

Morita, H., Taguchi, J., Kurihara, H., Kitaoka, M., Kaneda, H., Kurihara, Y., Maemura, K., Shindo, T., Minamino, T., Ohno, M., Yamaoki, K., Ogasawara, K., Aizawa, T., Suzuki, S. & Yazaki, Y. (1997) Genetic polymorphism of 5,10-methylenetetrahydrofolate reductase (MTHFR) as a risk factor for coronary artery disease. *Circulation*, **95**, 2032–6.

Morshed, K. M. & McMartin, K. E. (1997) Reabsorptive and secretory 5-methyltetrahydrofolate transport pathways in cultured human proximal tubule cells. *American Journal of Physiology*, **272**, F380–8.

Morshed, K. M., Ross, D. M. & McMartin, K. E. (1997) Folate transport proteins mediate the bidirectional transport of 5-methyltetrahydrofolate in cultured human proximal tubule cells. *Journal of Nutrition*, **127**, 1137–47.

MRC Vitamin Study Research Group (1991) Prevention of neural tube defects: results of the Medical Research Council Vitamin Study, *Lancet*, **338**, 131–7.

Mulinare, J. (1995) Public health perspectives on folic acid and neural tube defects. *Cereal Foods World*, **40**, 58–61.

Mulinare, J., Cordero, J. F., Erickson, J. D. & Berry, R. J. (1988) Periconceptional use of multivitamins and the occurrence of neural tube defects. *Journal of the American Medical Association*, **260**, 3141–5.

Nappo, F., De Rosa, N., Marfella, R., De Lucia, D., Ingrosso, D., Perna, A. F., Farzati, B. & Giugliano, D. (1999) Impairment of endothelial functions by acute hyperhomocysteinemia and reversal by antioxidant vitamins. *Journal of the American Medical Association*, **281**, 2113–18.

Naughton, C. A., Chandler, C. J., Duplantier, R. B. & Halsted, C. H. (1989) Folate absorption in alcoholic pigs: in vitro hydrolysis and transport at the intestinal brush border membrane. *American Journal of Clinical Nutrition*, **50**, 1436–41.

Nelen, W. L. D. M., Blom, H. J., Thomas, C. M. G., Steegers, E. A. P., Boers, G, H. J. & Eskes, T. K. A. B. (1998) Methylenetetrahydrofolate reductase polymorphism affects the change in homocysteine and folate concentrations resulting from low dose folic acid supplementation in women with unexplained recurrent miscarriages. *Journal of Nutrition*, **128**, 1336–41.

Neunteufl, T., Katzenschlager, R., Hassan, A., Klaar, U., Schwarzacher, S., Glogar, D., Bauer, P. & Weidinger, F. (1997) Systemic endothelial dysfunction is related to the extent and severity of coronary artery disease. *Atherosclerosis*, **129**, 111–18.

Ng, H.-H. & Bird, A. (1999) DNA methylation and chromatin modification. *Current Opinion in Genetics & Development*, **9**, 158–63.

Nguyen, T. T., Dyer, D. L., Dunning, D. D., Rubin, S. A., Grant, K. E. & Said, H. M. (1997) Human intestinal folate transport: cloning, expression, and distribution of complementary RNA. *Gastroenterology*, **112**, 783–91.

Nygård, O., Nordrehaug, J. E., Refsum, H., Ueland, P. M., Farstad, M. & Vollset, S. E. (1997) Plasma homocysteine levels and mortality in patients with coronary artery disease. *New England Journal of Medicine*, **337**, 230–6.

Okamura-Ikeda, K., Fujiwara, K. & Motokawa, Y. (1987) Mechanism of the glycine cleavage reaction. Properties of the reverse reaction catalyzed by T-protein. *Journal of Biological Chemistry*, **262**(14), 6746–9.

Perry, I. J., Refsum, H., Morris, R. W., Ebrahim, S. B., Ueland, P. M. & Shaper, A. G. (1995) Prospective study of serum total homocysteine concentration and risk of stroke in middle-aged British men. *Lancet*, **346**, 1395–8.

Pfeiffer, C. M., Rogers, L. M., Bailey, L. B. & Gregory, J. F. III (1997) Absorption of folate from fortified cereal-grain products and of supplemental folate consumed with or without food determined by using a dual-label stable-isotope protocol. *American Journal of Clinical Nutrition*, **66**, 1388–97.

Picciano, M. F., Green, T. & O'Connor, D. L. (1994) The folate status of women and health. *Nutrition Today*, **29**, 20–9.

Prasad, P. D., Ramamoorthy, S., Moe, A. J., Smith, C. H., Leibach, F. H. & Ganapathy, V. (1994a) Selective expression of the high-affinity isoform of the folate receptor (FR-α) in the human placental syncytiotrophoblast and choriocarcinoma cells. *Biochimica et Biophysica Acta*, **1223**, 71–5.

Prasad, P. D., Mahesh, V. B., Leibach, F. H. & Ganapathy, V. (1994b) Functional coupling between a bafilomycin A_1-sensitive proton pump and a probenecid-sensitive folate transporter in human placental choriocarcinoma cells. *Biochimica et Biophysica Acta*, **1222**, 309–14.

Prasad, P. D., Ramamoorthy, S., Leibach, F. H. & Ganapathy, V. (1995) Molecular cloning of the human placental folate transporter. *Biochemical and Biophysical Research Communications*, **206**, 681–7.

Rijnboutt, S., Jansen, G., Posthuma, G., Hynes, J. B., Schornagel, J. H. & Strous, G. J. (1996) Endocytosis of GPI-linked membrane folate receptor-α. *Journal of Cell Biology*, **132**, 35–47.

Rimm, E. B., Willett, W. C., Hu, F. B., Sampson, L., Colditz, G. A., Manson, J. E., Hennekens, C. & Stampfer, M. J. (1998) Folate and vitamin B_6 from diet and supplements in relation to risk of coronary heart disease among women. *Journal of the American Medical Association*, **279**, 359–64.

Rong, N., Selhub, J., Goldin, B. R. & Rosenberg, I. H. (1991) Bacterially synthesized folate in rat large intestine is incorporated into host tissue folyl polyglutamates. *Journal of Nutrition*, **121**, 1955–9.

Rosenquist, T. H., Ratashak, S. A. & Selhub, J. (1996) Homocysteine induces congenital defects of the heart and neural tube: effect of folic acid. *Proceedings of the National Academy of Sciences of the U.S.A.*, **93**, 15 227–32.

Ross, J. F., Chaudhuri, P. K. & Ratnam, M. (1994) Differential regulation of folate receptor isoforms in normal and malignant tissues in vivo and in established cell lines. *Cancer*, **73**, 2432–43.

Rothberg, K. G., Ying, Y. S., Kolhouse, J. F., Kamen, B. A. & Anderson, R. G. (1990) The glycophospholipid-linked folate receptor internalizes folate without entering the clathrin-coated pit endocytic pathway. *Journal of Cell Biology*, **110**, 637–41.

Rozen, R. (1997) Genetic predisposition to hyperhomocysteinemia: deficiency of methylenetetrahydrofolate reductase (MTHFR). *Thrombosis and Haemostasis*, **78**, 523–6.

Russell, R. M., Dhar, G. J., Dutta, S. K. & Rosenberg, I. H. (1979) Influence of intraluminal pH on folate absorption: studies in control subjects and in patients with pancreatic insufficiency. *Journal of Laboratory and Clinical Medicine*, **93**, 428–36.

Russell, R. M., Rosenberg, I. H., Wilson, P. D., Iber, F. L., Oaks, E. B., Giovetti, A. C. Otradovec, C. L., Karwoski, P. A. & Press, A. W. (1983) Increased urinary excretion and prolonged turnover time of folic acid during ethanol ingestion. *American Journal of Clinical Nutrition*, **38**, 64–70.

Said, H. M. & Redha, R. (1987) A carrier-mediated transport for folate in basolateral membrane vesicles of rat small intestine. *Biochemical Journal*, **247**, 141–6.

Said, H. M., Ghishan, F. K. & Redha, R. (1987) Folate transport by human intestinal brush-border membrane vesicles. *American Journal of Physiology*, **252**, G229–36.

Said, H. M., Ma, T Y., Ortiz, A., Tapia, A. & Valerio, C. K. (1997) Intracellular regulation of intestinal folate uptake: studies with cultured IEC-6 epithelial cells. *American Journal of Physiology*, **272**, C729–36.

Said, H. M., Chatterjee, N., ul Haq, R., Subramanian, V. S., Ortiz, A., Matherly, L. H., Sirotnak, F. M., Halsted, C. & Rubin, S. A. (2000) Adaptive regulation of intestinal folate uptake: effect of dietary folate deficiency. *American Journal of Physiology*, **279**, C1889–95.

Salomon, O., Rosenberg, N., Zivelin, A., Steinberg, D. M., Kornbrot, N., Dardik, R., Inbal, A. & Seligsohn, U. (2001) Methionine synthase A2756G and methylenetetrahydrofolate reductase A1298C polymorphisms are not risk factors for idiopathic venous thromboembolism. *Hematology Journal*, **2**, 38–41.

Salter, D. N. & Blakeborough, P. (1988) Influence of goat's-milk folate-binding protein on transport of 5-methyltetrahydrofolate in neonatal-goat small intestinal brush-border-membrane vesicles. *British Journal of Nutrition*, **59**, 497–507.

Salter, D. N. & Mowlem, A. (1983) Neonatal role of milk folate-binding protein: studies on the course of digestion of goat's milk folate binder in the 6-d-old kid. *British Journal of Nutrition*, **50**, 589–96.

Sauberlich, H. E., Kretch, M. J., Skala, J. H., Johnson, H. L. & Taylor, P. C. (1987) Folate requirement and metabolism in nonpregnant women. *American Journal of Clinical Nutrition*, **46**, 1016–28.

Schmitz, C., Lindpaintner, K., Verhoef, P., Gaziano, J. M. & Buring, J. (1996) Genetic polymorphism of methylenetetrahydrofolate reductase and myocardial infarction. A case-control study. *Circulation*, **94**, 1812–14.

Schorah, C. J., Devitt, H., Lucock, M. & Dowell, A. C. (1998) The responsiveness of plasma homocysteine to small increases in dietary folic acid: a primary care study. *European Journal of Clinical Nutrition*, **52**, 407–11.

Schron, C. M. (1991) pH modulation of the kinetics of rabbit jejunal, brush-border folate transport. *Journal of Membrane Biology*, **120**, 192–200.

Scott, J. M., Kirke, P. N. & Weir, D. G. (1990) The role of nutrition in neural tube defects. *Annual Review of Nutrition*, **10**, 277–95.

Selhub, J. & Franklin, W. A. (1984) The folate-binding protein of rat kidney. Purification, properties, and cellular distribution. *Journal of Biological Chemistry*, **259**(10), 6601–6.

Selhub, J. & Miller, J. W. (1992) The pathogenesis of homocysteinemia: interruption of the coordinate regulation by *S*-adenosylmethionine of the remethylation and transsulfuration of homocysteine. *American Journal of Clinical Nutrition*, **55**, 131–8.

Selhub, J. & Rosenberg, I. H. (1981) Folate transport in isolated brush border membrane vesicles from rat intestine. *Journal of Biological Chemistry*, **256**(9), 4489–93.

Selhub, J., Jacques, P. F., Bostom, A. G., D'Agostino, R. B., Wilson, P. W. F., Belanger, A. J., O'Leary, D. H., Wolf, P. A., Schaefer, E. J. & Rosenberg, I. H. (1995) Association between plasma homocysteine concentrations and extracranial carotid-artery stenosis. *New England Journal of Medicine*, **332**, 286–91.

Seyoum, E. & Selhub, J. (1998) Properties of food folates determined by stability and susceptibility to intestinal pteroylpolyglutamate hydrolase action. *Journal of Nutrition*, **128**, 1956–60.

Shane, B. (1989) Folylpolyglutamate synthesis and role in the regulation of one-carbon metabolism. *Vitamins and Hormones*, **45**, 263–335.

Shaw, G. M., Rozen, R., Finnell, R. H., Wasserman, C. R. & Lammer, E. J. (1998) Maternal vitamin use, genetic variation of infant methylenetetrahydrofolate reductase, and risk for spina bifida. *American Journal of Epidemiology*, **148**, 30–7.

Shields, D. C., Kirke, P. N., Mills, J. L., Ramsbottom, D., Molloy, A. M., Burke, H., Weir, D. G., Scott, J. M. & Whitehead, A. S. (1999) The 'thermolabile' variant of methylenetetrahydrofolate reductase and neural tube defects: an evaluation of genetic risk and the relative importance of the genotypes of the embryo and the mother. *American Journal of Human Genetics*, **64**, 1045–55.

Shin, H.-C., Takakuwa, F., Shimoda, M. & Kokue, E. (1995) Enterohepatic circulation kinetics of bile-active folate derivatives and folate homeostasis in rats. *American Journal of Physiology*, **269**, R421–5.

Simon, B. J., Kulanthaivel, P., Burckhardt, G., Ramamoorthy, S., Leibach, F. H. & Ganapathy, V. (1992) Characterization of an ATP-driven H+ pump in human placental brush-border membrane vesicles. *Biochemical Journal*, **287**, 423–30.

Spector, R. (1981) Megavitamin therapy and the central nervous system. In: *Vitamins in Human Biology and Medicine*. (Ed. M. H. Briggs), pp. 137–56. CRC Press, Inc., Boca Raton, Florida.

Spector, R. & Lorenzo, A. V. (1975a) Folate transport by the choroid plexus in vitro. *Science*, **187**, 540–2.

Spector, R. & Lorenzo, A. V. (1975b) Folate transport in the central nervous system. *American Journal of Physiology*, **229**, 777–82.

Spector, R., Coakley, G. & Blakely, R. (1980) Methionine recycling in brain: a role for folates and vitamin B_{12}. *Journal of Neurochemistry*, **34**, 132–7.

Stampfer, M. J., Malinow, M. R., Willett, W. C., Newcomer, L. M., Upson, B., Ullmann, D., Tishler, P. V. & Hennekens, C. H. (1992) A prospective study of plasma homocyst(e)ine and risk of myocardial infarction in US physicians. *Journal of the American Medical Association*, **268**, 877–81.

Steinberg, S. E. (1984) Mechanisms of folate homeostasis. *American Journal of Physiology*, **246**, G319–24.

Strum, W. B. (1979) Enzymatic reduction and methylation of folate following pH-dependent, carrier-mediated transport in rat jejunum. *Biochimica et Biophysica Acta*, **554**, 249–57.

Subar, A. F., Block, G. & James, L. D. (1989) Folate intake and food sources in the US population. *American Journal of Clinical Nutrition*, **50**, 508–16.

Tawakol, A., Omland, T., Gerhard, M., Wu, J. T. & Creager, M. A. (1997) Hyperhomocyst(e)inemia is associated with impaired endothelium-dependent vasodilation in humans. *Circulation*, **95**, 1119–21.

Tsai, J.-C., Perrella, M. A., Yoshizumi, M., Hsieh, C.-M., Haber, E., Schlegel, R. & Lee, M.-E. (1994) Promotion of vascular smooth muscle cell growth by homocysteine: a link to atherosclerosis. *Proceedings of the National Academy of Sciences of the U.S.A.*, **91**, 6369–73.

Undas, A., Domagala, T. B., Jankowski, M. & Szczeklik, A. (1999) Treatment of hyperhomocysteinemia with folic acid and vitamins B_{12} and B_6 attenuates thrombin generation. *Thrombosis Research*, **95**, 281–8.

Upchurch, G. R. Jr., Welch, G. N., Fabian, A. J., Pigazzi, A., Keaney, J. F. Jr. & Loscalzo, J. (1997) Stimulation of endothelial nitric oxide production by homocyst(e)ine. *Atherosclerosis*, **132**, 177–85.

van der Put, N. M. J., van der Molen, E. F., Kluijtmans, L. A. J., Heil, S. G., Trijbels, J. M. F., Eskes, T. K. A. B., van Oppenraaij-Emmerzaal, D., Banerjee, R. & Blom, H. J. (1997) Sequence analysis of the coding region of human methionine synthase: relevance to hyperhomocysteinaemia in neural-tube defects and vascular disease. *Quarterly Journal of Medicine*, **90**, 511–17.

van der Put, N. M. J., Gabreëls, F., Stevens, E. M. B., Smeitink, J. A. M., Trijbels, F. J. M., Eskes, T. K. A. B., van den Heuvel, L. P. & Blom, H. J. (1998) A second common mutation in the methylenetetrahydrofolate reductase gene: an additional risk factor for neural-tube defects? *American Journal of Human Genetics*, **62**, 1044–51.

van het Hof, K. H., Tijburg, L. B. M., Pietrzik, K. & Weststrate, J. A. (1999) Influence of feeding different vegetables on plasma levels of carotenoids, folate and vitamin C. Effect of disruption of the vegetable matrix. *British Journal of Nutrition*, **82**, 203–12.

Verhaar, M. C., Wever, R. M. F., Kastelein, J. J. P., van Dam, T., Koomans, H. A. & Rabelink, T. J. (1998) 5-Methyltetrahydrofolate, the active form of folic acid, restores endothelial function in familial hypercholesterolemia. *Circulation*, **97**, 237–41.

Verhaar, M. C., Wever, R. M. F., Kastelein, J. J. P., van Loon, D., Milstien, S., Koomans, H. A. & Rabelink, T. J. (1999) Effects of oral folic acid supplementation on endothelial function in familial hypercholesterolemia. A randomized placebo-controlled trial. *Circulation*, **100**, 335–8.

Wagner, C. (1996) Symposium on the subcellular compartmentation of folate metabolism. *Journal of Nutrition*, **126**, 1228S–34S.

Wang, X., Shen, F., Freisheim, J. H., Gentry, L. E. & Ratnam, M. (1992) Differential stereospecificities and affinities of folate receptor isoforms for folate compounds and antifolates. *Biochemical Pharmacology*, **44**, 1898–1901.

Ward, M., McNulty, H., McPartlin, J., Strain, J. J., Weir, D. G. & Scott, J. M. (1997) Plasma homocysteine, a risk factor for cardiovascular disease, is lowered by physiological doses of folic acid. *Quarterly Journal of Medicine*, **90**, 519–24.

Wei, M.-M. & Gregory, J. F. III (1998) Organic acids in selected foods inhibit intestinal brush border pteroylpolyglutamate hydrolase in vitro: potential mechanism affecting the bioavailability of dietary polyglutamyl folate. *Journal of Agricultural and Food Chemistry*, **46**, 211–19.

Weisberg, I., Tran, P., Christensen, B., Sibani, S. & Rozen, R. (1998) A second genetic polymorphism in methylenetetrahydrofolate reductase (MTHFR) associated with decreased enzyme activity. *Molecular Genetics and Metabolism*, **64**, 169–72.

Weitman, S. D., Weinberg, A. G., Coney, L. R., Zurawski, V. R., Jennings, D. S. & Kamen, B. A. (1992) Cellular localization of the folate receptor: potential role in drug toxicity and folate homeostasis. *Cancer Research*, **52**(23), 6708–11.

Wilcken, D. E. L., Wang, X. L., Sim, A. S. & McCredie, R. M. (1996) Distribution in healthy and coronary populations of the methylenetetrahydrofolate reductase (MTHFR) $C_{677}T$ mutation. *Arteriosclerosis, Thrombosis, and Vascular Biology*, **16**, 878–82.

Wild, J., Schorah, C. J. & Smithells, R. W. (1994) Investigation of folate intake and metabolism in women who have had two pregnancies complicated by neural tube defects. *British Journal of Obstetrics and Gynaecology*, **101**, 197–202.

Williams, W. M. & Huang, K. C. (1982) Renal tubular transport of folic acid and methotrexate in the monkey. *American Journal of Physiology*, **242**, F484–90.

Wilson, A., Platt, R., Wu, Q., Leclerc, D., Christensen, B., Yang, H., Gravel, R. A. & Rozen, R. (1999) A common variant in methionine synthase reductase combined with low cobalamin (vitamin B_{12}) increases risk for spina bifida. *Molecular Genetics and Metabolism*, **67**, 317–23.

Woo, K. S., Chook, P., Lolin, Y. I., Cheung, A. S. P., Chan, L. T., Sun, Y. Y., Sanderson, J. E., Metreweli, C. & Celermajer, D. S. (1997) Hyperhomocyst(e)inemia is a risk factor for arterial endothelial dysfunction in humans. *Circulation*, **96**, 2542–4.

Woo, K. S., Chook, P., Lolin, Y. I., Sanderson, J. E., Metreweli, C. & Celermajer, D. S. (1999) Folic acid improves arterial endothelial function in adults with hyperhomocysteinemia. *Journal of the American College of Cardiology*, **34**, 2002–6.

Yates, Z. & Lucock, M. (2002) Methionine synthase polymorphism A2756G is associated with susceptibility for thromboembolic events and altered B vitamin/thiol metabolism. *Haematologica*, **87**, 751–6.

Zimmerman, J., Selhub, J. & Rosenberg, I. H. (1986) Role of sodium ion in transport of folic acid in the small intestine. *American Journal of Physiology*, **251**, G218–22.

18
Vitamin B$_{12}$

Key discussion topics

- Vitamin B$_{12}$ requires the aid of a specific binding protein (intrinsic factor) secreted by the stomach before it can be absorbed by the ileum.
- Any impairment of the absorption and transport of vitamin B$_{12}$ can cause pernicious anaemia.

- Pernicious anaemia has two major components: a megaloblastic anaemia, which is clinically indistinguishable to that seen in folate deficiency, and neurological degeneration.
- Vitamin B$_{12}$ is a coenzyme for only two mammalian enzymes: methionine synthase and L-methylmalonyl-coenzyme A mutase.

18.1 Historical overview

A type of anaemia attributed to a digestive disorder was reported by Combe in 1822 and later recognized as pernicious anaemia by Addison in 1849. It was not until 1926 that Minot and Murphy started to cure patients suffering from pernicious anaemia by feeding them with large amounts of raw liver. The idea for this treatment originated from the discovery by Whipple that dietary liver improved haemoglobin production in iron-deficient dogs. In 1929, Castle showed that the intestinal absorption of the 'antipernicious anaemia principal' required prior binding to a specific protein (intrinsic factor) secreted by the stomach.

Research into isolating the active principal from liver was hampered by the inability to induce pernicious anaemia in animals. For many years, the only known bioassay was the haemopoietic response of patients with the disease. Eventually, in 1948, a red crystalline substance having the clinical activity of liver and designated as vitamin B_{12} was isolated by several independent scientific groups. The success of one group, headed by Folkers (Merck and Co., USA), was largely attributable to a microbiological assay developed by Shorb in 1947. The complicated structure of vitamin B_{12} was established by Hodgkin using X-ray crystallography in 1955. Its complete chemical synthesis was achieved in 1973, but because of the large number of stages required (over 70) the procedure is of no commercial interest.

18.2   Chemistry

In accordance with the literature on nutrition and pharmacology, the term vitamin B_{12} is used in this text as the generic descriptor for all cobalamins that exhibit antipernicious anaemia activity. Individual cobalamins will be referred to by their specific names (e.g. cyanocobalamin).

The cobalamin molecule depicted in Fig. 18.1 contains a corrin ring system and a cobalt atom, which may assume an oxidation state of (I), (II) or (III).

There are two vitamin B_{12} coenzymes with known metabolic activity in humans, namely methylcobalamin and 5′-deoxyadenosylcobalamin (frequently abbreviated to adenosylcobalamin and also known as coenzyme B_{12}). The methyl or adenosyl ligands of the coenzymes occupy the X position in the corrin structure. The coenzymes are bound intracellularly to their protein apoenzymes through a covalent peptide link, or in milk and plasma to specific transport proteins. The enzyme-bound cobalamins exist as cob(I)alamins.

Cyanocobalamin is the most stable of the vitamin B_{12}-active cobalamins and is the one mostly used in pharmaceutical preparations and food supplementation. Aqueous solutions of cyanocobalamin are stable in air at room temperature if protected from light. On exposure to light, the cyano group dissociates from cyanocobalamin and hydroxocobalamin is formed. In neutral and acid solution hydroxocobalamin exists in the form of aquocobalamin (Gräsbeck & Salonen, 1976). This photolytic reaction does not cause a loss of activity.

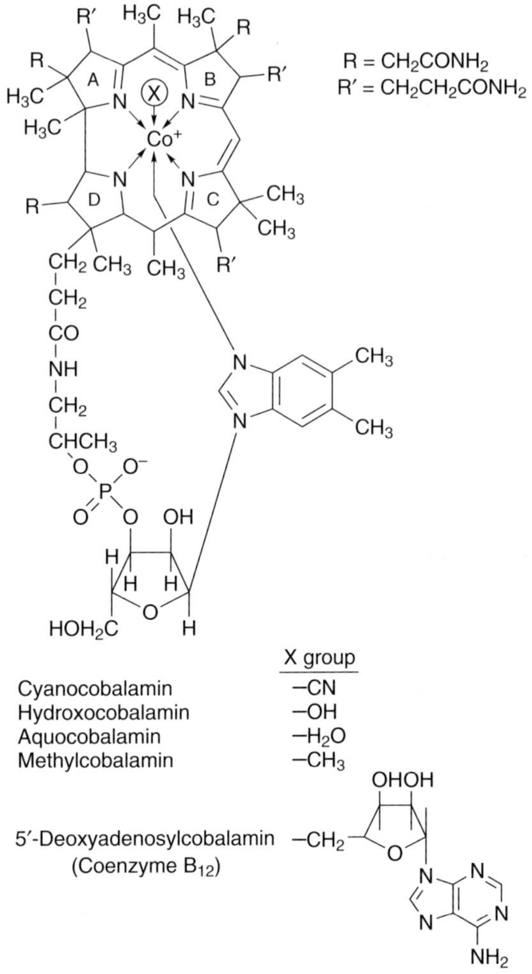

Fig. 18.1 Structures of vitamin B_{12} compounds.

18.3   Dietary sources and bioavailability

18.3.1   Dietary sources

Naturally occurring vitamin B_{12} originates solely from synthesis by bacteria and other microorganisms growing in soil or water, in sewage, and in the rumen and intestinal tract of animals. Any traces of the vitamin that may be detected in plants are due to microbial contamination from the soil or manure or, in the case of certain legumes, to bacterial synthesis in the root nodules.

Vitamin B_{12} is ubiquitous in foods of animal origin and is derived from the animal's ingestion of cobalamin-containing animal tissue or microbiologically contaminated plant material, in addition to vitamin absorbed from the animal's own digestive tract. Liver is the outstanding dietary source of the vitamin, followed by kidney and heart. Muscle meats, fish, eggs, cheese and milk are other important food sources. Vitamin B$_{12}$ activity has been reported in yeast, but this has since been attributed to the presence of non-cobalamin corrinoids or vitamin B$_{12}$ originating from the enriching medium (Herbert, 1988). About 5 to 30% of the reported vitamin B$_{12}$ in foods may be microbiologically active non-cobalamin corrinoids rather than true B$_{12}$ (National Research Council, 1989).

Vitamin B$_{12}$ in foods exists in several forms as reported by Farquharson & Adams (1976). Meat and fish contain mostly adenosyl- and hydroxocobalamins; these compounds, accompanied by methylcobalamin, also occur in dairy products, with hydroxocobalamin predominating in milk. Sulphitocobalamin is found in canned meats and fish. Cyancobalamin was only detected in small amounts in egg white, cheeses and boiled haddock.

18.3.2 Bioavailability

Humans appear to be entirely dependent on a dietary intake of vitamin B$_{12}$. Although microbial synthesis of the vitamin occurs in the human colon, it is apparently not absorbed. Strict vegetarians may obtain limited amounts of vitamin B$_{12}$ through ingestion of the vitamin-containing root nodules of certain legumes and from plant material contaminated with microorganisms.

The percentage of ingested vitamin B$_{12}$ that is absorbed decreases as the actual amount in the diet increases. At intakes of 0.5 µg or less, about 70% of the available vitamin B$_{12}$ is absorbed. At an intake of 5.0 µg, a mean of 28% is absorbed (range, 2–50%) while at a 10-µg intake the mean absorption is 16% (range, 0–34%) (Herbert, 1987). When 100 µg or more of crystalline vitamin B$_{12}$ is taken, the absorption efficiency drops to 1%, and the excess vitamin is excreted in the urine.

In normal human subjects, the vitamin B$_{12}$ in lean mutton (Heyssel *et al.*, 1966), chicken meat (Doscherholmen *et al.*, 1978) and fish (Doscherholmen *et al.*, 1981) is absorbed as efficiently as a comparable amount of crystalline cyanocobalamin administered orally in aqueous solution. In contrast, the vitamin B$_{12}$ in eggs is poorly absorbed (Doscherholmen *et al.*,

1975) owing to the presence of distinct vitamin B$_{12}$-binding proteins in egg white and egg yolk (Levine & Doscherholmen, 1983).

18.4 Absorption, transport and metabolism

The absorption and transport of the vitamin B$_{12}$ naturally present in foods takes place by specialized mechanisms that accumulate the vitamin and deliver it to cells that require it. The high efficiency of these mechanisms enables 50–90% of the minute amount of B$_{12}$ present in a typical omnivorous diet (approximately 10 µg) to be absorbed and delivered to cells. The specificity is such that all natural forms of vitamin B$_{12}$ are absorbed and transported in the same way; structurally similar but biologically inactive analogues, which are metabolically useless and possibly harmful, bypass the transport mechanisms and are eliminated from the body.

18.4.1 Digestion and absorption of dietary vitamin B$_{12}$

Ingested protein-bound cobalamins are released by the combined action of hydrochloric acid and pepsin in the stomach. Gastric juice also contains two functionally distinct cobalamin-binding proteins: (1) haptocorrin (there are actually several haptocorrins, which are also known as R binders or cobalophilin) and (2) intrinsic factor. Haptocorrin binds a wide variety of cobalamin analogues in addition to vitamin B$_{12}$, whereas intrinsic factor binds B$_{12}$ vitamers with high specificity and equal affinity. The 5,6-dimethylbenzimidazole moiety is essential for recognition by intrinsic factor (Seetharum & Alpers, 1991). The haptocorrin originates in saliva while intrinsic factor is synthesized and secreted directly into gastric juice by the parietal cells of the stomach. At the acid pH of the stomach, cobalamins have a greater affinity for haptocorrin than for intrinsic factor. Therefore cobalamins leave the stomach and enter the duodenum bound to haptocorrin and accompanied by free intrinsic factor. In the mildly alkaline environment of the jejunum, pancreatic proteases, particularly trypsin, partially degrade both free haptocorrin and haptocorrin complexed with cobalamins. Intrinsic factor, which is resistant to proteolysis by pancreatic enzymes, then binds avidly to the released B$_{12}$ vitamers.

The intrinsic factor–B$_{12}$ complex is carried down to the ileum where it binds avidly to specific receptors on the brush border of the ileal enterocyte. The presence of calcium ions and a pH above 5.5 are necessary to induce the appropriate configuration of the receptor for binding (Donaldson, 1987). The intrinsic factor–B$_{12}$ complex is absorbed intact (Seetharam *et al.*, 1985), but the precise mechanism of absorption and subsequent events within the enterocyte have yet to be elucidated. It is possible that ileal absorption of the intrinsic factor–B$_{12}$ complex is accomplished by receptor-mediated endocytosis (Donaldson, 1985), but clathrin-coated pits or vesicles have not been found. The B$_{12}$ is subsequently released at an intracellular site, possibly either in lysosomes or pre-lysosomal vesicles (endosomes), both of which are acidic (Seetharam, 1994). The intrinsic factor appears to be degraded by proteolysis after releasing its bound B$_{12}$, there being no apparent recycling of intrinsic factor to the brush-border membrane.

The intrinsic factor-mediated system is capable of handling between 1.5 and 3.0 µg of vitamin B$_{12}$. The limited capacity of the ileum to absorb B$_{12}$ can be explained by the limited number of receptor sites, there being only about one receptor per microvillus. Saturation of the system at one meal does not preclude absorption of normal amounts of the vitamin some hours later. The entire absorptive process, from ingestion of the vitamin to its appearance in the portal vein, takes 8–12 hours.

Absorption can also occur by simple diffusion across the entire small intestine. This process probably accounts for the absorption of only 1% to 3% of the vitamin consumed in ordinary diets, but can provide a physiologically significant source of the vitamin when it is administered as free cobalamin in pharmacological doses of 30 µg or more.

18.4.2   Post-absorptive metabolism, storage and excretion

An estimated 80% of the circulating vitamin B$_{12}$ (200–300 pg mL^{-1}) is bound to transcobalamin I. This protein, a plasma haptocorrin, serves no apparent physiological role in cellular uptake of B$_{12}$; however, it does prevent circulating B$_{12}$ from being filtered by the kidney, thus obviating the need for renal reabsorption. Vitamin B$_{12}$ destined for tissue uptake binds to a plasma β-globulin, transcobalamin II, with

the exclusion of most inactive cobalamin analogues that may have gained access to the circulation. The binding of B$_{12}$ to transcobalamin II takes place either within the ileal enterocyte or at its serosal surface. The transcobalamin II–B$_{12}$ complex is conveyed in the portal blood to the liver which takes up approximately 50% of the vitamin. The remainder is conveyed to other tissues, where cellular uptake of the complex is accomplished by receptor-mediated endocytosis. Following lysosomal degradation of transcobalamin II, the vitamin B$_{12}$ is released into the cytoplasm in the form of hydroxocobalamin. This compound is either converted directly to methylcobalamin in the cytoplasm or eventually to adenosylcobalamin in the mitochondria.

The body is extremely efficient at conserving vitamin B$_{12}$. Unlike the other water-soluble vitamins, vitamin B$_{12}$ is stored in the liver, primarily in the form of adenosylcobalamin. In an adult man, the total body store of vitamin B$_{12}$ is estimated to be 2000 to 5000 µg, of which about 80% is in the liver. The amount stored in the liver increases with age, more than doubling between the ages of 20 and 60. The remainder of the stored vitamin is located in muscle, skin and blood plasma. Only 2 to 5 µg of vitamin B$_{12}$ are lost daily through metabolic turnover, regardless of the amount stored in the body.

Approximately 0.5–5 µg of cobalamin is secreted into the jejunum daily, mainly in the bile. Of this, at least 65–75% is reabsorbed in the ileum along with dietary sources of the vitamin (Ellenbogen & Cooper, 1991). Reabsorption of biliary vitamin B$_{12}$ requires intrinsic factor: in the absence of intrinsic factor all the cobalamin is excreted with the faeces rather than recirculated. The enterohepatic cycle allows the excretion of unwanted non-vitamin cobalamin analogues, which constitute about 60% of the corrinoids secreted in bile, and returns vitamin B$_{12}$ relatively free of analogues.

The binding of vitamin B$_{12}$ with transcobalamins I and II prevents the vitamin molecule from being excreted in the urine as it passes through the kidney. Only if the circulating B$_{12}$ exceeds the vitamin binding capacity of the blood is the excess excreted; this typically occurs only after injection of cobalamin. The binding with plasma proteins, negligible urinary loss and an efficient enterohepatic circulation, together with the slow rate of turnover, explains why strict vegetarians, whose absorptive capacity is intact, take

20 years or more to develop signs of deficiency. People with absorptive malfunction develop deficiency signs within 2–3 years.

18.5   Biochemical functions

In humans, only two enzymes require a B$_{12}$ coenzyme: methionine synthase (EC 2.1.1.13) and L-methylmalonyl-coenzyme A (CoA) mutase (EC 5.4.99.2).

18.5.1   *Methionine synthase*

Methionine synthase catalyses the conversion of homocysteine to methionine and regenerates THF. A deficiency of vitamin B$_{12}$ lowers intracellular levels of 5,10-methylene-THF, which is required for DNA synthesis. The following two pathways suggest how this might happen.

The methyl trap hypothesis

It can be seen from Fig. 17.10 that a lack of methionine synthase activity resulting from vitamin B$_{12}$ deficiency leads to reduced synthesis of methionine and THF and accumulation of homocysteine and 5-methyl-THF. The reduction in THF leads to reduced availability of 5,10-methylene-THF, which is needed to convert deoxyuridine monophosphate (dUMP) to deoxythymidine monophosphate (dTMP) for DNA synthesis. 5-Methyl-THF does not directly participate in DNA synthesis. The deficiency in methionine means that less S-adenosylmethionine (SAM) is produced. SAM normally suppresses 5,10-methylene-THF reductase, so an impaired production of SAM will reduce this suppression and promote the conversion of 5,10-methylene-THF to 5-methyl-THF. The latter compound becomes metabolically trapped because (1) the reductase reaction is irreversible *in vivo* and (2) methionine synthase is rendered inactive by the lack of its coenzyme, methylcobalamin. This series of events is known as the methyl trap hypothesis.

A potential way of circumventing the methyl trap is provided by the following reactions in which BH$_4$ is tetrahydrobiopterin (Fig. 18.2), BH$_3$OH is 4a-hydroxytetrahydrobiopterin and qBH$_2$ is quinonoid dihydrobiopterin.

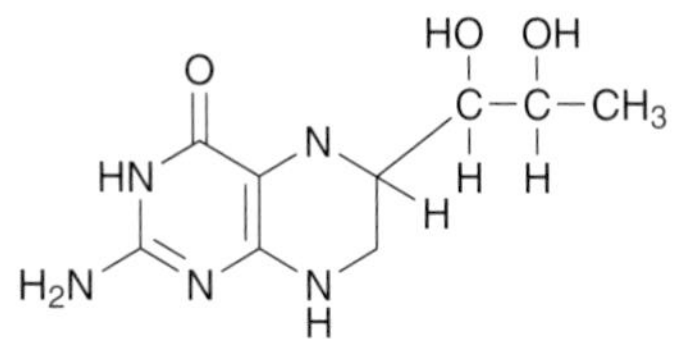

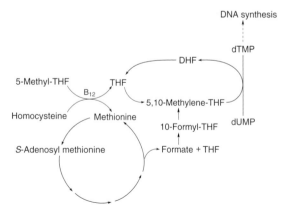

Fig. 18.2 Structure of tetrahydrobiopterin.

$$\text{phenylalanine} + O_2 + BH_4 \longrightarrow \text{tyrosine} + BH_3OH \tag{18.1}$$

$$BH_3OH \longrightarrow qBH_2 + H_2O \tag{18.2}$$

$$qBH_2 + NAD+ H^+ \longrightarrow BH_4 + NAD^+ \tag{18.3}$$

$$qBH_2 + \text{5-CH}_3\text{-THF} \longrightarrow BH_4 + \text{5,10-CH}_2\text{-THF} \tag{18.4}$$

It is evident that if adequate amounts of qBH$_2$ are present, reaction 18.4 can make 5,10-methylene-THF available for one-carbon metabolism. Whether this escape reaction from the methyl trap actually occurs will depend on the presence of the various enzymes and substrates required to sustain the above reactions (Kaufman, 1991).

The formate starvation hypothesis

According to this hypothesis, the lack of methionine caused by vitamin B$_{12}$ deficiency leads to impaired synthesis of 'active' formate (Fig. 18.3) and consequent reduced synthesis of 10-formyl-THF, a precursor of 5,10-methylene-THF. In support of this hypothesis, impaired deoxythymidine synthesis is

Fig. 18.3 Pathways showing how a lack of methionine can result in reduced synthesis of 5,10-methylene-THF.

either not improved or only marginally improved when THF is added to vitamin B_{12}-deficient bone marrow cells, but is corrected completely with formyl-THF (Chanarin *et al.*, 1989).

18.5.2 L-Methylmalonyl-coenzyme A mutase

L-Methylmalonyl-CoA mutase requires adenosylcobalamin for the conversion of L-methylmalonyl-CoA to succinyl-CoA, an important intermediary in the tricarboxylic acid cycle.

$$
\begin{array}{ccc}
 & & COOH \\
 & & | \\
COOH & & CH_2 \\
| & & | \\
H_3C-CH & \xrightarrow{B_{12}} & CH_2 \\
| & & | \\
C=O & & C=O \quad (18.5) \\
| & & | \\
S\sim CoA & & S\sim CoA \\
\end{array}
$$

L-Methylmalonyl-CoA   Succinyl-CoA

L-Methylmalonyl-CoA is generated from propionyl-CoA, which in turn arises from (1) the degradation of carbon skeletons of methionine, isoleucine, threonine and valine and (2) the beta-oxidation of fatty acids with odd-numbered chains. Propionyl-CoA is converted in a biotin-dependent reaction to D-methylmalonyl-CoA, which then undergoes racemization to L-methylmalonyl-CoA.

18.6 Vitamin B_{12} deficiency

The vitamin B_{12} deficiency disease pernicious anaemia manifests as a megaloblastic anaemia and a neuropathy. The megaloblastic anaemia is clinically indistinguishable from that induced by folate deficiency. About 12% of patients with pernicious anaemia present with neuropathy alone (Lindenbaum *et al.*, 1988). Unless treated, pernicious anaemia is fatal in 1 to 3 years following diagnosis.

18.6.1 Causes of vitamin B_{12} malabsorption

Vitamin B_{12} deficiency results from a failure of intestinal absorption or subsequent transport to the tissues;

it is rarely, if ever, caused by a lack of B_{12} in the diet. Disorders of vitamin B_{12} absorption and transport have been discussed by Kapadia & Donaldson (1985) and just a few examples of malabsorption are mentioned here.

- Elderly people are prone to atrophic gastritis, a condition in which the gastric oxyntic mucosa atrophies to such an extent that virtually no hydrochloric acid or intrinsic factor is secreted.
- In patients with diverticula, strictures and fistulas of the small intestine, stagnant regions of the lumen may become contaminated with colonic bacteria which can take up much of the dietary vitamin B_{12} passing by. Bacteria can take up vitamin B_{12} bound to intrinsic factor, although not as avidly as they can take up the free vitamin. Intrinsic factor and bacteria have a similar affinity for B_{12}, so it is possible that bacterial uptake could take place following the vitamin's release from haptocorrin but before its transfer to intrinsic factor.
- The fish tapeworm *Diphyllobothrium latum* competes with the host for B_{12}, making it less available for absorption.
- A common inherited disorder is an auto-immune reaction with formation of antibodies against intrinsic factor. Such cases involve two types of antibody: type I prevents intrinsic factor from binding to cobalamin and type II blocks the binding of the intrinsic factor–cobalamin complex to the ileal receptor.

18.6.2 Megaloblastic anaemia

Incoming dietary folate is converted mainly to monoglutamyl 5-methyl-THF, which circulates in the plasma. Normally, the 5-methyl-THF is demethylated by the action of methionine synthase and glutamate residues are attached to the resultant THF to facilitate cellular uptake. However, in the absence of vitamin B_{12}, demethylation cannot take place and the monoglutamyl 5-methyl-THF, being a poor substrate for folylpolyglutamate synthetase, is poorly incorporated into the B_{12}-deficient cell. Thus a deficiency in vitamin B_{12} results in an inability of cells to utilize folate for DNA synthesis and this leads to megaloblastic anaemia. This interrelationship between folate and vitamin B_{12} explains why dietary deficiencies of vitamin B_{12} and folate result in morphologically identical anaemias.

The direct cause of the megaloblastic anaemia that results from vitamin B$_{12}$ deficiency is a defective production of erythrocytes in the bone marrow due to impaired DNA synthesis. This impairment is a consequence of reduced intracellular levels of 5,10-methylene-THF, which is needed to synthesize deoxythymidine monophosphate, a precursor for DNA synthesis. The haematological changes and clinical signs of megaloblastic anaemia are described in Section 17.8.1.

18.6.3   Neurological changes

The neurological changes reflect the inability to manufacture the lipid component of myelin, which results in a generalized demyelinization of nerve tissue. The myelin sheath insulates axons, enabling them to conduct nerve impulses at very rapid rates. Neuropathy begins in the peripheral nerves and progresses to the spinal cord and brain. The earliest neurological symptoms are often a tingling, numbness and a feeling of muscle weakness in the limbs. There is a loss of vibratory and position sense in the feet and a feeling of walking on cotton wool. Motor disturbances are shown by incoordination of the legs and a loss of fine coordination of the fingers. Impaired bowel and bladder control are manifested by a sense of urinary urgency and constipation. An uncommon symptom, found mainly in carriers of the fish tapeworm, is impaired bilateral vision due to demyelination of the optic nerves. Neuropsychiatric symptoms appear when demyelination progresses to the deep white matter of the cerebral hemispheres. These symptoms may include irritability, memory disturbances, mild depression and apathy. Uncommonly, more serious mental problems such as psychosis and dementia develop. The response to treatment with vitamin B$_{12}$ depends on the duration of symptoms prior to diagnosis. Treatment will halt progression of neurological impairment, but much of the damage present will remain. If untreated, the patient will die.

The metabolic basis for the neuropathy of vitamin B$_{12}$ deficiency has been the subject of much debate. One plausible explanation proposed by Scott (1992) and Metz (1992) is based on the impaired synthesis of methionine that leads to a deficiency of S-adenosyl-methionine (SAM), a general donor of methyl groups in transmethylation reactions. Baldwin & Carnegie

(1971) demonstrated the specific methylation of an arginine residue in myelin basic protein, and so a deficiency of SAM could explain the demyelination of neural tissue. As shown in Fig. 17.4, methionine can be synthesized independently of vitamin B$_{12}$ by the reaction between betaine (a product of choline catabolism) and homocysteine that has accumulated as a result of impaired methionine synthase activity. This reaction takes place in the liver but in neural tissue of human, pig and rat there is a complete absence of betaine:homocysteine methyltransferase in the three species examined (McKeever et al., 1991). Thus, when vitamin B$_{12}$ becomes deficient, neural tissue becomes deprived of a vital substrate, SAM, required for myelination.

There is some evidence to support the above hypothesis that impairment of methionine synthase activity due to lack of vitamin B$_{12}$ leads to blocking of SAM production and consequent demyelination. The evidence is based on the inactivation of methionine synthase by the anaesthetic gas nitrous oxide (N$_2$O). Treatment of monkeys (Scott et al., 1981) and pigs (Weir et al., 1988) with nitrous oxide causes a neuropathy similar to that caused by vitamin B$_{12}$ deficiency; the neuropathy is alleviated by dietary supplementation with methionine. Further evidence comes from children with a deficiency of 5,10-methylenetetrahydrofolate reductase – an inborn error of metabolism associated with reduced concentrations of methionine and SAM in the cerebrospinal fluid. These patients exhibit demyelination in the brain and degeneration of the spinal cord, but there is no megaloblastic bone marrow or anaemia (Hyland et al., 1988).

18.6.4   Diagnosis of vitamin B$_{12}$ malabsorption and deficiency

It is of utmost importance to diagnose vitamin B$_{12}$ deficiency because deficiency causes irreversible damage to nerve tissue. In confirmed B$_{12}$ deficiency, whatever the cause, the vitamin must be injected into the bloodstream as soon as possible. Saturation of body stores of B$_{12}$ is accomplished rapidly with parenteral treatment. Patients with pernicious anaemia are usually given intramuscular injections of hydroxocobalamin every 2–3 months throughout life, once stores have been replenished (Beatty & Wickramasinghe, 1993).

The Schilling test for malabsorption

The classical procedure for defining the nature of vitamin B_{12} malabsorption in adult humans is the Schilling test. This test is based on the fact that free cobalamin does not occur in plasma unless all binding proteins are saturated. Once this is achieved the free cobalamin is then filtered through the glomerulus and excreted in the urine. The test procedure is as follows. A physiological (0.5 to 2.0 µg) quantity of cyanocobalamin labelled with ^{57}Co is given orally to the fasting subject. To release absorbed radioactivity from tissues so that it can be excreted in the urine, a 'flushing dose' of 1 mg of non-radioactive cyanocobalamin is administered by intramuscular injection within 2 hours of the oral dose. Under these conditions about one-third of the absorbed radioactivity is recovered from the urine, and healthy subjects generally excrete 10–20% of the administered radioactivity in a 24-hour collection of the urine. If <5% of the labelled dose is excreted, malabsorption is indicated and the test must be repeated to determine if a lack of endogenous intrinsic factor is the cause. In the re-test labelled cyanocobalamin is fed together with an excess of intrinsic factor, under conditions that assure that residual radioactivity from the first test will not be excreted in the urine. If the excretion is restored to normal by the co-administration of intrinsic factor, a simple lack of intrinsic factor is indicated. If the excretion is not restored, bacterial overgrowth may explain the lack of B_{12} absorption. The presence of bacterial overgrowth can be tested by antibiotic therapy.

The Schilling test can be shortened by using two different isotopes of cobalt to label free and intrinsic factor-bound cyanocobalamin and administering the mixture simultaneously. Absorption is determined by measuring the relative amounts of each isotope excreted in the urine.

The Schilling test provides evidence of vitamin B_{12} malabsorption, but it does not provide evidence of B_{12} deficiency. For example, strict vegetarians, who have low plasma B_{12} levels, will produce a normal result. On the other hand, patients with pernicious anaemia will produce an abnormal result, even though their plasma B_{12} levels are normal from treatment with the vitamin. Because vitamin B_{12} in food is protein-bound, the Schilling test only reflects true absorption if proteolysis in the subject is adequate. Subjects whose gastric acid and enzyme production are inadequate cannot absorb protein-bound cobalamins but, because there is still substantial intrinsic factor secretion, will be able to absorb the dose of free cyanocobalamin and thus produce a normal Schilling test.

Serum holotranscobalamin II as a marker for vitamin B_{12} malabsorption

The earliest serum marker of subnormal vitamin B_{12} absorption is low serum holotranscobalamin II despite normal total serum B_{12} level (Herzlich & Herbert, 1988).

Tests for vitamin B_{12} deficiency

A common procedure for determining vitamin B_{12} nutritional status has been the measurement of serum B_{12} levels. The lower limit is considered to be approximately 120 to 180 pmol L^{-1} for adults but varies with the analytical method used. However, B_{12} deficiency is not always accompanied by a low serum B_{12} level. Despite tissue depletion of B_{12}, serum B_{12} may be normal or even elevated in liver disease and leukaemia owing to the release into the plasma of large amounts of B_{12} binders from liver and leucocytes, which hold B_{12} in the plasma (Jacob et al., 1980). In addition to problems with diagnosis, the serum B_{12} concentration cannot be used to monitor response to therapy because it increases in all subjects who receive parenteral B_{12} regardless of whether they were deficient or not.

A more reliable indicator of B_{12} deficiency is the measurement of serum methylmalonic acid. This metabolite accumulates when L-methylmalonyl-CoA mutase activity is blocked by a deficiency of its coenzyme, adenosylcobalamin. Elevations of methylmalonic acid are very specific to vitamin B_{12} deficiency and are unrelated to folate deficiency (Stabler et al., 1996).

The detection of circulating antibodies to intrinsic factor will confirm auto-immune pernicious anaemia.

18.7   Dietary intake

18.7.1   Human requirement

The human need for vitamin B_{12} is extremely small, and for normal people does not exceed 1 µg daily. To ensure normal serum concentrations and adequate body stores, the RDA for adults is set at 2.4 µg per day.

The human placenta concentrates vitamin B$_{12}$ and newborns often have twice or more the serum B$_{12}$ concentrations of their mothers. Although maternal body stores are normally sufficient to meet the needs of pregnancy, the RDA during pregnancy is increased to 2.6 µg per day. During lactation, the RDA is further increased to 2.8 µg per day (Institute of Medicine, 1998).

18.7.2   Effects of high intake

Vitamin B$_{12}$ is non-toxic, even in doses that exceed the minimal daily adult human requirement by 10 000 times (Herbert & Das, 1994). Vitamin B$_{12}$ is not broken down within the body. Ingested amounts that exceed the limited binding capacity in plasma and tissues are excreted unchanged in the urine and faeces.

Further reading

Glusker, J. P. (1995) Vitamin B$_{12}$ and the B$_{12}$ coenzymes. *Vitamins and Hormones*, **50**, 1–76.

References

Baldwin, G. S. & Carnegie, P. R. (1971) Specific enzymatic methylation of an arginine in the experimental allergic encephalomyelitis protein from human myelin. *Science*, **171**, 579–81.

Beatty, C. & Wickramasinghe, S. N. (1993) Megaloblastic anaemias. In: *Encyclopaedia of Food Science, Food Technology and Nutrition*, Vol. 1. (Ed. R. Macrea, R. K. Robinson & M. J. Sadler), pp. 171–7. Academic Press, London.

Chanarin, I., Deacon, R., Lumb, M. & Perry, J. (1989) Cobalamin–folate interrelations. *Blood Reviews*, **3**, 211–15.

Donaldson, R. M. (1985) How does cobalamin (vitamin B$_{12}$) enter and traverse the ileal cell? *Gastroenterology*, **88**, 1069–71.

Donaldson, R. M. (1987) Intrinsic factor and the transport of cobalamins. In: *Physiology of the Gastrointestinal Tract*, 2nd edn. (Ed. L. R. Johnson), pp. 959–73. Raven Press, New York.

Doscherholmen, A., McMahon, J. & Ripley, D. (1975) Vitamin B$_{12}$ absorption from eggs. *Proceedings of the Society for Experimental Biology and Medicine*, **149**, 987–90.

Doscherholmen, A., McMahon, J. & Ripley, D. (1978) Vitamin B$_{12}$ assimilation from chicken meat. *American Journal of Clinical Nutrition*, **31**, 825–30.

Doscherholmen, A., McMahon, J. & Economon, P. (1981) Vitamin B$_{12}$ absorption from fish. *Proceedings of the Society for Experimental Biology and Medicine*, **167**, 480–4.

Ellenbogen, L. & Cooper, B. A. (1991) Vitamin B$_{12}$. In: *Handbook of Vitamins*, 2nd edn. (Ed. L. J. Machlin), pp. 491–536. Marcel Dekker, New York.

Farquharson, J. & Adams, J. F. (1976) The forms of vitamin B-12 in foods. *British Journal of Nutrition*, **36**, 127–36.

Gräsbeck, R. & Salonen, E.-M. (1976) Vitamin B$_{12}$. *Progress in Food and Nutrition Science*, **2**, 193–231.

Herbert, V. (1987) Recommended dietary intakes (RDI) of vitamin B-12 in humans. *American Journal of Clinical Nutrition*, **45**, 671–8.

Herbert, V. (1988) Vitamin B-12: plant sources, requirements, and assays. *American Journal of Clinical Nutrition*, **48**, 852–8.

Herbert, V. & Das, K. C. (1994) Folic acid and vitamin B$_{12}$. In: *Modern Nutrition in Health and Disease*, 8th edn, Vol. 1. (Ed. M. E. Shils, J. A. Olson & M. Shike), pp. 402–25. Lea & Febiger, Philadelphia.

Herzlich, B. & Herbert, V. (1988) Depletion of serum holotranscobalamin II: An early sign of negative vitamin B$_{12}$ balance. *Laboratory Investigation*, **58**, 332–7.

Heyssel, R. M., Bozian, R. C., Darby, W. J. & Bell, M. C. (1966) Vitamin B$_{12}$ turnover in man. The assimilation of vitamin B$_{12}$ from natural foodstuff by man and estimates of minimal daily dietary requirements. *American Journal of Clinical Nutrition*, **18**, 176–84.

Hyland, K., Smith, I., Bottiglieri, T., Perry, J., Wendel, U., Clayton, P. T. & Leonard, J. V. (1988) Demyelination and decreased S-adenosylmethionine in 5,10-methylenetetrahydrofolate reductase deficiency. *Neurology*, **38**, 459–62.

Institute of Medicine (1998) *Dietary Reference Intakes for Thiamin, Riboflavin, Niacin, Vitamin B$_6$, Folate, Vitamin B$_{12}$, Pantothenic Acid, Biotin, and Choline.* National Academy Press, Washington, D.C.

Jacob, E., Baker, S. J. & Herbert, V. (1980) Vitamin B$_{12}$-binding proteins. *Physiological Reviews*, **60**, 918–59.

Kapadia, C. R. & Donaldson, R. M. Jr. (1985) Disorders of cobalamin (vitamin B$_{12}$) absorption and transport. *Annual Review of Medicine*, **36**, 93–110.

Kaufman, S. (1991) Some metabolic relationships between biopterin and folate: implications for the 'methyl trap hypothesis'. *Neurochemical Research*, **16**, 1031–6.

Levine, A. S. & Doscherholmen, A. (1983) Vitamin B$_{12}$ bioavailability from egg yolk and egg white: relationship to binding proteins. *American Journal of Clinical Nutrition*, **38**, 436–9.

Lindenbaum, J., Healton, E. B., Savage, D. G., Brust, J. C. M., Garrett, T. J., Podell, E. R., Marcell, P. D., Stabler, S. P. & Allen, R. H. (1988) Neuropsychiatric disorders caused by cobalamin deficiency in the absence of anemia or macrocytosis. *New England Journal of Medicine*, **318**, 1720–8.

McKeever, M. P., Weir, D. G., Molloy, A. & Scott, J. M. (1991) Betaine–homocysteine methyltransferase: organ distribution in man, pig and rat and subcellular distribution in the rat. *Clinical Science*, **81**, 551–6.

Metz, J. (1992) Cobalamin deficiency and the pathogenesis of nervous system disease. *Annual Review of Nutrition*, **12**, 59–79.

National Research Council (1989) Water-soluble vitamins. In: *Recommended Dietary Allowances*, 10th edn, pp. 115–73. National Academy Press, Washington, D.C.

Scott, J. M. (1992) Folate–vitamin B$_{12}$ interrelationships in the central nervous system. *Proceedings of the Nutrition Society*, **51**, 219–24.

Scott, J. M., Dinn, J. J., Wilson, P. & Weir, D. G. (1981) Pathogenesis of subacute combined degeneration: a result of methyl group deficiency. *Lancet*, **II**(8242), 334–7.

Seetharam, B. (1994) Gastrointestinal absorption and transport of cobalamin (vitamin B$_{12}$). In: *Physiology of the Gastrointestinal Tract*, 3rd edn. (Ed. L. R. Johnson), pp. 1997–2026. Raven Press, New York.

Seetharam, B. & Alpers, D. H. (1991) Gastric intrinsic factor and cobalamin absorption. In: *Handbook of Physiology, Section 6: The Gastrointestinal System, Vol. IV. Intestinal Absorption and Secretion*, (Volume ed. M. Field & R. A. Frizzell), pp. 437–61. American Physiological Society, Bethesda, Maryland.

Seetharam, B., Presti, M., Frank, B., Tiruppathi, C. & Alpers, D. H. (1985) Intestinal uptake and release of cobalamin complexed with rat intrinsic factor. *American Journal of Physiology*, **248**, G326–31.

Stabler, S. P., Lindenbaum, J. & Allen, R. H. (1996) The use of homocysteine and other metabolites in the specific diagnosis of vitamin B-12 deficiency. *Journal of Nutrition*, **126**, 1266S–72S.

Weir, D. G., Keating, S., Molloy, A., McPartlin, J., Kennedy, S., Blanchflower, J., Kennedy, D. G., Rice, D. & Scott, J. M. (1988) Methylation deficiency causes vitamin B_{12}-associated neuropathy in the pig. *Journal of Neurochemistry*, **51**, 1949–52.

19
Vitamin C

Key discussion topics

- Vitamin C aids the intestinal absorption of dietary inorganic iron.
- Vitamin C inhibits the formation of carcinogenic *N*-nitroso compounds in the stomach.
- Vitamin C is a cofactor for several hydroxylating enzymes involved in the synthesis of collagen, carnitine and noradrenaline; it is also a cofactor for the amidation of peptides to hormones and hormone-releasing factors.

- Vitamin C modulates neurotransmitter systems in the brain.
- Vitamin C stimulates collagen synthesis, which is a requirement for muscle and bone formation.
- Vitamin C reduces potentially carcinogenic free radicals to harmless non-radical species.
- Vitamin C plays an important role in the biochemistry of the immune system.
- Vitamin C inhibits some of the steps involved in atherosclerosis and thrombosis.

19.1 Historical overview

The structure of vitamin C, designated as a hexuronic acid, was established in 1933 at the University of Birmingham in England by Walter Haworth and his associates, who also accomplished its synthesis. Szent-Györgyi and Haworth renamed hexuronic acid 'L-ascorbic acid' to convey its antiscorbutic properties; the new name was officially accepted in 1965. Both Szent-Györgyi and Haworth were to be awarded the Nobel Prize in 1937, the former for Physiology and Medicine and the latter for Chemistry. Synthetic ascorbic acid proved to have identical physicochemical and biological properties to the vitamin C isolated from plant or animal tissues, and there was no difference in biological potency between the synthetic and natural products. In 1934, Reichstein and Grüssner in Switzerland worked out a chemical route for synthesizing ascorbic acid commercially, starting from glucose.

19.2 Chemistry

The term 'vitamin C' refers to both ascorbic acid and dehydroascorbic acid, since the latter oxidation

product is reduced back to ascorbic acid in the body. The principal natural compound with vitamin C activity is L-ascorbic acid. There are two enantiomeric pairs (mirror images) of the 2-hexenono-1,4-lactone structure; namely, L- and D-ascorbic acid and L- and D-isoascorbic acid (Fig. 19.1). D-Ascorbic acid and L-isoascorbic acid are devoid of vitamin C activ-

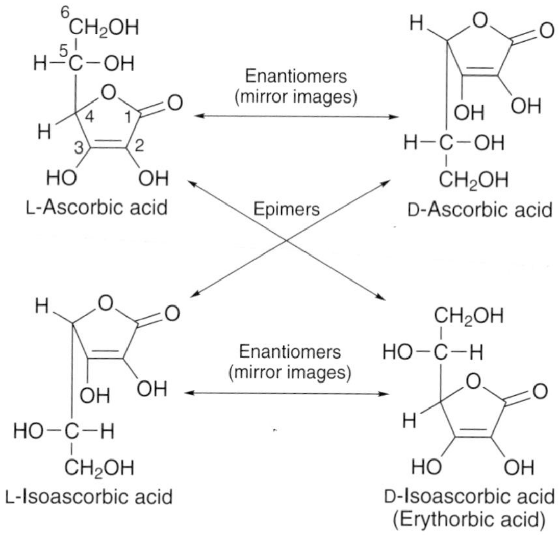

Fig. 19.1 Stereoisomers of 2-hexenono-1,4-lactone.

ity and do not occur in nature. D-Isoascorbic acid (commonly known as erythorbic acid) is an epimer of L-ascorbic acid, the structural difference being the orientation of the hydrogen and hydroxyl group at the fifth carbon atom. D-Isoascorbic acid is also not found in natural products, apart from its occurrence in certain microorganisms. It possesses similar reductive properties to L-ascorbic acid, but exhibits only 5% of the antiscorbutic activity of L-ascorbic acid in guinea pigs (Pelletier & Godin, 1969).

At around neutral pH, ascorbic acid exists as the ascorbate anion due to facile ionization of the hydroxyl group on C-3. Ascorbate is easily and reversibly oxidized to dehydro-L-ascorbic acid, forming the ascorbyl radical (also known as semidehydroascorbate) as an intermediate (Fig. 19.2). The delocalized nature of the unpaired electron in the ascorbyl radical makes it a relatively unreactive free radical and two ascorbyl radicals can react together non-enzymatically to produce ascorbate and dehydroascorbic acid. In the body, enzymes are available to reduce the ascorbyl radical and dehydroascorbic acid back to ascorbate. Dehydroascorbic acid is not a true organic acid as it contains no readily ionizable protons. In aqueous solution, dehydroascorbic acid exists not as the 2,3-diketo compound, but as the bicyclic hemiketal hydrate. In buffered solution at neutral or alkaline pH, dehydroascorbic acid undergoes a non-reversible oxidation in which the two rings open to give 2,3-diketogulonic acid in a straight-chain structure.

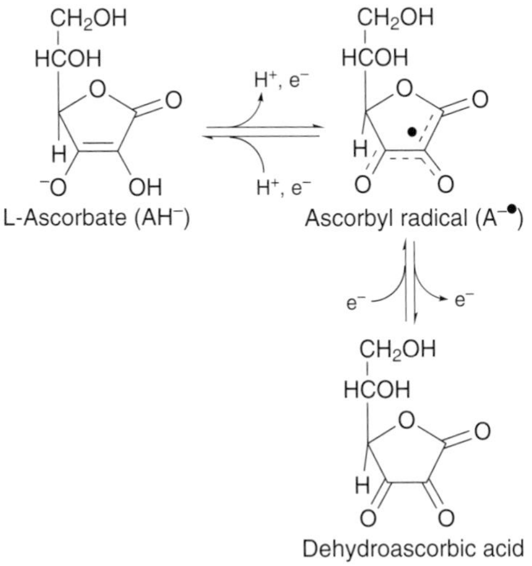

Fig. 19.2 Oxidation of ascorbate. Note the delocalized unpaired electron in the ascorbyl radical.

Humans and other primates, guinea pigs, fruit-eating bats, some exotic birds (e.g. the red-vented bulbul) and fish such as Coho salmon, rainbow trout and carp, lack the enzyme, L-gulono-γ-lactone oxidase, which catalyses the final step in the biosynthesis of ascorbic acid, and thus rely on their diet to provide vitamin C. Other animal species can synthesize ascorbic acid from glucose and have no need for dietary vitamin C.

19.3   Dietary sources and bioavailability

19.3.1   Dietary sources

Fresh fruits (especially citrus fruits and blackcurrants) and green vegetables constitute rich sources of vitamin C. Potatoes contain moderate amounts but, because of their high consumption, represent the most important source of the vitamin in the British diet. Liver (containing 10–40 mg per 100 g), kidney and heart are good sources, but muscle meats and cereal grains do not contain the vitamin in measurable amounts. Human milk provides enough ascorbic acid to prevent scurvy in breast-fed infants, but preparations of cow's milk are a poor source owing to oxidative losses incurred during processing.

19.3.2   Bioavailability

In a human study involving 68 adult male non-smokers (Mangels et al., 1993), ascorbic acid bioavailability from oranges, orange juice and cooked broccoli was not significantly different to that from synthetic ascorbic acid, indicating that the bioavailability of vitamin C in these natural food sources is high.

19.4   Absorption, transport and metabolism

Background information can be found in Sections 3.1.5, 3.5.2 and 3.5.3.

19.4.1   Vitamin C transport proteins

Both ascorbic acid and dehydroascorbic acid are transported into human cells, but by separate mechanisms (Welch et al., 1995). Two isoforms of the Na$^+$-dependent L-ascorbic acid transporter, SVCT1 and

SVCT2, have been cloned from rat kidney and rat brain, respectively, and characterized (Tsukaguchi *et al.*, 1999). Despite their close sequence homology and similar function, the two isoforms are discretely distributed (Table 19.1); SVCT1 is mainly confined to bulk-transporting epithelia (intestine, kidney, liver), whereas SVCT2 serves a host of metabolically active cells and specialized tissues in the brain, eye and other organs. The human SVCT1 isoform has also been cloned and shown to be expressed in intestine, kidney and liver (Wang *et al.*, 1999).

Dehydroascorbic acid can be transported by the sodium-independent facilitative glucose transporter isoforms GLUT1 and GLUT3 with an affinity similar to or lower than that for glucose (Rumsey *et al.*, 1997). GLUT1 has wide tissue distribution, while GLUT3 is primarily expressed in brain, placenta, testis and platelets. Dehydroascorbic acid uptake has been demonstrated in many human cells and tissues, including neutrophils, fibroblasts, erythrocytes, platelets, the blood–brain barrier and placenta, all of which express relatively high levels of either GLUT1 or GLUT3. In these cell and tissues, dehydroascorbic acid is transported across the cell membrane and accumulated in the reduced form, ascorbic acid, which is not transportable through the bi-directional glucose transporters (Vera *et al.*, 1995). The fact that these glucose transporters effectively mediate transport of dehydroascorbic acid does not imply that this is the preferred way of dehydroascorbic acid uptake in any tissue *in vivo*.

Table 19.1 Distribution of Na⁺-dependent L-ascorbic acid transporters (SVCT1 and SVCT2) in rat tissues.

Tissue	SVCT1	SVCT2
Intestine (enterocytes)	+	+
Liver (hepatocytes)	+	−
Kidney (proximal tubule)	+	−
Neurons throughout the central nervous system	−	+
Brain (meninges, choroid plexus)	−	+
Osteoblasts	−	+
Retina (inner nuclear layer)	−	+
Endocrine glands (various)	−	+
Stomach (gastric glands)	−	+
Immune system organs (spleen, thymus)	−	+
Testis (interstitial cells, spermatocytes)	−	+

+ indicates abundant expression; − indicates lack of expression or weak expression.
From Tsukaguchi *et al.* (1999).

19.4.2   *Intestinal absorption*

General principles

Approximately 80–90% of the vitamin C content of a given foodstuff exists in the reduced form, ascorbic acid; the remainder is in the oxidized form, dehydroascorbic acid. Ascorbic acid and dehydroascorbic acid are absorbed by separate transport mechanisms in animal species that depend upon dietary vitamin C (Fig. 19.3). Inside the absorptive cell (enterocyte) of the intestinal epithelium, dehydroascorbic acid is enzymatically reduced and the accumulated ascorbic acid is transported across the basolateral membrane to the bloodstream. In addition to uptake at the brush-border membrane, dehydroascorbic acid from the bloodstream can be taken up at the basolateral membrane, reduced within the cell, and returned to the circulation in the form of the useful and non-toxic ascorbic acid. The serosal uptake of dehydroascorbic acid from the bloodstream and intracellular reduction to ascorbic acid take place in animal species which do not have a dietary vitamin C requirement as well as those species that do. The ability of the enterocyte to absorb dehydroascorbic acid efficiently is important because, apart from the indigenous dehydroascorbic acid content of the diet, additional oxidation of ascorbic acid occurs in the gastrointestinal tract as the vitamin functions to maintain other nutrients such as iron in the reduced state. The intestinal uptake and reduction of dehydroascorbic acid explains why this compound, orally administered, maintains plasma concentrations of ascorbic acid and prevents scurvy. The overall system of intestinal transport and metabolism is designed to maximize the conservation of vitamin C and also to maintain the vitamin in its non-toxic reduced state, whether it is derived from the diet or from the circulation.

Transport mechanisms

Ascorbic acid

Absorption of physiological intakes of ascorbic acid by guinea pigs takes place mainly in the ileum and occurs as a result of specific carrier-mediated mechanisms in the brush-border and basolateral membranes of enterocytes (Mellors *et al.*, 1977; Patterson *et al.*, 1982; Bianchi *et al.*, 1986). Ascorbic acid is 99.9% ionized within the pH range of intestinal chyme, and therefore it is the ascorbate anion (specifically L-ascorbate⁻) that is transported across the brush-

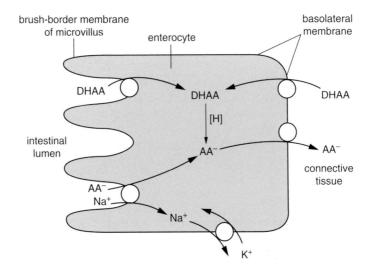

Fig. 19.3 Model of intestinal transport of the L-ascorbate anion (AA⁻) and uncharged dehydroascorbic acid (DHAA) in vitamin C-dependent animals. Thick arrowed lines indicate directional pathways; [H] signifies enzymatic reduction.

border membrane. The absorption mechanism is sodium-coupled, secondary active transport. Experiments using brush-border membrane vesicles from guinea pig small intestine have shown that ascorbate transport is unaffected by changes in the membrane potential (Siliprandi *et al.*, 1979). The transport system is therefore electrically neutral, indicating a 1:1 co-transport of ascorbate⁻ and Na⁺ by the same carrier. The immediate energy for the sodium-coupled transport of ascorbate is provided by the inward sodium concentration gradient, which in turn is created and maintained by the sodium pump at the basolateral membrane. Phloridzin, a well-known, fully competitive inhibitor of D-glucose transport across the small intestinal brush-border membrane, does not inhibit L-ascorbate uptake, demonstrating that D-glucose and L-ascorbate do not share the same carrier. Uptake of L-ascorbate is, however, competitively inhibited by D-isoascorbic acid, making the latter a potential antivitamin C.

Ascorbate leaves the enterocyte by sodium-independent, facilitated diffusion at the basolateral membrane (Bianchi *et al.*, 1986). Although the high intracellular concentration of ascorbate and the negative membrane potential are energetically favourable toward the exit of ascorbate, a carrier protein is required to facilitate transport of the hydrophobic anion across the lipid bilayer.

Dehydroascorbic acid

Dehydroascorbic acid, lacking the dissociable hydrogens at carbon atoms 2 and 3, does not ionize and is therefore unable to be co-transported with sodium. In the guinea pig intestine, intraluminal dehydroascorbic acid is transported across the brush-border membrane by facilitated diffusion, driven by the steep concentration gradient maintained by its intracellular reduction to ascorbate. In contrast, rat small intestine takes up dehydroascorbic acid from the lumen only very slowly. Dehydroascorbic acid is taken up from the blood across the basolateral membrane by facilitated diffusion in both guinea pig and rat (Rose *et al.*, 1988).

Efficiency of ascorbate absorption in humans

The usual dietary intake of vitamin C ranges from 30–180 mg per day and over this range the efficiency of absorption is 70–90% (Institute of Medicine, 2000). Brush-border uptake by the sodium-coupled, secondary active transport mechanism reaches its maximum rate at a relatively low luminal concentration. Beyond physiological intakes, absorption becomes progressively less efficient, falling from 75% of a single 1-g dose to 16% of a single 12-g dose (Table 19.2). This fall-off in efficiency occurs because absorption of high luminal concentrations of vitamin C takes place mainly by simple diffusion, and this passive movement proceeds at a very low rate.

The ingestion of eight 0.125-g doses of ascorbate spaced throughout the day produced a 72% increase in absorption compared to a single 1-g dose (Yung *et al.*, 1981). The absorption efficiency of a single dose can be improved if the ascorbate is ingested in the form of a sustained-release capsule (Sacharin *et al.*,

Table 19.2   Absorption of large, single, oral doses of ascorbic acid in humans.

Dose ingested (g)	Absorption efficiency (%)	
	Expt 1[a]	Expt 2[b]
1	75	–
1.5	–	50
2	44	–
3	39	36
4	28	–
5	20	–
6	–	26
12	–	16

[a]Hornig et al. (1980)
[b]Kübler & Gehler (1970)

1976). The ingestion of 1 g of ascorbate immediately after a fatty meal produced a 69% increase in absorption compared to the same dose given on an empty stomach (Yung et al., 1981). The divided dose effect is consistent with a saturable absorption mechanism, while the after-meal effect indicates a slowing of gastric emptying.

Adaptive regulation of ascorbate absorption in guinea pigs

In the guinea pig, intestinal absorption of ascorbate is adaptively regulated in a transient and reversible manner by the level of dietary ascorbate (Karasov et al., 1991). The mechanism of regulation is an increase or decrease in the number of carriers at both brush-border and basolateral membranes of enterocytes in response to low or high concentrations of ascorbate in the blood. The rationale for adaptive regulation is that carriers are most needed at low dietary ascorbate levels; at excessive levels the required amount of ascorbate can be absorbed by fewer carriers, aided by passive diffusion. As ascorbate does not provide metabolizable energy, there is nothing to gain from the cost of synthesizing and maintaining carriers when the vitamin supply is in excess. The issue of adaptive regulation has not been examined in humans.

19.4.3   Ascorbate in the circulation

Vitamin C in plasma occurs as free (non-protein-bound) ascorbate with concentrations ranging from 5 μM to 90 μM; dehydroascorbic acid is present at <2% of ascorbate and is often undetectable (Rumsey & Levine, 1998). Ascorbic acid is accumulated in millimolar concentrations in neutrophils, lymphocytes, monocytes and platelets. Uptake of ascorbate by human leucocytes is a stereospecific, sodium-dependent, active transport process that shows different transport kinetics for different cell types (Moser, 1987). Red cell levels of ascorbate are probably less than plasma levels (Rumsey & Levine, 1998).

19.4.4   Tissue distribution

Vitamin C is widely distributed to the cells of the body, which all take up and utilize the vitamin. Tissues with the greatest concentration of ascorbate include adrenal and pituitary glands with 30–50 mg per 100 g, followed by liver, spleen, eye lens, pancreas, kidney and brain with between 10 and 30 mg per 100 g (Rumsey & Levine, 1998). Liver has the greatest store by virtue of its size.

19.4.5   Ascorbic acid homeostasis in the central nervous system

Background information can be found in Section 3.2.1.

In vitamin C-deprived guinea pigs, the brain retains substantial amounts of ascorbic acid when other tissues are severely depleted. On the other hand, raising the plasma level of ascorbic acid does not markedly increase the concentration of ascorbate in the cerebrospinal fluid (CSF) or brain. The importance of ascorbic acid homeostasis in the brain lies in its functions as a neuromodulator and neuroprotective agent (Rebec & Pierce, 1994). The vitamin also enables Schwann cells to assemble a basal lamina, which is required for myelination to proceed (Eldridge et al., 1987, 1989).

Ascorbic acid concentrations in CSF and brain are maintained within a narrow range. The concentration of ascorbic acid in the brain exceeds that of plasma by more than ten-fold. Because ascorbic acid is not synthesized in the central nervous system or bound in the CSF or brain, there must be active (uphill) transport mechanisms for ascorbic acid at the blood–brain and/or blood–CSF barriers, and by brain cells themselves. Ascorbic acid is not able to pass through the blood–brain barrier, but its immediate oxidation product, dehydroascorbic acid, can do so by means of GLUT1

(Agus et al., 1997). Ascorbic acid enters the CSF by active transport via the choroid plexus and then diffuses into the extracellular space of the brain. It is then actively transported across the brain cell membrane and concentrated in the brain cell. Saturable ascorbic acid uptake by cultured rat cerebral astrocytes (a type of glial cell) was shown to be sodium-dependent and electrogenic with a Na^+/ascorbate$^-$ stoichiometry of 2:1 (Wilson, 1989; Wilson et al., 1991). Entry of ascorbic acid into CSF is half-saturated at the normal plasma level, whereas entry into brain is almost completely saturated at the normal CSF level (Spector, 1977). Thus the transport systems are ideally set for homeostasis.

19.4.6   Placental transport

Uptake of vitamin C in its oxidized form, dehydroascorbic acid, has been demonstrated in the isolated guinea pig placenta (Leichtweiss et al., 1987), the isolated human near-term placenta (Rybakowski et al., 1995), human placental membrane vesicles (Ingermann et al., 1986), and human placental tissue fragments (Choi & Rose, 1989). Placental uptake of dehydroascorbic acid proceeded much more rapidly than uptake of ascorbic acid. This can be explained by the high frequency of facilitative glucose transporters on the cell membrane coupled to the effective intracellular reduction of the transported dehydroascorbic acid to ascorbic acid. The finding of avid cellular uptake and reduction of dehydroascorbic acid supports the concept that the placenta clears this toxic compound from the maternal circulation and delivers the useful ascorbic acid to the fetus.

Prasad et al. (1998) measured the uptake of radioactive vitamin C by the human placental choriocarcinoma cell line, JAR, under conditions in which the vitamin existed either in the oxidized or reduced form. Both forms were transported into the cells, but by different mechanisms. Ascorbate was transported by a high-affinity/low-capacity active carrier with a binding constant (K_m) of 22 μM. Dehydroascorbic acid was transported by a low-affinity/high-capacity facilitative carrier that was sodium-independent and was inhibited by D-glucose. As both GLUT1 and GLUT3 are expressed in JAR cells, these glucose transporters are presumably responsible for the uptake of dehydroascorbic acid.

Rajan et al. (1999) isolated the human sodium-dependent vitamin C transporter (SVCT2) from placenta and found a Na^+:ascorbate$^-$ stoichiometry of 2:1. The functional characteristics of the induced transport activity were similar to those described for ascorbate transport in JAR cells.

19.4.7   Renal reabsorption

General principles

The kidney actively reabsorbs ascorbate present in the glomerular filtrate, thereby maximizing vitamin C conservation in the body and helping the intestine to maintain the circulating vitamin in its useful, reduced state. The kidneys of all mammals handle vitamin C in a similar manner. Renal reabsorption of vitamin C is an essential process for humans as, without it, urinary loss would far exceed the average daily intake of the vitamin. Although species that have the ability to synthesize ascorbic acid might be able to replace that lost in the urine, the metabolic costs would be high.

Transport mechanisms

Ascorbic acid

Renal uptake of the L-ascorbate anion at the brush-border membrane of the absorptive cell of the proximal convoluted tubule is, like intestinal uptake in the human or guinea pig, a sodium-coupled, secondary active transport system (Rose, 1986; Bowers-Komro & McCormick, 1991). Unlike the corresponding intestinal transport system, however, the renal system is electrogenic, indicating a Na^+/ascorbate$^-$ coupling ratio of 2:1 (Toggenburger et al., 1981). As the loaded carrier bears a net positive charge, its transport is accelerated by the negative membrane potential. Rapid renal reabsorption of ascorbate is essential considering that the transit time in the proximal tubule is only about 10 s. Ascorbate is transported across the basolateral membrane by sodium-independent facilitated diffusion (Bianchi & Rose, 1985a).

Dehydroascorbic acid

The mechanism of dehydroascorbic acid transport in renal brush-border (Bianchi & Rose, 1985b) and basolateral (Bianchi & Rose, 1985a) membrane vesicles appears to be facilitated diffusion. A favourable gradient for continued renal reabsorption is maintained by intracellular reduction of recently reabsorbed dehydroascorbic acid (Rose, 1989). Dehydroascorbic acid is taken up also from the blood across the basolateral cell membrane and subsequently reduced to ascorbate, which is then returned to the circulation (Rose, 1989). The kidney participates with the intestine and blood components in promoting reduction of dehydroascorbic acid derived from the blood.

19.4.8   Catabolism and excretion

In humans, the first step in the catabolism of ascorbic acid is reversible oxidation to dehydroascorbic acid by a variety of non-specific enzymatic and non-enzymatic reactions. Dehydroascorbic acid is hydrolysed enzymatically and irreversibly to 2,3-diketogulonic acid, which in turn is decomposed to a variety of compounds, including oxalic and threonic acids, L-xylose and ascorbate-2-sulphate. The major route for the elimination of catabolic products is urinary excretion; negligible amounts of ascorbic acid or its catabolites are excreted in faeces. The percentage of unmetabolized ascorbic acid excreted in urine relative to catabolic products increases with increasing dietary intake of vitamin C. When large amounts of vitamin C are ingested, appreciable amounts are broken down in the intestinal lumen to compounds that are degraded to carbon dioxide, which is eliminated by exhalation (Kallner et al., 1985). This pre-systemic formation of carbon dioxide may result from microbiological or chemical degradation of ascorbate.

19.5   Effect of ascorbic acid upon absorption of inorganic iron

19.5.1   Absorption, transport and storage of iron

The iron present in natural foodstuffs exists in two forms, haem iron and inorganic iron (referred to in the literature as non-haem iron). Haem iron is obtained from the haemoglobin and myoglobin present in the blood capillaries and muscle of meat, fish and poultry. Inorganic iron is found primarily in plant foods (cereals, nuts, pulses, fruits, vegetables). In addition, approximately half of the iron in meat, fish and poultry is inorganic; the other half is haem iron. Dairy products (milk, cheese, eggs) are poor sources of iron of either form. Inorganic iron provides 85% to 90%

of iron in a mixed diet and is the only source of iron in a vegetarian diet. The mechanisms of absorption of haem iron and inorganic iron differ. The absorption of inorganic iron ranges widely from 2% to 20% (Monsen, 1988). Unlike haem iron absorption, absorption of inorganic iron is affected by the presence of vitamin C and other constituents of the diet.

Inorganic iron bound to proteins within the food matrix is released by the action of gastric secretions, including hydrochloric acid and the protease pepsin. Once released, most inorganic iron is present as ferric (Fe^{3+}) iron in the acidic environment of the stomach, where it remains fairly soluble. Within the stomach, much of the ferric iron may be reduced to the ferrous (Fe^{2+}) state, which is also soluble. On arrival at the duodenum, which contains juices with an alkaline pH, the ferrous iron remains soluble and available for absorption. Ferric iron, mainly in the form of ferric hydroxide, is insoluble at alkaline pH and therefore potentially less available for absorption. In the body, however, the mucin of normal gastric juice chelates ferric iron, thereby reducing its propensity to precipitate in the alkaline environment of the small intestine (Conrad & Umbreit, 1993).

Absorption of inorganic iron takes place throughout the small intestine, but it is most efficient in the duodenum. It is probable that only ferrous iron can be absorbed. Uptake at the epithelial brush-border membrane is facilitated by one or more transmembrane proteins. Iron will only accumulate in the cell if there is free apo-ferritin in the cytoplasm to bind it and shift the equilibrium of the passive uptake system. Once inside the enterocyte, the iron binds to a cytoplasmic transport protein, mobilferrin, which delivers the iron to the serosal surface. Iron not being transported across the cell for release into the blood may be stored in the form of ferritin until needed. If not immediately needed, the iron remains in the enterocyte as ferritin and is excreted when the short-lived (2–3 days) cells are sloughed off into the lumen of the gastrointestinal tract. Little is known about iron transport across the basolateral membrane, but a receptor protein appears to be involved.

As ferrous iron enters the blood capillaries of the serosa, it is oxidized to the ferric state by ceruloplasmin, a copper-containing plasma enzyme. The ferric iron binds to apo-transferrin, the iron-transport protein in plasma, to form transferrin, which carries the iron first to the liver and then to all the tissues of the body. Cellular uptake of iron involves recognition of the transferrin by transferrin receptors on cell plasma membranes and internalization of the entire transferrin–transferrin receptor complex by endocytosis. Iron in excess of immediate need is stored in three principal sites: the liver, bone marrow and spleen. The hepatocytes of the liver contain about 60% of body iron; the remaining 40% is found in macrophage cells in the above three sites. Ferritin, the primary storage form of iron in cells, is constantly being degraded and resynthesized, thereby providing a pool of available iron.

The body lacks an effective means of excreting excess iron and, should iron overload occur for any reason, the result is widespread damage to vital organs such as the heart, liver and pancreas (Gordeuk et al., 1987). Tissue levels of iron are normally maintained within relatively narrow limits, despite wide variations in dietary levels. Iron absorption is controlled largely by the level of saturation of transferrin (Bendich & Cohen, 1990). That is, translocation of iron across the basolateral membrane of the enterocyte into the blood capillaries of the serosa depends on a supply of apo-transferrin in the plasma; once transferrin is saturated, iron will remain within the enterocyte in the form of ferritin. Furthermore, an increased concentration of intracellular iron results in decreased synthesis of cytosolic apo-ferritin and membrane-associated transferrin receptor; conversely, a decreased concentration of intracellular iron results in increased synthesis of these two proteins.

19.5.2   Effect of ascorbic acid supplementation on iron absorption

The amount of inorganic iron absorbed by the intestine is influenced by stimulatory and inhibitory factors of either dietary or endogenous origin. Inorganic iron absorption is enhanced by co-ingested low-molecular weight substances that combine with iron to form unstable chelates, thereby making the iron more soluble; such substances include ascorbic acid, citric acid, certain sugars and sulphur-containing amino acids. Some of these substances, including ascorbic acid, are reducing agents, which help to maintain the iron in the more soluble ferrous state. Meat, fish and poultry, besides providing well-absorbed haem iron, also enhance the absorption of inorganic iron,

apparently because of the binding of iron by cysteine-containing peptides that result from the digestion of muscle tissues (Taylor et al., 1986). In addition, the ingestion of meat may stimulate intestinal secretions which enhance iron absorption (Hurrell et al., 1988). Phytates which occur in cereals (especially in the bran fraction) bind inorganic iron and retard its absorption. The same is true for tannins (polyphenols) which are found in some vegetables and in tea.

Supplemental ascorbic acid consistently enhances absorption of inorganic iron from single meals, as indicated by incorporation of iron radioisotope into erythrocytes. In one study, 500 mg ascorbic acid taken with the meal increased iron absorption about sixfold (Cook & Monsen, 1977). When the indigenous ascorbic acid in a meal is fully or partially destroyed by prolonged warming, there is significant reduction in the absorption of iron (Hallberg et al., 1987). These observations suggest that the addition of vitamin C to meals may be considered a realistic alternative to iron fortification in cases of nutritional iron deficiency.

Ascorbic acid is thought to enhance iron absorption by both reducing and chelating iron to form soluble ferrous–ascorbate complexes which are readily absorbed (Hallberg, 1981). The most pronounced effects of ascorbic acid are found in meals containing a high content of phytates and/or tannins (Hallberg et al., 1986). This finding has led to the suggestion that ascorbic acid enhances iron absorption by counteracting the influence of inhibitory substances.

19.6   Inhibition of *N*-nitroso compound formation

The ingestion or endogenous formation of *N*-nitroso compounds is associated with an increased risk of gastric cancer (Mirvish, 1983). These compounds comprise *N*-nitrosamines and *N*-nitrosamides; they are formed in food matrices and in the human body by nitrosation reactions between nitrosating agents and secondary amines or *N*-substituted amides. Nitrosatable amines and amides may be ingested as drugs, food additives or natural constituents of foods.

Nitrous anhydride (N_2O_3), an important nitrosating agent in food matrices, forms readily from nitrite (NO_2^-) in aqueous acidic solution (Scanlan, 1983), as follows.

$$NO_2^- + H^+ \rightleftharpoons HNO_2 \qquad (19.1)$$

$$HNO_2 + H^+ \rightleftharpoons H_2NO_2^+ \qquad (19.2)$$

$$H_2NO_2^+ + NO_2^- \rightleftharpoons N_2O_3 + H_2O \qquad (19.3)$$

Nitrite is produced endogenously by bacterial reduction of ingested nitrate in the saliva. Vegetables contribute most of the nitrate ingested; other dietary sources include drinking water and fruit juices. Nitrite occurs naturally in some cereal grains and vegetables, and both nitrate and nitrite are used as preservatives in cured meat, meat products and fish.

Nitrosation reactions take place in the acidic medium of the stomach. The following example shows the nitrosation of a secondary amine (dimethylamine) to produce a nitrosamine (*N*-nitrosodimethylamine).

$$
\begin{array}{ccc}
CH_3 & & CH_3 \\
| & & | \\
NH + N_2O_3 & \rightleftharpoons & N{-}N{=}O + HNO_2 \\
| & & | \\
CH_3 & & CH_3
\end{array}
\qquad (19.4)
$$

Preformed nitrosamines can occur in trace amounts (parts per million) in smoked foods as well as foods cured with nitrite. The major dietary sources of preformed nitrosamines are cured meat products, especially bacon; other sources include some cheeses, non-fat dried milk, fish and beer. Nitrosamides (unlike nitrosamines) are chemically unstable; they probably do not persist in foods and thus may not be ingested as such (Mirvish, 1983).

Vitamin C reacts more rapidly with nitrosating agents than do amines or amides, and thus inhibits nitrosation by competing for these agents. Ascorbate (AH⁻) reacts with nitrous anhydride to form non-nitrosating nitric oxide (NO) and dehydroascorbate (A).

$$AH^- + N_2O_3 \rightleftharpoons A + 2NO + H_2O \qquad (19.5)$$

In the anaerobic conditions of the stomach, the nitric oxide is not oxidized to a nitrosating reagent such as nitrous anhydride. Thus, dietary vitamin C, at sufficient concentration, can prevent the formation of carcinogenic *N*-nitroso compounds in the stomach by exhausting the nitrosating capacity of the system (Tannenbaum & Wishnok, 1987).

The inhibitory action of vitamin C depends on the absence of oxygen. If oxygen is present, nitric oxide can be oxidized to nitrogen dioxide (NO_2), and these two species can combine to reform nitrous anhydride.

$$NO + NO_2 \rightleftharpoons N_2O_3 \qquad (19.6)$$

In the United States it is required to add ascorbic acid to the curing brine in the production of bacon in order to prevent the subsequent formation of *N*-nitroso compounds in the stomach (Scanlan, 1983). The formation of *N*-nitrosopyrrolidine is associated with the lipid portion of bacon and therefore a combination of α-tocopherol (vitamin E) and ascorbic acid has been suggested for nitrosamine inhibition (Fiddler *et al.*, 1978).

Mirvish (1994, 1996) reviewed the literature supporting the theory that the inverse relation between vitamin C consumption and the incidence of gastric cancer is due to the ability of ascorbate to inhibit *in vivo* formation of *N*-nitroso compounds, rather than to a direct inhibition of carcinogenesis. The ascorbate: nitrate ratio in foodstuffs is thus an important factor in determining the extent of gastric nitrosation.

Mirvish *et al.* (1998) used the nitrosoproline test to find what dose of ascorbate would inhibit nitrosamine formation in the human stomach when ascorbate and nitrosatable amines are given as part of the meal. Volunteers took a 400-mg dose of nitrate and, after 1 hour, ate a standard meal containing 500 mg L-proline and graded doses (120, 240 and 480 mg) of ascorbate. Urines were collected for 18 hours after the test meal and analysed for nitrosoproline. There is evidence that nitrosoproline is formed by the reaction of proline with gastric nitrite, which arises mainly from nitrate reduction by oral bacteria, and that the nitrosoproline is absorbed into the blood and quantitatively excreted in the urine. Therefore, the test serves as a measure of the potential for intragastric nitrosation of amines to form carcinogenic nitrosamines. The test is considered safe because nitrosoproline is not carcinogenic and is a normal constituent of urine. The ascorbic acid doses of 120, 240 and 480 mg were found to inhibit nitrosoproline by 28%, 62% and 60%, respectively. The authors concluded that taking 120 mg of ascorbic acid with every meal (total of 360 mg daily) would significantly inhibit the intragastric formation of carcinogenic nitrosamines.

19.7   Biochemical and neurochemical functions

Ascorbic acid acts as a cofactor for eight mammalian enzymes (Table 19.3) by keeping enzyme-bound iron or copper ions in the necessary reduced state. Other reducing agents are far less effective as cofactors *in vitro* and so these enzymes are considered to be ascorbic acid-dependent. The roles of such enzymes in four biochemical processes are discussed below (Sections 19.7.1–19.7.4). Ascorbic acid also enhances the synthesis of at least one of the prostaglandins.

Ascorbic acid modulates neurotransmitter systems by regulating neural receptor synthesis and facilitating the release of transmitters.

19.7.1   Biosynthesis of collagen

Collagen is the major macromolecule of most connective tissues. It is composed of three α chain subunits that are wound together to form a triple helix. Cross-linking gives the molecule a rigid and inextensible structure. There are over 25 different α chains that associate to yield 15 different types of collagen. Type I collagen, which is found in large quantities in skin and bone, comprises two $\alpha1(I)$-chains and one $\alpha2(I)$-chain. The amino acid composition of collagen is unusual among animal proteins in that it has an abundance of proline and 4-hydroxyproline and a few residues of 3-hydroxyproline and hydroxylysine. The hydroxyproline residues are necessary for proper structural conformation and stability; hydroxylysine residues take part in cross-linking and facilitate subsequent glycosylation and phosphorylation.

Collagen α chains are synthesized in a precursor form known as proα chains, which have additional non-collagenous amino acid sequences (propeptides) at both amino and carboxyl termini. The presence of hydroxyproline and hydroxylysine arises through the post-translational hydroxylation of particular proline and lysine residues in the polypeptide chain. Within the cisternae of the rough endoplasmic reticulum, the newly synthesized proα chains encounter three hydroxylating enzymes. Two of these enzymes, prolyl-4-hydroxylase and prolyl-3-hydroxylase, convert proline residues to 4-hydroxyproline or 3-hydroxyproline respectively, and the third, lysyl hydroxylase, converts lysine residues to hydroxylysine. Following amino acid modification, the propeptides at the carboxyl termini of two pro$\alpha1$ and one pro$\alpha2$ chains associate and bond through disulphide bridges. Triple helix formation then takes place as the protein passes through the endoplasmic reticulum. Following attachment of carbohydrate moieties to the carboxy terminal propeptides, the procollagen molecules are transported to the cell surface within secretory granules. Enzymatic removal of the propeptides during the process of extrusion allows the collagen molecules to spontaneously assemble into fibrils. These are then cross-linked by a series of covalent bonds and deposited into the extracellular matrix.

Ascorbic acid stimulates collagen synthesis through increased transcription of procollagen genes (Hitomi & Tsukagoshi, 1996). Also, ascorbic acid is an essential cofactor for the post-translational hydroxylation of proline and lysine residues in the polypeptide chain. Each of the enzymes concerned contains an iron ion (maintained in the ferrous state by ascorbate) and requires molecular oxygen and α-ketoglutarate as co-substrates (Prockop *et al.*, 1979) (Fig. 19.4). The absence of wound healing is one of the features of scurvy that can be attributed to impaired collagen synthesis arising from lack of vitamin C.

The pathway of collagen synthesis is tightly coupled through feedback regulation (Schwarz *et al.*, 1987). Proline hydroxylation stabilizes the triple helical

Table 19.3 Ascorbic acid-dependent mammalian enzymes.

Enzyme	Function
Prolyl-4-hydroxylase (EC 1.14.11.2)	Collagen synthesis
Prolyl-3-hydroxylase (EC 1.14.11.7)	Collagen synthesis
Lysyl hydroxylase (EC 1.14.11.4)	Collagen synthesis
ε-*N*-Trimethyllysine hydroxylase (EC 1.14.11.8)	Carnitine synthesis
γ-Butyrobetaine hydroxylase (EC 1.14.11.1)	Carnitine synthesis
Dopamine β-hydroxylase (EC 1.14.17.1)	Noradarenaline synthesis
Peptidylglycine α-amidating monooxygenase (EC 1.14.17.3)	Peptide amidation
4-Hydroxyphenylpyruvate hydroxylase (EC 1.13.11.27)	Tyrosine metabolism

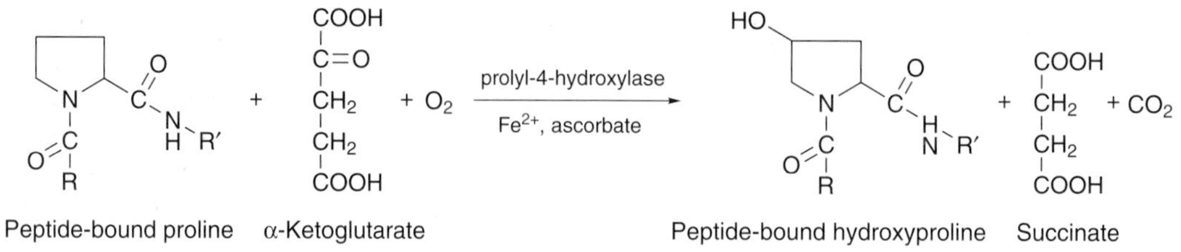

Fig. 19.4 Hydroxylation of proline.

conformation of the procollagen. This conformation increases the secretion rates by six-fold and this in turn leads to an increase in translational efficiency. Therefore ascorbate levels, solely by controlling the activity of the proline hydroxylation step, can control the chain of events through the whole pathway.

19.7.2 Biosynthesis of carnitine

Carnitine (3-hydroxy-4-*N*-trimethylaminobutyric acid) (Fig. 19.5) is essential for the β-oxidation of long-chain fatty acids, producing energy in the mitochondria. Neither free fatty acids nor fatty acyl coenzyme As can penetrate the inner membranes of mitochondria, but acylcarnitine can readily do so. The translocation of fatty acids from the cytosol to the β-oxidation site in the matrix of the mitochondrion is therefore dependent upon carnitine.

The synthesis of carnitine commences with the conversion of specific peptide-linked lysine residues to trimethyllysine within certain proteins. Proteins in which trimethyllysine has been found include histones, myosin, calmodulin and cytochrome c. Free trimethyllysine released by proteolytic cleavage is converted to carnitine in a number of steps which include two hydroxylations. The enzymes responsible for these hydroxylations are ε-*N*-trimethyllysine hydroxylase and γ-butyrobetaine hydroxylase. Like the hydroxylases involved in collagen biosynthesis, both enzymes contain ferrous iron and require molecular oxygen and α-ketoglutarate as co-substrates. Ascorbate is required as a cofactor to maintain the iron in the ferrous state (Rebouche, 1991).

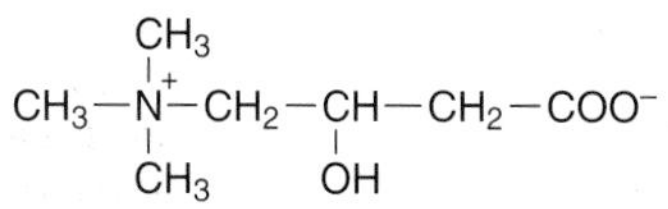

Fig. 19.5 L-Carnitine.

Vitamin C deficiency results in a variable decrease in carnitine levels of skeletal muscle, heart muscle, liver and kidney. Although it has never been systematically tested, investigators have postulated that the fatigue and muscle weakness observed in human scurvy is attributable to the lack of fatty acid-based energy production, resulting from depleted carnitine levels in skeletal muscle. Carnitine status depends on dietary carnitine intake, a modest rate of carnitine biosynthesis, and efficient conservation of carnitine by renal reabsorption (Rebouche, 1988). The rate of carnitine synthesis in scorbutic guinea pigs was shown to be much higher than the rate in normal guinea pigs (Rebouche, 1995a), thus impaired synthesis of carnitine does not appear to be responsible for carnitine depletion in scurvy. Further investigation (Rebouche, 1995b) showed that the factor responsible is increased urinary excretion of carnitine resulting from inefficient renal reabsorption. In support of the guinea pig studies, Jacob & Pianalto (1997) showed that urinary carnitine excretion increased in healthy men during experimental vitamin C depletion. However, the increased excretion had no substantial effect on carnitine status (plasma carnitine and serum triglycerides) over the 9-week period of vitamin C depletion. The mechanism by which vitamin C deficiency increases the rate of carnitine excretion is not known.

19.7.3 Biosynthesis of noradrenaline

As a neurotransmitter, noradrenaline (norepinephrine) is synthesized in the nerve terminals of postganglionic sympathetic neurons, referred to as adrenergic neurons. As a hormone, noradrenaline, along with adrenaline, is synthesized in the chromaffin cells of the adrenal medulla. The final and probably rate-limiting step in the biosynthetic pathway – the conversion of dopamine to noradrenaline (Fig. 19.6) – is catalysed by dopamine-β-hydroxylase in the pres-

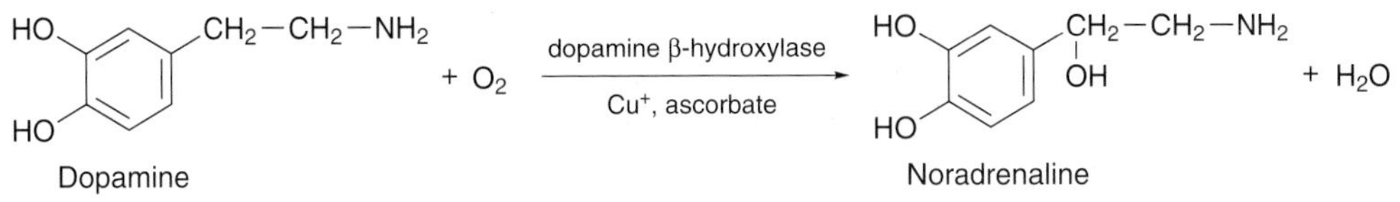

Fig. 19.6 Hydroxylation of dopamine.

ence of molecular oxygen. Dopamine-β-hydroxylase (EC 1.14.17.1) is a tetramer, each monomer containing two copper ions maintained in the cuprous (Cu$^+$) state by ascorbate. The enzyme is localized within storage vesicles in both adrenergic neurons and adrenomedullary chromaffin cells. Intravesicular ascorbate is maintained in the reduced state by electron transport across the vesicle membrane, cytosolic ascorbate being the most likely electron donor. Cytosolic semidehydroascorbate generated in the extra- to intra-vesicular electron transfer reaction may be reduced by the outer mitochondrial membrane enzyme, semidehydroascorbate reductase (EC 1.6.5.4), to complete the ascorbate regeneration cycle (Menniti *et al.*, 1986). In this manner, a stable rate of noradrenaline biosynthesis can be maintained in the absence of exogenous ascorbate.

19.7.4   Amidation of peptides to hormones and hormone-releasing factors

A large number of peptides act as hormones and hormone-releasing factors. The vast majority of these peptides are initially synthesized as larger, inactive precursor molecules, which are converted to their active forms through a series of post-translational modifications. One such final step of activation is carboxy-terminal α-amidation, which is essential for biological activity. Examples of α-amidated peptides include α- and γ-melanotropins, calcitonin, pro-ACTH, vasopressin, oxytocin, cholecystokinin, gastrin, gastrin-releasing peptide, and releasing fac-

tors for growth hormone, corticotropin and thyrotropin. Direct precursors to α-amidated peptides have glycine as the carboxy-terminal amino acid. The enzyme responsible for the amidation is the bifunctional peptidylglycine α-amidating monooxygenase (PAM), which is found in secretory granules in many neuroendocrine tissues. PAM is actually a precursor protein which undergoes endoproteolytic cleavage to generate two enzymes, peptidylglycine α-hydroxylating monooxygenase (PHM) and peptidyl-α-hydroxyglycine α-amidating lyase (PAL). The two-step nature of the amidation is shown in Fig. 19.7. Step 1 requires molecular oxygen, cuprous ion and ascorbate as the reductant (Eipper & Mains, 1991).

19.7.5   Enhancement of prostaglandin synthesis

The prostaglandins (PG) are a group of hormone-like lipids, which are formed in the body from derivatives of essential fatty acids, particularly arachidonic acid (20:4n-6). Prostaglandins have a vast range of effects and modulate cardiovascular, pulmonary, immune and reproductive functions. PGE$_1$, for example, is required for T-lymphocyte formation, regulation of collagen and cholesterol metabolism, and regulation of responsiveness to insulin; it is also an inhibitor of platelet aggregation (Horrobin *et al.*, 1979).

Physiological concentrations of vitamin C stimulate the formation of PGE$_1$ (but not PGE$_2$) from di-homo-γ-linolenic acid in human platelets (Manku *et al.*, 1979). In many vitamin C deficiency states, PGE$_1$

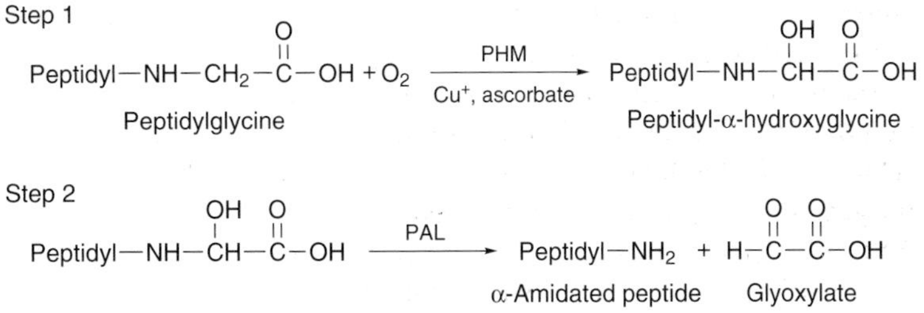

Fig. 19.7 Amidation of peptidylglycine.

has an action similar to that of vitamin C supplementation. It is therefore possible that ascorbate stimulation of PGE_1 biosynthesis could contribute to many well-known actions of vitamin C.

19.7.6   Modulation of neurotransmitter systems

Of the subcellular fractions of rat brain, the synaptosomal cytoplasm has the highest content of ascorbic acid (Kuo et al., 1979). This fraction contains the nerve terminals, where synthesis, storage and release of transmitters take place.

Regulation of acetylcholine receptor synthesis

The expression of cell-surface acetylcholine receptors involves transcription of the four constituent subunit mRNAs (α, β, γ, δ), their translation, post-translational processing, assembly of the subunit proteins, and receptor insertion into the cell membrane. Ascorbic acid increases the number of acetylcholine receptors in cultures of the L_5 muscle cell line. This effect is specific for ascorbic acid and is not a general property of reducing agents (Knaak et al., 1986). Ascorbic acid increases the mRNA for the α-subunit, but not the mRNAs for the other subunits (Horovitz et al., 1989). Thus increased expression of cell-surface acetylcholine receptors in response to ascorbic acid is controlled by the availability of the α-subunit mRNA.

Regulation of neurotransmitter release

Ascorbic acid stimulates the release of acetylcholine and noradrenaline from isolated synaptic vesicles (Kuo et al., 1979). Release of each transmitter requires the presence of ATP, Mg^{2+} and Ca^{2+}. Ascorbic acid also enhances the neurotransmitter-evoked release of luteinizing hormone-releasing hormone (LH-RH) from the mediobasal hypothalamus in vitro, probably by enhancing the activity of endogenous noradrenaline (Miller & Cicero, 1986). The neuropeptide, atrial natriuretic factor (ANF), acts in the brain to alter salt appetite and drinking behaviour among other functions. Ascorbic acid acts alone or in synergism with forskolin to stimulates the production and secretion of ANF in rat hypothalamic neurons in culture (Huang et al., 1993). The synergistic effect operates at the genomic level, with enhanced production of pro-ANF mRNA, and is mediated, at least in part, through the adenylyl cyclase–cyclic AMP signalling system.

The role of ascorbic acid in facilitating hypothalamic LH-RH and ANF release appears to be independent of its antioxidant properties.

19.8   Role of ascorbic acid in mesenchymal differentiation

Ascorbate is involved in the development of connective tissue cells, such as myoblasts, adipocytes, chondrocytes and osteoblasts, which all arise from a common mesenchymal precursor cell.

19.8.1   Myogenesis and adipogenesis

The formation of skeletal muscle (myogenesis) entails, among other events, the differentiation of myoblasts and their fusion to produce multinucleated myotubes. Fat is produced and stored in adipocytes. Collagen synthesis, and hence the presence of ascorbate, is an essential requirement for myogenesis and adipogenesis. This was demonstrated in vitro by the inhibition of myoblast differentiation and preadipocyte cell differentiation when collagen synthesis was inhibited by ethyl-3,4-dihydroxybenzoate; addition of ascorbate at high concentration partially reversed the drug's effect (Nandan et al., 1990; Ibrahimi et al., 1992). Ascorbate likely promotes myoblast differentiation through the increased expression of a myogenic regulatory protein, myogenin (Mitsumoto et al., 1994).

19.8.2   Chondrogenesis

During longitudinal bone growth, the cartilaginous structure of the epiphyseal growth plate is divided into distinct zones which define the different stages of chondrocyte differentiation. Resting chondrocytes in the growth plate undergo a sequential process of proliferation, hypertrophy and matrix production before finally differentiating into mineralizing cells. Specific changes in the expression of collagen genes take place during the process of chondrogenesis. A shift in production from type I to types II and IX collagens occurs when chondrogenesis begins, and a shift from types II and IX to type X collagens occurs when chondrocytes become hypertrophic (Castagnola et al., 1988).

Treatment of cultured prehypertropic chondrocytes with ascorbate induces the production of type X collagen mRNA after 24 hours (Leboy et al., 1989).

The same treatment also increases the activity of alkaline phosphatase. The delayed response implies that ascorbate does not activate transcription directly; rather it activates a pathway which leads to enhanced transcription. In control cultures grown in the absence of ascorbate, type X collagen mRNA production is markedly lower, alkaline phosphatase activity is insignificant, and there is no evidence of calcium deposition. The ability of ascorbate to modulate chondrocyte gene expression, unlike the osteoblast system, does not depend on production of a collagen-rich matrix (Sullivan *et al.*, 1994).

19.8.3   Osteogenesis

Osteoblasts play a key role in osteogenesis by secreting bone matrix components. During differentiation of cultured osteoblasts, a temporal sequence of expression of the genes encoding osteoblast marker proteins defines three distinct periods: (1) active proliferation, during which cell growth-related genes are actively expressed, and maximal levels of type I collagen mRNA are observed; (2) extracellular matrix maturation, when the alkaline phosphatase gene is maximally expressed; and (3) mineralization (Owen *et al.*, 1990). The transitions between the developmental periods represent restriction points beyond which cells cannot pass without the appropriate signals.

The importance of ascorbic acid for osteogenesis is evident from the defective bone extracellular matrix seen in vitamin C deficiency (scurvy) and the presence of a specific transport system for ascorbate in osteoblasts (Wilson & Dixon, 1989). *In vivo*, administered [^{14}C]ascorbate accumulates preferentially in sites of active osteogenesis (Hammarström, 1966). Preosteoblast culture systems require the addition of ascorbic acid in order to induce the expression of osteoblast marker proteins (alkaline phosphatase and osteocalcin) and to form a mineralized extracellular matrix (Franceschi & Iyer, 1992).

Franceschi & Iyer (1992) investigated the role of collagen synthesis in osteoblast differentiation using the MC3T3-E1 cell line as a model system. These cells display a time-dependent and sequential expression of osteoblast characteristics analogous to *in vivo* bone formation (Quarles *et al.*, 1992). Within 24 hours of ascorbic acid addition to cell cultures, cells had increased levels of type I collagen mRNA and had begun synthesizing a collagen-containing extracellular matrix. After 2 to 3 days, the cells had increased alkaline phosphatase mRNA and enzyme activity, followed by osteocalcin mRNA after 4 to 6 days. Mineralization of the collagen matrix began after 6 to 8 days. Ascorbate also stimulated cell proliferation, the cells becoming incorporated into the collagen matrix to form multilayered structures with a discrete zone of mineral. Blocking collagen synthesis with specific inhibitors prevented ascorbic acid-dependent cell proliferation and expression of osteoblast marker genes without affecting non-collagen protein synthesis or basal proliferation rates.

In a discussion of the above work, Franceschi (1992) considered that once vitamin C has formed some critical amount of collagen matrix, an extracellular environment is established that is permissive for subsequent expression of osteoblast marker genes. They speculated that collagen or some other extracellular matrix protein may interact with cell-surface adhesion receptors, thereby generating a signal that stimulates proliferation and marker gene expression. Harada *et al.* (1991) reported that peptides containing the sequence Arg-Gly-Asp completely blocked the proliferative activity of ascorbate. This finding suggests that integrins may be the signalling receptors. Integrins are known to interact with proteins via an Arg-Gly-Asp sequence (among other sequences) and can act as true signalling receptors in a variety of cell types (Hynes, 1992). The Arg-Gly-Asp sequence is present in type I collagen and also in fibronectin (Dedhar *et al.*, 1987).

19.9   Antioxidant role

Background information can be found in Section 4.3.

Ascorbate is an effective scavenger of all aggressive reactive oxygen species within the aqueous environment of the cytosol and extracellular fluids. These species include hydroxyl, superoxide anion and non-lipid peroxyl radicals together with the non-radicals singlet oxygen and hydrogen peroxide (Sies & Stahl, 1995). Ascorbate reacts with free radicals to produce the ascorbyl radical and detoxified product through a single-electron transfer. Fig. 19.8 shows a possible scheme in which ascorbate can be recycled during the scavenging process.

Ascorbate is not the only antioxidant in aqueous systems: other water-soluble antioxidants such as

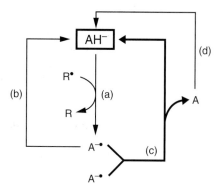

Fig. 19.8 Possible scheme for recycling of ascorbate during the process of free radical scavenging. Ascorbate (AH⁻) donates an electron to the free radical (R•), forming detoxified product (R) and is itself oxidized to the ascorbyl radical (A⁻•), also known as semidehydroascorbate (reaction a). Ascorbyl radical is converted to ascorbate by semidehydroascorbate reductase (reaction b). In addition, pairs of ascorbyl radicals disproportionate non-enzymatically to form one molecule each of dehydroascorbic acid (A) and ascorbate (reaction c). The rapid rate of disproportionation of the ascorbyl radical prevents substantial interactions with other substances. Dehydroascorbic acid can be reduced to ascorbate by either a glutathione-dependent or an NADPH-dependent reductase (reaction d).

protein thiols and urate are also present. However, ascorbate is the only endogenous antioxidant that effectively protects the lipids in blood plasma (and also low-density lipoprotein) against oxidative damage initiated by non-lipid peroxyl radicals generated in the aqueous phase. This is observed as a complete cessation of lipid peroxidation when ascorbate is added to plasma; other endogenous antioxidants, including α-tocopherol, do not have this effect (Frei, 1991). Apparently, ascorbate traps virtually all peroxyl radicals generated in the aqueous phase before they can diffuse into the lipid phase. Thus, ascorbate acts as the first and major line of antioxidant defence in the protection of lipoidal plasma constituents and low-density lipoprotein. In this action, ascorbate spares vitamin E, the chain-breaking antioxidant in the lipid phase (Doba et al., 1985).

In its role as a lipid-soluble, chain-breaking antioxidant in biomembranes and lipoproteins (see Section 9.5), vitamin E (tocopherol, T-OH) scavenges lipid peroxyl free radicals and itself is converted to the tocopheroxyl radical (T-O•). Lipid peroxyl radicals, because of their location in lipid environments, cannot be scavenged by ascorbate anion. However, in vitro studies using phospholipid liposomes as model biomembranes have shown that ascorbate (AH⁻) restores the antioxidant activity of vitamin E by converting the tocopheroxyl radical back to the phenolic tocopherol (reaction 19.7). Ascorbate works at the lipid–water interface of membranes, very close to the polar head groups of tocopherol.

$$\text{T-O}^• + \text{AH}^- \rightarrow \text{T-OH} + \text{A}^{-•} \qquad (19.7)$$

Whether vitamin C regenerates vitamin E in vivo is debatable. Burton et al. (1990) found no evidence for an interaction between the two vitamins in guinea pigs and concluded that any such interaction must be negligible in comparison with the normal turnover of vitamin E.

As discussed above, ascorbate is an excellent antioxidant but, paradoxically, it can also behave as a pro-oxidant at lower concentrations (Buettner & Jurkiewicz, 1996). This crossover effect from pro-oxidant to antioxidant is dependent on the ability of transition metals in their reduced forms (e.g. Fe^{2+} and Cu^+) to catalyse the generation of free radicals. Ascorbate, being a powerful reducing agent, maintains transition metals in their catalytic reduced forms. At a high concentration of ascorbate, the length of free radical chain reactions will be small owing to ascorbate's free radical scavenging action. As the concentration of ascorbate is lowered, there will come a point where its antioxidant action is negligible but its capacity to reduce catalytic metals is still sufficient. At this crossover point ascorbate switches from being an antioxidant to a pro-oxidant. The antioxidant/pro-oxidant behaviour of ascorbate has implications in the protection of plasma LDL from oxidative modification (Section 19.11.3).

The antioxidant action of vitamin C has a wide variety of protective roles in the body. For example:

- the DNA in human sperm is protected from free radical damage (Fraga et al., 1991);
- lung tissue is protected from free radical damage resulting from inhalation of tobacco smoke, pollutants and ozone;
- ocular tissue is protected from photo-oxidative damage that can ultimately result in cataract formation;
- the high concentrations of ascorbate in neutrophils and macrophages and its release on stimulation protect these phagocytes and host tissue during the respiratory burst in which reactive oxygen species are produced to kill phagocytosed pathogens.

19.10   Immune function

Background information can be found in Chapter 5.

19.10.1   Introduction

There is a large body of evidence that vitamin C plays an important role in the biochemistry of the human immune system, particularly in the stimulation of phagocytosis. Leucocytes accumulate ascorbic acid after uptake from the plasma by active transport (Moser, 1987), suggesting an involvement of the vitamin in the normal function of these cells. The concentration of ascorbate in monocytes, for example, is over 80 times higher than that in plasma (Evans *et al.*, 1982) and macrophages contain about twice as much ascorbate as neutrophils and monocytes (Schmidt & Moser, 1985). Vitamin C accumulation in activated human neutrophils is increased as much as ten-fold above the concentrations present in resting neutrophils as a result of a novel vitamin recycling mechanism. Extracellular ascorbate is oxidized to dehydroascorbic acid by oxidants generated by the activated neutrophil. The dehydroascorbic acid is preferentially taken up by the neutrophil and reduced intracellularly to ascorbate within minutes (Washko *et al.*, 1993). Ascorbate, as an antioxidant, protects phagocytes from self-destruction by reactive oxidants (Muggli, 1993). It also neutralizes reactive oxidants released extracellularly by activated phagocytes, thereby preventing damage to surrounding host tissue (Anderson & Lukey, 1987).

19.10.2   Effects of ascorbic acid on metabolic pathways in phagocytes

Cooper *et al.* (1971) reported that the *in vitro* addition of ascorbic acid markedly stimulated the hexose monophosphate shunt (HMS) in human neutrophils, rabbit alveolar macrophages, and in neutrophils from a patient with chronic granulomatous disease. DeChatelet *et al.* (1972) suggested the following sequence of reactions to explain the ascorbate-induced HMS activity.

$$\text{ascorbate} + O_2 \xrightarrow{Cu^{2+}} \text{dehydroascorbic acid} + H_2O_2 \tag{19.8}$$

$$\text{ascorbate} + H_2O_2 + 2H^+ \rightarrow \\ \text{dehydroascorbic acid} + 2H_2O \tag{19.9}$$

$$\text{dehydroascorbic acid} + 2GSH \rightarrow \\ \text{ascorbate} + GSSG \tag{19.10}$$

$$GSSG + NADPH + H^+ \rightarrow 2GSH + NADP \tag{19.11}$$

$$\text{glucose-6-phosphate} + NADP \rightarrow \\ \text{initiation of HMS} \tag{19.12}$$

Antimicrobial activity may be apparent during both reactions 19.8 and 19.9 in which ascorbate is oxidized to dehydroascorbic acid. The oxidation of ascorbic acid by a peroxide plus copper ions is accompanied by a strong bactericidal, fungicidal and virucidal effect (Ericsson & Lundbeck, 1955). Miller (1969) demonstrated that a mixture of ascorbic acid and hydrogen peroxide is bactericidal *in vitro* and renders Gram-negative bacteria sensitive to lysis by lysozyme. DeChatelet *et al.* (1972) also observed bactericidal activity of ascorbic acid and hydrogen peroxide *in vitro*. The remaining reactions (reaction 19.10 to 19.12) serve to explain the HMS stimulation by ascorbate. Dehydroascorbic acid is reduced by reduced glutathione (GSH) (reaction 19.10) and the oxidized glutathione (GSSG) thus formed is reduced by NADPH to produce NADP (reaction 19.11). The NADP in turn reacts with glucose-6-phosphate to initiate the HMS (reaction 19.12).

Ascorbic acid was shown to inhibit the myeloperoxidase-H_2O_2-halide reaction, which has been implicated in the bactericidal activity of neutrophils (Section 5.2.3) but, despite this inhibition, the neutrophils were still able to kill bacteria (McCall *et al.*, 1971). This finding supports the concept that the capacity of the neutrophil to destroy bacteria does not depend solely on a single mechanism.

Shilotri (1977) assessed the effects of vitamin C on phagocytosis by studying metabolic changes in neutrophils isolated from ascorbic acid-deficient guinea pigs, using *Escherichia coli* as the test organism. Activities of the glycolytic and HMS pathways were decreased during phagocytosis and bactericidal activity was low compared with these activities in control neutrophils. These findings showed that bacterial engulfment by neutrophils (as indicated by glycolytic activity) and also bacterial destruction (as indicated by HMS activity) are impaired in vitamin C activity.

19.10.3   Neutralization of harmful extracellular oxidants and proteases

Reactive oxidants

Phagocytes are susceptible to attack by the reactive oxidants that they produce and their ability to accumulate ascorbate affords them some protection. There are notable differences in the degree of protection afforded to neutrophils and macrophages. Neutrophils die after phagocytosis and so they only need to be protected from oxidation in processes leading up to this event. Their ascorbate content is low relative to that of macrophages and their intracellular ascorbate pool does not show a decline during phagocytosis (Oberritter *et al.*, 1986). Macrophages, on the other hand, can perform repeated phagocytosis and are thus better protected against self-destruction. Three independent observations provide evidence for the role of ascorbate as an antioxidant in protecting macrophages.

- Firstly, the ascorbate content of macrophages is twice that of neutrophils and monocytes (Schmidt & Moser, 1985).
- Secondly, macrophages increase their consumption of ascorbate during phagocytosis (Oberritter *et al.*, 1986); the intracellular pool of ascorbate can be replenished afterwards by uptake from plasma.
- Thirdly, ascorbate offers partial protection to macrophages against phagocytosis-induced destruction *in vitro* (McGee & Myrvik, 1979).

Elastase

The lysosomes of neutrophils contain large quantities of elastase, an enzyme capable of degrading almost all components of the host's extracellular matrix. Plasma and interstitial fluids contain a series of antiproteinases, including α_1-proteinase, that can limit the destructive effects of elastase on extracellular substrates by forming an enzyme–inhibitor complex. Hypochlorous acid released by neutrophils during phagocytosis inactivates the protective antiproteinases, allowing unregulated elastase and other proteolytic enzymes to attack and degrade host tissues (Weiss, 1989).

Ascorbic acid at physiological concentrations can scavenge the myeloperoxidase-derived hypochlorous acid at rates sufficient to protect α_1-proteinase against inactivation by this oxidant (Halliwell *et al.*, 1987). Lunec & Blake (1985) reported a decreased level of ascorbate and increased level of dehydroascorbate in

the synovial fluid and sera of patients with rheumatoid arthritis compared with normal fluid and sera. This presumably reflects the increased antioxidant activity of vitamin C at inflammatory sites. This depletion of ascorbic acid may give hypochlorous acid free rein to destroy the antiproteinases that protect inflamed tissues from attack by proteases; in short, ascorbic acid depletion may allow proteolytic damage.

19.10.4   Antihistamine activity

Histamine stimulates the early phase inflammatory response by causing localized vasodilation and increased capillary permeability, thereby enhancing the flow of immune factors to the site of inflammation. After a while, the increasing histamine concentration reaches a level at which the amine begins to suppress the immune response (Section 5.6).

Histamine is degraded non-enzymatically by ascorbic acid *in vitro* (Uchida *et al.*, 1989) and an inverse relationship between blood histamine and vitamin C status has been demonstrated (Clemetson, 1980; Johnston *et al.*, 1996). In view of this antihistamine activity, an elevated consumption of vitamin C-rich foods may be particularly valuable in allergy-prone individuals.

19.10.5   Enhancement of microtubule assembly in neutrophils

Boxer *et al.* (1979) reported that exposure of thin sections of human neutrophils to ascorbic acid resulted in an increase in assembled microtubules. This response was diminished by prior incubation of the neutrophils to colchicine, a compound known to promote disassembly of microtubules. In addition, ascorbic acid directly enhanced the assembly of microtubules from purified tubulin *in vitro*. Microtubules may be involved not only in the internal organization of cells, but also in phagocyte chemotaxis and degranulation (Schmidt & Moser, 1985).

19.10.6   Stimulation of neutrophil chemotaxis

The incubation of human leucocytes with ascorbic acid at concentrations achievable in normal tissues increased chemotactic migration of the cells: the enhanced mobility correlated with the cells' ability to assemble microtubules (Boxer *et al.*, 1979). Stimulation of neutrophil chemotaxis *in vivo* has been reported in normal adult volunteers following the daily ingestion of 1 g (Boxer *et al.*, 1976) or 2–3 g of vitamin C (Anderson *et al.*, 1980). Ganguly *et al.* (1976) reported a reduced migration of macrophages from vitamin C-deficient guinea pigs.

Johnston *et al.* (1992) examined the effect of supplemental vitamin C on blood histamine levels and neutrophil chemotaxis in healthy men and women. The data indicated that chronic oral administration of the vitamin (2 g ascorbic acid per day for 2 weeks) significantly lowered blood histamine levels, and that this fall in histamine was directly related to a rise in neutrophil chemotaxis. There was no *direct* effect of ascorbate on chemotaxis. Blood histamine and neutrophil chemotaxis did not change 4 hours following a single 2-g dose of ascorbic acid, although plasma ascorbate rose 150%. Thus oral administration of ascorbate reduced blood histamine levels only when taken chronically. Johnston *et al.* (1996) reported that blood histamine levels were not significantly affected until mean plasma vitamin C concentrations rose over 20 μmol L^{-1}, a level three-fold greater than that associated with overt scurvy.

19.10.7 Natural killer cell activity

An *in vivo* effect of ascorbic acid on enhancement of human natural killer cell activity has been reported at a dosage of 60 mg per kg body weight (Vojdani & Ghoneum, 1993).

19.10.8 Regulation of the complement component C1q

When guinea pigs were fed tissue-saturating amounts of vitamin C, plasma C1q concentrations were significantly higher than in those animals fed only enough ascorbate for adequate growth and for the prevention of scurvy (Haskell & Johnston, 1991). When healthy men and women were given 500 mg ascorbate three times daily with meals for 4 weeks, their plasma C1q levels were not significantly altered (Johnston, 1991). Hence, significantly enhanced C1q production may occur only during activation of the immune system, and not in healthy, non-infected individuals.

19.10.9 Enhancement of lymphocyte blastogenesis

Using cultured spleen cells from an inbred strain of rat that does not synthesize vitamin C, Oh & Nakano (1988) observed that ascorbic acid enhanced lymphocyte blastogenesis through inhibition of the biosynthesis of immunosuppressive histamine.

19.10.10 Enhancement of interferon synthesis

The participation of vitamin C in protection against some viral infections may be in the enhancement of interferon biosynthesis as demonstrated *in vivo* and *in vitro*. The level of circulating interferon induced in mice by inoculation with leukaemia virus was enhanced by the addition of ascorbate to the drinking water (Siegel, 1974). Ascorbate also enhanced the interferon levels produced by cultured human embryo fibroblasts in response to Newcastle Disease virus (Dahl & Degré, 1976; Karpińska *et al.*, 1982).

19.10.11 Regulation of cytokines

Vitamin C has an indirect effect on lymphocyte proliferation through its action on cytokines, as shown *in vitro* by Cunningham-Rundles *et al.* (1993). Ascorbic acid suppressed proliferation response to interleukin-2, suggesting a basis for the vitamin's inhibitory effect on mitogen-induced lymphocyte proliferation. In contrast, ascorbic acid enhanced the proliferative response to interferon-γ, without inhibiting the production of interferon-γ that accompanied the response to influenza A (Table 19.4).

19.10.12 Clinical application to immunodeficiency diseases

Anderson (1981) administered a single oral daily dose of 1 g sodium ascorbate to three children suffering from chronic granulomatous disease as a supplement to prophylactic trimethoprim–sulphamethoxazole therapy for 2 years. In all three patients, introduction of ascorbate to the therapeutic regimen resulted in the correction of defective neutrophil motility and increased activity against staphylococci. These responses were accompanied by a decrease in the frequency of infection and increased weight and growth rate.

Culture	Culture condition	Counts per min (mean triplicate)	Interferon-γ (units per mL)
1	Cells alone	230	0
2	Influenza A	2300	58
3	Influenza A + ascorbic acid	4100	59
4	Interferon-γ	3800	–
5	Interferon-γ + ascorbic acid	6800	–
6	Ascorbic acid	200	0

Table 19.4 Effect of ascorbic acid (8 μg mL⁻¹) on interferon-γ production and lymphocyte proliferation.

Reproduced with permission of Marcel Dekker, Inc., from Cunningham-Rundles *et al.* (1993).

Boxer *et al.* (1976) administered a daily oral supplement of 200 mg ascorbic acid to an 11-month-old child afflicted with Chediak–Higashi syndrome. After ascorbate treatment, the chemotactic migration of the patient's leucocytes was improved and bactericidal activity of the leucocytes was enhanced to that of normal controls.

19.10.13 Viruses and the common cold

Vitamin C supplementation has been suggested for the prevention of the common cold and the alleviation of its symptoms. Reviews of numerous studies generally conclude that vitamin C mega-doses have no consistent effect on reducing the incidence of colds in people in general. However, in four studies with British male schoolchildren and students, a statistically highly significant reduction in common cold incidence was found in vitamin C-supplemented groups (Hemilä, 1997). This could be interpreted as a correction of a marginal deficiency in the study subjects, rather than an effect of the high dosage. Placebo-controlled studies have consistently shown that high doses of vitamin C alleviate common cold symptoms, although the validity of some of these studies has been questioned.

19.11 Vitamin C and cardiovascular disease

Ascorbic acid through its numerous metabolic and antioxidant effects may inhibit some of the steps involved in atherosclerosis and thrombosis, thus reducing the risk of cardiovascular disease. In a case-control study, Ramirez & Flowers (1980) reported significantly lower ($p < 0.001$) leucocyte vitamin C levels in 101 cases of angiographically documented cardiovascular disease.

19.11.1 Cholesterol metabolism

Studies of animals that either synthesize (rat, rabbit) or do not synthesize (guinea pig, monkey) vitamin C have shown that vitamin C is intimately involved in cholesterol metabolism. Guinea pigs subjected to chronic vitamin C deficiency exhibit increased cholesterol levels in blood plasma and liver due to slower conversion of cholesterol to bile acids (Ginter *et al.*, 1971; Ginter, 1973). The impaired conversion results from a decreased activity of the rate-limiting liver enzyme cholesterol 7α-hydroxylase (Horio *et al.*, 1989). When guinea pigs, rats and rabbits are rendered hypercholesterolaemic by feeding a high-cholesterol diet, vitamin C supplementation lowers their blood cholesterol levels.

19.11.2 Lipoprotein profile

Diets low in vitamin C lead to a redistribution of cholesterol among the various plasma lipoproteins. Vitamin C deficiency in ODS rats (rats with an hereditary inability to synthesize ascorbic acid) leads to an increase in potentially pro-atherogenic LDL cholesterol and a decrease in HDL cholesterol, resulting in hypercholesterolaemia (Uchida *et al.*, 1990).

19.11.3 Protection of LDL against peroxidative modification

Physiological concentrations of ascorbic acid protect LDL against copper-catalysed peroxidative modification *in vitro*, maintaining the ability of LDL to be recognized by appropriate LDL receptors and not by the scavenger receptor of macrophages (Sakuma et al., 2001). This protective action preserves LDL's indigenous lipid-soluble antioxidants, except for ubiquinol, the reduced form of coenzyme Q (Retsky & Frei, 1995). Ascorbic acid spares, rather than regenerates, LDL-associated α-tocopherol, i.e. prevents α-tocopherol oxidation in the first place. The dilemma of whether ascorbate acts as a pro-oxidant or as an antioxidant when interacting with LDL has been addressed by Lynch et al. (1996). Ascorbate protects native or mildly oxidized LDL against further metal ion-dependent oxidation; only if LDL becomes extensively oxidized does ascorbate acts as a pro-oxidant.

19.11.4   Effects on nitric oxide-mediated arterial relaxation

Several studies have shown that an acute application of ascorbic acid enhanced endothelium-dependent vasodilation in patients with diabetes, coronary artery disease, hypertension, hypercholesterolaemia, or chronic heart failure, and in cigarette smokers (Heitzer et al., 1996; Levine et al., 1996; Ting et al., 1996; Solzbach et al., 1997; Ting et al., 1997; Hornig et al., 1998). Long-term ascorbic acid treatment (500 mg per day) produced a sustained improvement in endothelium-dependent vasodilation in patients with coronary artery disease (Gokce et al., 1999). Kanani et al. (1999) demonstrated that administration of ascorbic acid prevents induction of endothelial dysfunction by homocysteine. These findings may be attributable to the scavenging of superoxide by ascorbate, thus preventing the reaction between superoxide and nitric oxide to form hydroxyl radicals and nitrogen dioxide, both of which can initiate lipid peroxidation.

Heller et al. (1999) demonstrated that pre-incubation of cultured endothelial cells with ascorbic acid led to a three-fold increase of the cellular production of nitric oxide after stimulation with ionomycin or thrombin. Ascorbate did not induce the expression of nitric oxide synthase and appeared to act through an effect on the availability or affinity of the enzyme cofactor tetrahydrobiopterin. The findings suggest that saturation of the vascular tissue with ascorbate provides the optimum reaction conditions for adequate nitric oxide synthesis and that a decrease in intracellular ascorbate leads to endothelial dysfunction.

19.11.5   Enhancement of prostacyclin formation

The formation of prostacyclin (PGI_2), a member of the prostaglandin family which protects the arterial wall against deposition of platelets, is inhibited by hydroperoxides of unsaturated fatty acids. In vitro studies have shown that physiological concentrations of ascorbic acid enhance the formation of prostacyclin by aortic rings by protecting the cyclooxygenase and PGI-synthase (Beetens & Herman, 1983).

19.11.6   Effects of vitamin C supplementation

Rifici & Khachadurian (1993) administered vitamin C (1 g per day) and vitamin E (800 IU per day), both separately and in combination, to healthy female and male subjects and examined oxidation of lipoproteins in vitro. Vitamin E administration alone produced a 52% inhibition and vitamin C alone a 15% inhibition of copper-catalysed thiobarbituric acid reactive substances production; the combination of vitamins produced a 63% inhibition. Harats et al. (1998) reported that in young healthy male subjects consuming a diet high in saturated fats, supplementation with citrus fruits containing an estimated 500 mg per day of vitamin C reduced the in vitro susceptibility of LDL to oxidation. Mosca et al. (1997) reported that antioxidant supplementation with a combination of 800 IU of vitamin E, 1000 mg of vitamin C and 24 mg of β-carotene significantly reduced the susceptibility of LDL to oxidation in patients with coronary artery disease. The response produced by a similar combination containing half the amounts of each antioxidant was non-significant.

19.11.7   Epidemiological studies

Current evidence from epidemiological studies on the role of vitamin C in the prevention of cardiovascular disease is inconclusive, with some studies showing a very strong correlation between vitamin C intake and incidence of cardiovascular events and other studies showing no correlation at all (Lynch et al., 1996; Institute of Medicine, 2000).

19.12 Vitamin C deficiency

19.12.1 Deficiency in humans

A deficiency of vitamin C results in scurvy. Fully developed scurvy is rarely seen nowadays, but clinical signs of mild scurvy are found quite frequently in alcoholics and drug addicts. The symptoms described below have been observed in patients with scurvy (Chazan & Mistilis, 1963) and in experimentally induced scurvy (Hodges *et al.*, 1971).

Early symptoms in adults are weakness, easy fatigue and listlessness, followed by shortness of breath and aching bones, joints and muscles. Progressive changes in the skin then appear after about 4 months of complete vitamin C deprivation. A horny material piles up around the openings of hair follicles, and the hair becomes fragmented and coiled. Red spots of pinpoint to pinhead size caused by the rupture of small blood vessels appear first on the feet and ankles, and then spread upwards. Thereafter, bruises appear over large areas of skin, particularly on the legs. Bruising is the manifestation of haemorrhages in subcutaneous tissue, beneath the periosteum of bones and in the synovia of joints. The gums become swollen and bleeding, especially where there is advanced dental caries. Haemorrhages are caused by rupture of capillaries, which are fragile because of impaired ascorbic acid-dependent synthesis of vascular basement membrane (Priest, 1970). Wounds fail to heal and old wounds reopen. The sufferer is visibly anaemic due in part to haemolysis caused by peroxidative damage to the erythrocyte plasma membrane (Goldberg, 1963). Vitamin C deficiency in adults may cause osteoporosis due to a diminished production of organic matrix in bones. The corresponding symptoms in infantile scurvy are impaired ossification and bone growth.

Kinsman & Hood (1971) studied the psychological aspects of vitamin C deficiency in healthy volunteers. They measured four behavioural areas: physical fitness (strength, coordination and balance), mental functions (memory, vigilance and problem solving), psychomotor performance tasks (reaction time, manipulative skills and hand–arm steadiness), and personality. Three areas of change associated with vitamin C deficiency were found: physical fitness involving bending or twisting of the legs, psychomotor tasks, and measures of personality. The changes in the physical fitness could be accounted for by the pro-nounced joint pain in the legs that occurred during the deficiency period. The decrements in psychomotor performance were attributed to a reduced motivational level. The personality changes corresponded to the classical 'neurotic triad' of the Minnesota Multiphasic Personality Inventory, i.e. hypochondriasis, depression and hysteria. Elevation of this triad is also found in prolonged semi-starvation and deficiencies of B-complex vitamins.

In fully developed scurvy, as witnessed and recorded at sea by James Lind in 1752, the body is covered with spots and bruises, and the skin overlying the joints becomes discoloured from the haemolysed blood in and around them. There may be bleeding into the peritoneal cavity and pericardial sac as well as into joints. The gums become swollen, spongy and of a livid blue-red colour. The swelling can develop to such an extent that the gum tissue completely encases and hides the teeth. The spongy gums bleed on the slightest touch and become secondarily infected, leading to loosening of the teeth and gangrene. Death preceded by dyspnoea, cyanosis and convulsions is inevitable in the continuing absence of vitamin C.

19.12.2 Rebound scurvy

Theoretically, the absorption of ascorbic acid could be impaired on resumption of normal vitamin C inputs following mega-dosing (>1 g per day), because of insufficient carriers in the enterocyte cell membranes. Based on experiments with guinea pigs, it is considered likely that, in humans, renewed synthesis of carriers will take place well before the onset of scurvy. During mega-dosing, reduced ascorbate absorption is accompanied by increased rates of ascorbate catabolism. In adult guinea pigs, the accelerated catabolism is not reversible after more than 2 months on subnormal uptake of ascorbate (Sorensen *et al.*, 1974). Guinea pigs are thus susceptible to a systemic conditioning effect known as rebound scurvy, caused by an induction of ascorbic acid-metabolizing enzymes by high dietary vitamin C. The body stores of vitamin C are depleted more rapidly in juvenile guinea pigs than in adults, increasing the likelihood of rebound scurvy in juveniles. Solid evidence for the existence of rebound scurvy in humans is tenuous (Gerster & Moser, 1988), and reports by Schrauzer & Rhead (1973) and Siegel *et al.* (1982) describe only single cases.

19.13   Dietary intake

19.13.1   Human requirement

In the United States the Recommended Dietary Allowance (RDA) for vitamin C is 90 mg per day for adult men and 75 mg per day for adult non-pregnant women (Institute of Medicine, 2000). These values are based on the vitamin C intake to maintain near-maximal neutrophil concentration with minimal urinary excretion of ascorbate. Because smoking increases oxidative stress and metabolic turnover of vitamin C, the requirement for smokers is increased by 35 mg per day.

19.13.2   Effects of high intake

Herbert *et al.* (1996) expressed strong opinions against mega-dosing with vitamin C because of its effects upon iron. Excess vitamin C can promote repetitive free radical generation by iron and, in the presence of iron overload, can mobilize such an enormous amount of iron from high body iron stores that the binding capacity of iron-binding proteins is overwhelmed and potentially lethal free iron is released into the circulation.

The fact that oxalic acid is a normal product of ascorbic acid catabolism prompts concern about the possible formation of calcium oxalate stones in the kidneys. Excess ascorbic acid is mostly excreted in the urine unchanged, and the amount metabolized to oxalate is normally limited, regardless of vitamin C intake. So for most people, high intakes of vitamin C do not pose a risk for kidney stone formation. Individuals who are prone to kidney stones have some metabolic abnormality and excrete unusually high amounts of oxalate. These individuals and patients with kidney disorders are advised not to take pharmacological doses of vitamin C (Sauberlich, 1994).

Dehydroascorbic acid is non-toxic when given by mouth because it is reduced to ascorbic acid in the tissues of the gastrointestinal tract. However, dehydroascorbic acid itself disrupts membrane structure and, if given intravenously, causes a diabetic condition by increasing the permeability of pancreatic B-cells, resulting in loss of insulin (Bianchi & Rose *et al.*, 1986).

19.13.3   Assessment of vitamin C status

Out of the various blood components (whole blood, erythrocytes, plasma and leucocytes), measurement of the ascorbate present in leucocytes has the best correlation to liver stores of the vitamin and to the total body pool. Plasma ascorbate levels are usually more reflective of recent intakes of vitamin C than of total body stores. After consuming vitamin C, plasma values rise rapidly within 1 or 2 hours, reaching a peak concentration in about 3 to 6 hours. When the vitamin intake is poor, the plasma concentration can become depleted even when tissue reserves remain adequate (Omaye *et al.*, 1987).

Further reading

Bendich, A., Machlin, L. J., Scandurra, O., Burton, G. W. & Wayner, D. D. M. (1986) The antioxidant role of vitamin C. *Advances in Free Radical Biology and Medicine*, **2**, 419–44.
Franceschi, R. T. (1992) The role of ascorbic acid in mesenchymal differentiation. *Nutrition Reviews*, **50**, 65–70.
Frei, B. (1994) Reactive oxygen species and antioxidant vitamins: mechanisms of action. *American Journal of Medicine*, **97** (suppl. 3A), 5S–13S.
Goldenberg, H. & Schweinzer, E. (1994) Transport of vitamin C in animal and human cells. *Journal of Bioenergetics and Biomembranes*, **26**, 359–67.
Ronchetti, I. P., Quaglino, D. Jr. & Bergamini, G. (1996) Ascorbic acid and connective tissue. In: *Subcellular Biochemistry, Vol. 25. Ascorbic Acid: Biochemistry and Biomedical Cell Biology.* (Ed. J. R. Harris), pp. 249–64. Plenum Press, New York.
Rumsey, S. C. & Levine, M. (1998) Absorption, transport, and disposition of ascorbic acid in humans. *Journal of Nutritional Biochemistry*, **9**, 116–30.
Siegel, B. V. (1993) Vitamin C and the immune response in health and disease. In: *Nutrition and Immunology.* (Ed. D. M. Klurfeld), pp. 167–96. Plenum Press, New York.

References

Agus, D. B., Gambhir, S. S., Pardridge, W. M., Spielholz, C., Baselga, J., Vera, J. C. & Golde, D. W. (1997) Vitamin C crosses the blood–brain barrier in the oxidized form through the glucose transporters. *Journal of Clinical Investigation*, **100**, 2842–8.
Anderson, R. (1981) Ascorbate-mediated stimulation of neutrophil motility and lymphocyte transformation by inhibition of the peroxidase/H_2O_2/halide system in vitro and in vivo. *American Journal of Clinical Nutrition*, **34**, 1906–11.
Anderson, R. & Lukey, P. T. (1987) A biological role for ascorbate in the selective neutralization of extracellular phagocyte-derived oxidants. *Annals of the New York Academy of Sciences*, **498**, 229–47.

Anderson, R., Oosthuizen, R., Maritz, R., Theron, A. & Van Rensburg, A. J. (1980) The effects of increasing weekly doses of ascorbate on certain cellular and humoral immune functions in normal volunteers. *American Journal of Clinical Nutrition*, **33**, 71–6.

Beetens, J. R. & Herman, A. G. (1983) Vitamin C increases the formation of prostacyclin by aortic rings from various species and neutralizes the inhibitory effect of 15-hydroperoxy-arachidonic acid. *British Journal of Pharmacology*, **80**, 249–54.

Bendich, A. & Cohen, C. (1990) Ascorbic acid safety: analysis of factors affecting iron absorption. *Toxicology Letters*, **51**, 189–201.

Bianchi, J. & Rose, R. C. (1985a) Transport of L-ascorbic acid and dehydro-L-ascorbic acid across renal cortical basolateral membrane vesicles. *Biochimica et Biophysica Acta*, **820**, 265–73.

Bianchi, J. & Rose, R. C. (1985b) Na⁺-independent dehydro-L-ascorbic acid uptake in renal brush-border membrane vesicles. *Biochimica et Biophysica Acta*, **819**, 75–82.

Bianchi, J. & Rose, R. C. (1986) Dehydroascorbic acid and cell membranes: possible disruptive effects. *Toxicology*, **40**, 75–82.

Bianchi, J., Wilson, F. A. & Rose, R. C. (1986) Dehydroascorbic acid and ascorbic acid transport systems in the guinea pig ileum. *American Journal of Physiology*, **250**, G461–8.

Bowers-Komro, D. M. & McCormick, D. B. (1991) Characterization of ascorbic acid uptake by isolated rat kidney cells. *Journal of Nutrition*, **121**, 57–64.

Boxer, L. A., Watanabe, A. M., Rister, M., Besch, H. R. Jr., Allen, J. & Baehner, R. L. (1976) Correction of leukocyte function in Chediak–Higashi syndrome by ascorbate. *New England Journal of Medicine*, **295**, 1041–5.

Boxer, L. A., Vanderbilt, B., Bonsib, S., Jersild, R., Yang, H.-H. & Baehner, R. L. (1979) Enhancement of chemotactic responses and microtubule assembly in human leukocytes by ascorbic acid. *Journal of Cellular Physiology*, **100**, 119–26.

Buettner, G. R. & Jurkiewicz, B. A. (1996) Catalytic metals, ascorbate and free radicals: combinations to avoid. *Radiation Research*, **145**, 532–41.

Burton, G. W., Wronska, U., Stone, L., Foster, D. O. & Ingold, K. U. (1990) Biokinetics of dietary *RRR*-α-tocopherol in the male guinea pig at three dietary levels of vitamin C and two levels of vitamin E. Evidence that vitamin C does not "spare" vitamin E *in vivo*. *Lipids*, **25**, 199–210.

Castagnola, P., Dozin, B., Moro, G. & Cancedda, R. (1988) Changes in the expression of collagen genes show two stages in chondrocyte differentiation in vitro. *Journal of Cell Biology*, **106**, 461–7.

Chazan, J. A. & Mistilis, S. P. (1963) The pathophysiology of scurvy. A report of seven cases. *American Journal of Medicine*, **34**, 350–8.

Choi, J.-L. & Rose, R. C. (1989) Transport and metabolism of ascorbic acid in human placenta. *American Journal of Physiology*, **257**, C110–13.

Clemetson, C. A. B. (1980) Histamine and ascorbic acid in human blood. *Journal of Nutrition*, **110**, 662–8.

Cook, J. D. & Monsen, E. R. (1977) Vitamin C, the common cold, and iron absorption. *American Journal of Clinical Nutrition*, **30**, 235–41.

Cooper, M. R., McCall, C. E. & DeChatelet, L. R. (1971) Stimulation of leukocyte hexose monophosphate shunt activity by ascorbic acid. *Infection and Immunity*, **3**, 851–3.

Conrad, M. E. & Umbreit, J. N. (1993) A concise review: iron absorption – the mucin–mobilferrin–integrin pathway. A competitive pathway for metal absorption. *American Journal of Hematology*, **42**, 67–73.

Cunningham-Rundles, W. F., Berner, Y. & Cunningham-Rundles, S. (1993) Interaction of vitamin C in lymphocyte activation: current status and possible mechanisms of action. In: *Nutrient Modulation of the Immune Response*. (Ed. S. Cunningham-Rundles), pp. 91–103. Marcel Dekker, Inc., New York.

Dahl, H. & Degré, M. (1976) The effect of ascorbic acid on production of human interferon and the antiviral activity *in vitro*. *Acta Pathologica et Microbiologica Scandinavica*, Section B, **84**, 280–4.

DeChatelet, L. R., Cooper, M. R. & McCall, C. E. (1972) Stimulation of the hexose monophosphate shunt in human neutrophils by ascorbic acid: mechanism of action. *Antimicrobial Agents and Chemotherapy*, **1**, 12–16.

Dedhar, S., Ruoslahti, E. & Pierschbacher, M. D. (1987) A cell surface receptor complex for collagen type I recognizes the Arg-Gly-Asp sequence. *Journal of Cell Biology*, **104**, 585–93.

Doba, T., Burton, G. W. & Ingold, K. U. (1985) Antioxidant and co-antioxidant activity of vitamin C. The effect of vitamin C, either alone or in the presence of vitamin E or a water-soluble vitamin E analogue, upon the peroxidation of aqueous multilamellar phospholipid liposomes. *Biochimica et Biophysica Acta*, **835**, 298–303.

Eipper, B. A. & Mains, R. E. (1991) The role of ascorbate in the biosynthesis of neuroendocrine peptides. *American Journal of Clinical Nutrition*, **54**, 1153S–6S.

Eldridge, C. F., Bunge, M. B., Bunge, R. P. & Wood, P. M. (1987) Differentiation of axon-related Schwann cells in vitro. I. Ascorbic acid regulates basal lamina assembly and myelin formation. *Journal of Cell Biology*, **105**, 1023–34.

Eldridge, C. F., Bunge, M. B. & Bunge, R. P. (1989) Differentiation of axon-related Schwann cells *in vitro*. II. Control of myelin formation by basal lamina. *Journal of Neuroscience*, **9**, 625–38.

Ericsson, Y. & Lundbeck, H. (1955) Antimicrobial effect in vitro of the ascorbic acid oxidation. I. Effect on bacteria, fungi and viruses in pure cultures. *Acta Pathologica et Microbiologica Scandinavica*, **37**, 493–506.

Evans, R. M., Currie, L. & Campbell, A. (1982) The distribution of ascorbic acid between various cellular components of blood, in normal individuals, and its relation to the plasma concentration. *British Journal of Nutrition*, **47**, 473–82.

Fiddler, W., Pensabene, J. W., Piotrowski, E. G., Phillips, J. G., Keating, J., Mergens, W. J. & Newark, H. L. (1978) Inhibition of formation of volatile nitrosamines in fried bacon by the use of cure-solubilized α-tocopherol. *Journal of Agricultural and Food Chemistry*, **26**, 653–6.

Fraga, C. G., Motchnik, P. A., Shigenaga, M. K., Helbock, H. J., Jacob, R. A. & Ames, B. N. (1991) Ascorbic acid protects against endogenous oxidative DNA damage in human sperm. *Proceedings of the National Academy of Sciences of the U.S.A.*, **88**, 11 003–6.

Franceschi, R. T. (1992) The role of ascorbic acid in mesenchymal differentiation. *Nutrition Reviews*, **50**, 65–70.

Franceschi, R. T. & Iyer, B. S. (1992) Relationship between collagen synthesis and expression of the osteoblast phenotype in MC3T3-E1 cells. *Journal of Bone and Mineral Research*, **7**, 235–46.

Frei, B. (1991) Ascorbic acid protects lipids in human plasma and low-density lipoprotein against oxidative damage. *American Journal of Clinical Nutrition*, **54**, 1113S–18S.

Ganguly, R., Durieux, M.-F. & Waldman, R. H. (1976) Macrophage function in vitamin C-deficient guinea pigs. *American Journal of Clinical Nutrition*, **29**, 762–5.

Gerster, H. & Moser, U. (1988) Is high-dose vitamin C intake associated with systemic conditioning? *Nutrition Research*, **8**, 1327–32.

Ginter, E. (1973) Cholesterol: vitamin C controls its transformation to bile acids. *Science*, **179**, 702–4.

Ginter, E., Červeň, J., Nemec, R. & Mikuš, L. (1971) Lowered cholesterol catabolism in guinea pigs with chronic ascorbic acid deficiency. *American Journal of Clinical Nutrition*, **24**, 1238–45.

Gokce, N., Keaney, J. F. Jr., Frei, B., Holbrook, M., Olesiak, M., Zachariah, B. J., Leeuwenburgh, C., Heinecke, J. W. & Vita, J. A. (1999) Long-term ascorbic acid administration reverses endothelial vasomotor dysfunction in patients with coronary artery diseases. *Circulation*, 99, 3234–40.

Goldberg, A. (1963) The anaemia of scurvy. *Quarterly Journal of Medicine*, 32, 51–64.

Gordeuk, V. R., Bacon, B. R. & Brittenham, G. M. (1987) Iron overload: causes and consequences. *Annual Review of Nutrition*, 7, 485–508.

Hallberg, L. (1981) Bioavailability of dietary iron in man. *Annual Review of Nutrition*, 1, 123–47.

Hallberg, L., Brune, M. & Rossander, L. (1986) Effect of ascorbic acid on iron absorption from different types of meals. *Human Nutrition: Applied Nutrition*, 40A, 97–113.

Hallberg, L., Brune, M. & Rossander-Hulthén, L. (1987) Is there a physiological role of vitamin C in iron absorption? *Annals of the New York Academy of Sciences*, 498, 324–32.

Halliwell, B., Wasil, M. & Grootveld, M. (1987) Biologically significant scavenging of the myeloperoxidase-derived oxidant hypochlorous acid by ascorbic acid. Implications for antioxidant protection in the inflamed rheumatoid joint. *FEBS Letters*, 213, 15–17.

Hammarström, L. (1966) Autoradiographic studies on the distribution of C^{14}-labelled ascorbic acid and dehydroascorbic acid. *Acta Physiologica Scandinavica*, 70 (Supplementum 289), 1–84.

Harada, S., Matsumoto, T. & Ogata, E. (1991) Role of ascorbic acid in the regulation of proliferation in osteoblast-like MC3T3-E1 cells. *Journal of Bone and Mineral Research*, 6, 903–8.

Harats, D., Chevion, S., Nahir, M., Norman, Y., Sagee, O. & Berry, E. M. (1998) Citrus fruit supplementation reduces lipoprotein oxidation in young men ingesting a diet high in saturated fat: presumptive evidence for an interaction between vitamins C and E in vivo. *American Journal of Clinical Nutrition*, 67, 240–5.

Haskell, B. E. & Johnston, C. S. (1991) Complement component C1q activity and ascorbic acid nutriture in guinea pigs. *American Journal of Clinical Nutrition*, 54, 1228S–30S.

Heitzer, T., Just, H. & Münzel, T. (1996) Antioxidant vitamin C improves endothelial dysfunction in chronic smokers. *Circulation*, 94, 6–9.

Heller, R., Münscher-Paulig, F., Gräbner, R. & Till, U. (1999) L-Ascorbic acid potentiates nitric oxide synthesis in endothelial cells. *Journal of Biological Chemistry*, 274(12), 8254–60.

Hemilä, H. (1997) Vitamin C intake and susceptibility to the common cold. *British Journal of Nutrition*, 77, 59–72.

Herbert, V., Shaw, S. & Jayatilleke, E. (1996) Vitamin C-driven free radical generation from iron. *Journal of Nutrition*, 126, 1213S–20S.

Hitomi, K. & Tsukagoshi, N. (1996) Role of ascorbic acid in modulation of gene expression. In: *Subcellular Biochemistry, Vol. 25. Ascorbic Acid: Biochemistry and Biomedical Cell Biology*. (Ed. J. R. Harris), pp. 41–56. Plenum Press, New York.

Hodges, R. E., Hood, J., Canham, J. E., Sauberlich, H. E. & Baker, E. M. (1971) Clinical manifestations of ascorbic acid deficiency in man. *American Journal of Clinical Nutrition*, 24, 432–43.

Horio, F., Ozaki, K., Oda, H., Makino, S., Hayashi, Y. & Yoshida, A. (1989) Effect of dietary ascorbic acid, cholesterol and PCB on cholesterol and bile acid metabolism in a rat mutant unable to synthesize ascorbic acid. *Journal of Nutrition*, 119, 409–15.

Hornig, B., Arakawa, N., Kohler, C. & Drexler, H. (1998) Vitamin C improves endothelial function of conduit arteries in patients with chronic heart failure. *Circulation*, 97, 363–8.

Hornig, D., Vuilleumier, J.-P. & Hartmann, D. (1980) Absorption of large, single, oral intakes of ascorbic acid. *International Journal for Vitamin and Nutrition Research*, 50, 309–14.

Horovitz, O., Knaak, D., Podleski, T. R. & Salpeter, M. M. (1989) Acetylcholine receptor α-subunit mRNA is increased by ascorbic acid in cloned L5 muscle cells; Northern blot analysis and in situ hybridization. *Journal of Cell Biology*, 108, 1823–32.

Horrobin, D. F., Oka, M. & Manku, M. S. (1979) The regulation of prostaglandin E1 formation: a candidate for one of the fundamental mechanisms involved in the actions of vitamin C. *Medical Hypotheses*, 5, 849–58.

Huang, W., Yang, Z., Lee, D., Copolov, D. L. & Y Lim, A. T. (1993) Ascorbic acid enhances forskolin-induced cyclic AMP production and pro-ANF mRNA expression of hypothalamic neurons in culture. *Endocrinology*, 132, 2271–3.

Hurrell, R. F., Lynch, S. R., Trinidad, T. P., Dassenko, S. A. & Cook, J. D. (1988) Iron absorption in humans: bovine serum albumin compared with beef muscle and egg white. *American Journal of Clinical Nutrition*, 47, 102–7.

Hynes, R. O. (1992) Integrins: versatility, modulation, and signaling in cell adhesion. *Cell*, 69, 11–25.

Ibrahimi, A., Bonino, F., Bardon, S., Ailhaud, G. & Dani, C. (1992) Essential role of collagens for terminal differentiation of preadipocytes. *Biochemical and Biophysical Research Communications*, 187, 1314–22.

Ingermann, R. L., Stankova, L. & Bigley, R. H. (1986) Role of monosaccharide transporter in vitamin C uptake by placental membrane vesicles. *American Journal of Physiology*, 250, C637–41.

Institute of Medicine (2000) *Dietary Reference Intakes for Vitamin C, Vitamin E, Selenium, and Carotenoids*. National Academy Press, Washington, D.C.

Jacob, R. A. & Pianalto, F. S. (1997) Urinary carnitine excretion increases during experimental vitamin C depletion of healthy men. *Journal of Nutritional Biochemistry*, 8, 265–9.

Johnston, C. S. (1991) Complement component C1q unaltered by ascorbate supplementation in healthy men and women. *Journal of Nutritional Biochemistry*, 2, 499–501.

Johnston, C. S., Martin, L. J. & Cai, X. (1992) Antihistamine effect of supplemental ascorbic acid and neutrophil chemotaxis. *Journal of the American College of Nutrition*, 11, 172–6.

Johnston, C. S., Solomon, R. E. & Corte, C. (1996) Vitamin C depletion is associated with alterations in blood histamine and plasma free carnitine in adults. *Journal of the American College of Nutrition*, 15, 586–91.

Kallner, A., Hornig, D. & Pellikka, R. (1985) Formation of carbon dioxide from ascorbate in man. *American Journal of Clinical Nutrition*, 41, 609–13.

Kanani, P. M., Sinkey, C. A., Browning, R. L., Allaman, M., Knapp, H. R. & Haynes, W. G. (1999) Role of oxidant stress in endothelial dysfunction produced by experimental hyperhomocyst(e)inemia in humans. *Circulation*, 100, 1161–8.

Karasov, W. H., Darken, B. W. & Bottum, M. C. (1991) Dietary regulation of intestinal ascorbate uptake in guinea pigs. *American Journal of Physiology*, 260, G108–18.

Karpińska, T., Kawecki, Z. & Kandefer-Szerszeń, M. (1982) The influence of ultraviolet irradiation, L-ascorbic acid and calcium chloride on the induction of interferon in human embryo fibroblasts. *Archivum Immunologiae et Therapiae Experimentalis*, 30, 33–7.

Kinsman, R. A. & Hood, J. (1971) Some behavioral effects of ascorbic acid deficiency. *American Journal of Clinical Nutrition*, 24, 455–64.

Knaak, D., Shen, I., Salpeter, M. M. & Podleski, T. R. (1986) Selective effects of ascorbic acid on acetylcholine receptor number and distribution. *Journal of Cell Biology*, 102, 795–802.

Kübler, W. & Gehler, J. (1970) On the kinetics of the intestinal absorption of ascorbic acid: a contribution to the calculation of an absorption process that is not proportional to the dose.

International Journal for Vitamin and Nutrition Research, **40**, 442–53. (In German)

Kuo, C.-H., Hata, F., Yoshida, H., Yamatodani, A. & Wada, H. (1979) Effect of ascorbic acid on release of acetylcholine from synaptic vesicles prepared from different species of animals and release of noradrenaline from synaptic vesicles of rat brain. *Life Sciences*, **24**, 911–16.

Leboy, P. S., Vaias, L., Uschmann, B., Golub, E., Adams, S. L. & Pacifici, M. (1989) Ascorbic acid induces alkaline phosphatase, type X collagen, and calcium deposition in cultured chick chondrocytes. *Journal of Biological Chemistry*, **264**(29), 17 281–6.

Leichtweiss, H.-P., Lisbôa, B. & Steinborn, C. (1987) Uptake of ascorbic acid and its oxidized products in the isolated guinea pig placenta. *Trophoblast Research*, **2**, 501–14.

Levine, G. N., Frei, B., Koulouris, S. N., Gerhard, M. D., Keaney, J. F. Jr. & Vita, J. A. (1996) Ascorbic acid reverses endothelial vasomotor dysfunction in patients with coronary artery disease. *Circulation*, **93**, 1107–13.

Lunec, J. & Blake, D. R. (1985) The determination of dehydroascorbic acid and ascorbic acid in the serum and synovial fluid of patients with rheumatoid arthritis. *Free Radical Research Communications*, **1**, 31–9.

Lynch, S. M., Gaziano, J. M. & Frei, B. (1996) Ascorbic acid and atherosclerotic cardiovascular disease. In: *Subcellular Biochemistry, Vol. 25. Ascorbic Acid: Biochemistry and Biomedical Cell Biology*. (Ed. J. R. Harris), pp. 331–67. Plenum Press, New York.

McCall, C. E., DeChatelet, L. R., Cooper, M. R. & Ashburn, P. (1971) The effects of ascorbic acid on bactericidal mechanisms of neutrophils. *Journal of Infectious Diseases*, **124**, 194–8.

McGee, M. P. & Myrvik, Q. N. (1979) Phagocytosis-induced injury of normal and activated alveolar macrophages. *Infection and Immunity*, **26**, 910–15.

Mangels, A. R., Block, G., Frey, C. M., Patterson, B. H., Taylor, P. R., Norkus, E. P. & Levander, O. A. (1993) The bioavailability to humans of ascorbic acid from oranges, orange juice and cooked broccoli is similar to that of synthetic ascorbic acid. *Journal of Nutrition*, **123**, 1054–61.

Manku, M. S., Oka, M. & Horrobin, D. F. (1979) Differential regulation of the formation of prostaglandins and related substances from arachidonic acid and from dihomogammalinolenic acid. II. Effects of vitamin C. *Prostaglandins and Medicine*, **3**, 129–37.

Mellors, A. J., Nahrwold, D. L. & Rose, R. C. (1977) Ascorbic acid flux across mucosal border of guinea pig and human ileum. *American Journal of Physiology*, **233**, E374–9.

Menniti, F. S., Knoth, J. & Diliberto, E. J. Jr. (1986) Role of ascorbic acid in dopamine β-hydroxylation. *Journal of Biological Chemistry*, **261**(36), 16 901–8.

Miller, T. E. (1969) Killing and lysis of gram-negative bacteria through the synergistic effect of hydrogen peroxide, ascorbic acid, and lysozyme. *Journal of Bacteriology*, **98**, 949–55.

Miller, B. T. & Cicero, T. J. (1986) Ascorbic acid enhances the release of luteinizing hormone-releasing hormone from the mediobasal hypothalamus *in vitro*. *Life Sciences*, **39**, 2447–54.

Mirvish, S. S. (1983) The etiology of gastric cancer: intragastric nitrosamide formation and other theories. *Journal of the National Cancer Institute*, **71**, 629–47.

Mirvish, S. S. (1994) Experimental evidence for inhibition of *N*-nitroso compound formation as a factor in the negative correlation between vitamin C consumption and the incidence of certain cancers. *Cancer Research*, **54**, 1948s–51s.

Mirvish, S. S. (1996) Inhibition by vitamins C and E of *in vivo* nitrosation and vitamin C occurrence in the stomach. *European Journal of Cancer Prevention*, **5** (Supplement 1), 131–6.

Mirvish, S. S., Grandjean, A. C., Reimers, K. J., Connelly, B. J., Chen, S. C., Morris, C. R., Wang, X., Haorah, J. & Lyden, E. R. (1998)

Effect of ascorbic acid dose taken with a meal on nitrosoproline excretion in subjects ingesting nitrate and proline. *Nutrition and Cancer*, **31**, 106–10.

Mitsumoto, Y., Liu, Z. & Klip, A. (1994) A long-lasting vitamin C derivative, ascorbic acid 2-phosphate, increases myogenin gene expression and promotes differentiation in L6 muscle cells. *Biochemical and Biophysical Research Communications*, **199**, 394–402.

Monsen, E. R. (1988) Iron nutrition and absorption: dietary factors which impact iron bioavailability. *Journal of the American Dietetic Association*, **88**, 786–90.

Mosca, L., Rubenfire, M., Mandel. C., Rock, C., Tarshis, T., Tsai, A. & Pearson, T. (1997) Antioxidant nutrient supplementation reduces the susceptibility of low density lipoprotein to oxidation in patients with coronary artery disease. *Journal of the American College of Cardiology*, **30**, 392–9.

Moser, U. (1987) Uptake of ascorbic acid by leukocytes. *Annals of the New York Academy of Sciences*, **498**, 200–15.

Muggli, R. (1993) Vitamin C and phagocytes. In: *Nutrient Modulation of the Immune Response*. (Ed. S. Cunningham-Rundles), pp. 75–90. Marcel Dekker, Inc., New York.

Nandan, D., Clarke, E. P., Ball, E. H. & Sanwal, B. D. (1990) Ethyl-3,4-dihydroxybenzoate inhibits myoblast differentiation: evidence for an essential role of collagen. *Journal of Cell Biology*, **110**, 1673–9.

Oberritter, H., Glatthaar, B., Moser, U. & Schmidt, K. H. (1986) Effect of functional stimulation on ascorbate content in phagocytes under physiological and pathological conditions. *International Archives of Allergy and Applied Immunology*, **81**, 46–50.

Oh, C. & Nakano, K. (1988) Reversal by ascorbic acid of suppression by endogenous histamine of rat lymphocyte blastogenesis. *Journal of Nutrition*, **118**, 639–44.

Omaye, S. T., Schaus, E. E., Kutnink, M. A. & Hawkes, W. C. (1987) Measurement of vitamin C in blood components by high-performance liquid chromatography. Implication in assessing vitamin C status. *Annals of the New York Academy of Sciences*, **498**, 389–401.

Owen, T. A., Aronow, M., Shalhoub, V., Barone, L. M., Wilming, L., Tassinari, M. S., Kennedy, M. B., Pockwinse, S., Lian, J. B. & Stein, G. S. (1990) Progressive development of the rat osteoblast phenotype in vitro: reciprocal relationships in expression of genes associated with osteoblast proliferation and differentiation during the formation of the bone extracellular matrix. *Journal of Cellular Physiology*, **143**, 420–30.

Patterson, L. T., Nahrwold, D. L. & Rose, R. C. (1982) Ascorbic acid uptake in guinea pig intestinal mucosa. *Life Sciences*, **31**, 2783–91.

Pelletier, O. & Godin, C. (1969) Vitamin C activity of D-isoascorbic acid for the guinea pig. *Canadian Journal of Physiology and Pharmacology*, **47**, 985–91.

Prasad, P. D., Huang, W., Wang, H., Leibach, F. H. & Ganapathy, V. (1998) Transport mechanisms for vitamin C in the JAR human placental choriocarcinoma cell line. *Biochimica et Biophysica Acta*, **1369**, 141–51.

Priest, R. E. (1970) Formation of epithelial basement membrane is restricted by scurvy *in vitro* and is stimulated by vitamin C. *Nature*, **225**, 744–5.

Prockop, D. J., Kivirikko, K. I., Tuderman, L. & Guzman, N. A. (1979) The biosynthesis of collagen and its disorders. *New England Journal of Medicine*, **301**, 13–23.

Quarles, L. D., Yohay, D. A., Lever, L. W., Caton, R. & Wenstrup, R. J. (1992) Distinct proliferative and differentiated stages of murine MC3T3-E1 cells in culture: an in vitro model of osteoblast development. *Journal of Bone and Mineral Research*, **7**, 683–92.

Rajan, D. P., Huang, W., Dutta, B., Devoe, L. D., Leibach, F. H.,

Ganapathy, V. & Prasad, P. D. (1999) Human placental sodium-dependent vitamin C transporter (SVCT2): molecular cloning and transport function. *Biochemical and Biophysical Research Communications*, **262**, 762–8.

Ramirez, J. & Flowers, N. C. (1980) Leukocyte ascorbic acid and its relationship to coronary heart disease in man. *American Journal of Clinical Nutrition*, **33**, 2079–87.

Rebec, G. V. & Pierce, R. C. (1994) A vitamin as neuromodulator: ascorbate release into the extracellular fluid of the brain regulates dopaminergic and glutamatergic transmission. *Progress in Neurobiology*, **43**, 537–65.

Rebouche, C. J. (1988) Carnitine metabolism and human nutrition. *Journal of Applied Nutrition*, **40**, 99–111.

Rebouche, C. J. (1991) Ascorbic acid and carnitine biosynthesis. *American Journal of Clinical Nutrition*, **54**, 1147S–52S.

Rebouche, C. J. (1995a) The ability of guinea pigs to synthesize carnitine at a normal rate from ε-*N*-trimethyllysine or γ-butyrobetaine in vivo is not compromised by experimental vitamin C deficiency. *Metabolism, Clinical and Experimental*, **44**, 624–9.

Rebouche, C. J. (1995b) Renal handling of carnitine in experimental vitamin C deficiency. *Metabolism, Clinical and Experimental*, **44**, 1639–43.

Retsky, K. L. & Frei, B. (1995) Vitamin C prevents metal ion-dependent initiation and propagation of lipid peroxidation in human low-density lipoprotein. *Biochimica et Biophysica Acta*, **1257**, 279–87.

Rifici, V. A. & Khachadurian, A. K. (1993) Dietary supplementation with vitamins C and E inhibits in vitro oxidation of lipoproteins. *Journal of the American College of Nutrition*, **12**, 631–7.

Rose, R. C. (1986) Ascorbic acid transport in mammalian kidney. *American Journal of Physiology*, **250**, F627–32.

Rose, R. C. (1989) Renal metabolism of the oxidized form of ascorbic acid (dehydro-L-ascorbic acid). *American Journal of Physiology*, **256**, F52–6.

Rose, R. C., Choi, J.-L. & Koch, M. J. (1988) Intestinal transport and metabolism of oxidized ascorbic acid (dehydroascorbic acid). *American Journal of Physiology*, **254**, G824–8.

Rumsey, S. C. & Levine, M. (1998) Absorption, transport, and disposition of ascorbic acid in humans. *Journal of Nutritional Biochemistry*, **9**, 116–30.

Rumsey, S. C., Kwon, O., Xu, G. W., Burant, C. F., Simpson, I. & Levine, M. (1997) Glucose transporter isoforms GLUT1 and GLUT3 transport dehydroascorbic acid. *Journal of Biological Chemistry*, **272**(30), 18 982–9.

Rybakowski, C., Mohar, B., Wohlers, S., Leichtweiss, H.-P. & Schröder, H. (1995) The transport of vitamin C in the isolated near-term placenta. *European Journal of Obstetrics & Gynecology and Reproductive Biology*, **62**, 107–14.

Sacharin, R., Taylor, T. & Chasseaud, L. F. (1976) Blood levels and bioavailability of ascorbic acid after administration of a sustained-release formulation to humans. *International Journal for Vitamin and Nutrition Research*, **47**, 68–74.

Sakuma, N., Yoshikawa, M., Hibino, T., Sato, T., Kamiya, Y., Ohte, N., Tamai, N., Kunimatsu, M., Kimura, G. & Inoue, M. (2001) Ascorbic acid protects against peroxidative modification of low-density lipoprotein, maintaining its recognition by LDL receptors. *Journal of Nutritional Science and Vitaminology*, **47**, 28–31.

Sauberlich, H. E. (1994) Pharmacology of vitamin C. *Annual Review of Nutrition*, **14**, 371–91.

Scanlan, R. A. (1983) Formation and occurrence of nitrosamines in food. *Cancer Research* (Supplement), **43**, 2435s–40s.

Schmidt, K. & Moser, U. (1985) Vitamin C – a modulator of host defense mechanisms. *International Journal for Vitamin and Nutrition Research*, Supplement No. 27, 363–79.

Schrauzer, G. N. & Rhead, W. J. (1973) Ascorbic acid abuse: effects

of long term ingestion of excessive amounts on blood levels and urinary excretion. *International Journal for Vitamin and Nutrition Research*, **43**, 201–11.

Schwarz, R. I., Kleinman, P. & Owens, N. (1987) Ascorbate can act as an inducer of the collagen pathway because most steps are tightly coupled. *Annals of the New York Academy of Sciences*, **498**, 172–85.

Shilotri, P. G. (1977) Glycolytic, hexose monophosphate shunt and bactericidal activities of leukocytes in ascorbic acid deficient guinea pigs. *Journal of Nutrition*, **107**, 1507–12.

Siegel, B. V. (1974) Enhanced interferon response to murine leukemia virus by ascorbic acid. *Infection and Immunity*, **10**, 409–10.

Siegel, C., Barker, B. & Kunstadter, M. (1982) Conditioned oral scurvy due to megavitamin C withdrawal. *Journal of Periodontology*, **53**, 453–5.

Sies, H. & Stahl, W. (1995) Vitamins E and C, β-carotene, and other carotenoids as antioxidants. *American Journal of Clinical Nutrition*, **62**, 1315S–21S.

Siliprandi, L., Vanni, P., Kessler, M. & Semenza, G. (1979) Na⁺-dependent, electroneutral L-ascorbate transport across brush border membrane vesicles from guinea pig small intestine. *Biochimica et Biophysica Acta*, **552**, 129–42.

Solzbach, U., Hornig, B., Jeserich, M. & Just, H. (1997) Vitamin C improves endothelial dysfunction of epicardial coronary arteries in hypertensive patients. *Circulation*, **96**, 1513–19.

Sorensen, D. I., Devine, M. M. & Rivers, J. M. (1974) Catabolism and tissue levels of ascorbic acid following long-term massive doses in the guinea pig. *Journal of Nutrition*, **104**, 1041–8.

Spector, R. (1977) Vitamin homeostasis in the central nervous system. *New England Journal of Medicine*, **296**, 1393–8.

Sullivan, T. A., Uschmann, B., Hough, R. & Leboy, P. S. (1994) Ascorbate modulation of chondrocyte gene expression is independent of its role in collagen secretion. *Journal of Biological Chemistry*, **269**(36), 22 500–6.

Tannenbaum, S. R. & Wishnok, J. S. (1987) Inhibition of nitrosamine formation by ascorbic acid. *Annals of the New York Academy of Sciences*, **498**, 354–63.

Taylor, P. G., Martínez-Torres, C., Romano, E. L. & Layrisse, M. (1986) The effect of cysteine-containing peptides released during meat digestion on iron absorption in humans. *American Journal of Clinical Nutrition*, **43**, 68–71.

Ting, H. H., Timimi, F. K., Boles, K. S., Creager, S. J., Ganz, P. & Creager, M. A. (1996) Vitamin C improves endothelium-dependent vasodilation in patients with non-insulin-dependent diabetes mellitus. *Journal of Clinical Investigation*, **97**, 22–8.

Ting, H. H., Timimi, F. K., Haley, E. A., Roddy, M.-A., Ganz, P. & Creager, M. A. (1997) Vitamin C improves endothelium-dependent vasodilation in forearm resistance vessels of humans with hypercholesterolemia. *Circulation*, **95**, 2617–22.

Toggenburger, G., Häusermann, M., Mütsch, B., Genoni, G., Kessler, M., Weber, F., Hornig, D., O'Neill, B. & Semenza, G. (1981) Na⁺-dependent, potential-sensitive L-ascorbate transport across brush border membrane vesicles from kidney cortex. *Biochimica et Biophysica Acta*, **646**, 433–43.

Tsukaguchi, H., Tokui, T., Mackenzie, B., Berger, U. V., Chen, X.-Z., Wang, Y., Brubaker, R. F. & Hediger, M. A. (1999) A family of mammalian Na⁺-dependent L-ascorbic acid transporters. *Nature*, **399**, 70–75.

Uchida, K., Mitsui, M. & Kawakishi, S. (1989) Monooxygenation of *N*-acetylhistamine mediated by L-ascorbic acid. *Biochimica et Biophysica Acta*, **991**, 377–9.

Uchida, K., Nomura, Y., Takase, H., Tasaki, T., Seo, S., Hayashi, Y. & Takeuchi, N. (1990) Effect of vitamin C depletion on serum cholesterol and lipoprotein levels in ODS (*od/od*) rats unable to synthesize ascorbic acid. *Journal of Nutrition*, **120**, 1140–7.

Vera, J. C., Rivas, C. I., Velásquez, F. V., Zhang, R. H., Concha, I. I. & Golde, D. W. (1995) Resolution of the facilitated transport of dehydroascorbic acid from its intracellular accumulation as ascorbic acid. *Journal of Biological Chemistry*, **270**(40), 23 706–12.

Vojdani, A. & Ghoneum, M. (1993) In vivo effect of ascorbic acid on enhancement of human natural killer cell activity. *Nutrition Research*, **13**, 753–64.

Wang, H., Dutta, B., Huang, W., Sevoe, L. D., Leibach, F. H., Ganapathy, V. & Prasad, P. P. (1999) Human Na$^+$-dependent vitamin C transporter 1 (hSVCT1): primary structure, functional characteristics and evidence for a non-functional splice variant. *Biochimica et Biophysica Acta*, **1461**, 1–9.

Washko, P. W., Wang, Y. & Levine, M. (1993) Ascorbic acid recycling in human neutrophils. *Journal of Biological Chemistry*, **268**(21), 15 531–5.

Weiss, S. J. (1989) Tissue destruction by neutrophils. *New England Journal of Medicine*, **320**, 365–76.

Welch, R. W., Wang, Y., Crossman, A. Jr., Park, J. B., Kirk, K. L. & Levine, M. (1995) Accumulation of vitamin C (ascorbate) and its oxidized metabolite dehydroascorbic acid occurs by separate mechanisms. *Journal of Biological Chemistry*, **270**(21), 12 584–92.

Wilson, J. X. (1989) Ascorbic acid uptake by a high-affinity sodium-dependent mechanism in cultured astrocytes. *Journal of Neurochemistry*, **53**, 1064–71.

Wilson, J. X. & Dixon, S. J. (1989) High-affinity sodium-dependent uptake of ascorbic acid by rat osteoblasts. *Journal of Membrane Biology*, **111**, 83–91.

Wilson, J. X., Jaworski, E. M. & Dixon, S. J. (1991) Evidence for electrogenic sodium-dependent ascorbate transport in rat astroglia. *Neurochemical Research*, **16**, 73–8.

Yung, S., Mayersohn, M. & Robinson, J. B. (1981) Ascorbic acid absorption in man: influence of divided dose and food. *Life Sciences*, **28**, 2505–11.

Abbreviations

ACTH	adrenocorticotrophic hormone	EAR	Estimated Average Requirement
ACTR	activator of nuclear receptors	EDTA	ethylenediaminetetraacetic acid
AF-1 and AF-2	activation function 1/2 (formerly called TAF-1/2)	EGF-R	epidermal growth factor receptor
		ELAM-1	endothelial leucocyte adhesion molecule-1 (= E-selectin)
AP-1/2	activator protein-1/2		
AR	androgen receptor	ER	(o)estrogen receptor
ARAT	acyl coenzyme A:retinol acyltransferase	ERA-1	early retinoic acid-1
		E-selectin	see ELAM-1
ARP-1	apoAI regulatory protein-1 (a homologue of COUP-TF II)	FBP	folate-binding protein
		FMLP	f-Met-Leu-Phe (a chemotactic peptide)
ATF-1	activating transcription factor-1		
cyclic AMP	3′,5′-cyclic adenosine monophosphate (cAMP)	FXR	farnesoid X-activated receptor
		GABA	γ-aminobutyric acid
cyclic GMP	3′,5′-cyclic guanosine monophosphate (cGMP)	Gla	γ-carboxyglutamate
		Glu	glutamate
CBP	CREB-binding protein	GR	glucocorticoid receptor
CD	cluster of differentiation (e.g. CD4 and CD8 molecules)	GRE	glucocorticoid receptor response element
cDNA	complementary DNA	GRIP-1	glucocorticoid receptor-interacting protein
CoA	coenzyme A		
CoQ	coenzyme Q (ubiquinone)	HAT	histone acetyltransferase
CoR box	co-repressor box	HDAC	histone deacetylase
COUP-TF	chicken ovalbumin upstream promoter transcription factor	HDL	high-density lipoprotein
		HNF-4	hepatic nuclear factor-4 (an orphan nuclear receptor)
CRABP	cellular retinoic acid-binding protein		
		hox gene	homeobox gene
CRBP	cellular retinol-binding protein	HRPE	human retinal pigment epithelium
CRE	cyclic AMP response element	ICAM-1	intracellular adhesion molecule-1
CREB	cyclic AMP response element-binding protein	IDL	intermediate-density lipoprotein
		IFN	interferon (e.g. IFN-γ)
CSF	cerebrospinal fluid	Ig	immunoglobulin
Da	Dalton – a unit of molecular weight	IGF-I	insulin-like growth factor-I
DBP	vitamin D-binding protein	IL	interleukin (e.g. IL-1β)
DIDS	4.4′-diisothiocyanostilbene-2,2′-disulphonic acid	Inr	initiator
		IU	international unit
DPPD	N,N^1-diphenyl-p-phenylenediamine	kDa	kiloDalton (Da $\times$ 10^3)
DRIP	vitamin D$_3$ receptor interacting protein	LDL	low-density lipoprotein

LFA-1	leucocyte function associated antigen-1
LPS	lipopolysaccharide
LRAT	lecithin:retinol acyltransferase
LXR	an orphan nuclear receptor initially isolated from liver
MAC-1	$\alpha M\beta$-2 integrin
MCP-1	monocyte chemotactic protein-1
M-CSF	macrophage-colony stimulating factor
MGP	matrix Gla protein
MHC	major histocompatibility complex
MR	mineralocorticoid receptor
mRNA	messenger RNA
NAC	*N*-acetyl-L-cysteine
NCoA-62	nuclear receptor coactivator 62 kDa
N-CoR	nuclear receptor co-repressor
NF-1	nuclear factor 1
NFAT	nuclear factor of activated T cells
NF-κB	nuclear factor-κB
NGFI-B	nerve growth factor I-B (an orphan nuclear receptor; also termed nur77)
nurr-1	nur-related factor 1 (an orphan nuclear receptor)
OC box	osteocalcin box
PCAF	p300/CBP associating factor
PDGF	platelet-derived growth factor
Pit-1	pituitary-specific transcription factor
PKA	protein kinase A
PKC	protein kinase C
PMA	phorbol 12-myristate 13-acetate
PPAR	peroxisome proliferator-activated receptor
PR	progesterone receptor
PTH	parathyroid hormone
PUFA	polyunsaturated fatty acid
RAC3	receptor-associated coactivator 3
RAR	retinoic acid receptor
RARE	retinoic acid response element
RBP	retinol-binding protein
RCP	riboflavin carrier protein
RDA	Recommended Dietary Allowance
RXR	retinoid X receptor
RXRE	retinoid X response element
SAGA	Spt-Ada-Gcn5-acetyltransferase
SMRT	silencing mediator for retinoic acid receptor and thyroid hormone receptor
SMVT	sodium-dependent multivitamin transporter
Snf	transcription factor (sucrose non-fermenting)
Srb proteins	suppressor of RNA polymerase B regulatory proteins
SRC-1	steroid receptor coactivator-1
Swi	transcription factor (switching mating type)
TAF	TBP-associated factor
TBP	TATA box-binding protein
TCA cycle	tricarboxylic acid cycle
TGF-α/β	transforming growth factor-α/β
TIF-1	transcriptional intermediary factor-1
TNF-α/β	tumour necrosis factor-α/β
TPA	12-*O*-tetradecanoylphorbol-13-acetate
TR	thyroid hormone receptor
TRAC	thyroid hormone receptor- and retinoic acid receptor-associated co-repressors
TRAP	thyroid hormone receptor associated protein
TRE	thyroid hormone response element
TRL	triglyceride-rich lipoprotein
VCAM-1	vascular cell adhesion molecule-1
VDR	vitamin D receptor
VDRE	vitamin D response element
VLA-4	very late antigen-4
VLDL	very-low-density lipoprotein
YY1	Yin Yang-1 (identical to nuclear matrix protein-1, NMP-1)

Glossary

actinomycin D: An inhibitor of **transcription** (mRNA synthesis). Inhibits RNA polymerase.

activator: *Genetics*. A protein that binds to an **enhancer** element on the DNA and stimulates the basal level of **transcription**.

adjuvant: *Immunology*. A vehicle used to enhance antigenicity.

alleles: Two or more alternate forms of a gene that occupy the same site (locus) on homologous chromosomes.

allograft: A graft transplanted between genetically non-identical individuals of the same species.

allosteric enzyme: An enzyme whose activity can be regulated. Binding of an **activator** to an allosteric site changes the three-dimensional conformation of the enzyme, thereby allowing the catalytic site to bind the intended substrate.

alopecia: Hair loss.

amenorrhoea: Absence or abnormal cessation of menstruation.

amphipathic (amphiphilic): Describes a molecule containing both hydrophilic and hydrophobic regions.

ampholyte: A substance that can ionize to form either an anion or a cation and thus may act as either an acid or a base.

angina: Usually refers to angina pectoris, a severe constricting pain in the chest due to **ischaemia** of the heart muscle.

angiography: Radiography of blood vessels after the injection of a radiopaque contrast material.

angiospasm: See **vasospasm**.

anorexia: Diminished appetite; aversion to food.

antibody: An immunoglobulin capable of binding with a specific **antigen** through its antigen-binding sites.

antigen: Any material that is recognized as foreign by the acquired immune system.

antioxidant: *Biochemistry*. A dietary antioxidant is a substance in food that significantly decreases the adverse effects of reactive oxygen/nitrogen species on biochemical functions.

apoenzyme: The protein portion of an enzyme; an enzyme with its **coenzyme** or **prosthetic group** removed.

apoptosis: Programmed cell death characterized by DNA fragmentation. It plays a key role in the development and regulation of many tissues.

ataxia: A nervous disorder characterized by a staggering gait.

atony: Lack of tone or tension; relaxation, flaccidity. *See also* **gastric atony**.

autocrine: Situations in which hormones act on the very same cell from which they were secreted. *See also* **endocrine**, **paracrine**.

autoimmunity: An immune response to 'self' tissues or components. Such an immune response may have pathological consequences leading to autoimmune diseases.

autosomal: If a gene is described as autosomal, the cell contains two copies of that gene – one maternally derived and the other paternally derived.

blebbing: Release of microvesicles by a cell.

cardiocyte: Heart muscle cell.

catecholamines: The catecholamines of biochemical interest are noradrenaline, adrenaline and dopamine.

caveolae: Invaginations in the plasma membrane, which are involved in **potocytosis**.

cell cycle: The life cycle of a cell is the period from cell reproduction (**mitosis**) to the next reproduction.

chemokinesis: Stimulated random motility of cells.

chemotaxis: The directed migration of cells up a concentration gradient of a chemotactic molecule.

cholestasis: An arrest in the flow of bile due to obstruction of the bile ducts.

chondrocyte: A non-dividing cartilage cell.

cirrhosis: Endstage liver disease resulting ultimately in biochemical and functional signs of liver failure. In Laënnec cirrhosis, normal liver lobules are replaced by small regeneration nodules, sometimes containing fat, separated by a framework of fine fibrous tissue strands. This 'hob-nail liver' is usually due to chronic alcoholism.

cis-**acting elements:** *Genetics.* Regulatory elements comprising DNA sequences which are located on the same DNA molecule as the gene whose expression is being regulated. *See also* ***trans*-acting factors**.

cisternae of endoplasmic reticulum: The tubular elements of the **endoplasmic reticulum**.

coactivator: *Genetics.* A protein which is required for activated transcription, i.e. **transcription** above the basal rate. Coactivators form a molecular bridge linking a distal DNA-bound **activator** to the **general transcription machinery**.

codon: A triplet of nucleotide bases in a messenger RNA molecule that codes for a specific amino acid or for polypeptide chain termination during protein synthesis.

coenzyme: An organic non-protein molecule, frequently a derivative of a B-group vitamin, that binds with a protein molecule (**apoenzyme**) to form an active enzyme (which is then known as a **holoenzyme**).

cofactor: A substance such as a **coenzyme** or a metal ion with which an enzyme must unite in order to become catalytically active.

combinatorial control: *Genetics.* A regulatory phenomenon in which a gene is turned on by combinations of **activators** or multiple molecules of a particular activator.

constitutive expression: *Genetics.* Expression as a function of the interaction of RNA polymerase with the **promoter**, without additional regulation.

co-repressor: *Genetics.* A protein that bridges the **repressor** to the histone deacetylase.

cyanosis: A condition in which the skin appears blue due to insufficient oxygenation of the blood.

cycloheximide: An inhibitor of **translation** (polypeptide synthesis).

cytokines: Short-acting signalling molecules which affect cellular function.

cytokinesis: Division of the **cytoplasm** cell, after division of the nucleus, to form two daughter cells.

cytoplasm: The cellular region within the plasma membrane, including the cytosol and the **organelles**, but excluding the nucleus. *See also* **cytosol**.

cytosol: The clear fluid portion of the cytoplasm. It contains mainly dissolved proteins, electrolytes, glucose and minute quantities of lipid compounds. It also includes cytoskeletal fibres and small particles such as ribosomes, but excludes the membrane-enclosed **organelles**. *See also* **cytoplasm**.

dexamethasone: A synthetic glucocorticoid analogue.

diastereoisomers: In molecules that contain more than one asymmetric carbon atom, any two stereoisomers that constitute an enantiomeric pair (mirror image isomers) will be stereoisomeric with, but not mirror images of, the remaining stereoisomers. They are related to the remaining stereoisomers as diastereoisomers.

diuresis: Excretion in urine.

dysarthria: Incoordination of the muscles used for speaking.

dysmorphogenesis: The process of abnormal tissue formation.

dyspnoea: The sensation of breathlessness and respiratory distress which occurs if the airways are obstructed.

EAR-2: A nuclear receptor closely related to COUP-TF.

electrophoresis: A separation technique in which charged particles in solution migrate in an electric field gradient.

enantiomer: One of a pair of mirror image optical isomers. They are designated according to the configuration of the molecule, the D isomer standing for dextro (right-hand) and the L isomer for levo (left-hand). Enantiomers, by virtue of their asymmetric carbon atoms, have the ability to rotate a plane of polarized light in a clockwise or anticlockwise direction. The D and L designations do not indicate the actual rotation; the latter is represented by the symbols + (clockwise direction) and − (anticlockwise direction).

endocrine: Situations in which hormones act at sites distant from their tissues of origin, generally being carried in the blood to reach their target tissues. *See also* **autocrine**, **paracrine**.

endocytosis: A collective term for the variety of different mechanisms by which mammalian cells take up extracellular particles or specific macromolecules by trapping them within inward foldings of the cell membrane that pinch off from the surface to form intracellular **vesicles**. These mechanisms are dependent on ATP as a source of energy.

endoplasmic reticulum: A cytoplasmic **organelle** consisting of a network of membranes, vesicles and tubules.

endorphins: Peptides produced by the pituitary gland and the brain that have pain-killing properties and are thought to regulate emotional responses.

endosome: A cytoplasmic **vesicle** formed from endocytic vesicles that have shed their clathrin coats.

endothelin: A vasoconstrictor peptide with **mitogenic** properties that is important in the regulation of vascular tone.

enhancer: *Genetics*. A DNA sequence that is a binding site for a transcriptional **activator**.

enterohepatic circulation (cycle): Reabsorption by the small intestine of nutrients excreted in bile.

epimer: An epimer of a particular compound differs in the configuration at a single asymmetric carbon atom.

epitope: *Immunology*. Characteristic, three-dimensional chemical group on the surface of a microorganism or foreign body that serves as a recognition site in an acquired immune response.

erythema: Increased redness of the skin that is caused by capillary dilatation.

erythroid: Reddish in colour.

eukaryotes: Organisms above the primitive prokaryotic level that contain a true nucleus enclosed within a membrane.

exocrine: Denoting a glandular secretion delivered to an apical or luminal surface via a secretory duct.

exocytosis: The reverse sequence of **endocytosis**. A membranous intracellular **vesicle** fuses with the plasma membrane and creates an opening through which the packaged substance is discharged into the extracellular space. Exocytosis is dependent on ATP as a source of energy.

extravasate: To exude from or pass out of a vessel into the tissues.

fenestration: Circular opening.

fibroblasts: Spindle-shaped cells present in areolar (loose) connective tissue.

forskolin: an activator of the adenylyl cyclase–cyclic AMP signalling pathway.

free energy: Energy that is available to do work.

gastric atony: Lack of tone in the smooth muscle of the stomach and intestine.

gene expression: The conversion of genetic information encoded within chromosomal DNA into a protein molecule.

general transcription machinery: The general transcription factors and associated proteins that assemble at the DNA **promoter** to form the pre-initiation complex.

genetic code: The set of 64 triplets of bases (**codons**) corresponding to the 20 amino acids in proteins and the signals for initiation and termination of polypeptide synthesis.

genome: The total genetic information stored in the chromosomes.

genotype: A description of the genetic composition of an organism.

germ cell: A cell that gives rise to reproductive cells (ova or spermatozoa).

gingivitis: Inflammation of the gums.

glycocalyx: A loose carbohydrate coat covering the entire surface of cells.

Golgi apparatus: A cellular **organelle** involved in intracellular transport.

haemopoietic: Blood-forming.

haemostasis: Prevention of blood loss.

heat shock proteins: These proteins are produced by the body in response to many environmental stresses including temperature changes, inflammation, fever and viral infections.

holoenzyme: The entire enzyme (**apoenzyme** plus **coenzyme** or **prosthetic group**).

housekeeping genes: Genes that are expressed at a basal level of transcription in all tissues. The gene products are assumed to be involved in key steps in cellular metabolism.

humoral: Pertaining to the extracellular fluids, including the serum and lymph.

hydropic: Containing an excess of water or of watery fluid.

hypercalciuria: Excretion of abnormally large amounts of calcium in the urine.

hyperplasia: Increase in the total number of cells.

hypertonia: Extreme tension of the muscles or arteries.

hypochlorohydria: Insufficient production of hydrochloric acid in the stomach.

hypophysectomy: Surgical removal of the pituitary gland.

hypotonia: Reduced tension of the muscles or arteries.

idiopathic: Denoting a disease of unknown origin.

inanition: State of lack of nourishment.

insulin: The internal secretion from the pancreas. It enables the muscles and other tissues to take up sugar from the blood, sugar being required for their activity. When insulin is deficient, as in diabetes mellitus, the sugar derived from the diet accumulates in the blood and is wastefully excreted in the urine.

ischaemia: Inadequate blood flow and thus oxygen supply due mainly to arterial narrowing.

jaundice: Yellowing of the skin indicating excess bilirubin (a bile pigment) in the blood.

keratosis: A benign horny **lesion**.

kwashiorkor: Severe protein deficiency.

lesion: A pathological alteration in the structure or function of a tissue or organ.

ligand: The molecule that binds to a specific receptor.

liposome: An artificial biological membrane.

lysis: Destruction of cells by disintegration of their plasma membrane; e.g. haemolysis is lysis of red blood cells.

lysosome: Cellular **organelle** consisting of a unit membrane enclosing a matrix containing about 40 hydrolytic enzymes.

macrolide: A class of antibiotics which inhibit protein synthesis.

meiosis: Reduction division resulting in **germ cells** containing half the number of chromosomes found in somatic (non-germ) cells.

meningitis: Inflammation of the membranes of the brain or spinal cord.

mesenchymal cells: Cells which have the potential to differentiate along several different lines to produce many different kinds of connective tissue cells.

microsome: A spherical microvesicle derived from the **endoplasmic reticulum** after disruption of cells and ultracentrifugation.

micturition: Urination.

mitogen: A molecule that induces cells (particularly lymphocytes) to proliferate (i.e. undergo cell division).

mitogenic: Causing or inducing cellular **mitosis**.

mitosis: The process of nuclear division and subsequent cell division (cytokinesis) that results in two daughter cells having a diploid complement (two similar sets) of chromosomes identical with that of the parent cell.

muscarinic receptor: One of two main types of receptor activated by acetylcholine; the other is the nicotinic receptor.

myocardial infarction: Sudden insufficiency of blood to an area of the heart muscle, usually as a result of occlusion of a coronary artery.

myocardium: The middle layer of the heart; cardiac muscle.

myopathy: A general term for degenerative damage to skeletal muscle.

naked DNA: DNA with no attached proteins.

necrosis: Death of cells in a portion of tissue or organ.

neonate: An infant aged 1 month or less.

neoplasm: A mass of benign or malignant tissue arising from an abnormally rapid rate of cellular proliferation which continues after the instigating factor is no longer present.

neuropathy: A general term for degenerative damage to the nerve fibres of neurons.

neurotransmitter: A chemical substance which transmits the electrical action of a nerve to a cell. Examples are acetylcholine, noradrenaline and dopamine.

oedema: Abnormal accumulation of fluid in body tissues.

oestrogens: A generic term for a group of female steroid hormones comprising β-oestradiol, oestrone and oestriol. *See also* **progestins**.

oncogene: Mutant version of a **proto-oncogene** that is excessively or inappropriately active, leading to uncontrolled cell proliferation and to malignant transformation, i.e. cancer.

ophthalmoplegia: Paralysis of one or more of the eye muscles.

organelles: Subcellular structures (e.g. **endoplasmic reticulum**, **Golgi apparatus**, **lysosomes**, mitochondria).

oropharynx: The portion of the pharynx that lies posterior to the mouth.

osteomalacia: A bone disease that results from a prolonged deficiency of vitamin D. During bone remodelling, the newly formed uncalcified bone tissue gradually takes the place of the older bone tissue, thereby weakening the skeleton.

osteopenia: Severely reduced bone mass.

osteopetrosis: An inherited disease characterized by an increase in bone mass due to decreased bone resorption.

osteoporosis: A common bone disease in the elderly that results from diminished organic bone matrix rather than from poor calcification.

otitis media: Inflammation of the middle ear.

oxidative stress: A disturbance in the pro-oxidant–antioxidant balance in favour of the former, leading to potential cell damage.

paracrine: Situations in which hormones act locally on different cells from which they were secreted. *See also* **autocrine**, **endocrine**.

parenteral: The introduction of substances into the body by means other than through the gastrointestinal tract (e.g. by intravenous injection).

paresthesia: An abnormal sensation, such as burning, pricking, tickling or tingling.

peroxisome: A membrane-bound **organelle** thought to be important in detoxifying various molecules and in catalysing the breakdown of fatty acids to acetyl-CoA.

phenotype: The observable characteristics displayed by a cell or organism as a result of its **genotype** and its environment.

pluripotent: The ability of stem cells to differentiate into several cell types.

polydipsia: Frequent drinking because of extreme thirst.

polymorphism: *Genetics*. The existence of multiple **alleles** at a particular gene locus.

polyuria: Copious production of watery urine.

post-prandial: After a meal.

potocytosis: Receptor-mediated uptake of small molecules via **caveolae**.

precordial: Pertaining to the **precordium**.

precordium: The area on the anterior surface of the body overlying the heart and lower part of the thorax.

primary transcript: The initial RNA product of gene **transcription**, subsequently processed to give messenger RNA.

probenecid: An anion transport inhibitor.

progestins: A generic term for two female steroid hormones, primarily progesterone with small amounts of 17-α-hydroxyprogesterone. *See also* **oestrogens**.

promoter: *Genetics*. A group of transcriptional control modules located immediately upstream of the transcription start site on a DNA molecule.

prosthetic group: Non-amino organic cofactors that are tightly bound to the **apoenzyme** and that are required for the enzyme to be catalytically active.

proteoglycans: Carbohydrate structures protruding from the surface of a cell.

proto-oncogene: A normal cellular gene that controls cell proliferation. The 'normal' counterpart of an **oncogene**.

racemic: A term describing an organic compound in which equal parts of dextro- and levo-rotatory isomers are blended. As a result, the molecule is not optically active, as the two opposite rotations cancel each other.

rachitic: Afflicted with rickets.

repression: *Genetics*. The inhibition of gene **transcription** by a **repressor**.

repressor: *Genetics*. A protein that binds to a **silencer** element on the DNA and mediates transcriptional **repression**.

rheological: Pertaining to the flow of materials.

scission: *Chemistry*. Splitting of a molecule to give two reaction products.

seborrhoea: Overactivity of the sebaceous glands.

seborrhoeic: Relating to **seborrhoea**.

silencer: *Genetics*. A DNA sequence that is a binding site for a transcriptional **repressor**.

solvent drag: The net movement of solute in the same direction as the flow of water due to frictional interaction.

sprue: A chronic form of malabsorption syndrome occurring in both tropical and non-tropical forms.

squame: An epidermal scale, i.e. a small thin plate of horny epithelium cast off from the skin.

stenosis: Narrowing of a duct, especially a narrowing of a heart valve.

stoichiometry: The quantitative relationship between interacting chemical substances.

stroma: Framework of a tissue.

synovial fluid: A fluid which lubricates the articular surfaces of joints.

tachycardia: A very rapid heart rate.

TATA box: *Genetics*. A short A/T-rich sequence (consensus 5′-TATAAA-3′) located within the DNA about 30 base pairs upstream of the transcription start site. The TATA box is a recognition site for general transcription factors that assemble to eventually form the pre-initiation complex.

temporal: Of or relating to time.

thrombus: Blood clot in the cardiovascular system.

thymus: A primary lymphoid organ lying in the thoracic cavity over the heart.

***trans*-acting factors**: *Genetics*. Endogenous factors, usually proteins, which bind to *cis*-acting DNA regulatory elements and alter the rate of gene transcription. The proteins are termed *trans*-acting because they are products of separate genes, which may be located on different chromosomes to the ones they are acting upon. Examples are steroid hormone–receptor protein complexes and general transcription factors. *See also **cis*-acting elements**.

transactivation: *Genetics*. Activation of gene transcription by ***trans*-acting factors**.

transcription: *Genetics*. The process by which an RNA polymerase produces single-stranded RNA complementary to one strand of a DNA template.

translation: *Genetics*. The process by which ribosomes and transfer RNA decipher the **genetic code** in a messenger RNA in order to synthesize a specific polypeptide.

turnover: *Biochemistry*. The rate at which atoms or molecules in a living system are replaced.

vasospasm: Contraction or **hypertonia** of the muscular coats of the blood vessels. (Syn. **angiospasm**).

vesicle: *Biology*. A microscopic sac.

warfarin: Warfarin is used for the treatment and prophylaxis of thromboembolic diseases. It exhibits anticoagulant activity by inhibiting the effective recycling of vitamin K.

Index